Physiology, Stress, and Malnutrition

Functional Correlates, Nutritional Intervention

Physiology, Stress, and Malnutrition

Functional Correlates, Nutritional Intervention

Editors

John M. Kinney, M.D.

Visiting Professor and Physician
The Hirsch-Leibel Laboratories
The Rockefeller University
New York, New York

Hugh N. Tucker, Ph.D.

Nestlé Clinical Nutrition and
Baxter Healthcare Corporation
Deerfield, Illinois

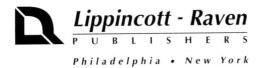

Lippincott - Raven
P U B L I S H E R S
Philadelphia • New York

Acquisitions Editors: Joyce-Rachel John and Bernadine Richey
Developmental Editor: Xenia Golovchenko
Manufacturing Manager: Dennis Teston
Production Manager: Lawrence Bernstein
Production Editor: Daniel Kulkosky
Cover Designer: Patricia Gast
Indexer: Mary Coughlin
Compositor: Lippincott–Raven Electronic Production
Printer: Quebecor Kingsport

Printed in the United States of America

9 8 7 6 5 4 3 2 1

Library of Congress Cataloging-in-Publication Data
Physiology, stress, and malnutrition: functional correlates, nutritional intervention/editors, John M. Kinney, Hugh N. Tucker.
    p. cm.
  Based on the proceedings of the Third Clintec International Horizons Conference held in Amsterdam in June 1996.
  Includes bibliographical references and index.
  ISBN 0-397-58763-5 (hardcover)
  1. Stress (Physiology)—Pathophysiology—Congresses.
2. Malnutrition—Pathophysiology—Congresses. I. Kinney, John M., 1921–   .II. Tucker, Hugh N.
III. Clintec International Horizons Conference (3rd: 1996: Amsterdam, Netherlands)
  [DNLM: 1. Nutrition—congresses. 2. Nutrition disorders—complications—congresses. 3. Stress—prevention & control—congresses. 4. Stress, Psychological—prevention & control—congresses.
5. Metabolism—physiology—congresses. QU 145 P5785 1997]
RB112.P48 1997
616.9'8—dc21
DNLM/DLC
for Library of Congress

Contents

Contributing Authors

Torbjörn Åkerstedt, Ph.D.
Department of Public Health Sciences
Karolinska Institute
Tomtebodavagen 11F
S-171 77 Stockholm, Sweden

Simon P. Allison, M.D., F.R.C.P.
Consultant Physician
Department of Medicine
University Hospital
Queens Medical Centre
Nottingham NG7 2UH, United Kingdom

Josephine Arendt, Ph.D.,
   F.R.C.Path.
School of Biological Sciences
University of Surrey
Guildford, Surrey GU2 5XH,
   United Kingdom

Peter Arner, M.D., Ph.D.
Department of Medicine
Karolinska Institute
Huddinge University Hospital
MK Division
S–141 86 Huddinge, Sweden

Tobias Bäckström
Department of Physiology and
   Pharmacology
Karolinska Institute
S-171 77 Stockholm, Sweden

George L. Brenglemann, Ph.D.
Department of Physiology and
   Biophysics
Box 357290
University of Washington
Seattle, Washington 98195

Tomas Brundin, M.D., Ph.D.
Department of Clinical Physiology
Karolinska Hospital
S-171 76 Stockholm, Sweden

Francesco Carli, M.D., M.Phil.,
   F.R.C.A.
Department of Anesthesia
McGill University
Royal Victoria Hospital
687 Pine Avenue West
Montreal, Quebec H3A 1A1
Canada

Anna Casey, M.Sc., Ph.D.
Departments of Physiology and
   Pharmacology
University of Nottingham Medical School
Nottingham NG7 2UH, United Kingdom

Charmaine Childs, Ph.D.
Regional Pediatric Burns Unit
Booth Hall Children's Hospital
Charlestown Road
Blackley, Manchester M9 2AA,
   United Kingdom

Deepak K. Chugh, M.D.
Unit for Experimental Psychiatry
Department of Psychiatry
University of Pennsylvania
School of Medicine
1013 Blockley Hall
423 Guardian Drive
Philadelphia, Pennsylvania 19104-6021

Michael G. Clark, Ph.D., D.Sc.
Department of Biochemistry
University of Tasmania
GPO Box 252
Hobart TAS 7001, Tasmania
Australia

D. Constantin-Teodosiu
Departments of Physiology and
Pharmacology
Queen's Medical Centre
University of Nottingham
Nottingham NG7 2UH, United Kingdom

Stephen J. Deacon, Ph.D.
School of Biological Sciences
University of Surrey
Guildford, Surrey GU2 5XH,
United Kingdom

Derk-Jan Dijk, Ph.D.
Department of Medicine
Brigham and Women's Hospital
Harvard Medical School
221 Longwood Ave.
Boston, Massachusetts 02115

David F. Dinges, M.S., Ph.D.
Unit for Experimental Psychiatry
Department of Psychiatry
University of Pennsylvania School of
Medicine
1013 Blockley Hall
423 Guardian Drive
Philadelphia, Pennsylvania 19104-6021

Kim A. Dora
Division of Biochemistry
University of Tasmania
GPO Box 252
Hobart TAS 7001, Tasmania
Australia

Marinos Elia, M.D., F.R.C.P.
Medical Research Council Dunn Clinical
Nutrition Centre
Hills Road
Cambridge CB2 2DH, United Kingdom

Arny A. Ferrando, Ph.D.
Department of Surgery/Metabolism
University of Texas Medical Branch
815 Market Street
Galveston, TX 77550

Barbara A. Fielding
Oxford Lipid Metabolism Group
Radcliffe Infirmary
Woodstock Road
Oxford OX2 6HE, United Kingdom

Simon Folkard, Ph.D., D.Sc.
Medical Research Council Body Rhythms
and Shiftwork Centre
Department of Psychology
University of Wales, Swansea
Singleton Park
Swansea SA2 8PP, United Kingdom

Keith N. Frayn, Ph.D.
Oxford Lipid Metabolism Group
Radcliffe Infirmary
Woodstock Road
Oxford OX2 6HE, United Kingdom

Karl E. Friedl, Ph.D.
Army Operational Medicine Research
Program
U.S. Army Medical Research and Materiel
Command
Fort Detrick
Frederick, Maryland 21702-5012

Per-Olof Grände, M.D., Ph.D.
Department of Anesthesia and Intensive
Care
University Hospital of Lund
S-221 85 Lund, Sweden

Allison L. Green, B.Pharm., Ph.D.
Departments of Physiology and
Pharmacology
University Hospital, Nottingham
Medical School, Queens Medical Centre
Nottingham NG7 2UH, United Kingdom

Paul L. Greenhaff, Ph.D.
Departments of Physiology and
Pharmacology
University of Nottingham Medical School
Queen's Medical Centre
Nottingham NG7 2UH, United Kingdom

E. M. M. A. Habas
Departments of Physiology and
Pharmacology
University of Nottingham Medical School
Queen's Medical Centre
Nottingham NG7 2UH, United Kingdom

Åse Hallström
Department of Physiology and
Pharmacology
Karolinska Institute
S–171 77 Stockholm, Sweden

Shelagh M. Hampton, M.I.Biol., Ph.D.
School of Biological Sciences
University of Surrey
Guildford, Surrey, GU2 5XH,
    United Kingdom

Johan Hellmér, M.D.
Division of Endocrinology
Huddinge University Hospital
S–141 86 Huddinge, Sweden

Jules Hirsch, M.D.
Laboratory of Human Behavior and
    Metabolism
The Rockefeller University and
Rockefeller University Hospital
1230 York Avenue
New York, New York 10021-6399

E. Hultman
Departments of Physiology and
    Pharmacology
Queen's Medical Centre
University of Nottingham
Nottingham NG7 2UH, United Kingdom

Susan A. Jebb, Ph.D.
Medical Research Council Dunn Clinical
    Nutrition Centre
Hills Road
Cambridge, CB2 2DH United Kingdom

Bodil Nielsen Johannsen, Ph.D.
August Krogh Institute
Copenhagen University
Universitetsparken 13
DK 2100 Copenhagen, Denmark

Mark T. Kearney, M.B.B.S.
Departments of Physiology and
    Pharmacology
University of Nottingham Medical School
Clifton Boulevard
Nottingham NG7 2UH, United Kingdom

Henrik Kehlet, M.D., Ph.D.
Department of Surgical Gastroenterology
Hvidovre University Hospital
Kettegårds Allé 30
2650 Hvidovre, Denmark

John M. Kinney, M.D.
Hirsch/Leibel Laboratory
Rockefeller University
1230 York Ave.
New York, New York 10021-6399

Matthew J. Kluger, Ph.D.
Pathophysiology Division
Lovelace Respiratory Research Institute
2425 Ridgecrest Drive, SE
Albuquerque, New Mexico 87108

Ian A. Macdonald, Ph.D.
Departments of Physiology and
    Pharmacology
University of Nottingham Medical School
Clifton Boulevard
Nottingham NG7 2UH, United Kingdom

Willy J. Malaisse, M.D., Ph.D.
Laboratory of Experimental Medicine
Brussels Free University, CP618
808 Route de Lennik
Brussels B-1070, Belgium

Bruce S. McEwen, Ph.D.
Laboratory of Neuroendocrinology
Box 165
Rockefeller University
1230 York Avenue
New York, New York 10021

Dennis J. McGinty, Ph.D.
Department of Neurophysiology Research
Sepulveda Veterans Administration
    Medical Center
16111 Plummer St.
Los Angeles, California 91343

Pekka Mellergård
Department of Physiology and
    Pharmacology
Karolinska Institute
S-171 77 Stockholm, Sweden

Kelly A. Miller, B.Sc.
Division of Biochemistry
University of Tasmania
GPO Box 252-58
Hobart TAS 7001, Tasmania
Australia

Linda M. Morgan, M.Sc., Ph.D., M.R.C.Path.
School of Biological Sciences
University of Surrey
Guildford, Surrey GU2 5XH,
 United Kingdom

John M. B. Newman, B.Sc.
Department of Biochemistry
University of Tasmania
GPO Box 252-28
Hobart, TAS 7001, Tasmania
Australia

Carl-Henrik Nordström
Department of Neurosurgery
Lund's University Hospital
Lund, Sweden

Deborah S. Owens, Ph.D.
Medical Research Council Body Rhythms
 and Shiftwork Centre
Department of Psychology
University of Wales, Swansea
Singleton Park, Swansea SA2 8PP,
United Kingdom

Stephen Rattigan
Department of Biochemistry
University of Tasmania
GPO Box 252
Hobart TAS 7001, Tasmania
Australia

David C. O. Ribeiro, M.Sc.
School of Biological Sciences
University of Surrey
Guildford, Surrey GU2 5XH,
 United Kingdom

Jacob Rosenberg, M.D., D.M.Sc.
Department of Surgical Gastroenterology
Hvidovre University Hospital
DK-2650 Hvidovre, Denmark

Jaswinder Singh Samra, M.B., D.Phil., F.R.C.S
Neufield Department of Clinical Medicine
Oxford University
Woodstock Road
Oxford OX2 6EH,
 United Kingdom

William H. M. Saris, M.D., Ph.D.
Nutrition Research Institute "NUTRIM"
University of Maastricht
PO Box 616
Maastricht 6200 MD, The Netherlands

Margaret V. Savage, M.Sc., M.Ed., Ph.D.
Department of Physiology, Biophysics
University of Washington
Box 357290
Seattle, Washington 98195; and
School of Kinesiology
Simon Fraser University
Burnaby, British Columbia
V5A 156 Canada

K. Soderlund
Departments of Physiology and
 Pharmacology
Queen's Medical Centre
University of Nottingham
Nottingham NG7 2UH, United Kingdom

John T. Steen
Division of Biochemistry
University of Tasmania
GPO Box 252
Hobart TAS 7001, Tasmania
Australia

Mike A. Stroud, M.D.
Department of Nutrition
Southampton General Hospital
Tremona Road
Southampton SO16 6YD, United Kingdom

Tracy A. Stubbs, R.G.N.
Departments of Physiology and
 Pharmacology
University of Nottingham Medical School
Clifton Boulevard
Nottingham NG7 2UH, United Kingdom

Lucinda K. M. Summers
Radcliffe Infirmary
Woodstock Road
Oxford OX2 6HE, United Kingdom

James A. Timmons, Ph.D.
*Departments of Physiology and
    Pharmacology
Queen's Medical Centre
University of Nottingham
Nottingham NG7 2UH, United Kingdom*

Hugh N. Tucker, Ph.D.
*Healthcare Consultant
55 Blanche Street
Barrington, Illinois 60010-2276*

Urban Ungerstedt, Ph.D.
*Department of Physiology and
    Pharmacology
Karolinska Institute
S-171 77 Stockholm, Sweden*

Michelle A. Vincent, B.Sc.
*Department of Biochemistry
University of Tasmania
GPO Box 252C-58
Hobart TAS 7001, Tasmania
Australia*

John Wahren, M.D., Ph.D.
*Section of Clinical Physiology
Department of Surgical Sciences
Karolinska Hospital
S-171 77 Stockholm, Sweden*

Robert R. Wolfe, Ph.D.
*Departments of Surgery, Anesthesiology,
    and Biochemistry
University of Texas Medical Branch
815 Market Street
Galveston, Texas 77550*

Preface

This volume is the most recent in a series of three texts generated from the proceedings of the Clintec International Horizons Conferences. Once again we returned to Amsterdam in June with arrangements for a conference and an environment that encouraged free comment and communication among the 34 invited participants. As with the past conferences, the objective of the third conference was to provide the opportunity for multidisciplinary researchers to present their latest scientific and clinical studies and to have the results discussed from very different perspectives by researchers from divergent but related fields. Our goal was to repeat the successes of the previous two conferences by generating a novel structure and substance of thought, research direction, and collaboration. Dr. John Kinney's selection and organization of the subject matter—combined with the opportunity for this type of creative interchange—created remarkable results. This type of unusual and creative interchange strengthens the understanding of scientific direction to directly improve nutrition care for critically ill patients. As evidenced by the experience of the previous conferences, this forum results in a more rapid and appropriate incorporation of technical and clinical advances into patient care.

The Grand Hotel Amsterdam was a perfect setting for the four days of presentations and discussion. The conference, *Physiology, Stress and Malnutrition: Functional Correlates and Nutritional Intervention*, was organized into six sessions. Each session was organized around individual oral presentations by the participants and group discussions of the presubmitted manuscripts. The session chair provided an integrated overview of the five papers presented during the session and added perspective from his own unique research and clinical interests. Each chair also provided an overview chapter for each section of the text after reviewing the manuscripts comprising each section.

The first volume, *Energy Metabolism: Tissue Determinants and Cellular Corollaries*, presented work on human energy metabolism, energy stores, and energy balance with a focus on the cellular mechanisms. The second volume, *Organ Metabolism and Nutrition: Ideas for Future Critical Care*, continued the discussion to the level of organ systems and began speculation on the role of nutrition in organ failure and nutritional support strategies.

The evolution of healthcare has continued toward a managed care environment worldwide. Regardless of any particular healthcare system, every country is experiencing an ever-growing crisis in escalating healthcare costs. In the United States, the financial risk of healthcare is being shifted away from the third-party payers and moved to the healthcare providers through managed care plans or capitation. The pressure to reduce burgeoning healthcare costs has resulted in an overwhelming emphasis on calculating the financial implications of each therapy. As the cost-containment trend deepens, there will be an increasing need for reliable measures of outcome performance that will demonstrate a cost-effective relationship between the care provided and the clinical result.

In this third volume we place the subject matter of the first two into perspective with whole body metabolism, and we begin to address the challenging issues of whole body outcome measures.

Over the years since the first conference there have been many changes, both within industry and among healthcare practitioners. On the industry front, Baxter Healthcare Corporation and Nestlé S. A. have embarked this year on new directions for their clinical nutrition businesses. The former partnership, Clintec Nutrition Company—the sponsor for the Horizons Conference Series— has been divided into two separate business entities. This decision provides each of the parent companies—Baxter and Nestlé—the opportunity to dedicate incremental resources and to lend its own separate focus to separate worldwide parenteral and enteral nutrition businesses, respectively. Both Baxter and Nestlé will continue to emphasize the importance of multidisciplinary interchange fostering creative thinking about new areas for clinical nutrition development and will encourage fundamental and applied research to move clinical nutrition technology and science forward.

The three conferences and resulting texts exemplify the unique abilities and dedication of Dr. John Kinney. Clintec Nutrition Company, and now Baxter and Nestlé, continue to be indebted to Dr. Kinney and his wife, Mimi, for their untiring efforts and dedication to the Horizons Conferences.

Hugh N. Tucker, Ph.D.
NESTLÉ CLINICAL NUTRITION
BAXTER HEALTHCARE CORPORATION

Introduction

This volume completes a series derived from the Clintec International Horizons conferences. The first conference (1991) was devoted to *Energy Metabolism*, with an effort to look for common ground between whole body and cellular physiology. The second conference (1993) was devoted to *Organ Metabolism*, with attention to how failure in one organ could predispose to failure in other organs. The third conference on *Physiology, Stress, and Malnutrition* was held in Amsterdam on June 9-13, 1996. This volume covers the subjects presented and discussed at that conference. Each chairman of the five sessions was invited to write an overview of his session and to provide a personal perspective on the present status of our understanding in a particular subject area.

The laboratory science of nutrition has largely been directed toward the biochemical behavior of individual nutrients. Nutritional biochemistry is usually seen as important for clinical practice only when it relates to the physiological performance of organs and tissues. Yet our knowledge of nutritional physiology lags behind our knowledge of nutritional biochemistry. This is generally true for the normal body, and is particularly notable in the presence of injury, infection, or other forms of stress.

Certain areas of physiology are obviously important in the routine care of patients while other areas seldom influence decisions in patient care. Therefore this conference has been devoted to selected areas of physiology in which stress and malnutrition are thought to play important but poorly defined roles in human convalescence. These areas include: sleep, energetics of organs and tissue during weight loss, the microcirculation and metabolic regulation, the limits of muscle performance, and thermal metabolism during conditions of stress or malnutrition.

It is common knowledge that sleep is disturbed by severe illness or injury. The patient will often point to a favorable turning point in convalescence by volunteering that "last night I slept for the first time." Can physiologically meaningful sleep be understood well enough in the future to become a marker of metabolic recovery from stress?

Interest has recently turned to extracellular sites, particularly the microcirculation, which may provide metabolic regulation formerly assumed to be the result of intracellular control. Insulin provides an example, as it has been identified as a vasoactive hormone. Since stress states are often accompanied by insulin resistance, this new knowledge contributes to the many new questions about extracellular metabolic regulation.

Physical exercise appears to have various metabolic benefits in addition to the preservation of muscle mass. What are the limits to the metabolic benefits of exercise in conditions of weight loss? Are these limits modified in the presence of stress as well as malnutrition?

Energy exchange is a balance of intake and output. Yet the clinical view of energy exchange is almost entirely restricted to the intake of calories and the gas exchange requirements for fuel oxidation. The associated production and handling of body heat is seldom considered in quantitative terms. Yet there is evidence that in the malnourished state, thermoregulation becomes impaired, particularly in the elderly. Likewise, the return of normal thermoregulation appears to be associated with the restoration of tissue in the depleted patient. Thus in the future the study of human thermal metabolism may assume greater importance in the nutritional care of patients.

The most difficult clinical conditions in which to overcome weight loss by nutritional means are those complicated by stress. Supranormal intake of calories and nitrogen to restore tissue seems to be of limited value until the catabolic influences of stress can be reduced. A better understanding of the abnormal physiology of the stressed patient undergoing weight loss may establish more specific guidelines for the use of nutritional support in such cases. While the appropriate physiologic studies are conducted, nutritional support must be subjected to more discerning outcomes research, as exemplified in the concluding paper of this conference.

John M. Kinney, M.D.

Physiology, Stress, and Malnutrition: Functional Correlates, Nutritional Intervention, edited by J.M. Kinney and H.N. Tucker. Lippincott–Raven Publishers © 1997.

Physiologic Correlates of Sleep Deprivation

David F. Dinges and Deepak K. Chugh

Unit for Experimental Psychiatry, Department of Psychiatry, University of Pennsylvania School of Medicine, Philadelphia, Pennsylvania 19104

Sleep, like food, is a biologic imperative that occurs in all humans. By 70 years of age, the average person will have spent a cumulative total of approximately 20 years asleep. However, sleep deprivation (SD) is also pervasive in modern human societies owing to unrecognized and untreated disorders of sleep (e.g., obstructive sleep apnea) and poor sleep hygiene (1). Sleep disturbance and SD accompany stressful life experiences (1a), many painful disorders (2), and debilitating infectious diseases (3), and sleep loss can result from medical practices and procedures necessary in the treatment of the critically ill patient (4). Identifying the effects of SD can enhance understanding of how sleep loss compromises human health and of ways to prevent such effects. In the past 15 years, in particular, total SD (TSD) and partial SD have been used to experimentally probe the physiologic functions of sleep and of specific sleep stages in animals and humans. After first briefly summarizing relevant comparative and neurobiologic evidence on the functions of sleep, we review the major physiologic correlates of SD, with special emphasis on human data and on a provocative animal model showing the lethal effects from SD (5).

MAMMALIAN SLEEP FUNCTIONS

Evolutionary Perspective: Endothermy and Energy Conservation

Although there are species-specific differences in the timing parameters of sleep, human sleep is remarkably similar to sleep in most other mammals in terms of brain activity, body posture, and reduced environmental responsivity. Given the pervasiveness of sleep within and between species, it is surprising that the physiologic function(s) of sleep have been difficult to identify. This has begun to change in recent years, as an increasing number of lines of investigation converge on a formulation of the role of sleep in survival. An evaluation of sleep from the perspective of evolutionary history suggests that mammalian sleep developed in association with endothermy and that sleep may serve a fundamental role in energy conservation (6). Among mammals, body weight and

1

metabolic rate together account for 35% of the variance in daily sleep time. It appears that as body weight increases across mammalian species, sleep time decreases (6–8). The reduced pressure for sleep in larger mammalian species may be due to their greater energy reserves as a result of the increase in the ratio of fat to body mass as size increases (6). Sleep time also has a negative correlation with metabolic rate (6,7), however, which may be the result of including some species that have high sleep quotas, low metabolic rates for their size, and relatively poor diets (e.g., marsupials, edentates). In such animals, sleep is thought to relieve the metabolic pressure of wake activity (6). Consequently, there is evidence for greater requirements for sleep in species with low energy reserves, as defined either endogenously (body fat) or ecologically (nutritional availability).

Mammalian sleep consists of two physiologically distinct, alternating types of sleep. Paradoxical sleep is comparable with human rapid eye movement (REM) sleep, during which there is activation of the electroencephalogram (EEG) and other physiologic markers, as well as skeletal muscle atonia. Non-REM (NREM), or quiet sleep, varies on an intensity continuum from low- to high-amplitude EEG sleep [human delta or slow-wave sleep (SWS)], during which there is synchronous EEG, muscle tone, and low physiologic activation. Inter-species analyses have shown that, like total sleep time, quiet sleep time (NREM sleep) varies inversely with body size (8). In contrast, the amount of paradoxical sleep (REM sleep) has been found to be negatively associated with ethologic factors such as danger (8), as well as with developmental factors such as gestational age and the altricial–precocial dimension (6). Altricial species, or those born immature (e.g., rat, human), tend to have REM sleep, and altriciality evolved in mammals in conjunction with endothermy (6). Therefore, sleep, both from the standpoint of daily amount as well as amounts of specific stages, appears to have a correlative if not causal connection to the evolution of endothermy and the maintenance of energy balance in mammals. Putative endothermic and energy conservation functions for sleep are consistent with the results reviewed below on the prolonged effects of total SD in rats (5,9).

Neurobiologic Perspective: Brain Homeostasis and Energy Balance

The daily occurrence of sleep in relation to waking is conceptualized as involving two interactive neurobiologic processes: a sleep drive and a temporal control process (10–12). Neither process substitutes for the other, and both appear essential for effective survival. The neurobiology of the temporal component includes an endogenous circadian pacemaker located in the suprachiasmatic nuclei (SCN) of the hypothalamus, which when lesioned results in loss of circadian organization of sleep and waking (e.g., shorter bouts of waking), and increased total sleep time, suggesting that the SCN actively facilitates the initiation and maintenance of wakefulness and opposes the homeostatic sleep drive at certain circadian times (13). In contrast, deprivation of sleep in humans and other species does not prevent the circadian rhythm in core body temperature and many other biologic functions (14), but it quickly leads to an elevated pressure for sleep that appears to override the endogenous, wake-promoting, circadian opposition to sleep (15). If the elevations in sleepiness, sleep propensity, and involuntary sleep onsets induced by TSD are considered an expression of the neurobiology of sleep, then in a fundamental sense sleep cannot be totally deprived in either humans or animals [e.g., TSD in rats typically results in loss of 90% of sleep time, rather than 100% (9)]. On the other hand, there is ample evidence reviewed in this article that deprivation of a majority of sleep time in healthy mammals leads to a number of neurobehavioral and physiologic changes that reflect deficiencies in the regulation of both brain and body.

Such deficiencies suggest that sleep also has a basic role in physiologic recovery from waking metabolic costs, especially in relation to the brain (16,17). Neurobiologic theories of sleep function have derived from progress on the neural mechanisms involved in sleep regulation (18–21). This research indicates that the alternation of sleep and waking, and between NREM and REM sleep states, is neuroanatomically and neurophysiologically diffusely regulated within the isodendritic core of the mammalian brain, extending rostrally from the medulla through the brain stem and hypothalamus to the basal forebrain (21). Although specific areas within this core are more critically important for some elements of sleep (e.g., regulation of REM sleep muscle atonia in the pontine tegmentum), it appears that no structure within this core is the sole regulator of sleep (21). Similarly, the neurochemical regulation of sleep and sleep states appears to involve a diversity of substances, including neurotransmitters (e.g., adenosine, γ-aminobutyric acid); amine neuromodulators (e.g., catecholamines, serotonin, histamine); neurohormones (e.g., growth hormone–releasing factor; somatostatin); neuropeptides (e.g., delta sleep–inducing peptide, muramyl peptides); and neuroimmunomodulating proteins [e.g., interleukin-1β (IL-1β), interferon-α (IFN-α)] (21–24). In addition, temperature and thermoregulatory processes in warm-sensitive neurons in the preoptic anterior hypothalamus are thought to participate in the regulation of sleep, especially SWS (25), and thermoregulation has been theorized to be a key function of sleep (26).

The diversity of structures, interconnections, and chemical agents capable of mediating sleep have led to recent theories of sleep function that emphasize that sleep homeostasis (i.e., accumulation of sleep need after waking) can occur in different brain areas, at different rates, until eventually the whole brain changes state (27,28). For example, Bennington and Heller (28) emphasize the role sleep might have in restoration of brain energy metabolism, especially restoration of glycogen stores that are depleted during waking. Krueger et al. (29) posited that sleep preserves a constancy of synaptic superstructure that is a brain manifestation of a wider growth function of sleep. Many recent neurobiologic theories, therefore, emphasize two primary purposes for sleep: (a) maintenance of waking brain function, and (b) energy-saving, anabolic functions for brain. There is considerable evidence that the primary disruptive effects of SD, especially short-term SD, are on homeostatic maintenance and anabolic functions of the brain. However, studies of prolonged SD in rats also suggest a role for sleep in whole-body energy balance. When considering the effects of SD, we begin with the most dramatic results.

LETHAL EFFECTS FROM PROLONGED SD

SD in Rats Using the Disk-Over-Water Method

If sleep serves vital physiologic functions, SD should be life threatening. There are two lines of evidence suggesting that prolonged SD may be lethal. The first derives from experimental evidence of forced sleep loss in animals. Although a number of studies from 1894 to 1962 have reported lethal outcomes from TSD in dogs, rabbits, and rats (30), these investigations have been disregarded for lack of controls for the procedures used to keep animals awake (e.g., stimulation, forced ambulation) (16). In 1983, however, Rechtschaffen et al. (5) at the University of Chicago published the first of a series of experiments on prolonged TSD, and later on selective sleep stage deprivation, in Sprague-Dawley rats, using a novel disk-over-water methodology and yoked control procedure (31,32). In this paradigm, sleep in the rat, as continuously monitored by EEG, results in disk rotation, forcing the experimental animal to ambulate to avoid being carried into shallow water. The control rat on the opposite side of the divided disk receives the same physical stimulation (EEG monitoring, forced ambulation with disk rotation), but the animal can sleep ad libitum when the disk is stationary. The results obtained from this paradigm have supported the claims of the earlier studies of lethal effects from prolonged TSD in animals by establishing that with the disk-over-water method mortality is high in the SD experimental rats, but not in either yoked control or home cage control rats. In fact, during the 13 years since the paradigm was first described, Rechtschaffen and Bergmann (9) observed that "no rat survived unrelenting deprivation of sleep."

Because the disk-over-water paradigm involves excellent control procedures, and use of the technique has yielded a wide range of physiologic effects from SD in rats, which have been systematically reported in a series of papers, results from this paradigm for studying SD will be a major focus of this review. Table 1 summarizes the range of biobehavioral effects obtained in rats sleep deprived using the disk-over-water method, whereas Table 2 summarizes those parameters that showed no differences, and Table 3 summarizes the effects of various interventions used to probe the effects of SD by this method. Listed first in Table 1 is the average time to lethal outcome from TSD and from two forms of selective partial SD in rats: paradoxical SD (PSD) and high EEG amplitude SD (HSD). In this paradigm, TSD was lethal on average within 2–3 weeks (mean= 17 days), whereas lethality from either form of partial SD was approximately

TABLE 1. *Effects observed in sleep-deprived (SD) rats relative to yoked control rats using disk-over-water method*

Observed effects	References
Lethal outcome	
Death in 5–33 days of TSD (M = 17 days)	5,9,36,38–41
Death in 16–54 days of PSD (M = 36 days)	42
Death in 28–66 days of HSD (M = 44 days)	43
Brain activity decreased	
50% loss of EEG amplitude	5
Reduced cerebral glucose utilization in hypothalamus, thalamus, limbic system, and occipital cortex by quantitative autoradiographic 2-^{14}C-deoxyglucose method	44
Altered appearance and behavior	
Bilateral ulcerative and keratotic skin lesions on tails and paws	5,9,37,38,42,43, 45–47
Ataxia and severe motor weakness	5
Debilitated appearance (scrawny, fur color change from creamy white to brownish yellow, fur disheveled and stuck together in clumps as if oily, patches of skin visible between clumps)	5,9,37,38,42,46
Sensitive to touch and aggressive (PSD rats)	42
Negative energy balance	
Weight loss	5,9,37,38,41–43, 46–48
Increased energy expenditure	9,35,37,38,41–43, 46,48,49
Hyperphagia	9,37,38,41–43, 46–48
Increased brown adipose tissue type II 5′-deiodinase activity	35
Absence of observable body fat	38,42,46
Calorie malnutrition	41
Increased water intake	38,42
Lower weight spleen and liver	5
Plasma albumin decreased (TSD rats, not in PSD rats)	38,42
Plasma urea nitrogen increased	38,42
Thermoregulatory changes	
Body temperature increased early in deprivation (TSD and HSD, not PSD)	37,39,40,43,46,49
Accelerating decline in body temperature later in deprivation	37,39,43,49–51
Hypothalamic temperature initial increase prolonged relative to body temperature	40
Hypothalamic temperature decrease late in deprivation less than body temperature decrease	40
Wake-to-sleep body temperature drop reduced or reversed during recovery sleep	9,121
Amplitude of diurnal body temperature rhythm declined over course of TSD	37
Behavioral preference for increasingly warmer ambient temperature (up to 50°C)	39,46,50,118)
Neuroendocrine changes	
Adrenal hypertrophy	5,38,42,43
Plasma thyroxine (total T_4 and free T_4) decreased	9,49,51
Plasma triiodothyronine (total T_3 and free T_3) decreased	49,51
T_3/T_4 ratio increased	49
Plasma epinephrine increased	49
Plasma norepinephrine increased	9,49
Elevated heart rate	38,42

TABLE 1. *Continued.*

Observed effects	References
Hematologic changes	
Plasma white blood cell counts increased	38,42
Plasma red blood cell counts, hemoglobin, and hematocrit decreased	38
Plasma globulins increased	42
Brown–maroon cast to mesenteric, inguinal nodes, adrenal and	
thymus glands	38
Blending of mesenteric lymph nodes	38
Less prominent germinal centers with sinus histiocytosis in spleen	
and mesenteric nodes	34
Immune responses	
Lower mitotic index in the jejunum	45
Common lethal opportunistic microbes in heart blood late in	
deprivation, but no fever or host response to systemic infection,	
on examination	47
W256 tumor growth reduced faster in TSD rats	9, 52, 52a
Recovery sleep	
Recovery sleep promotes survival if permitted early enough	36,37
Paradoxical sleep rebounds during recovery sleep	36,37
Recovery sleep reverses negative energy balance on the first	
recovery day	9
Recovery sleep reverses other physiologic effects of SD	9

TSD, total SD; PSD paradoxical SD; HSD, high EEG amplitude SD.

twice as long (mean 36–44 days). Debate over the mechanisms of lethality using this method of SD have continued for more than a decade (9,33). Surprisingly, lethal outcome does not appear to involve whole organ failure. Postmortem examinations of organs from sleep-deprived rats have shown only a few apparently modest morphologic changes in internal organs (e.g., lymphoid tissues of the spleen and mesenteric nodes). Although heart tissue was not mentioned, histologic analyses have thus far failed to identify differences in brain, liver, kidney, duodenum, stomach, thyroid, parathyroid glands, thymus, or lungs between SD and yoked control rats (Table 2), suggesting that a biochemical or functional change was responsible for death (34). Consistent with this conclusion, as summarized in Table 1, the lethal progression of SD was correlated with disturbances of a range of behavioral, brain, and bodily functions, especially physiologic systems involved in regulation of metabolism, thermogenesis, and immunity. In general, sleep-deprived rats show a progressive syndrome that includes debilitated appearance, core body temperature decreases, heat-seeking behavior, hyperphagia, weight loss, increased metabolic rate, elevated levels of plasma norepinephrine, decreased plasma thyroxine, and an increase of an enzyme that mediates thermogenesis by brown adipose tissue (9,35). The complexity of these effects, debates over which physiologic events could be producing the lethal outcome (9,33), and differences in interpretations of the significance of the findings relative to both stress (9,16) and results of SD in other

TABLE 2. *Failure to find differences between sleep-deprived (SD) rats and yoked control rats using disk-over-water method*

Observed Effects	References
Brain	
Brain histologic abnormalities (vacuolization, increased eosinophilia, and shrinkage of neuronal perikarya present in both SD and yoked control rats)	34
Brain monoamine (serotonin, dopamine, norepinephrine) and their metabolites (5HIAA, DOPAC, homovanillic acid, respectively)	48
Cerebral glucose utilization in cerebral cortex, basal ganglia, mesencephalic and pontine region by quantitative autoradiographic 2-^{14}C-deoxyglucose method	44
Microstructure of neuronal organelles and synaptic density for neurons in the cortex, preoptic anterior hypothalamus, and dorsolateral pons	63
Appearance and behavior	
Hair growth and regrowth	42
Grooming behavior	38
Nutritional parameters	
Serum iron, potassium, and sodium levels	38,42
Urinary urobilinogen, nitrite, bilirubin, glucose, ketone, specific gravity, pH, protein, and blood	38,42
Body hydration	64
Absorption of nutrients	64
Glucose uptake	38,42
Energy expended	
Gross motor activity	49
Efficiency of energy utilization by bomb calorimetry of wastes	49
Internal organs	
Weights of spleen, liver, lungs, and brain	38,42,43
Number of splenic cells	43
Histology of liver, kidney, duodenum, stomach, thyroid, parathyroid, thymus, and lungs	34
Neuroendocrine parameters	
Plasma ACTH	9,49
Plasma corticosterone	5,9,36,49,51
Plasma TSH (unstimulated)	51
Immune function	
Splenic lymphocyte proliferation responses to Con-A and LPS	65
In vitro splenic B lymphocyte PFC response to thymus-independent antigen phosphorylcholine and thymus-dependent antigen SRC	65
Recovery sleep	
NREM during recovery sleep	36

species, necessitate separate discussions of a number of the major areas outlined in Table 1 and the extent to which these same effects are observed in SD experiments in humans.

The final section of Table 1, however, highlights a critical outcome of these experiments that strengthens the likelihood that the ultimately lethal physiologic effects observed in these experiments are due to SD per se. If rats are permitted to sleep after many days of SD, and after development of the full syndrome described above but before hypothermia is too great (i.e., >1°C decline from baseline), then they survive and recover (9,36,37).

TABLE 3. *Effects of interventions in totally sleep-deprived (TSD) rats*

Intervention and purpose	Results	References

High protein ($\uparrow$P) vs. high calorie ($\uparrow$C) diets
  Test if diet composition altered
  malnutrition and negative energy
  balance in TSD
	$\uparrow$P diet prevented TSD
	  hyperphagia; $\uparrow$C diet caused
	  marked TSD hyperphagia
	$\uparrow$C diet did not result in abnormal
	  plasma levels of cholesterol,
	  triglycerides, glucose
	$\uparrow$P diet caused accelerated TSD
	  weight loss; $\uparrow$C diet prevented
	  TSD weight loss
	$\uparrow$P diet hastened TSD skin lesions;
	  $\uparrow$C diet delayed TSD skin lesions
	$\uparrow$P diet shortened TSD life span by
	  40% relative to $\uparrow$C diet
		41

Propylthiouracil-induced hypothyroidism
  Test if prevention of $\uparrow$EE by
  hypothyroidism changed T_b responses
  in TSD
	Hypothyroidism prevented $\uparrow$EE in
	  TSD and control rats
	
	Hypothyroid TSD rats had no
	  initial rise in T_b and greater fall in
	  T_b (severe hypothermia)
	Hypothyroidism reduced skin
	  lesions and debilitated
	  appearance from TSD
	Hypothyroidism did not change
	  occurrence or timing of TSD-
	  induced mortality
		100

Thyroxine (T_4) administration to increase
  metabolic rate
  Test if thyroxine-induced increases in
  metabolic rate alter TSD effects
	T_4 rats had higher metabolic rates,
	  higher T_b, reduced warming
	  behavior during TSD
	T_4 rats had shortened life span by
	  37% relative TSD control rats
		46

Thyrotropin-releasing hormone (TRH)
  administration to test HPT axis
  Test plasma levels of free T_4 [FT_4],
  free T_3 [FT_3], and how TRH affects
  TSH, FT_4, FT_3
	Plasma FT_4 and FT_3 decreased
	  with TSD comparable to total
	  T_4 and T_3
	Plasma TSH was unchanged by
	  TSD
	TRH increased plasma TSH
	  similarly in TSD rats and
	  controls
	TRH-stimulated TSH release
	  increased FT_4 and FT_3 to
	  control values
		51

Guanethidine (GU)-induced sympathetic
  blockade
  Test if norepinephrine (NE) resulted in
  $\uparrow$EE in TSD
	GU reduced NE response but
	  did not change $\uparrow$EE response to TSD
	Plasma epinephrine increased
	  above levels seen in other
	  TSD studies
	GU did not change TSD
	  syndrome or mortality
		101

TABLE 3. *Continued*

Intervention and purpose	Results	References
TSD effects in light–dark (12:12) cycle		37
Test if TSD effects on rats were due to flattened circadian rhythms from constant light	Amplitude of diurnal T_b rhythm declined over TSD course	
	Amplitude of diurnal T_b rhythm recovered on first recovery day	
	Light–dark cycle did not change TSD syndrome or mortality	
Aspirin effects on body temperature		102
Test if TSD-induced ↑T_b (increased thermal set point) is mediated by prostaglandins	Aspirin decreased T_b during TSD relative to its effects at baseline	
Preoptic/anterior hypothalamic (POAH) lesions		103
Test if bilateral POAH lesions produce or alter TSD effects	POAH lesions produced more rapid decline in T_b during TSD	
	POAH lesions did not prevent TSD effects on ↑EE, skin lesions, or mortality	
Antibiotic treatment to block bacteremia		103a
Test if prophylactic antibiotics prevent bacterial invasion in TSD	Trend for bacterial invasion early in TSD (day 4) even in rats treated with antibiotic	
	Antibiotic treatment did not prevent late TSD decline in T_b or mortality	
Walker 256 rat carcinoma cell implantation		52a
Test if host defense against subdermal implantation of tumor cells was changed by TSD	Tumor size was significantly smaller in TSD rats compared to controls	
	Tumor size predicted by change in sleep time during TSD, not by weight loss	

EE, increased energy expenditure; T_b, body temperature.

Fatal Familial Insomnia

The second line of evidence that SD may be lethal, even in humans, is far less direct than the experimental data on rats. It comes from discovery of a rare inherited prion disease termed fatal familial insomnia (FFI) (53). This disease is caused by an abnormal isoform of the prion protein in the brain (54) and is transmitted in an autosomal-dominant manner. Prion protein is encoded by a gene located in the short arm of human chromosome 20; it is highly conserved in evolution as a membrane-associated protein, but its function remains unknown. The age of onset of FFI is between 36 and 62 years of age (55). Insomnia develops in the form of gradually decreasing nocturnal sleep, with frequent awakenings, and progresses to total inability to sleep. After a few weeks or months, wakefulness is interspersed with dreamlike states and diminished environmental contact, which may indicate that in some cases the disease involves severe chronic partial SD rather than TSD. During the disease there are symptoms of increased autonomic activation, including sweating, elevated heart rate and blood pressure, and slightly increased body temperature, as well as increased levels of norepinephrine in urine, plasma, and cerebrospinal fluid (56). Although adrenocorticotrophic hormone (ACTH) levels are normal, plasma levels of cortisol tend to be high. There appears to be a loss of circadian variation in body temperature and melatonin secretion. Although magnetic resonance imaging shows only mild brain atrophy in patients, findings on fluorodeoxyglucose positron emission tomography (PET) scans show profound reductions in the metabolism of the thalamus (57). As the disease becomes prolonged, ataxia and motor abnormalities develop and progress to total inability to stand and walk. The disease is uniformly fatal, leading to death after 7–9 months in acute cases, or 25–30 months when it takes a chronic course (55). Postmortem brain studies confirm the loss of neurons and reactive astrogliosis in the anteroventral and dorsomedial thalamic nuclei.

Some of the clinical characteristics and physiologic correlates of FFI appear to be similar to the effects of SD in rats (Table 1). These include loss of slow-wave sleep, enhanced sympathetic activation, motor ataxia, and a chronic stress syndrome, which have been attributed to a failure of the neurobiologic controls of metabolic energy restoration in FFI (55). However, it is not known whether the lethal mechanism of FFI is the same as that in sleep-deprived rats or even whether SD is the primary cause of death in FFI (58). Nevertheless, FFI remains a potentially important link between animal SD and human SD because laboratory experiments on the effects of TSD on healthy humans have not extended beyond 11 days (59,60), and nearly all have been limited to 2–5 days, which is well below the duration of SD seen in patients with FFI or the duration capable of producing the syndromal effects seen in rats using the disk-over-water method. Although there are references to lethal outcomes in persons with mania (61,62), studies of 1–11 days of SD in healthy humans have not turned up a single case of mortality and have provided no evidence of serious risk to health. On the other hand, human safety may be imperiled by SD (e.g., drowsy driving accidents) because such short-term human SD studies consistently find evidence of diminished brain activation and impaired neurobehavioral functions.

ALTERED BRAIN ACTIVITY DURING SD

Neurobehavioral Changes with SD

Although animal studies of SD have quantified neurobehavioral functions associated with such phenomena as the role of REM SD in memory consolidation and the effects of SD on behavior (e.g., increased irritability) (42,66), neurobehavioral effects of SD have not been the focus of most animal investigations of SD. In contrast, the neurobehavioral effects of SD have been the primary focus in hundreds of experiments on humans. These studies consistently demonstrate that human brain function is sensitive to sleep loss. The clinical manifestations of a number of neurologic and neuropsychiatric disorders are altered by a single night of TSD. For example, SD has a transient antidepressant effect in many patients with depression (67); it can switch a patient with bipolar disorder from depression to mania (68); it has been reported to improve motor deficits in patients with Parkinson's disease (69); and it can lower the seizure threshold in patients with seizure disorders (70).

In healthy human adults, the most immediate and measurable neurobehavioral effects of TSD are increases in subjective sleepiness and fatigue, diminished alertness, and cognitive performance deficits characterized by increases in response variability, lapses, vigilance decrements, errors, cognitive disorganization and perseveration, and decreases in cognitive and motor speed, and short-term memory accuracy (15,16,71–73). These effects are cumulative, increasing with each consecutive day of TSD until days 3–5, when neurobehavioral output is characterized by nearly continuous lability of attention, diminished responding, overwhelming sleepiness, and a characteristic semi-waking state. With the exception of the periodically timed promotion of waking by the endogenous circadian pacemaker, the brain appears be unable to sustain wakefulness during SD, at least not without nearly continuous external stimulation. The same effects can occur with partial SD below 5 hours per night, but relative to TSD they take longer to develop and may be less severe, depending on the amount of sleep obtained (74a). Persons sleep deprived for more than a day report that it requires increasing amounts of compensatory effort to continue in the experiment and that such compensatory effort has diminished returns, especially after 48 hours without sleep. Although rarely considered as a factor in SD effects, humans must be kept awake with stimulation, which in SD experiments typically takes the form of ambulation, interesting activity, and social stimulation. Aversive stimuli of the kind used to keep animals ambulating and therefore awake in SD experiments are generally not used in human laboratory experiments, although field studies of military operations have combined other aversive elements (physical work, caloric deficits) with SD (75–78).

Neurophysiologic Changes with SD

The physiologic bases of the neurobehavioral changes associated with SD appear to result from an increasing inability of the sleep-deprived brain to sustain a stable waking state. A wide variety of EEG analyses in humans and animals indicate that SD leads to lability of the neurophysiologic state and increasing pressure for sleep. After even moderate TSD (24–48 hours) in humans, the voluntary latency from wake to sleep (considered to reflect sleep propensity) shortens from its normal range of 8–20 minutes to 0.5–3 minutes (79). Involuntary sleep onsets also begin to occur as TSD progresses, along with microsleep intrusions into waking EEG (15). There is diminution and eventual loss of waking EEG alpha activity in sleep-deprived humans (80), a finding that may be analogous to the observation of a 50% reduction in EEG amplitude during TSD in rats (5). Power spectral analyses of the waking EEG in humans show an increase in theta frequency power as TSD progresses (81,82). Evoked brain potentials in TSD subjects show diminished amplitudes and increasing latencies (83). A host of other psychophysiologic and neurologic changes are evident during human TSD, including constricted pupil size, loss of contingent negative variation, reduced ability to maintain coordination and postural balance (84), and undulating slow eye movements (80).

Studies have used neuroimaging of regional cerebral glucose metabolism to determine specific areas of the brain that are affected by SD. Positron emission tomography (PET) with F-18 deoxyglucose has shown decreases in absolute glucose metabolism in prefrontal cortex, thalamic, basal ganglia, limbic, cerebellar, and brain stem regions in young adults undergoing 32–72 hours of TSD (85,86). As noted above, PET scans of patients with FFI also showed reductions in thalamic metabolism (57). In TSD rats, use of quantitative autoradiographic $2\text{-}^{14}C$-deoxyglucose method for measuring regional cerebral glucose utilization ($ICMR_{glc}$) has shown regional metabolic decreases in hypothalamus, thalamus, limbic system and central gray area (Table 1), but not in cerebral cortex, basal ganglia, or most mesencephalic and pontine regions (Table 2) (44). Although there is not complete agreement on whether SD makes the brain hypo- or hypermetabolic (87), all studies of neuroimaging of cerebral metabolism in sleep-deprived rats, humans, and patients with FFI, have observed only regional hypometabolism in brain areas, especially in the thalamus. These hypometabolic effects of SD on the brain are in stark contrast to the apparently hypermetabolic effects of SD on the rest of the body, reviewed below.

As in rats, recovery sleep in humans after TSD does not reclaim all the lost sleep (88), but rather it is marked by increased sleep intensity (i.e., reduced latencies, greater consolidation, reduced arousal threshold, and elevations in specific sleep stages). Although recovery sleep in sleep-deprived rats is marked by paradoxical sleep rebounds in particular (Table 1) (36,37,89), SWS is elevated in humans in response to acute TSD. This is evident in a number of ways: the latency from light NREM sleep to SWS accelerates markedly (90), and the recovery sleep contains increased amounts of SWS (91) and EEG slow-wave activity (92,93). Despite the differences in sleep stages during recovery sleep in humans and rats, in both species a single night of recovery sleep after days of TSD results in substantial re-establishment of waking physiologic functions. This suggests that up to some point in time (in rats this appears to be just before severe hypothermia develops), SD does not produce permanent changes or irreversible damage, and that whatever neurophysiologic deficits SD may create at cellular or extracellular levels in brain and/or body, they can be reversed through the sleep process.

Monoamines have been consistently linked to the neurobiologic regulation of sleep, and several studies have examined the effects of TSD or PSD on indicators of brain monoamine metabolism in rats (48). In one of the more extensive, controlled studies in this area (48), the caudate, frontal cortex, hippocampus, hypothalamus, mid-brain, and pons-medulla of TSD rats (11–20) days were compared with yoked and home cage controls for concentrations of serotonin (5HT), its metabolite 5-hydroxyindoleactic acid (5HIAA), dopamine (DA), its metabolite 3,4-dihydroxyphenylacetic acid (DOPAC), and either norepinephrine or the dopamine metabolite homovanillic acid. The ratios of metabolites to monoamines (DOPAC/DA, 5HIAA/5HT) also were calculated. TSD rats did not have either significantly higher or lower values of any monoamine or metabolite in any brain region relative to control rats (Table 2). Thus, prolonged SD in the rat did not reliably produce regional changes in the levels of major brain monoamines or their metabolites, although the results do not preclude the possibility that TSD leads to monoaminergically mediated changes in neuronal firing rates, receptor sensitivity, or in more fundamental cellular mechanisms (48). Increased dopamine receptor density and decreased receptor affinity in the anteromedial frontal cortex has been reported in REM sleep-deprived rats (94).

There have been a number of recent studies of cellular and molecular changes in rat brain tissue during SD (95). Consistent with the lack of histologic evidence of organ failure during prolonged TSD (Table 2), it was recently reported that 8 days of TSD in rats did not produce changes detectable by electron miscroscopy on either the microstructure of neuronal organelles or the synaptic density for neurons in the cortex, preoptic anterior hypothalamus, or dorsolateral pons (63). More short-term SD studies in rats have shown physiologic reactions to SD. In a study of immediate early gene expression, up to 6 hours of TSD produced higher expression of c-*fos* messenger RNA (mRNA) (but not *junB* mRNA) in cortex, thalamus, cerebellum, pons, and hypothalamus (96). After 24 hours, TSD in rats, mRNA and protein levels of the 17-kDa protein neurogranin (NG), a postsynaptic substrate of the protein kinase C were reduced in subcortical areas and cerebral cortex, respectively (97). During 24 hours of PSD, mRNA and protein levels of glutamine synthetase (GS), an enzyme located in astrocytes, increased in the cortex and then decreased with 4 hours of recovery sleep (98). Induction of galanin gene expression in the rat brain preoptic and periventricular areas by 24 hours of REM SD also has been reported (99). These studies indicate immediate cellular and molecular changes in brain tissue in response to SD in rats. It remains uncertain to what extent such changes reflect sleep loss, sleep-initiating mechanisms, or more general stress effects, or how the effects observed thus far relate to changes in brain function, metabolism, thermoregulation, and immune function observed with more prolonged SD.

DISTURBANCE OF ENERGY BALANCE DURING SLEEP DEPRIVATION

Metabolic Changes During SD: Energy Expenditure, Diet, and Physical Activity

Energy Expenditure

Among the most consistent changes induced by prolonged TSD, PSD, and HSD in the rat using the disk-over-water method are those indicative of whole-body hypermetabolism (5,9,38,41–43,46,47,49). In these studies, sleep-deprived rats developed a negative energy balance through a doubling of energy expenditure (EE) (mean 210–270% of baseline), based on increased food intake (hyperphagia) accompanied by weight loss (Table 1). Loss of weight in sleep-deprived rats could not be explained by dehydration, malabsorption, or gross perturbations in intermediary metabolism (Table 2) (64), and the increased EE could not be explained by the metabolic cost of increased wakefulness, water exposure, or motor activity (38,49). Thus, it appears the sleep-deprived animals undergo an increase in basal EE not evident in work, waste, or weight (9,45). The heightened catabolism is associated with signs of malnutrition (e.g., reduced plasma albumin, cachexic appearance, and absence of observable body fat) and appears to involve a 100-fold increase in thermogenesis of brown adipose tissue, which in mammals is the site of facultative thermogenesis in response to overfeeding and cold exposure (35,51). The hormone profiles of sleep-deprived rats [increased plasma levels of norepinephrine (NE) and an elevated ratio of triiodothyronine (T_3) to thyroxine (T_4), reviewed below] are also consistent with compensatory thermogenesis.

Diet

Whether malnutrition secondary to heightened catabolism is the lethal mechanism of SD in rats remains unclear (9,41). TSD effects in rats have been likened to the sustained sleep loss, elevated energy expenditure, malnutrition, and life-threatening state of many critically ill patients (41). Although TSD effects in rats suggest protein malnutrition, an experiment on the effects of protein-rich versus calorie-rich diets on TSD rats yielded surprising results (Table 3). Contrary to expectation, TSD rats fed diets high in protein-to-calorie ratio had accelerated body weight loss, developed skin lesions sooner (Table 1), and had markedly reduced life spans compared with TSD rats fed calorie-augmented (fat) diets (41). Food consumption remained normal throughout TSD in the rats fed protein-rich diets, but increased by 250% during TSD in the rats fed calorie-rich diets. However, the latter exhibited no evidence of weight gain or abnormal levels of cholesterol, triglycerides, or glucose, indicating accelerated turnover of nutrients, consistent with the elevated EE. Calorie intake in the first 14 days of TSD was significantly correlated with length of survival ($r = 0.84$), but protein intake and carbohydrate intake during these same 14 days did not predict survival time (41). This experiment established that diet composition interacts with prolonged SD effects in rats, altering the time course and development of pathologies. Importantly, however, dietary fat and calorie augmentation (rather than protein augmentation), was beneficial for health and longevity but did not prevent the elevated EE and lethal effects of TSD. On the other hand, a single night of recovery sleep appears to reverse the negative energy balance resulting from SD (9).

Unfortunately, there are few systematic controlled studies of metabolism, energy utilization, or nutritional effects during short-term TSD in humans. What little information exists in healthy human subjects is consistent with the whole-body hypermetabolic demands seen in sleep-deprived rats (80,104–106). Metabolism (O_2 uptake relative to CO_2 output) has been reported to increase in healthy young men during consecutive nights of experimental disruption of sleep (arousal every 3 minutes) and to decrease below baseline sleep levels on the recovery night (107). Protein metabolism was reported to be increased by 12% on the second day of TSD in six healthy young adults (108). Anecdotally, we have observed increased food intake in adult subjects permitted ad libitum access to food and water during 3 days of TSD, and consistent with the rat TSD studies, there are claims in the literature that SD creates a preference in humans to use lipids over carbohydrates as a source of energy (80). In the only double-blind experiment on the effect of nutrition on SD in healthy humans, 150 mg/kg tyrosine, a large neutral amino acid found in dietary proteins, was reported to significantly improve psychomotor and vigilance performance throughout a nighttime work period (one night of SD) (109). The effect lasted for approximately 3 hours and was attributed to the role of tyrosine as a precursor to catecholamine neurotransmitters and its beneficial effects in countering the depletion of brain norepinephrine associated with exposure to physical stressors (109).

Physical Activity

Studies on the capacity to perform physical work or exercise during TSD have produced equivocal results. These studies generally suggest that although TSD might erode physical performance (110), it does not alter maximal physiologic performance capacity associated with exercise or physical work. However, it does lead to neurobehavioral, perceptual, and motivational changes, including reduced endurance (i.e., time to feel exhausted and/or quit the exercise) and perceptions of greater effort and exertion during TSD (16,110–112). TSD (24–60 hours) appears to have no net effect on the factors that reflect energy substrates used during acute, intermittent exercise or the physiologic stress response to

exercise in humans (113,114). There is evidence that the major metabolic perturbation during TSD with physical work is an increase in insulin resistance and
a decrease in glucose tolerance (115). It is possible that the metabolic costs of
acute TSD in healthy humans may not be fully apparent until recovery sleep is
taken. It has been reported that physical fitness of healthy human subjects who
had undergone 5 days of TSD was decreased after recovery sleep (116,117),
prompting Naitoh (80) to suggest that the "metabolic debts incurred, due to a
stepped-up catabolism during SD, were paid back by an intense recuperative
anabolism which used all the resources during the recovery period."

Thermoregulatory Changes with SD

A number of thermoregulatory responses have been documented to occur in
prolonged TSD of rats. Core body temperature (both intraperitoneal and hypothalamic) increased early in both TSD and HSD, although this effect was not
seen during PSD (37,39,40,43,46,49). The effect has been interpreted as reflecting an elevated temperature set point in response to NREM sleep loss (common
to both TSD and HSD), which accounts for why it did not occur in PSD rats
allowed NREM sleep (9). The second thermoregulatory response is most evident
later in SD (all forms) and involves an accelerating decline in body temperature
(toward hypothermia), indicating excessive heat loss as SD progresses
(37,39,43,49,50). Although an elevated temperature set point is most evident
early in SD and excessive heat loss later in SD, it is believed that both of these
thermoregulatory changes occur throughout SD in the rat (9,40). Consistent with
the excessive heat loss induced by SD, rats showed a behavioral preference for
increasingly warmer ambient temperatures on a thermal gradient (50°C) (39)
and increased operant responding for ambient heat (37°C) (118), relative to
baseline ambient temperature preference (26°C), prompting Rechtschaffen and
Bergmann (9) to conclude that "in both TSD and PSD rats, the positive correlation between EE and preferred ambient temperature is consistent with an elevation of thermogenesis and behavioral warming in response to a heat retention
deficit. If the primary pathology had been an increase in EE, then one would
have expected behavioral cooling." The increased plasma levels of NE (49), elevated T_3:T_4 ratio (49), and increased brown adipose tissue enzyme (35), as well
as the responses of sleep-deprived rats made hypothyroid by administration of
propylthiouracil (100), are consistent with compensatory thermogenesis driving,
at least in part, the increased EE of SD (9). It remains uncertain, however, how
SD-induced thermoregulatory changes are mediated (9) because noradrenergi-
cally mediated vasoconstriction appears normal (119), neither blockade of
prostaglandins (102) nor blockade of opioids (120) eliminated the elevated temperature set point in sleep-deprived rats, and lesions in the preoptic anterior
hypothalamus did not produce substantial changes in body temperature or elevated EE (103).

In addition to elevated thermal set point and increased heat loss (leading to hypothermia), sleep-deprived rats had reductions in the amplitude of the diurnal body temperature rhythm over the course of TSD, with complete recovery of the amplitude after the first day of recovery sleep (37). This effect is likely a reflection of increased heat loss. However, sleep-deprived rats also did not have a normal decrease in core body temperature accompanying recovery sleep (121). The wake-to-sleep body temperature decrease typically seen in non–sleep-deprived rats was reduced or reversed during recovery sleep in sleep-deprived rats (121). Although most dramatic on the first recovery sleep, this change continued across recovery days, in proportion to the length of TSD (9), suggesting that SD had long-term effects on thermogenesis and prompting the conclusion that recovery sleep was not serving either energy reduction or body cooling functions (121).

Body temperature responses in humans undergoing acute TSD for 1–11 days have been reported to show no changes, or to show changes similar to those seen in rats, but far more modest. For example, sleep-deprived humans typically show normal circadian variation in body temperature, but the amplitude of the circadian temperature rhythm can be reduced, an effect often attributed to the masking effects of ambulation on temperature. Human body temperature also has been reported to decrease across days of TSD, and subjects often complain of feeling cold even though the room temperature is held constant during SD experiments (115,122). However, there have been no reports of elevated temperature set points or serious hypothermia during SD in humans or of a failure of body temperature to decline during recovery sleep.

NEUROENDOCRINOLOGIC CHANGES WITH SD

There is a growing body of evidence that every hypothalamic–pituitary axis is influenced by both sleep and circadian rhythmicity (123). Similarly, SD with and without physical stressors affects many hormone secretion profiles (77), including growth hormone (115), prolactin (124), melatonin (125,127), and gonadal steroids (126). However, the most extensively investigated effects of SD in laboratory experiments are on sections of glucocorticoids, thyroid hormones, and catecholamines.

Hypothalamic–Pituitary–Adrenal Axis During SD

Upregulation of the hypothalamic–pituitary–adrenal (HPA) axis is established as the classic stress response. SD has long been considered to be stressful, yet controlled experiments have consistently failed to find elevated plasma or urinary levels of glucocorticoids (ACTH, corticosterone) during TSD in humans (61,106,115,127,144). In fact, there are even reports of reduced levels of corticosteroid levels as SD progressed (126). Surprisingly, similar negative results have been reported for prolonged SD in rats (Table 2) (5,9,36,49,51). Although adrenal hypertrophy has been found in sleep-deprived rats (Table 1) (5,36,42,43), in general, the classic physiologic markers of stress, including increased plasma levels of glucocorticoids, adrenal hypertrophy, and stomach ulcers, have either been absent, minimal, or uncorrelated with physiologic changes in sleep-deprived rats (64). It appears that experimentally induced SD under controlled laboratory conditions does not produce a classic HPA activation stress response in either humans or rats.

Thyroid Hormones During SD

In contrast to the HPA axis, changes in the hypothalamic–pituitary–thyroid (HPT) axis consistently accompany SD. Rats have been observed to develop central hypothyroidism during prolonged SD (9,51). Although plasma levels of unstimulated TSH were not changed by SD in rats (51), plasma thyroxine levels (total T_4 and free T_4) were decreased (9,35,51), as were plasma levels of triiodothyronine (total T_3 and free T_3) (49,51). Because the T_4 reductions with SD were greater than the T_3 decreases, the T_3/T_4 ratio increased (35). The changes in peripheral levels of thyroid hormones accompanying SD in rats are thought to reflect a compensatory thermogenesis (9). A number of experiments have been performed to probe thyroid function in sleep-deprived rats (Table 3). Induction of hypothyroidism by administration of propylthiouracil showed that the thyroid responses to TSD contributed to the increased EE, thermoregulatory set point increase and excessive heat loss, and development of skin lesions and debilitated appearance in TSD rats but did not change occurrence or timing of mortality (100). Administration of TRH to sleep-deprived rats increased circulating levels of TSH, free T_4, and free T_3 to levels found in control animals, suggesting that thyroid responses during TSD are intact (51). Administration of thyroxine (T_4) to sleep-deprived rats increased metabolic rates, elevated body temperature, and reduced warming behaviors, but it also shortened life span by 37% (46).

In contrast, to the effects in rats, in humans SD is associated with elevated levels of TSH (128–130) and elevated circulating levels of T_4 and T_3 (130). The latter show a dose-dependent response to TSD, and the increases appear to be due in part to sustained physical and cognitive activity demands during TSD (130–132). The basis for the differences in thyroid responses of humans and rats to SD remain unclear, but as noted above, experiments in humans typically involve many fewer days of SD than the rat studies. Increases in T_4 and T_3 in both rat serum and frontal cortex after 24 hours of SD have been found (133), suggesting that the differential thyroid hormone profiles of SD in humans and rats may indeed be due to the duration of SD studied.

Catecholamines and SD

One of the more consistent effects of prolonged SD in rats is elevated plasma levels of norepinephrine (49), which is thought to reflect sympathetic activation

(9). Blockade of sympathetic activation by guanethidine (GU) in TSD rats reduced plasma NE levels but resulted in elevations of plasma epinephrine above levels seen in other TSD rat studies (Table 3) (101). GU administration did not alter either increased energy expenditure or the typical syndromal and lethal effects of TSD, prompting the conclusion that GU resulted in "substitution of one calorigenic mediator (epinephrine) for another (NE) in response to an abnormally elevated *need* for energy" (9).

In humans, urinary excretion of NE and epinephrine have not been found to be increased during controlled laboratory studies of SD (131,134,135), and similar results have been obtained for plasma NE (136). However, one study has reported increased vanilylmandelic acid (a catecholamine metabolite) excretion during SD (105). In studies of SD combined with continuous heavy physical activities and an almost total lack of food, plasma levels of NE have been reported to increase significantly across days (77). Thus, it appears that in humans, catecholamine activation is modest during SD, unless the deprivation is accompanied by other physical stressors.

NEUROIMMUNE FUNCTION DURING SD

There is a growing scientific literature on the regulation of sleep by cytokines (IL-β, IFN-α) and related neuroimmunomodulators (23,24) and the role of sleep in immune enhancement (137–139). The effects of SD on immunologic parameters have been the focus of a growing number of experiments in recent years (140–142, 142a). In rats sleep deprived by the disk-over-water method, immune function has not been extensively studied, and what has been found is not entirely consistent. Studies of splenic lymphocytes from rats undergoing prolonged TSD found no significant in vitro effects of SD on T-lymphocyte blastogenesis to stimulation by mitogens [concanavalin A (Con-A) and lipopolysaccharide (LPS)], and no altered B-lymphocyte antibody response to stimulation (Table 2) (65). However, Everson (47) found bacteremia and septicemia from common opportunistic microbes in TSD rats in the terminal stages of debilitation (Table 1). These animals had no febrile response. She concluded that prolonged SD involves a breakdown of host defense against indigenous and pathogenic microorganisms (47) and that it is the adverse effects SD immune function that leads to most of the other physiologic effects of SD (33,47,142a). For example, she posits that if SD compromises host defense, then the ensuing infection would trigger release of cytokines, which could mediate the hypercatabolism, weight loss, cachexia, hypothermia, skins lesions, and neuroendocrine responses found in sleep-deprived rats (33,142a). However, two recent experiments cast doubt on the likelihood that compromised host defense is a necessary condition for the lethal effects of SD in rats (Table 3) (9). In the first of these, antibiotics were administered to TSD rats, and although there was a nonsignificant trend for bacterial invasion early in TSD, as Everson (33) would have predicted, antibiotic treatment did not prevent the hypothermia or lethality of TSD (103a). In the second study, TSD rats and controls were implanted with Walker 256 rat carcinoma cells to test if host defense against subdermal implantation of tumor cells was changed by TSD (52,52a). Tumor size was reduced faster in TSD rats than controls (Tables 1 and 3), and change in sleep time during TSD, not weight loss, predicted tumor size, prompting the conclusion that compromised host defense is unlikely to be the primary physiologic effect of SD. The issue remains open to inquiry, however, because other experiments of shorter durations of SD in rats (143) and mice (140) have reported immune deficits, especially in animals that had been immunologically challenged (139,142a).

Experiments on human neuroimmune responses to SD have been as infrequent and inconclusive as the animal studies (141,142a). One consistent finding is that TSD in humans is associated with elevated plasma levels of leukocytes, granulocytes, and monocytes (105,141,144), suggesting an upregulation during TSD in human nonspecific host defense. The basis for this upregulation and its significance for immune function and possible host defense compromise remain to be elucidated. Lymphocyte counts have been found to both increase and decrease in sleep-deprived humans, with no consistent outcomes concerning in vitro lymphocyte responses to mitogens or plasma levels of cytokines (141). There is also no evidence to date that acute TSD in healthy humans results in elevated physiologic markers of infection or illness (141,144). On the other hand, experiments on the immune effects of SD have been performed in healthy young adults who have not been challenged immunologically; consequently, the functional capability of human immune responses during SD remains to be more thoroughly examined.

CONCLUSIONS

Based on an evaluation of the physiologic correlates of SD, there is evidence that sleep serves a fundamental role in the maintenance of balanced energy expenditure for the whole organism, with a possible executive role in this process based in brain activity. Service to this energy balance function would explain why SD does not result in apparent failure of any one organ in the body or any one specific area of the brain, but rather results in a range of deficits throughout the body. Although sleep may ultimately serve energy balance, it also appears to do this on two markedly different time scales: one for the brain and another for the body. The effects of SD on the brain are surprisingly immediate relative to those on the body and include rapid development of sleepiness, diminished waking brain functions, and heightening homeostatic response during recovery sleep. Early onset of neurobehavioral and neurophysiologic changes in response to SD have been found in humans and other animals, suggesting that these early brain responses either indicate deficits from SD or compensatory mechanisms that engage to promote sleep behavior in advance of more serious consequences for the body. As SD progresses, it is possible that the metabolic costs of sustained wakefulness and the behavioral processes required to maintain it take a cumulative toll.

The biologic basis for the increased metabolic demand may reside in thermoregulatory changes, but the mechanisms remain unknown. Whatever the source, the hypermetabolism the sleep-deprived rats undergo does not show up in weight, waste, or work. Food is being burned at a higher rate, but the body does not appear to benefit thermally from this increased consumption. It is as though the SD rat cannot regulate its daily metabolic needs within an energy utilization range that ensures survival but instead continues to metabolically upregulate as SD progresses, either because of an as yet unrecognized energy demand or because metabolism has become fixed in an upwardly spiraling cycle in response to each prior level of hypermetabolism. In this second possibility, sleep serves to reset the daily waking metabolic rate slightly above the sleep rate.

These conclusions rely on the findings of the experiments of SD in rats using the disk-over-water method developed by Rechtschaffen et al. (5). We do not believe that this paradigm can be dismissed based on arguments that it is lethal merely by virtue of being stressful, or that it simply reflects a unique species-specific response of rats to SD. Although certain details of the SD effects obtained with the paradigm may not translate to humans (e.g., skin lesions, REM vs. SWS rebound), the results of the paradigm are consistent with data on the relationship between sleep, endothermy, and energy conservation. Moreover, this animal model of prolonged SD effects is comparable with human SD effects in one fundamental way. A single night of recovery sleep reverses the major effects of days of SD on brain function in humans and weeks of SD on metabolic disturbance in rats (assuming hypothermia has not gone too far). This remarkable reversal occurs for physiologic effects that have shown cumulative increases to debilitating levels. In both humans and rats, recovery sleep responds by an intensity function. Thus, the first recovery sleep after TSD is not characterized by a duration that reclaims all or even most of the lost sleep, but rather by a very deep, sustained sleep. That a single recovery sleep pulse can reverse the negative energy balance that the sleep-deprived rats experience suggests (a) that short of severe hypothermia, SD effects are not due to irreversible changes and (b) that recovery sleep and its accompanying anabolism serve to somehow recalibrate waking metabolic demands. A similar rapid resetting of neurobehavioral functions deteriorated by SD characterizes recovery sleep in humans. On the other hand, critically ill humans and those unable to acquire adequate recovery sleep may be more vulnerable to SD effects, especially if their energy compensatory systems (i.e., nutritional status, thermoregulatory capacity, immune function) are diminished by illness or medical procedures. Clearly there is much more to be discovered about how SD leads to physiologic changes and how sleep promotes recovery from illness.

ACKNOWLEDGMENTS

The substantive evaluation on which this article is based was supported in part by grants from the National Institutes of Health (HL42236, NR04281, HL07713), U.S. Public Health Service, National Aeronautics and Space Administration (NCC-2-599), U.S. Air Force Office of Scientific Research (F49620-95-1-0388), and Institute for Experimental Psychiatry Research Foundation. We thank Sheelu Samuel for help in preparing the manuscript.

REFERENCES

1. National Commission on Sleep Disorders Research. *Wake up America: a national sleep alert.* Washington, DC: Sup. of Docs., US Govt Off, 1993:1–76.
1a. Whitehouse WG, Dinges DF, Orne EC, Keller SE, Bates BL, Bauer NK, Morahan P, Haupt BA, Carlin MM, Bloom PB, Zaugg L, Orne MT. Psychosocial and immune effects of self-hypnosis training for stress management throughout the first semester of medical school. *Psychosom Med* 1996;58(3)249–263.
2. Leventhal L, Freundlich B, Lewis J, et al. Controlled study of sleep parameters in patients with fibromyalgia. *J Clin Rheumatol* 1995;1:110–113.
3. Darko DF, McCutchan JA, Kripke DF, et al. Fatigue, sleep disturbance, disability, and indices of progression of HIV infection. *Am J Psychiatry* 1992;149:514–520.
4. Schwab RJ. Disturbances of sleep in the intensive care unit. *Crit Care Clin* 1994;10:681–694.
5. Rechtschaffen A, Gilliland MA, Bergmann BM, Winter JB. Physiological correlates of prolonged sleep deprivation in rats. *Science* 1983;221:182–184.
6. Zepelin H. Mammalian sleep. In: Kryger MH, Roth T, Dement WC, eds. *Principles and Practice of Sleep Medicine. 2nd ed.* London:WB Saunders; 1994:69–80.
7. Elgar MA, Pagel MD, Harvey PH. Sleep in mammals. *Animal Behaviour* 1988;36:1407–1419.
8. Allison T, Cicchetti DV. Sleep in mammals: ecological and constitutional correlates. *Science* 1976; 194:732–734.
9. Rechtschaffen A, Bergmann BM. Sleep deprivation in the rat by the disk-over-water method. *Behav Brain Res* 1995;69:55–63.
10. Borbely AA. A two-process model of sleep regulation. *Hum Neurobiol* 1982;1:195–204.
11. Daan S, Beersma DGM, Borbely AA. Timing of human sleep: recovery process gated by a circadian pacemaker. *Am J Physiol* 1984;246:R161–R178.
12. Dijk D, Duffy JF, Czeisler CA. Circadian and sleep/wake dependent aspects of subjective alertness and cognitive performance. *J Sleep Res* 1992;1:112–117.
13. Edgar DM, Dement WC, Fuller CA. Effect of SCN lesions on sleep in squirrel monkeys: evidence for opponent processes in sleep-wake regulation. *J Neurosci* 1993;13:1065–1079.
14. Babkoff H, Caspy T, Mikulincer M. Monotonic and rhythmic influences: a challenge for sleep deprivation research. *Psychol Bull* 1991;109:411–428.
15. Dinges DF, Kribbs NB. Performing while sleepy: effects of experimentally-induced sleepiness. In: Monk TH, ed. *Sleep, Sleepiness and Performance.* Chichester: Wiley; 1991:97–128.
16. Horne JA. *Why we sleep: the functions of sleep in humans and other mammals.* New York: Oxford University Press; 1988.
17. Horne JA. Human sleep, sleep loss and behaviour: implications for the prefrontal cortex and psychiatric disorder. *Br J Psychiatry* 1993;162:413–419.
18. Steriade M, McCormick DA, Sejnowski TJ. Thalamocortical oscillations in the sleeping and aroused brain. *Science* 1993;262:679–685.
19. Steriade M. Brain electrical activity and sensory processing during waking and sleep states. In: Kryger MH, Roth T, Dement WC, eds. *Principles and practice of sleep medicine. 2nd ed.* London: WB Saunders; 1994:105–124.
20. Siegel JM. Brainstem mechanisms generating REM sleep. In: Kryger MH, Roth T, Dement WC, eds. *Principles and practice of sleep medicine. 2nd ed.* London: WB Saunders; 1994:125–144.

21. Jones BE. Basic mechanisms of sleep-wake states. In: Kryger MH, Roth T, Dement WC, eds. *Priniciples and practice of sleep medicine.* 2nd ed. London: WB Saunders; 1994:145–162.
22. Borbely AA, Tobler I. Endogenous sleep-promoting substances and sleep regulation. *Physiol Rev* 1989;69:605–670.
23. Krueger JM, Majde JA. Microbial products and cytokines in sleep and fever regulation. *Crit Rev Immunol* 1994;14:355–379.
24. Krueger JM, Toth LA, Floyd R, et al. Sleep, microbes and cytokines. *Neuroimmunomodulation* 1994;1:100–109.
25. McGinty DJ, Szymusiak RS. Keeping cool: a hypothesis about the mechanisms and functions of slow wave sleep. *Trends Neurosci* 1990;13:480–487.
26. Berger RJ, Phillips NH. Regulation of energy metabolism and body temperature during sleep and circadian torpor. In: Lydic R, Biebuyck JF, eds. *Clinical physiology of sleep.* Bethesda, MD: American Physiological Society; 1988:171–198.
27. Krueger JM, Obal F Jr. Growth hormone-releasing hormone and interleukin-1 in sleep regulation. *FASEB J* 1993;7:645–652.
28. Benington JH, Heller HC. Restoration of brain energy metabolism as the function of sleep. *Prog Neurobiol* 1995;45:347–360.
29. Krueger JM, Obal F Jr, Kapas L, Fang J. Brain organization and sleep function. *Behav Brain Res* 1995;69:177–185.
30. Kleitman N. *Sleep and wakefulness.* Chicago: University of Chicago Press; 1963.
31. Rechtschaffen A, Bergmann BM, Everson CA, et al. Sleep deprivation in the rat. I. Conceptual issues. *Sleep* 1989;12:1–4.
32. Bergmann BM, Kushida CA, Everson CA, et al. Sleep deprivation in the rat. II. Methodology. *Sleep* 1989;12:5–12.
33. Everson CA. Functional consequences of sustained sleep deprivation in the rat. *Behav Brain Res* 1995;69:43–54.
34. Gilliland MA, Wold L, Wollmann R, et al. Pathology in sleep deprived rats is not reflected in histologic abnormalities [Abstract]. *Sleep Res* 1984;13:190.
35. Balzano S, Bergmann BM, Gilliland MA, et al. Effect of total sleep deprivation on 58-deiodinase activity of rat brown adipose tissue. *Endocrinology* 1990;127:882–890.
36. Everson CA, Gilliland MA, Kushida CA, et al. Sleep deprivation in the rat. IX. Recovery. *Sleep* 1989;12:60–67.
37. Tsai L, Bergmann BM, Rechtschaffen A. Sleep deprivation in the rat. XVI. Effects in a light-dark cycle. *Sleep* 1992;15:537–544.
38. Everson CA, Bergmann BM, Rechtschaffen A. Sleep deprivation in the rat. III. Total sleep deprivation. *Sleep* 1989;12:13–21.
39. Prete FR, Bergmann BM, Holtzman P, et al. Sleep deprivation in the rat. XII. Effect on ambient temperature choice. *Sleep* 1991;14:109–115.
40. Obermeyer W, Bergmann BM, Rechtschaffen A. Sleep deprivation in the rat. XIV. Comparison of waking hypothalamic and peritoneal temperatures. *Sleep* 1991;14:285–93.
41. Everson CA, Wehr TA. Nutritional and metabolic adaptations to prolonged sleep deprivation in the rat. *Am J Physiol* 1993;264:R376–R387.
42. Kushida CA, Bergmann BM, Rechtschaffen A. Sleep deprivation in the rat. IV. Paradoxical sleep deprivation. *Sleep* 1989;12:22–30.
43. Gilliland MA, Bergmann BM, Rechtschaffen A. Sleep deprivation in the rat. VIII. High EEG amplitude sleep deprivation. *Sleep* 1989;12:53–59.
44. Everson CA, Smith SB, Sokoloff L. Effects of prolonged sleep deprivation on local rates of cerebral energy metabolism in freely moving rats. *J Neurosci* 1994;14:6769–6778.
45. Kushida CA, Everson CA, Suthipinittharm P, et al. Sleep deprivation in the rat. VI. Skin changes. *Sleep* 1989;12:42–46.
46. Bergmann BM, Gilliland MA, Balzano S, et al. Sleep deprivation in the rat. XIX. Effects of thyroxine administration. *Sleep* 1995;18:317–324.
47. Everson CA. Sustained sleep deprivation impairs host defense. *Am J Physiol* 1993;265: R1148–R1154.
48. Bergmann BM, Seidan LS, Landis CA, et al. Sleep deprivation in the rat. XVIII. Regional brain levels of monoamines and their metabolites. *Sleep* 1994;17:583–589.
49. Bergmann BM, Everson CA, Kushida CA, et al. Sleep deprivation in the rat. V. Energy use and mediation. *Sleep* 1989;12:31–41.

50. Landis CA, Bergmann BM, Ismail MM, Rechtschaffen A. Sleep deprivation in the rat. XV. Ambient temperature choice in paradoxical sleep-deprived rats. *Sleep* 1992;15:13–20.
51. Everson CA, Reed HL. Pituitary and peripheral thyroid hormone responses to thyrotropin-releasing hormone during sustained sleep deprivation in freely moving rats. *Endocrinology* 1995;136: 1426–1434.
52. Bergmann BM, Kovar S, Rechtschaffen A, Quintans J. Effect of brief sleep deprivation on tumor growth in the rat [Abstract]. *Sleep Res* 1994;23:403.
52a. Bergmann BM, Rechtschaffen A, Gilliland MA, Qunitans J. Effect of extended sleep-deprivation on tumor-growth in rats. *Am J Physiol* 1996;40(5)R1460–R1464.
53. Lugaresi ER, Medori R, Montagna P, et al. Fatal familial insomnia and dysautonomia with selective degeneration of thalamic nuclei. *N Engl J Med* 1986;315:997–1003.
54. Medori R, Tritschler HJ, LeBlanc A, et al. Fatal familial insomnia:a prion disease with a mutation at codon 178 of the prion protein gene. *N Engl J Med* 1992;326:444–487.
55. Montagna P, Cortelli P, Gambetti P, Lugaresi ER. Fatal familial insomnia: sleep, neuroendocrine and vegetative alterations. *Adv Neuroimmunol* 1995;5:13–21.
56. Montagna P, Cortelli P, Tinuper P, et al. Fatal familial insomnia: a disease that emphasizes the role of the thalamus in regulation of sleep and vegetative functions. In: Guilleminault C, Lugaresi E, Montagna P, Gambetti P, eds. *Fatal familial insomnia: inherited prion diseases, sleep, and the thalamus.* New York: Raven; 1994:1–14.
57. Perani D, Cortelli P, Lucignani G, et al. [18F] FDG PET in fatal familial insomnia: the functional effects of thalamic lesions. *Neurology* 1993;43:2565–2569.
58. Lugaresi E, Montagna P. Thalamus, sleep, and circadian functions. In: Guilleminault C, Lugaresi E, Montagna P, Gambetti P, eds. *Fatal familial insomnia: inherited prion diseases, sleep, and the thalamus.* New York: Raven; 1994:215–219.
59. Johnson LC, Slye ES, Dement WC. Electroencephalographic and autonomic activity during and after prolonged sleep deprivation. *Psychosomatic Med* 1965;27:415–423.
60. Gulevich G, Dement WC, Johnson LC. Psychiatric and EEG observations on a case of prolonged (264 hours) wakefulness. *Arch Gene Psychiatry* 1966;15:29–35.
61. Kollar EJ, Slater GR, Palmer JO, et al. Stress in subjects undergoing sleep deprivation. *Psychosomat Med* 1966;28:101–113.
62. Wehr TA. Sleep loss: a preventable cause of mania and other excited states. *J Clin Psychiatry* 1989;50(suppl):8–16.
63. Feng P, Bergmann BM, Rechtschaffen A. Effect of total sleep deprivation on neuronal ultrastructure in the rat [Abstract]. *Sleep Res* 1996;25:466.
64. Rechtschaffen A, Bergmann BM, Everson CA, et al. Sleep deprivation in the rat. X. Integration and discussion of the findings. *Sleep* 1989;12:68–87.
65. Benca RM, Kushida CA, Everson CA, et al. Sleep deprivation in the rat. VII. Immune function. *Sleep* 1989;12:47–52.
66. Licklider JCR, Bunch ME. Effects of enforced wakefulness upon the growth and the maze-learning performance of white rats. *J Compar Psychol* 1946;39:339–350.
67. Ebert D, Kaschka WP, Loew T, Beck G. Cortisol and beta-endorphin responses to sleep deprivation in major depression—the hyperarousal theories of sleep deprivation. *Neuropsychobiology* 1994;29:64–68.
68. Wehr TA. Effects of sleep and wakefulness on depression and mania. In: Montplaisir J, Godbout R, eds. *Sleep and biological rhythms.* London: Oxford Press; 1991
69. Reist C, Sokolski KN, Chen C, et al. The effect of sleep deprivation on motor impairment and retinal adaptation in Parkinson's disease. *Prog Neuropsychopharmacol Biol Psychiatry* 1995;19: 445–454.
70. Tartara A, Moglia A, Manni R, Corbellini C. EEG findings and sleep deprivation. *Eur Neurol* 1980;19:330–334.
71. Johnson LC. Sleep deprivation and performance. In: Webb WB, ed. *Biological rhythms, sleep and performance.* New York: Wiley; 1982:111–141.
72. Dinges DF. Probing the limits of functional capability: the effects of sleep loss on short-duration tasks. In: Broughton RJ, Ogilvie RD, eds. *Sleep, arousal, and performance.* Boston: Birkhauser; 1992:176–188.
73. Bonnet MH. Sleep deprivation. In: Kryger MH, Roth T, Dement WC, eds. *Principles and practice of sleep medicine.* Philadelphia: WB Saunders; 1994:50–67.
74. Carskadon MA, Roth T. Sleep restriction. In: Monk TH, ed. *Sleep, sleepiness and performance.* New York: Wiley; 1991:155–167.

74a. Dinges DF, Pack F, Williams K, Gillen KA, Powell JA, Ott GE, Aptowicz C, Pack AI. Cumulative sleepiness, mood disturbance, and psychomotor vigilance performance decrements during a week of sleep restricted to 4–5 hours per night. *Sleep* (in press).

75. Opstad PK, Aakvaag A, Rognum TO. Altered hormonal response to short-term bicycle exercise in young men after prolonged physical strain, caloric deficit, and sleep deprivation. *Eur J Appl Physiol* 1980;45:51–62.

76. Opstad PK, Aakvaag A. The effect of a high calorie diet on hormonal changes in young men during prolonged physical strain and sleep deprivation. *Eur J Applied Physiol* 1981;46:31–39.

77. Opstad PK. Circadian rhythm of hormones is extinguished during prolonged physical stress, sleep and energy deficiency in young men. *Eur J Endocrinol* 1994;131:56–55.

78. Opstad PK, Haugen AH, Sejersted OM, et al. Atrial natriuretic peptide in plasma after prolonged physical strain, energy deficiency and sleep deprivation. *Eur J Appl Physiol* 1994;68:122–126.

79. Carskadon MA, Dement WC. Daytime sleepiness: quantification of a behavioral state. *Neurosci Biobehav Rev* 1987;11:307–317.

80. Naitoh P. Sleep deprivation in human subjects: a reappraisal. *Waking Sleeping* 1976;1:53–60.

81. Lorenzo I, Ramos J, Arce C, et al. Effect of total sleep deprivation on reaction time and waking EEG activity in man. *Sleep* 1995;18:346–354.

82. Cajochen C, Brunner DP, Krauchi K, et al. Power density in theta/alpha frequencies of the waking EEG progressively increases during sustained wakefulness. *Sleep* 1995;18:890–894.

83. Humphrey DG, Kramer AF, Stanny RR. Influence of extended wakefulness on automatic and nonautomatic processing. *Hum Factors* 1994;36:652–669.

84. Schlesinger A, Dahl R, Redfern M, Jennings R. Sleep deprivation impairs the control of postural balance while performing a cognitive task [Abstract]. *Sleep Res* 1996;25:477.

85. Wu JC, Gillin JC, Buchsbaum MS, et al. The effect of sleep deprivation on cerebral glucose metabolic rate in normal humans assessed with positron emission tomography. *Sleep* 1991;14:155–162.

86. Thomas ML, Sing HC, Belenky G, et al. Cerebral glucose utilization during task performance and prolonged sleep loss [Abstract]. *J Cereb Blood Flow Metab* 1993;13:S531.

87. Thakkar M, Mallick BN. Rapid eye movement sleep-deprivation–induced changes in glucose metabolic enzymes in rat brain. *Sleep* 1993;16:691–694.

88. Rosenthal L, Merlotti L, Roehrs TA, Roth T. Enforced 24-hour recovery following sleep deprivation. *Sleep* 1991;14:448–453.

89. Feinberg I, March JD. Observations on delta homeostasis, the one-stimulus model of NREM-REM alternation and the neurobiologic implications of experimental dream studies. *Behav Brain Res* 1995;69:97–108.

90. Dinges DF. Differential effects of prior wakefulness and circadian phase on nap sleep. *Electroencephalogr Clin Neurophysiol* 1986;64:224–227.

91. Feinberg I. Changes in sleep cycle patterns with age. *J Psychiatr Res* 1974;10:283–306.

92. Borbely AA, Baumann F, Brandeis D, et al. Sleep deprivation: effect on sleep stages and EEG power density in man. *Electroencephalogr Clin Neurophysiol* 1981;51:483–493.

93. Achermann P, Dijk D, Brunner DP, Borbely AA. A model of human sleep homeostasis based on EEG slow-wave activity: quantitative comparison of data and simulations. *Brain Res Bull* 1993; 31:97–113.

94. Brock JW, Hamdi A, Ross K, et al. REM sleep deprivation alters dopamine D2 receptor in the rat frontal cortex. *Pharmacol Biochem Behav* 1995;52:43–48.

95. Mallick BN, Thakkar M, Gangabhagirathi R. Rapid eye movement sleep deprivation decreases membrane fluidity in the rat brain. *Neurosci Res* 1995;22:117–122.

96. O'Hara BF, Young KA FL, et al. Immediate early gene expression in brain during sleep deprivation: preliminary observations. *Sleep* 1993;16:1–7.

97. Neuner-Jehle M, Rhyner TA, Borbely AA. Sleep deprivation differentially alters the mRNA and protein levels of neurogranin in rat brain. *Brain Res* 1995;685:143–153.

98. Sallanon-Moulin M, Touret M, Didier-Bazes M, et al. Glutamine synthetase modulation in the brain of rats subjected to deprivation of paradoxical sleep. *Mol Brain Res* 1994;22:113–120.

99. Toppila J, Stenberg D, Alanko L, et al. REM sleep deprivation induces galanin gene expression in the rat brain. *Neurosci Lett* 1995;183:171–174.

100. Pilcher JJ, Bergmann BM, Refetoff S, et al. Sleep deprivation in the rat. XIII. The effect of hypothyroidism on sleep deprivation symptoms. *Sleep* 1991;14:201–210.

101. Pilcher JJ, Bergmann BM, Fang VS, et al. Sleep deprivation in the rat. XI. The effect of guanethidine-induced sympathetic blockade on the sleep deprivation syndrome. *Sleep* 1990;13: 218–231.

102. Bergmann BM, Landis CA, Zenko CE. Sleep deprivation in the rat. XVII. Effect of aspirin on elevated body temperature. *Sleep* 1993;16:221–225.

103. Feng P, Bergmann BM, Rechtschaffen A. Sleep deprivation in rats with preoptic/anterior hypothalamic lesions [Abstract]. *Sleep Res* 1994;23:411.

103a. Bermann BM, Gilliland MA, Feng PF, et al. Are physiological effects of sleep-deprivation in the rat mediated by bacterial invasion. *Sleep* 1996;19(7):554–562.

104. Fiorica V, Higgins EA, Iampietro PF, et al. Physiological responses of men during sleep deprivation. *J Appl Physiol* 1968;24:167–176.

105. Kuhn E, Brodan V, Brodanova M, Rysanek K. Metabolic reflection of sleep deprivation. *Activitas Nervosa Superior* 1969;11:165–174.

106. Kant GJ, Genser SG, Thorne DR, et al. Effects of 72 hour sleep deprivation on urinary cortisol and indices of metabolism. *Sleep* 1984;7:142–146.

107. Bonnet MH, Berry RB, Arand DL. Metabolism during normal, fragmented, and recovery sleep. *J Appl Physiol* 1991;71:1112–1118.

108. Scrimshaw NS, Habicht JP, Pellet P, et al. Effects of sleep deprivation and reversal of diurnal activity on protein metabolism of young men. *Am J Clin Nutr* 1966;19:313–319.

109. Neri DF, Wiegmann D, Stanny RR, et al. The effects of tyrosine on cognitive performance during extended wakefulness. *Aviat Space Environ Med* 1995;66:313–319.

110. Rodgers CD, Paterson DH, Cunningham DA, et al. Sleep deprivation: effects on work capacity, self-paced walking, contractile properties and perceived exertion. *Sleep* 1995;18:30–38.

111. Angus RG, Heslegrave RJ, Myles WS. Effects of prolonged sleep deprivation, with and without chronic physical exercise, on mood and performance. *Psychophysiology* 1985;22:276–282.

112. Hill DW, Borden DO, Darnaby KM, Hendricks DN. Aerobic and anaerobic contributions to exhaustive high-intensity exercise after sleep deprivation. *J Sports Sci* 1994;12:455–461.

113. Symons JD, Vanhelder T, Myles WS. Physical performance and physiological responses following 60 hours of sleep deprivation. *Med Sci Sports Exerc* 1988;20:374–380.

114. Martin BJ, Bender PR, Chen H. Stress hormonal response to exercise after sleep loss. *Eur J Appl Physiol Occup Physiol* 1986;55:210–214.

115. VanHelder T, Radomski MW. Sleep deprivation and the effect on exercise performance. *Sports Med* 1989;7:235–247.

116. Brodan V, Kuhn E. Physical performance in man during sleep deprivation. *J Sports Med Phys Fit* 1967;7:28–30.

117. Brodan V, Vojtechovsky M, Kuhn E, Cepelak J. Changes of mental and physical performance in sleep deprived healthy volunteers. *Activ Nerv Super* (Praha) 1969;11:175–181.

118. Shaw P, Bergmann BM, Rechtschaffen A. Operant control of ambient temperature during sleep deprivation [Abstract]. *Sleep Res* 1994;23:424.

119. Obermeyer WH, Bergmann BM, Rechtschaffen A. The effect of sleep deprivation on the thermoregulatory response of rats to phentolamine [Abstract]. *Sleep Res* 1993;22:340.

120. Zenko CE, Bergmann BM, Rechtschaffen A. The effects of naltrexone on the regulated rise in body temperature in sleep deprived rats [Abstract]. *Sleep Res* 1993;22:351.

121. Feng P, Shaw P, Bergmann BM, et al. Sleep deprivation in the rat. XX. Differences in wake and sleep temperatures during recovery. *Sleep* 1995;18:797–804.

122. Dinges DF, Orne MT, Whitehouse WG, Orne EC. Temporal placement of a nap for alertness: contributions of circadian phase and prior wakefulness. *Sleep* 1987;10:313–329.

123. Van Cauter E. Diurnal and ultradian rhythms in human endocrine function: a minireview. *Hormone Res* 1990;34:45–53.

124. Kasper S, Sack DA, Wehr TA, et al. Nocturnal TSH and prolactin secretion during sleep deprivation and prediction of antidepressant response in patients with major depression. *Biol Psychiatry* 1988;24:631–641.

125. Åkerstedt T, Fröberg JE, Friberg Y, Wetterberg L. Melatonin excretion, body temperature and subjective arousal during 64 hours of sleep deprivation. *Psychoneuroendocrinology* 1979;4:219–225.

126. Åkerstedt T, Palmblad J, de la Torre B, et al. Adrenocortical and gonadal steroids during sleep deprivation. *Sleep* 1980;3:23–40.

127. Salin-Pascual RJ, Ortega-Soto H, Huerto-Delgadillo L, et al. The effect of total sleep deprivation on plasma melatonin and cortisol in healthy human volunteers. *Sleep* 1988;11:362–369.

128. Parker DC, Rossman LG, Pekary AE, Hershman JM. Effect of 64-hour sleep deprivation on the circadian waveform of thyrotropin (TSH): further evidence of sleep-related inhibition of TSH release. *J Clin Endocrinol Metab* 1987;64:157–161.

129. Allan JS, Czeisler CA. Persistence of the circadian thyrotropin rhythm under constant conditions and after light-induced shifts of circadian phase. *J Clin Endocrinol Metab* 1994;79:508–512.
130. Gary KA, Winokur A, Douglas SD, et al. Total sleep deprivation and the thyroid axis: effects of sleep and waking activity. *Aviat Space Environ Med* 1996;67:513–519.
131. Palmblad J, Åkerstedt T, Fröberg JE, et al. Thyroid and adrenomedullary reactions during sleep deprivation. *Acta Endorinol* 1979;90:233–239.
132. Radomski MW, Hart LEM, Goodman JM, Plyley MJ. Aerobic fitness and hormonal responses to prolonged sleep deprivation and sustained mental work. *Aviat Space Environ Med* 1992;63: 101–106.
133. Campos-Barros A, Kohler R, Muller F, et al. The influence of sleep deprivation on thyroid hormone metabolism in rat frontal cortex. *Neurosci Lett* 1993;162:145–148.
134. Fröberg JE, Karlsson C, Levi L, Lidberg L. Circadian rhythms of catecholamine excretion, shooting range performance and self-ratings of fatigue during sleep deprivation. *Biol Psychol* 1975;2: 175–188.
135. Åkerstedt T, Fröberg JE. Sleep, stress and sleep deprivation in relation to circadian rhythms in catecholamine excretion. *Biol Psychol* 1979;8:69–80.
136. Candito M, Pringuey D, Jacomet Y, et al. Circadian rhythm in plasma noradrenaline of healthy sleep-deprived subjects. *Chronobiol Int* 1992;9:444–447.
137. Toth LA, Tolley EA, Krueger JM. Sleep as a prognostic indicator during infectious disease in rabbits. *Proc Soc Exp Biol Med* 1993;203:179–192.
138. Kimura-Takeuchi M, Majde JA, Toth LA, Krueger JM. Influenza virus-induced changes in rabbit sleep and acute phase responses. *Am J Physiol* 1992;263:R1115–R1121.
139. Toth LA, Opp MR, Mao L. Somnogenic effects of sleep deprivation and Escherichia coli inoculation in rabbits. *J Sleep Res* 1995;4:30–40.
140. Brown R, Pang G, Husband AJ, et al. Sleep deprivation and the immune response to pathogenic and non-pathogenic antigens. In: Husband AJ, ed. *Behaviour and Immunity.* Boca Raton, FL: CRC Press; 1992:127–133.
141. Dinges DF, Douglas SD, Hamarman S, et al. Sleep deprivation and human immune function. *Adv Neuroimmunol* 1995;5:97–110.
142. Toth LA. Sleep deprivation and infectious disease: studies in animals. *Adv Neuroimmunol* 1995;5:79–92.
142a. Everson CA. Sleep deprivation and the immue system. In: Pressman MR, Orr WC, eds. *Understanding Sleep: The Evaluation and Treatment of Sleep Disorders.* Washington, DC: American Psychological Association; (in press).
143. Brown R, Price RJ, King MG, Husband AJ. Interleukin-1 β and muramyl dipeptide can prevent decreased antibody response associated with sleep deprivation. *Brain Behav Immun* 1989;3: 320–330.
144. Dinges DF, Douglas SD, Zaugg L, et al. Leukocytosis and natural killer cell function parallel neurobehavioral fatigue induced by 64 hours of sleep deprivation. *J Clin Invest* 1994;93:1930–1939.

Physiology, Stress, and Malnutrition: Functional Correlates, Nutritional Intervention,
edited by J.M. Kinney and H.N. Tucker.
Lippincott–Raven Publishers © 1997.

Thermoregulatory Control of Non-REM Sleep

Dennis J. McGinty

Sepulveda Veterans Administration Medical Center, Los Angeles, California 91343

It is widely believed that sleep is restorative, providing some process essential for physiologic health and, therefore, for waking function. The hypothesis that sleep is restorative is supported by several findings. Studies summarized here show that deprivation of sleep, like deprivation of feeding, drinking, and breathing, is lethal. All homeotherms that have been studied exhibit sleep, and many physiologic correlates of sleep are similar among about 100 mammalian and avian species (1). Sleep is clearly a basic behavior of higher animals. Despite this evidence for the critical importance of sleep, there is little agreement among scientists concerning the essential role of sleep in the sustenance of life. This is one of the major unanswered questions in biology.

Additional arguments of the need for sleep include the fact that, as a survival strategy, sleep is a costly process, preventing the foraging for food. Sensory thresholds are elevated during sleep, exposing the animal to dangers such as predation. Of course, sleep "enforces" a period of inactivity in a nest; it has been argued that sleep is primarily a process that keeps a species in the circadian characteristic of its ecologic niche (2). But animals could remain in relatively secure nests without sleeping, and some species do not use nests. Also, this theory does not explain why sleep deprivation is lethal. It is doubtful that a ubiquitous essential-for-life homeothermic behavior exists only to ensure nesting or circadian regulation. It is possible that sleep may serve several functions, like other complex processes. For example, breathing provides gas exchange, phonation, and heat exchange. By analogy, sleep may serve multiple functions. However, also by analogy with the gas exchange provided by breathing, we might expect that some essential physiologic process is at the root of the need for sleep. We present evidence for one such basic function, bearing in mind that additional functions are likely. Our studies extend work by previous investigators that links sleep and thermoregulation as a basis for energy conservation and other temperature-dependent functions (3,4). In this model, sleep reduces energy use by lowering of body temperature, metabolic rate (MR), and heat loss to the environment.

As to other possible sleep functions, Horne (5) has argued that sleep in small mammals may serve energy conservation but that in larger animals with greater neocortical development sleep is likely to be important for brain function. A mechanistic basis of a role for sleep in support of brain function is not yet established. A recent hypothesis that brain energy storage may be depleted during waking and that sleep is facilitated by adenosine production resulting from elevated adenosine diphosphate levels is currently under investigation (6).

The following discussion applies primarily to so-called non–rapid eye movement (NREM) sleep, which is the predominant sleep state of homeotherms. This corresponds to stages 2, 3, and 4 in humans and is denoted by increased amplitude in lower frequency electroencephalography (EEG) waves, particularly 0.5–4.0 Hz slow waves (delta activity), sleep spindles (12–15 Hz), and intermediate frequencies. Sleep in nearly all mammals and birds includes two distinct types of sleep. Another state, REM sleep, usually makes up 5–25% of sleep and is characterized by an "activated" EEG. Readers are referred to a recent review (7) for discussion of the physiology and functions of REM sleep. The present discussion is concerned primarily with NREM sleep.

SLEEP DEPRIVATION

Among the methods that can be applied on the problem of the function of sleep, the study of sleep deprivation is potentially fruitful. In a recent series of studies, Rechtschaffen et al. (8) found that rats die after 2–3 weeks of automated total sleep deprivation; yoked control rats receiving the identical physical stimuli and having partial sleep loss show few deficits. The survival time is roughly comparable with that seen with total food deprivation. Earlier, less systematic animal studies had also reported mortality after prolonged sleep deprivation. REM sleep deprivation and high-voltage sleep deprivation are also lethal, with somewhat longer survival times.

Carefully controlled studies based on this method have not demonstrated a clear cause of death, although there are suggestive findings. Sleep-deprived rats lose fat reserves and eventually become mildly hypothermic, even while doubling their food intake. Food absorption is normal or enhanced. It is as if they are starved, even while consuming large mounts of food. Like starved animals, some sleep-deprived animals may develop bacteremia suggestive of host response deficiency (9). But after aggressive antibiotic treatment, rats died during sleep deprivation without signs of bacteremia (8). Although stress is an element of sleep deprivation experiments, Rechtschaffen has argued that prolonged stress and sleep deprivation produce quite different syndromes (8). Indeed, in the Rechtschaffen apparatus, chronic sleep-deprived rats show minimal hypothalamic–adrenal axis activation. Some other explanation is required.

Sleep-deprived rats show additional evidence of having thermoregulatory disturbances. Given a choice of different ambient temperatures, rats choose a dangerously hot environment (10). This and other evidence shows that sleep-deprived rats have an elevated temperature set point, although such an elevation is not a necessary antecedent of death. These findings indicate that one primary effect of sleep deprivation is the dysregulation of temperature control and/or energy exchange. Sleep-deprived rats fail to conserve heat, so much energy is "wasted" in the form of heat exchange with the environment. Alpha-adrenergic vasoconstrictive responses are present, as tested by alpha-receptor antagonists (11). One obvious loss during sleep deprivation is the insulation resulting from sleep postures and nesting. However, the increased heat lost with sleep deprivation seems to be greater than the heat conserved during sleep. Thus, the mechanisms by which sleep helps conserve heat involves physiology as well as insulation.

Sleep-deprived rats could be in a catabolic state despite high food intake. Although body temperature is elevated, cerebral MR is reduced particularly in the hypothalamus, the critical site for energy exchange regulation (12). Jejunal mitosis and serum albumin were reduced in sleep-deprived rats. Survival time is shortened in hyperthyroid animals (8). High-calorie diets prolong survival (13). Energy loss during sleep deprivation may deplete substrates or through some more subtle mechanism produce a catabolic state. It is possible that certain critical "high-turnover" proteins could be depleted by energy supply limitations during sleep deprivation. It has been proposed that membrane proteins in the gut and other sites could be defective, permitting breakdown of immunologic barriers (8).

SPECIES COMPARISONS

A second clue to the functional importance of sleep is provided by results of studies of the sleep required of various mammalian species. Sleep data have been collated for about 80 mammalian species, and these have been related to other physiologic and ecologic parameters (1). Amounts of sleep in 24 hours vary widely across species, from 19 hours in the bat to 3–4 hours in the elephant. These studies showed that the best correlate across species is body mass; small animals sleep more. Body mass is also correlated with weight-specific MR, but partial correlational analysis showed that body mass rather than MR is the best correlate of sleep amounts across species. Borrowing from the model provided by the sleep deprivation experiments described above, a likely explanation is that small animals have a greater surface to mass ratio, and greater potential mass-specific heat loss through the skin. Thus, these two fundamental approaches to function converge in suggesting that sleep may provide homeotherms with mechanisms for heat conservation.

Sleeplike or torporlike states are also recognized in ectothermic animals. However, ectothermic animals go in and out of sleep-like torpor slowly. Sleep in mammals and birds has emergent properties, including the capacity for rapid transitions between waking and sleep. Within certain limits, the timing of sleep in homeotherms can be independent of environmental temperature cycles. As noted above, homeothermic sleep is characterized by the occurrence during sleep of distinctive low-frequency electrical phenomena in the cortical neuronal network, known as the EEG. The low-frequency EEG signals generated by masses of cortical neurons are the summation of the fluctuations of neuronal membrane potentials. The occurrence of increased low-frequency, high-amplitude EEG waves is a key marker of sleep in homeotherms. The EEG synchrony that characterizes homeothermic sleep has not been found in several studies in reptiles and limited work in amphibians (14). The detection of slow-wave EEG signals may require synchronization of neural activity in large masses of neurons that do not exist in ectotherms. Despite the differences with homeotherms, the sleeplike state of reptiles is a likely evolutionary precursor of sleep in homeotherms and may have energy-conserving properties.

Because mammals and birds have separate evolutionary histories, it is likely that some aspect of the shared survival strategies of homeotherms produced selective pressure favoring evolution of slow-wave sleep. Two possibilities are homeothermy itself or cortical development. From the energy conservation perspective, NREM sleep is hypothesized to have evolved in mammals and birds to help compensate for the approximately ten times higher mass-specific MR required by endothermy. Sleep would be understood as one of several interrelated adaptations found in endotherms, ranging from development of insulating fur to large increases in aerobic capacity. These adaptations serve to generate heat, maintain a relatively constant body temperature, while minimizing heat loss.

The lowering of body temperature during sleep is understood as providing energy conservation through Q_{10} effects, the reduction in cellular energy use at lower temperatures. There seems to be little controversy that hibernation occurs to minimize energy utilization when the food supply is reduced. It also has been shown that hibernation is initiated as an extension of a primarily NREM sleep episode (4). Indeed, daily torpor, in which the temperature decrease is limited to several degrees, consists primarily of an NREM-like state. From this perspective, the specific distinctions between sleep, daily torpor, and hibernation lie in the degree of temperature decrease during the episode. Arousal from torpor or hibernation is slow, depending on initial body warming through heat production. The relatively small temperature decrease during sleep permits a rapid arousal. Given the similarities between sleep and hibernation and evidence that, at least in some species, sleep and hibernation slow similar responses to food restriction and season (15), it would seem reasonable to conclude that sleep and hibernation are related processes.

Hibernation is punctuated by euthermic awakenings. Two recent studies (16,17) have shown that animals sleep during euthermic bouts within seasonal hibernation, suggesting that sleep debt develops during hibernation. However, if there is another function for these awakenings, then sleep during the awakening conserves energy. If food is available, animals also eat during the awakenings from hibernation, but this does not mean that hibernation does not function to reduce the overall need to eat.

There are important differences between sleep and hibernation. First, sleep is not normally triggered seasonally. Judging by the deficits produced by one or a few days of sleep deprivation, sleep seems to serve a more immediate daily need than long-term energy stores. In humans, there is a reduction of about 20% in MR during sleep, or about 120 Kcal, although savings may be proportionally greater in small animals. Some have questioned the idea that a behavior as dramatic as sleep would be created to save the energy in a slice of bread. However, Berger and Phillips (4) have argued that during cold stress, savings would be greater. Sleep provides proportionally greater energy savings in small animals. In pigeons, fasting increases the amount of NREM sleep and the temperature drop during sleep. Fasted humans slightly decrease nocturnal body temperature and increase stage 3–4 sleep.

In summary, evolutionary considerations, sleep deprivation studies, species comparisons, and similarities between sleep and daily torpor and hibernation suggest a link between sleep and energy exchange regulation. The behaviors and physiology of sleep, suppression of motor activity, reduction in cerebral MR, initial body cooling, coupled with body insulation and subsequent vasoconstriction and a reduction in cortisol secretion are all considered as elements of an energy conservation strategy. The mechanisms controlling these processes have been localized in the preoptic/anterior hypothalamus (POAH) and closely adjacent brain structures and are coupled to regulation of body temperature. We use the term "thermoregulatory" to refer to these several interrelated processes, although this term may be modified as cellular mechanisms are clarified.

SLEEP AND THERMOREGULATION

Neural Control of Sleep: A Brief Overview

The role of thermoregulatory mechanisms in sleep regulation should be placed in the context of the history of the study of sleep mechanisms. The identification of NREM-, REM-, and wake-promoting neuronal systems has been a major occupation of sleep researchers for the past 50 years (18). The goal has been to identify specific neuronal systems that are critical for the occurrence of specific states, using lesion, local electrical and chemical stimulation, and neuronal unit recording methods. These studies showed that sleep and wake states are facilitated by several interacting neuronal systems, none of which seems to be essential for any state. Arousal from sleep and the maintenance of waking are enhanced by activation of several distinct brain stem neuronal systems, including cholinergic, serotoninergic, histaminergic, noradrenergic, and probably glutaminergic systems. All of these neural systems are localized in subregions of the reticular activating system first described by Moruzzi and Magoun (19). Lesions of these systems individually produce transient hypersomnia followed by rapid recovery of normal EEG-defined wake amounts within 1–3 days. Thus, there seems to be considerable redundancy in the wake-promoting systems. Each of these neuronal systems projects to thalamic and neocortical neurons that control the EEG activation. In thalamus, acetylcholine, serotonin, histamine, and noradrenaline induce the neuronal depolarization that is necessary for the activated EEG (20). Withdrawal of these activating inputs leads to thalamic neuronal hyperpolarization. EEG synchrony depends on hyperpolarization of thalamic and cortical neurons, which "deinactivates" a slow depolarizing calcium current, I_t, leading to spike bursts and a slow potassium-mediated after-hyperpolarization (21). Intrathalamic and thalamocorticothalamic circuitry reinforces and synchronizes these slow oscillations. The summation of these slow membrane potential waves produces the slow-wave EEG.

Multiple NREM sleep-promoting systems also have been suggested, including lower brain stem, dorsomedial (DM) thalamus, and POAH area. The DM thalamus was implicated in humans on the basis of an exceedingly rare genetic neurodegenerative disease, fatal familial insomnia (22,23). This disease is caused by expression of an abnormal isoform of the prion protein and may involve diffuse degeneration and autonomic and cognitive abnormalities. In one case, degeneration was restricted to the DM but was more often diffuse. DM lesions in cats reduce sleep for only 3–5 days.

The lower brain stem site was suggested on the basis of reduced EEG synchronization after complete transections at the mid-pontine level. Animals with slightly higher transections may have normal amounts of wake- and sleeplike EEG states in the forebrain, indicating the presence of a wake-promoting mechanism at the rostral pontine level and a sleep-promoting mechanism above the transections. The cholinergic neurons in the rostral pons are a possible substrate of the wake-promoting effect (18). The localization of the lower brain stem hypnogenic site is not established. The lower brain stem mechanism may be a substrate of more primitive rest–activity cycles.

Of the NREM sleep-promoting sites, the POAH is best documented. Large (3–5 mm) bilateral POAH lesions or transections produce complete insomnia, sometimes leading to death (24). Stimulation and unit recording studies support the hypothesis of a POAH hypnogenic site.

Some wake-promoting and sleep-promoting systems are found to be mutually antagonistic, both functionally and neurophysiologically. This is demonstrated by findings that insomnia induced by POAH lesions can be reversed by lesions of a posterior hypothalamic (PH) wake-promoting area that includes histaminergic neurons (25). Synchronous EEG patterns after midbrain lesions can be reversed by POAH lesions (26). Thus, deficits in an arousal system are balanced by deficits in a sleep-promoting system, and vice versa. Sleep–wake regulation may depend on the tonic balance between the activities of wake- and sleep-promoting systems. At a neurophysiologic level, this antagonistic interaction has been clarified for one system. POAH neurons projecting to the posterior hypothalamus including the histaminergic neurons contain the inhibitory neurotransmitter gamma-aminobutyric acid (GABA) (27). POAH activation inhibits histaminergic neurons (28).

A number of substances also have been identified that can increase sleep after being microinjected into the brain. These putative endogenous sleep factors include prostaglandin D2 (PGD2) (29), interleukin-1 (IL-1) and other cytokines (30), uridine (31), and adenosine (32). The effective sites for adenosine and PGD2 are in or near the POAH (30,33), and effects of uridine are blocked by POAH lesions (31). The medial POAH also seems to be a site for the hypnogenic action of the benzodiazepine triazolam (33). IL-1 and other cytokines are found to modulate the activity of temperature-sensitive neurons, which are particularly numerous in the POAH (34). These studies show that some endogenous hypnogens act through the POAH.

A thermoregulatory model of sleep starts with the idea that sleep is an integrated thermoeffector process supporting energy conservation and additional temperature-related functions. The term "integrated" refers to the fact that sleep includes behavioral, autonomic, endocrine, and cerebroregulatory elements. Sleep onset is associated with body cooling, but at the same time, in neutral and lower ambient temperatures, heat loss in minimized by behaviors such as nesting and piloerection. Later during sustained sleep, temperature may be relatively constant, and will increase slightly before awakening. The body cooling at sleep onset is independent of circadian phase and of postural changes at sleep onset (35). Mechanisms underlying circadian modulation of sleep are discussed below. Body cooling is brought about by the reductions of whole body and cerebral MR at sleep onset, combined with increased evaporative, conductive, and convective heat loss, depending on ambient conditions (36). It is important to emphasize that body cooling is only one component of the energy conservation strategy associated with sleep. Body cooling may not always occur at sleep onset after prolonged sleep deprivation (37), but other processes promoting energy conservation could be maintained.

Brain Mechanisms Serving Thermoregulatory Control of Sleep

Our studies have focused on a hypothesis that NREM sleep is controlled by thermoregulatory mechanisms localized in the POAH and adjacent structures. If sleep consists of a set of thermoregulatory processes promoting heat loss and energy conservation, we can apply to sleep the model of thermoregulatory control of body temperature itself. Thermoeffector processes promoting heat loss are hypothesized to be controlled by a neuronal network that initiates responses when local hypothalamic temperature is higher than temperature thresholds, or set points, that are intrinsic to the network. Set points may be modulated by circadian processes, by motor behaviors such as exercise, and by skin temperature. Heat loss effector processes, including sleep, are triggered when brain temperature increases above the set point or when the set point is lowered by circadian or other processes. In the case of spontaneous sleep, the lowering of the set point rather than the elevation of hypothalamic temperature would be the determining event. The intensity of a thermoeffector process may be determined by the temperature "error signal," that is, the difference between the set point and the temperature or by the slope of the temperature-response function.

Different thermoeffector processes have distinct set points, providing a hierarchy of processes, depending on the intensity of the POAH or peripheral thermal stimulus. For example, vasomotor responses have low threshold for early activation during thermal challenges. Vasomotor activities play a major role in regulating circadian rhythms in body temperature in the absence of thermal challenges (38). At sleep onset, heat loss processes including sweating and vasodilation are activated, suggesting that the set point for these processes has been lowered below the brain temperature. In a landmark study, Glotzbach and Heller (39) estimated the set point and response rate for heat production, showing that these parameters were reduced in NREM sleep compared with waking. In the pigeon, the set point for panting appears to change immediately at state transitions (40). We have found that the thermosensitivity of individual hypothalamic warm-sensitive neurons is increased during NREM sleep. Such neuronal sensitivity changes are a substrate for increased thermosensitivity or lowered response thresholds and have the effect of amplifying heat loss processes, explaining why body temperature decreases at sleep onset.

In the absence of sleep deprivation or circadian manipulations, the timing of sleep is determined primarily by circadian processes, with timing signals originating in the suprachiasmatic nucleus (SCN) (41,42). It is also known that there are circadian rhythms in the temperature set point for several thermoeffector processes, with a lower set point during the night in diurnal species. Thus, it is possible to hypothesize that the hypnogenic set point is lowered by the circadian clock before sleep onset, leading to the triggering of sleep onset. In humans, sleep propensity is greatest and sleep is most often initiated in the middle to late descending phases of the circadian temperature rhythm (35,43). Earlier in the temperature cycle, sleep may be inhibited. In the context of the thermoregulatory model, we postulate that hypnogenic temperature-sensitive neurons would be inhibited by the circadian oscillator until the midpoint of the temperature cycle. In circadian entrained subjects the sleep-evoked and circadian regulated decrease in body temperature are superimposed. It has been estimated that about half of the total circadian temperature range is due to sleep, the rest to circadian processes (36). In this model, sleep effects thermoregulation, and thermoregulation effects sleep. A formal model of this interaction is presented below.

Preoptic/Anterior Hypothalamic Thermoregulatory Modulation of Sleep

The POAH has been a focus of research on thermoregulation. Local POAH warming and cooling elicit appropriate thermoeffector responses such as vaso-motor activity, shivering and panting, and non-shivering thermogenesis, such as ambient warming and cooling (44).

What is the evidence that POAH temperature-sensitive neurons (TSNs) may regulate sleep? POAH warming has been found to trigger sleep onset in several species, including dogs, cats, opossums, rats, and kangaroo rats (36,45). During sustained POAH warming, the amount of sleep was found to be proportional to the elevation of POAH temperature (T_{hy}) elevation above the set point temperature threshold (T_{set}) for increased MR (45). This threshold is related to the regulated body temperature, analogous to the temperature threshold on the thermostat that controls a heating system. The activation of thermoeffector responses by POAH temperature changes is also proportional to the elevation of T_{hy} above T_{set}.

Thus, in this respect, NREM sleep induction by POAH warming is like other thermoeffector responses. POAH warming also induces several other correlates of sleep, including heat loss, motor suppression, and inhibition of the HPA axis (46). Thus, the idea that sleep can be a response to activation of hypothalamic warm-sensitive neurons is well justified.

Within NREM sleep, the intensity of sleep is correlated with the relative density of low-frequency, or delta (0.5–4.0 Hz), EEG frequencies. The amount of delta activity is increased at the beginning of the sleep period when sleep need is greatest and declines progressively across the night. Delta activity is also increased during recovery sleep after sleep deprivation (47).

Our study (48) examined the effect of POAH warming on the quantitative properties of the EEG within sleep. During sustained NREM sleep episodes, POAH warming increased the amount of delta activity (Fig. 1).

Other EEG frequencies were not effected by POAH warming. Both peak and average delta activity were increased by POAH warming. This effect was not due to changes in the duration of NREM sleep. We concluded that the intensity of sleep, as represented in EEG frequencies, could be regulated by the activation of POAH thermosensitive neurons.

Delta activity also was increased during a recovery period after warming. This result was consistent with studies in humans (49,50) and rats (51), showing that deep slow-wave sleep within NREM sleep could be increased during sleep that follows whole-body warming. POAH or whole-body warming seems to induce a "memory" for the heating, which is expressed by enhancement of subsequent NREM sleep. Tobler et al. (52) found only marginally significant increases in slow-wave activity after whole-body warming in rats. However, this study attempted to show increased slow-wave activity after mild body warming at the circadian time of peak delta activity. In addition, animals were recovering from sleep deprivation and had control delta activity levels about 150–200% above the

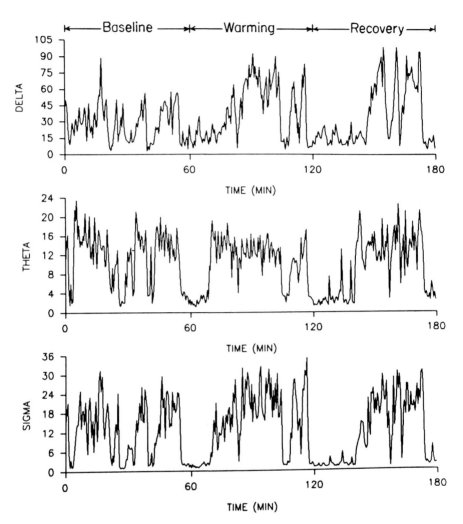

FIG. 1. Effects of POAH warming on EEG patterns within sustained sleep episodes in the cat. EEG activity was recorded during baseline, POAH warming, and recovery periods lasting 1 hour each. Cats were sleeping most of the time during the studies. During warming, POAH temperature was "clamped" at the highest level seen during normal waking. Control treatments, without warming, and POAH cooling trials were also done. EEG patterns were analyzed by power spectral analysis and summed into delta, theta, and sigma bands. **Upper panel:** Continuous record of spectral values in one animal. During warming peak delta values were higher. Higher values were also seen during the recovery period. **Lower panel:** Pooled data from five animals showing significant changes in the delta band, but not other frequency bands during warming. Mild cooling did not produce significant changes. Reprinted with permission (48).

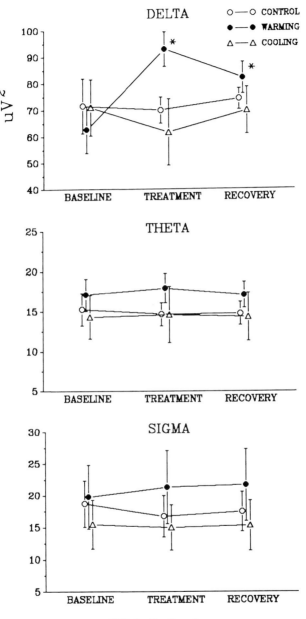

FIG. 1. *Continued*

high circadian baseline. Thus, further increases in delta activity may have been difficult to find because of a ceiling effect. A later study replicated and extended our original findings (53).

The neuronal mechanisms that mediate the effects of POAH warming were suggested by additional studies in which we recorded neuronal discharge in unrestrained cats and rats. In this experiment we characterized subsets of neurons in several brain sites on the basis of their activity changes during the sleep–wake cycle and responses to antidromic and orthodromic stimulation (54,55). Most of the sites we have studied contain mixtures of neurons and have multiple functions. As noted above, the posterior hypothalamus (PH) contains a subset of neurons that are thought to promote waking; these neurons exhibit increased discharge during waking compared with NREM sleep. We found that POAH warming induced suppression of discharge in the subset of PH arousal-related neurons (56). Other PH neurons were not systematically affected by POAH warming. In these studies the behavioral state of the animal is carefully monitored during the warming to ensure that discharge rate changes do not reflect drowsiness or sleep onset. The inhibitory effects of POAH warming may be mediated by a strong GABAergic projection to PH originating in the POAH and adjacent structures (27).

A similar study examined the effects of POAH warming on magnocellular basal forebrain (mBF) neurons. The mBF contains a well-characterized set of cholinergic neurons that project to cortical sites and intermixed non-cholinergic neurons, including GABAergic neurons (27). The mBF cholinergic system is hypothesized to be an important cortical arousal system. We previously described subsets of neurons with increased discharge with behavioral arousal, increased discharge in NREM sleep (sleep-active), and state-indifferent neurons. The wake-active and sleep-active neuronal groups had different antidromic conduction velocities (54). POAH warming had differential effects on these neuronal groups (57) (Fig. 2). The sleep-active neuronal group was facilitated during warming, and the wake-active group was inhibited. These types of studies show that POAH neurons responsive to local temperature can regulate the activity of arousal- and sleep-promoting neurons in other brain sites. The motor and autonomic events of sleep also can be controlled though these mechanisms.

Activity of POAH Thermosensitive Neurons During Sleep-Waking

The POAH contains a population of neurons that are responsive to local warming and cooling over a narrow temperature range, $\pm2.0°C$. In chronic or anesthetized animals, neuronal activity is recorded adjacent to a water-perfused thermode, and local temperature is measured close to the site of recording using a microthermocouple. By perfusing the thermode, local temperature is regulated. Given the effects of temperature on biochemical processes, it could be expected that all neurons would be responsive to even small changes in local temperature changes. However, only a minority of neurons in POAH or other

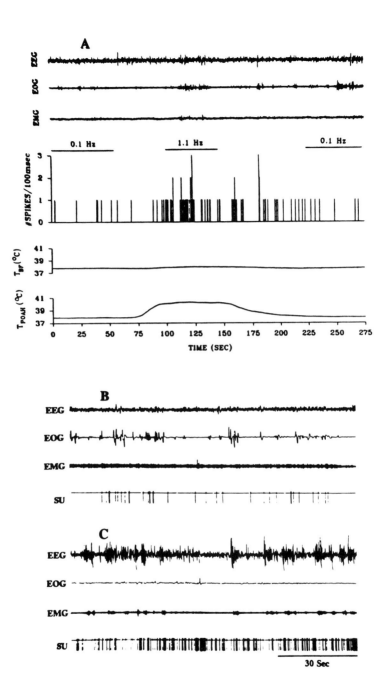

FIG. 2. Effects of POAH warming on neuronal discharge in the basal forebrain (BF). Neuronal activity was recorded in the freely moving cat along with polygraphic parameters, EEG, eye movements (EOG), and neck muscle activity (EMG). Neurons were first classified as waking-active, sleep-active, or state-indifferent as described previously (54). The neuron shown here exhibited higher discharge rates during NREM sleep (**C**) than in waking (**B**) and was sleep-active. **A:** POAH warming activated such sleep-active neurons but inhibited wake-active neurons in the same site. The POAH thermal stimulus did not reach the recording site (T_{BF}). Reprinted with permission (57).

sites respond to local warming or cooling with brisk responses, defined by standard criteria. This has been shown in anesthetized and awake animals and in living tissue slice preparations (44). In tissue slices, some POAH neurons are temperature-sensitive after blockade of synaptic input (58). Such neurons are denoted as primary or inherent thermodetectors.

During the experiments described above, POAH temperature was artificially elevated by a local thermode. These studies showed that the activation of warm-sensitive neurons (WSNs) or the deactivation of cold-sensitive neurons (CSNs) can inhibit putative arousal-related neurons in PH and BF and activate sleep-promoting neurons. Through such mechanisms the POAH can trigger NREM sleep and increase EEG delta activity during sleep. However, brain temperature tends to be decreasing rather than increasing before sleep onset. Therefore, we would have to predict that discharge of WSNs would slow at sleep onset and CSNs would accelerate.

We recorded the activity of POAH WSNs and CSNs in relation to spontaneously occurring sleep cycles in both cats (59) and rats (60). These neurons were defined by each of several standardized criteria for thermosensitivity; the results obtained were the same for all criteria. In both species 21–25% of POAH neurons were thermosensitive.

In both species, about 60% of WSNs exhibited increased discharge in NREM sleep as compared with waking (Fig. 3). About 70% of CSNs showed decreased discharge in NREM sleep. The changes in discharge usually preceded the appearance of EEG synchrony at sleep onset transitions. Therefore, these changes in neuronal activity may initiate the state transition. The magnitude of the spontaneous discharge changes at sleep onset was quantitatively equivalent to that produced by a 2.0°C local warming stimulus during waking. Such a local POAH stimulus is easily sufficient to induce or maintain NREM sleep.

Because it has been established that activation of WSNs and/or deactivation of CSNs by local POAH warming is sufficient to induce NREM sleep, and the neurons responsive to local warming show changes spontaneously at NREM onset like those induced by local warming, it is parsimonious to hypothesize that the changes in discharge of these neurons play a primary role in spontaneous NREM onset and maintenance as well as NREM induced by local warming.

The hypothesis that TSNs are necessary for sleep can be assessed in another way. We can predict that deactivation of WSNs and activation of CSNs can prevent sleep. We examined this by attempting to block NREM sleep by local POAH cooling, remembering that this type of stimulus affects only the subset of temperature-sensitive neurons. The test was conducted in the early part of the light period in rats acclimated to a fixed 12:12-hour light–dark cycle. Under these conditions, nocturnal rats normally sleep most of the time.

During a 3-hour test, POAH cooling by about 2.0°C suppressed spontaneous sleep and suppressed EEG frequency spectral power changes associated with sleep, particularly increased delta frequencies (Fig. 4). The termination of cooling was followed by a rebound increase in delta activity. Thus, selective deactivation

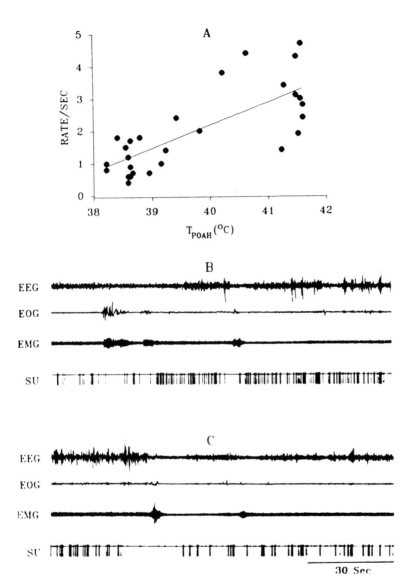

FIG. 3. POAH warm-sensitive neuron (WSN) in the freely moving cat. **A**: WSNs were identified on the basis of changes in discharge rate in response to local warming and cooling. Most WSNs exhibited increased discharge during naturally occurring NREM sleep. **B**: Discharge clearly increased before the occurrence of EEG synchrony at sleep onset transitions. **C**: Discharge usually decreased before transient arousals from NREM sleep. Reprinted with permission (59).

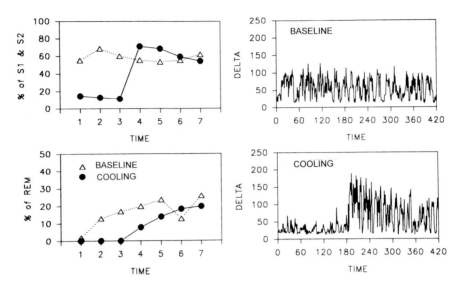

FIG. 4. Effects of POAH cooling on sleep and EEG delta activity. The POAH was cooled by about 2.0°C during a 3-hour period beginning 2.5 hours after light onset. Rats normally sleep during this period. POAH cooling (•) suppressed combined light (S1) and deep (S2) NREM sleep and REM sleep compared with control values (△). The amplitude of delta EEG activity was also greatly reduced. After termination of cooling there was a strong "rebound" of delta activity (unpublished data).

of POAH WSNs and/or activation of CSNs was sufficient to prevent sleep. Both NREM and REM were suppressed; REM suppression is typically associated with NREM suppression, probably because sustained NREM acts as a trigger for REM sleep. We chose 2.0°C because the change in activity of WSNs and CSNs during NREM sleep compared with waking corresponded to that induced by a 2.0°C stimulus during waking. Thus, this stimulus magnitude would be required to neutralize the changes in activity that normally occur during sleep. The suppression of sleep did not depend on the induction of shivering. As expected, shivering and body temperature elevation sometimes occurred with a 2.0°C stimulus, but a slightly reduced stimulus could suppress sleep without induction of shivering or body temperature elevation. A final point concerns the extent of the brain affected by the cooling stimulus. The thermal field around the thermode tip extends 4–5 mm. We refer to a POAH thermal stimulus, but the stimulus field would include adjacent basal forebrain and hypothalamic sites as well.

   In summary, we and others have made the following assertions about the role of POAH and adjacent neurons:

   1. Selective activation of POAH WSNs and/or deactivation of CSNs by local POAH warming facilitates NREM sleep, increases the amount of NREM sleep over several hours, and increases the delta wave EEG content of sustained NREM sleep.

2. Selective deactivation of POAH WSNs and/or activation of CSNs suppresses sleep at a time of peak circadian sleep propensity. Thus, selective modulation of TSNs either blocks or counteracts circadian regulation of sleep propensity. Nonselective lesions of the POAH produce long-lasting insomnia.

3. Activation of WSNs and deactivation of CSNs inhibits putative wake-promoting neurons in the posterior hypothalamus and basal forebrain. An anatomic substrate for these inhibitory influences has been demonstrated. This shows the part of the mechanisms by which POAH temperature-sensitive neurons can regulate other brain sites involved in sleep control.

4. Activation of POAH WSNs and deactivation of CSNs occurs spontaneously during the sleep onset transition and during sustained NREM sleep in both cats and rats. Because we have established that such neuronal discharge changes are sufficient to regulate NREM sleep, we can conclude that these spontaneous events must play a crucial role in the control of natural sleep. Recently, Sherin et al. (61) showed increased *c-fos* protein expression in the ventrolateral POAH that increased progressively during NREM sleep. Other hypothalamic sites failed to exhibit this expression. *c-fos* is a marker of increased neuronal activation.

5. Whole-body or local POAH warming induces delayed increases in sleep amounts, much like sleep deprivation. Normally body and brain temperature are elevated during waking. We may hypothesize that tissue warming during waking may play a role in the development of sleep debt. However, local POAH cooling that suppressed sleep was followed by a rebound in sleep. Thus, local POAH cooling does not prevent the development of sleep debt. The site of action in which warming contributes to sleep debt must be outside of the POAH.

CIRCADIAN CONTROL OF HUMAN SLEEP: A THERMOREGULATORY MODEL

The regulation of sleep parameters relative to the 24-hour (circadian) day has been confirmed in many species (41). It is this mechanism that induces sleep in the dark in diurnal animals and sleep in the light in nocturnal animals. The circadian distribution of sleep continues under constant environmental light and other potentially periodic stimuli, although the period of this free-running rhythm normally deviates slightly from 24 hours. This regulation is controlled by an internal biologic clock that, in mammals, has been localized in the suprachiasmatic nucleus (SCN). This nucleus is found in the ventromedial hypothalamus adjacent to the POAH. SCN lesions abolish the circadian distribution of sleep as well as circadian temperature, hormonal, and behavioral rhythms (41). After such lesions, rhythms can be reintroduced by implanting bits of SCN tissue from a donor animal in the third ventricle adjacent to the normal location of the SCN.

The distribution of human sleep propensity within the 24-hour day has been described in several studies (35,62). In such studies, sleep propensity is studied under conditions in which subjects have no clues about true clock time. Typically, sleep rhythms are described relative to the ongoing near 24-hour temperature rhythm that persists under these constant conditions. These studies have shown that there is a strong interaction between sleep parameters and the temperature rhythm. Most important findings from this literature have been confirmed recently using a paradigm called forced desynchronization, which allows separation of the effects of prior sleep duration and the phase position of sleep onset relative to the ongoing circadian temperature rhythm (35). The basic results are listed as follows:

1. Sleep propensity is increased rapidly in the mid-descending phase of the temperature cycle. This phase position corresponds to the initial part of the sleep period under entrained conditions. Sleep onset may occur in the steepest part of the temperature decrease, but sleep is maintained though the low phase of temperature. There is a second point of weak facilitation of sleep propensity just before the peak of the temperature rhythm, corresponding to mid-afternoon under entrained conditions. A biphasic sleep propensity with a secondary peak in mid-afternoon also has been shown in other paradigms (63). There is a wake-maintenance zone from the peak of the temperature rhythm to the mid-descending phase.
2. The propensity for slow-wave sleep (stages 3–4 sleep) declines across the sleep period and is primarily sleep dependent, but there is circadian facilitation of slow-wave sleep just before the peak of the temperature rhythm.
3. REM sleep propensity is strongly increased at the nadir of the temperature rhythm.

Conventionally, in the circadian research field, the temperature rhythm has been viewed as a convenient marker of circadian phase, but having no physiologic significance. However, we can hypothesize that the close coupling of sleep parameters to this rhythm reflects properties of the thermoregulatory hypnogenic control process. In particular, the coupling of high sleep propensity to descending phase of the temperature rhythm could reflect the fact that mechanisms that drive temperature down also facilitate sleep. That is, activation of POAH warm-sensitive neurons could mediate both the circadian decrease in body temperature beginning in the early evening and the onset of sleep late in the evening. The idea that hypnogenic neurons are a subset of temperature-sensitive neurons was supported by the neurophysiologic data presented above. Because sleep is initiated only at the midpoint of the circadian decrease in body temperature, we must hypothesize that the hypnogenic WSNs are modulated by another process. We hypothesize that the SCN circadian clock modulates sleep by modulating the activity or excitability of POAH thermosensitive neurons. The POAH receives many fibers emanating from the SCN (64).

Based on these considerations, we constructed a formal mathematical model of human sleep control in which sleep propensity is regulated as a thermoregulatory effector process (65). In this model, sleep is controlled as a thermoeffector process through the interaction of hypothalamic temperature and a set point ($T_{hypo} - T_{set}$). The set point is determined by a circadian oscillator, called the X oscillator. A second oscillator, Y, with a fixed phase relationship to the temperature rhythm was required to produce biphasic sleepiness. Sleep itself induces a decrease in temperature, waking induces an increase in temperature; these transients provide part of the feedback signal to the hypothalamus. The homeostatic component of sleep is induced by the integration of the waking heat load, as suggested by the whole-body and POAH warming studies summarized above. The output of the hypothalamic mechanisms is sleepiness. Sleep would normally occur when sleepiness reaches a threshold. Figure 5 shows the form of the

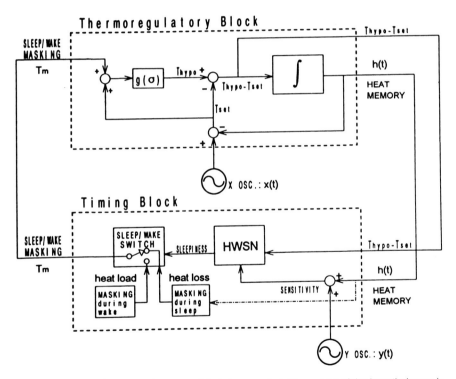

FIG. 5. Design of a thermoregulatory model of sleep control. The output of the hypothalamus is determined by the difference $T_{hypo} - T_{set}$. T_{set} is strongly modulated by a circadian oscillator (X). In addition, $T_{hypo} - T_{set}$ is integrated to produce the homeostatic component of sleep. These two outputs regulate the activity of hypnogenic warm-sensitive neurons (HWSN). The HWSN is also modulated by a second circadian oscillator (Y), representing a separate output of the SCN. The output of the HWSN is sleepiness. Sleep and waking are triggered at certain thresholds of sleepiness. Sleep and waking induce masking effects on temperature that are fed back to the hypothalamus. The mathematical representation of the model was solved with differential equations. Reprinted with permission (65).

model, which was determined by use of differential equations. Fixed parameters of the model were set only to produce 8 hours of sleep and sleep onset at the appropriate phase of the temperature rhythm. The model was evaluated through various simulations such as delaying sleep onset and sleep deprivation. Most of the features of the model summarized below were not specifically incorporated into the model and can be considered to be model predictions.

Figure 6 shows the parameters and output of the working model. The X oscillator closely corresponds to the temperature rhythm; this is modulated by the masking effects of sleep and waking. The Y oscillator exhibits a low point in mid-evening and increases throughout sleep, peaking at about the time of morning awakening. The sensitivity of WSNs is controlled by the Y oscillator. The low point of this oscillation produces the evening wake-maintenance zone, opposing the facilitation of sleep by the X oscillator at this point of the circadian cycle. In this respect our model is similar to that of Edgar et al. (41). Interestingly, the Y oscillator helps maintain sleep at the end of the night when thermoregulatory drive is reduced. T_{set} falls below T_{hypo} in mid-afternoon, driving temperature down and inducing the secondary mid-afternoon peak in sleepiness. The $T_{hypo} - T_{set}$ difference is greatest early in the sleep period. This could account for increased sleep depth at that time. Sleepiness increases after sleep onset, corresponding to the common experience of increasing sleepiness associated with voluntary wakefulness at that time.

The heat load driving the homeostatic component of sleep begins increasing only in the afternoon, suggesting a prediction that sleep deprivation restricted to the morning would produce no addition to sleep homeostatic drive. This aspect

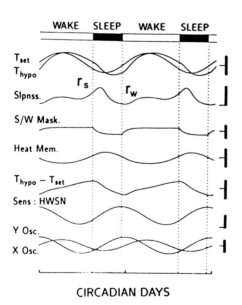

FIG. 6. Behavior of the variables derived from the model in Fig. 5 during 2 consecutive days. Sleep onset occurs on the middle descending phase of the circadian temperature rhythm. Sleepiness continues to increase in the early part of the sleep period. Reprinted with permission (65).

could explain the ability in some individuals and persons with mania to get along on little sleep. Other simulations show that awakening is associated with the ascending phase of the temperature rhythm.

Figure 7 shows simulations of short and sustained sleep deprivation based on the model. During sleep deprivation, circadian patterns of increasing and decreasing sleepiness and temperature persist, but average body temperature decreases. These results are consistent with previous results. Figure 8 shows recovery sleep after sleep deprivation. With 4–12 hours of deprivation, the first

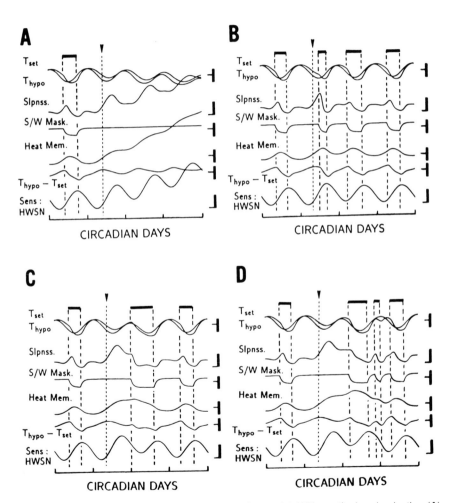

FIG. 7. Simulations of sleep deprivation based on the model. With continuing deprivation (**A**), sleepiness increases but exhibits circadian oscillations. Body temperature also oscillates, but gradually decreases. B, C, and D show aftereffects of 4, 16, and 20 hours of deprivation, respectively. Recovery sleep duration is maximal after 16 hours of deprivation. Reprinted with permission (65).

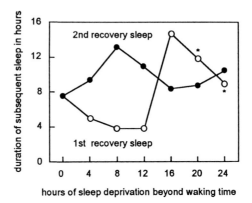

FIG. 8. Sleep durations during recovery sleep after deprivations of varying duration derived from the simulations shown in Fig. 7. The resulting first recovery sleep durations closely fit available data (66). Second recovery sleep durations have not been reported. Reprinted with permission (65).

recovery sleep is actually shorter than normal sleep. With 16 hours of deprivation, a long sleep occurs. These findings exactly fit previous experimental work (66). We also make predictions about the duration of the second recovery sleep, but this prediction has not been tested. Other simulations show that changing the phase angle between the X and Y oscillators strongly regulates sleep duration. In this way, the phenomenon of "internal desynchronization" can be simulated.

In thermoregulatory models, sleep is controlled by the relationship of body temperature and a set point. As our simulation clearly shows, this type of model does not predict that any absolute measurement of temperature will be correlated with sleep propensity. Because the lack of such correlations has been presented as evidence against the model (67), this requires further explanation. It is generally accepted that body temperature is controlled by a thermostatic process with feedback (and feed-forward) control. Control is achieved by thermoeffector processes. For example, vasodilation and heat conductance increase abruptly at the peak of the circadian rhythm, helping to produce subsequent cooling (38). Vasodilation is strong at both high and low absolute temperatures, and there is no general correlation between the two variables. What is predicted is that vasodilation induces lowering of body temperature within the next time block. A similar prediction applies to sleep. Indeed, it has been shown that the rate of change in body temperature is correlated with the amount of delta activity in the subsequent time block (68).

In summary, a model of human sleep regulation based on thermoregulatory control with powerful circadian modulation can simulate several subtle features of human sleep behavior. We have used two oscillators to achieve this goal. Some investigators have suggested that two oscillators are not required to achieve biphasic sleepiness or internal desynchronization. In fact, our model satisfies the analysis of Zulley and Campbell (69), showing that during internal desynchronization, sleep propensity remains in phase with the ongoing temperature rhythm. Our two oscillators could be two outputs of the SCN, one directly regulating temperature, the other suppressing sleep in the mid-evening to produce the wake-maintenance zone, and increasing sleep in the late portion of the sleep period. We have not completed modeling of detailed features of sleep such as the distribution of stages 3–4 sleep and the NREM–REM cycle.

CURRENT STATUS OF THE THERMOREGULATORY MODEL

We have summarized biologic, neurophysiologic, and modeling data supporting the application of the thermoregulatory hypothesis of sleep control. Several issues pertaining to this hypothesis are unresolved. The concept that sleep is for energy conservation is difficult to rationalize with the relative insensitivity of sleep to manipulations of availability of energy substrates. We may go to sleep either well fed or hungry. In larger animals, sleep saves a small percentage of the daily energy requirement. To help understand these issues, a comparison between control of sleep and control of eating may be useful. There would seem to be little doubt that eating is regulated by mechanisms that are sensitive to nutritional substrates and that the function of this behavior is to maintain nutrition. However, the prevalence of obesity and anorexia indicates that this regulation is "sloppy." Much eating follows daily rhythms rather than need. The nutritional status of the individual is a poor predictor of eating. Probably both sleep and eating control systems are genetically programmed (a) to anticipate their functional goals without strong feedback control and (b) to provide a reserve that can preserve life during deprivation.

The sleep deprivation experiments summarized above seem to show that energy substrates are depleted by sleep deprivation, but the underlying mechanisms involve physiologic processes beyond simple caloric intake and use. Rather, the physiologic capacity to conserve heat seems to be enhanced by sleep. What is suggested is that sleep may serve energy conservation in subtle ways, perhaps involving neurologic processes. Further studies of the exact mechanisms are required.

In humans, subjective level of arousal, psychomotor performance, and cognitive function performance are positively correlated with body temperature, except for a slight dip just before the peak in the daily temperature rhythm (70). The temperature rhythm may facilitate arousability directly, perhaps modulating neuronal excitability. It is adaptive to sleep when nervous system excitability is lower. It is possible that a variety of neurochemical processes are interwoven with temperature cycles and have functional linkages.

APPLICATION TO THE ACUTELY ILL PATIENT

The sleep disturbance found in most acutely ill patients is likely to have an impact on the energy balance. Prolonged sleep deprivation contributes to bacteremia in rats, probably as a result of their starved quality, even when food intake is adequate. A catabolic state may be produced. Bonnet et al. (71,72) have shown that sleep fragmentation prevents the normal decrease in MR during sleep and that daytime disturbances in insomnia are related to the interference in MR decrease in sleep. Clearly, one goal in patient management should be an attempt to minimize sleep disturbance. This can be achieved in several ways: minimizing nocturnal nursing interventions, recognition of the need for control of pain during sleep, and use of hypnotic agents. The importance of maintaining circadian rhythmicity and the use of room lighting control to assist in circadian regulation is discussed in chapters 3 and 4 of this volume. From the nutritional viewpoint, it is possible that, because of sleep disturbance, the caloric needs of the patient far exceed those that are expected on the basis of norms. In this context, high-fat diets may be useful.

ACKNOWLEDGMENTS

This work was supported by the Department of Veterans Affairs and U.S. Public Health Service Grant MH47480.

REFERENCES

1. Zepelin H. Mammalian sleep. In: Kryger MH, Roth T, Dement WC, eds. *Principles and practice of sleep medicine.* Philadelphia: WB Saunders; 1994:69–80.
2. Meddis R. On the function of sleep. *Animal Behav* 1975;23:676–691.
3. Allison T, Van Twyver H. The evolution of sleep. *Nat Hist* 1970;79:56–65.
4. Berger RJ, Phillips NH. Energy conservation and sleep. *Behav Brain Res* 1995;69:65–73.
5. Horne, JA. Factors relating to energy conservation during sleep in mammals. *Physiol Psychol* 1977; 5:403–408.
6. Benington JH, Heller HC. Restoration of brain energy metabolism as the function of sleep. *Prog Neurobiol* 1995;45:347–360.
7. Wehr TA. A brain-warming function for REM sleep. *Neurosci Biobehav Rev* 1992;16:379–397.
8. Rechtschaffen A, Bergmann BM. Sleep deprivation in the rat by the disk-over-water method. *Behav Brain Res* 1995;69:55–63.
9. Everson CA. Sustained sleep deprivation impairs host defense. *Am J Physiol* 1993;265:R1148–R1154.
10. Prete F, Bergmann BM, Holtzman P, Obermeyer WH, Rechstchaffen A. Sleep deprivation in the rat. XII. Effect on ambient temperature choice. *Sleep* 1991;14:109–115.
11. Obermeyer WH, Bergmann BM, Rechtschaffen A. The effect of sleep deprivation on the thermoregulatory response of rats to phentolamine. *Sleep Res* 1993;22:340.
12. Everson CA. Effects of prolonged sleep deprivation on local rates of cerebral energy metabolism in freely moving rats. *J Neurosci* 1994;14:6769–6778.
13. Everson CA. Nutritional and metabolic adaptations to prolonged sleep deprivation in the rat. *Am J Physiol* 1993;264:R376–R387.
14. McGinty D. Amphibians. In: Carkadon MA, Rechtschaffen A, Richardson G, Roth T, Siegel J, eds. *Encyclopedia of sleep and dreaming.* New York: MacMillan; 1993:34–35.
15. Berger RJ, Phillips NH. Comparative aspects of energy metabolism, body temperature, and sleep. *Acta Physiol Scand* 1988;133:21–27.
16. Daan S, Barnes BM, Strijkstra AM. Warming up for sleep? Ground squirrels sleep during arousals from hibernation. *Neurosci Lett* 1991;128:265–268.
17. Trachsel L, Edgar DM, Heller HC. Are ground squirrels sleep deprived during hibernation? *Am J Physiol* 1991;260:R1123–R1129.

18. Jones BE. Basic mechanisms of sleep-wake states. In: Kryger MH, Roth T, Dement WC, eds. *Principles and practice of sleep medicine*. Philadelphia: WB Saunders; 1994:145–162.
19. Moruzzi G, Magoun HW. Brain stem reticular formation and activation of the EEG. *Electroencephalogr Clin Neurophysiol* 1949;1:455–473.
20. McCormick DA. Neurotransmitter actions in the thalamus and cerebral cortex and their role in neuromodulation of thalamocortical activity. *Prog Neurobiol* 1992;39:337–388.
21. Steriade M, McCormack DA, Sejnowski TJ. Thalamocortical oscillations in the sleeping and aroused brain. *Science* 1993;162:679–685.
22. Lugaresi E, Medori R, Montagna P, et al. Fatal familial insomnia and dysautonomia with selective degeneration of thalamic nuclei. *N Engl J Med* 1986;315:997–1003.
23. Mancia M, Marini G. Thalamic nuclei and sleep-wake organization. In: Guilleminault C, Lugaresi E, Montagna P, Gambetti PL, eds. *Fatal familial insomnia:inherited prion diseases, sleep, and the thalamus*. New York: Raven; 1994:135–142.
24. McGinty D, Szymusiak R. Keeping cool: a hypothesis about the mechanisms and functions of slow wave sleep. *Trends Neurosci* 1990;13:480–487.
25. Sallanon M, Sakai K, Denoyer M, Jouvet M. Long lasting insomnia induced by preoptic neuron lesions and its transient reversal by muscimol injection into the posterior hypothalamus. *J Neurosci* 1989;32:669–683.
26. Nakata K, Kawamura H. ECoG sleep-waking rhythms and bodily activity in the cerveau isole rat. *Physiol Behav* 1986;36:1167–1172.
27. Gritti I, Mainville L, Jones BE. Projections of GABAergic and cholinergic basal forebrain and GABAergic peroptic-anterior hypothalamic neurons to the posterior lateral hypothalamus of the rat. *J Comp Neurol* 1994;339:251–268.
28. Yang OZ, Hatton GI. Excitatory and inhibitory inputs to histaminergic tuberomammillary nucleus (TM) in rat. *Soc Neuro Abstr* 1994;20:346.
29. Matsumura H, Nakajima T, Osaka T, et al. Prostaglandin D2-sensitive, sleep-promoting zone defined in the ventral surface of the rostral basal forebrain, *Proc Natl Acad Sci U S A* 1994;91:11998–12002.
30. Kreuger JM, Opp M, Toth LA, Johannsen L, Cady AB. Somnogenic cytokines and models concerning their effects on sleep. *Yale J Biol Med* 1990;63:157–172.
31. Ticho SR, Radulovacki M. Role of adenosine in sleep and temperature regulation in the preoptic area of rats. *Pharmacol Biochem Behav* 1991;40:33–40.
32. Kimura-Takeuchi M, Inoue S. Lateral preoptic lesions void slow-wave sleep enhanced by uridine but not by muramyl dipeptide in rats, *Neurosci Lett* 1993;157:17–20.
33. Mendelson WB, Martin JV, Perlis M, Wagner R. Enhancement of sleep by microinjection of triazolam into the medial preoptic area. *Neuropsychopharmacology* 1989;2:61–66.
34. Shibata M, Blatteis CM. Lack of mimocry between the effects of pyrogenic cytokines and monoamines on the activities of hypothalamic thermosensitive neurons. *Intern J Neurosci* 1990;51:291–293.
35. Dijk DJ, Czeisler CA. Contribution of the circadian pacemaker and the sleep homeostat to sleep propensity, sleep structure, electroencephalic slow waves, and sleep spindle activity in humans, *J Neurosci* 1995;15:3526–3538.
36. Glotzbach SF, Heller HC. Temperature regulation. In: Kryger MH, Roth T, Dement WC, eds. *Priciples and practice of sleep medicine*. Philadelphia: WB Saunders; 1994:260–276.
37. Feng P-F, Obermeyer WH, Tsai LL, Zenko CE, Bergmann BM, Rechtschaffen A. Changes in temperature during recovery from sleep deprivation in the rat. *Sleep Res* 1994;23:412.
38. Aschoff J. Circadian control of body temperature. *J Therm Biol* 1983;8:143–147.
39. Glotzbach SF, Heller HC. Central nervous regulation of body temperature during sleep. *Science* 1976;194:537–539.
40. Parmeggiani PL, Franzini C, Lenzi PL, Zamboni G. Threshold of respiratory responses to preoptic heating during sleep in freely moving cats. *Brain Res* 1973;52:189–201.
41. Edgar DM, Dement WC, Fuller CA. Effect of SCN lesions on sleep in squirrel monkeys: evidence for opponent processes in sleep-wake regulation. *J Neurosci* 1993;13:1065–1079.
42. Ibuka N, Kawamura H. Loss of circadian rhythm in sleep-wakefulness cycle in the rat by suprachiasmatic nucleus lesions. *Brain Res* 1975;96:76–81.
43. Campbell SS, Broughton RJ. Rapid decline in body temperature before sleep: fluffing the physiological pillow? *Chronobiol Int* 1994;11:126–131.
44. Boulant JA. Hypothalamic control of thermoregulation: neurophysiological basis. In: Morgane PJ, Panksepp J, eds. *Handbook of the hypothalamus*. New York: Dekker; 1980:1–82.
45. Sakaguchi S, Glotzbach SF, Heller HC. Influence of hypothalamic and ambient temperatures on sleep in kangaroo rats, *Am J Physiol* 1979;237:R80–R88.

46. Proppe DW, Gale CC. Endocrine thermoregulatory responses to local hypothalamic warming in unanesthetized baboons. *Am J Physiol* 1970;219:202–207.
47. Dijk DJ, Brunner DP, Beersma DGM, Borbely AA. EEG power density and slow wave sleep as a function of prior waking and circadian phase. *Sleep* 1990;13:430–440.
48. McGinty D, Szymusiak R, Thomson D. Preoptic/anterior hypothalamic warming increases EEG delta frequency activity within non-rapid eye movement sleep. *Brain Res* 1994;667:273–277.
49. Horne JA, Reid AJ. Night-time sleep EEG changes following body heating in a warm bath. *Electroencephalogr Clin Neurophysiol* 1985;60:154–157.
50. Jordan J, Montgomery I, Trinder J. The effect of afternoon body heating on body temperature and slow wave sleep. *Psychophysiology* 1990;27:560–566.
51. Morairty S, Szymusiak R, Thomson D, McGinty D. Selective increases in nonrapid eye movement sleep following whole body heating in rats. *Brain Res* 1993;617:10–16.
52. Tobler I, Franken P, Gao B, Jaggi K, Borbely AA. Sleep deprivation in the rat at different ambient temperatures: effect on sleep, EEG spectra and brain temperature. *Arch Ital Biol* 1994;132:39–52.
53. Obal F Jr, Alfoldi P, Rubicsek G. Promotion of sleep by heat in young rats. *Pflugers Arch* 1995;430:729–738.
54. Szymusiak R, Iriye T, McGinty D. Sleep-waking discharge of neurons in the posterior lateral hypothalamic area of cats. *Brain Res Bull* 1989;23:111–120.
55. Szymusiak R, McGinty D. Sleep-waking discharge of basal forebrain projection neurons in cats. *Brain Res Bull* 1989;22:423–430.
56. Krilowicz BL, Szymusiak R, McGinty D. Regulation of posterior lateral hypothalamic arousal related neuronal discharge by preoptic anterior hypothalamic warming. *Brain Res* 1995;668:30–38.
57. Alam MN, Szymusiak R, Mcginty D. Local preoptic/anteror hypothalamic warming alters spontaneous and evoked neuronal activity in the magno-cellular basal forebrain. *Brain Res* 1995;696:221–230.
58. Kelso SR, Boulant JA. Effect of synaptic blockade on thermosensitive neurons in hypothalamic tissue slices. *Am J Physiol* 1982;243:R480–R490.
59. Alam MN, McGinty D, Szymusiak R. Neuronal discharge of preoptic/anterior hypothalamic neurons: relation to NREM sleep. *Am J Physiol* 1995;269:R1240–R1249.
60. Alam MN, McGinty D, Steininger T, McGinty D. Discharge during wakefulness and sleep of rat preoptic/anterior hypothalamic (POAH) neurons. *Soc Neurol Abstr* 1995;21:955.
61. Sherin JE, Shiromani PJ, McCarley RW, Saper CB. Activation of ventrolateral preoptic neurons during sleep. *Science* 1966;271:216–219.
62. Czeisler CA, Weitzman ED, Moore-Ede MC, Zimmerman JC. Human sleep: its duration and organization depend on its circadian phase. *Science* 1980;210:1264–1267.
63. Lavie P. Ultradian rhythms: gates of sleep and wakefulness. In: Schulz H, Lavie P, eds. *Ultradian rhythms in physiology and behavior*. New York: Springer-Verlag; 1985:148–164.
64. Watts AG, Swanson LW, Sanchez-Watts G. Efferent projections of the suprachiasmatic nucleus. I. Studies using autograde transport of *Phaseolus vulgaris* leucagglutinin in the rat. *J Comp Neurol* 1987;258:240–229.
65. Nakao M, McGinty D, Szymusiak R, Yamamoto MA. Thermoregulatory model of sleep control. *Jpn J Physiol* 1995;45:291–309.
66. Akerstedt T, Gillberg M. The circadian variation of experimentally displaced sleep. *Sleep* 1981;4; 159–169.
67. Franken P, Tobler I, Borbely AA. Cortical temperature and EEG slow wave activity in the rat: analysis of vigilance state related changes. *Pflugers Arch* 1992;420:500–507.
68. Eder DN, Vitiello MV, Avery DH. Links between delta EEG intensity and decreases in core temperature. *Sleep Res* 1994;23:493.
69. Zulley J, Campbell SS. Napping behavior during "spontaneous internal desynchronization": sleep remains in synchrony with body temperature. *Hum Neurobiol* 1985;4:123–126.
70. Johnson MP, Duffy JF, Dijk DJ, Ronda JM, Dyal CM, Czeisler CA. Short-term memory, alertness, and performance: a reappraisal of their relationship to body temperature. *J Sleep Res* 1992;1:24–29.
71. Bonnett MH, Berry RB, Arand DL. Metabolism during normal sleep, fragmented sleep, and recovery sleep. *J Appl Physiol* 1991;71:1112–1118.
72. Bonnet MH, Arand DL. 24-hour metabolic rate in insomniacs and matched normal subjects. *Sleep* 1995;18:581–588.

Physiology, Stress, and Malnutrition: Functional Correlates, Nutritional Intervention,
edited by J.M. Kinney and H.N. Tucker.
Lippincott–Raven Publishers © 1997.

Light, Circadian Rhythms, and the Homeostatic Regulation of Human Sleep

Derk-Jan Dijk

Department of Medicine, Brigham and Women's Hospital, Harvard Medical School, Boston, Massachusetts 02115

Sleep and the changes in consciousness that accompany it have fascinated mankind for centuries. This interest may have contributed to the multitude of scientific theories on the neural basis of sleep and on its function. The wide array of theories also indicates that, despite the continuing interest and progress in our knowledge about sleep, no consensus has been reached on either the physiologic function of sleep or the neurophysiologic basis of the alternation of the three vigilance states: wakefulness, non–rapid eye movement (non-REM) sleep, and REM sleep.

In this chapter, I briefly summarize our current understanding of two aspects of sleep regulation: (a) the effect of light on the human circadian pacemaker and (b) the role of the circadian pacemaker and the sleep homeostat in the regulation of sleep timing and sleep structure.

These aspects of sleep regulation and circadian rhythms have been investigated intensively, and there has been remarkable progress in the understanding of the neurophysiologic basis of the generation of circadian rhythms. Furthermore, over the past 15 years a considerable number of experiments have addressed the effect of light on the human circadian pacemaker, and these experiments have conclusively demonstrated the impact of light on human circadian physiology. More recently, the role of the circadian pacemaker in the regulation of sleep timing and sleep structure, as well as its interaction with the homeostatic regulation of sleep, have been reinvestigated. Combining these approaches may allow for an understanding of how the effects of light on the circadian pacemaker result in changes in the timing and structure of sleep.

PHYSIOLOGY OF SLEEP

Phenomenology of Normal Human Sleep

In the adult human a nocturnal sleep episode, which is typically initiated about 6 hours before the nadir of the endogenous circadian rhythm of core body

55

temperature and approximately 1 hour after the evening increase of plasma melatonin, is characterized by a cyclic alternation between non-REM sleep and REM sleep with a period of approximately 90 minutes. In the course of the four to five nightly non-REM–REM sleep cycles, the duration of the non-REM sleep episodes become progressively shorter and the duration of REM sleep episodes increases. Within REM sleep, the density of phasic events such as the rapid eye movements and muscle twitches become more abundant over consecutive REM episodes.

Analysis of the electroencephalogram (EEG), by visual scoring or computerized analyses of wave amplitude, density, or power density, showed that in non-REM sleep low-frequency components of the EEG exhibit marked changes. Power density in the 0.75–4.5 Hz range [slow-wave activity (SWA)] and visually scored slow-wave sleep (SWS) decline exponentially over consecutive non-REM sleep episodes until a lower limit is reached (1). Within non-REM sleep episodes, SWA gradually increases until it decreases suddenly shortly before REM sleep. The increase rate of SWA in the initial part of non-REM sleep episodes becomes progressively lower over consecutive non-REM episodes (2,3).

Changes in the EEG are not limited to slow waves. A decrease of power density over consecutive sleep cycles has been described repeatedly for frequencies up to approximately 10 Hz in EEGs derived from the sensorimotor cortex, and all of these frequencies exhibit a time course that is qualitatively similar to the time course of slow waves (1,4). Sleep spindles and power density in the frequency range of sleep spindles (12–15 Hz) exhibit a time course that is clearly different from the time course of SWA. It is characterized by a U-shaped time-course over a single non-REM sleep episode, with the minimum coinciding with the maximum of SWA. On average, spindle activity increases over consecutive non-REM sleep episodes, even though the increase rate declines (2,3). The sleep-related changes in field potentials derived from scalp electrodes also can be observed in intracranial recordings from various cortical and subcortical structures in both humans (5) and cats (6), indicating that these changes in the macroscopic EEG reflect changes that occur in various brain areas.

Sleep Homeostasis

The concept of sleep homeostasis implies that compensation for loss of sleep is achieved either by variations in the duration of sleep states or by variations in the intensity of sleep (7). Early studies indicated that loss of sleep was not recovered by a substantial increase (>20%) in the duration of sleep, and this observation added to the notion that sleep did not serve an important function. However, in many of these early studies the impact of time of day, i.e., the circadian pacemaker, on sleep propensity and termination was not taken into account and often subjects were studied in laboratories not shielded from external time cues. Furthermore, in many of these studies long-term regulation of sleep duration was not studied; therefore, it could not be ruled out that recovery took place over more than just one or two recovery sleep episodes (7). More recent studies have demonstrated that when subjects are given ample opportunity to sleep, up to 60% of sleep time lost is recovered over a period of 24 hours of enforced bed rest (8).

In most total sleep deprivation studies, no selective increase of REM sleep has been observed. In some selective REM sleep deprivation studies and in partial REM sleep deprivation studies, a rebound of REM sleep was observed, although the REM sleep loss incurred was not fully recovered. Although from these studies it appears that REM sleep is not under strict homeostatic control, it should be noted that in many of these studies sleep duration was restricted and the number of recovery sleep episodes recorded were limited. This may have precluded homeostatic regulation of REM sleep to be observed (7).

The propensity to initiate sleep, as measured by sleep latency, responds in a predictive way to sleep loss (9). This variable thus indicates that sleep propensity is under homeostatic control. Similarly, total sleep deprivation studies and partial sleep deprivation studies have demonstrated a dose-response relationship between SWS, i.e., stages 3 and 4 of non-REM sleep, or SWA, and the duration of prior sleep. This quantitative dose-response relationship, which spans a range of durations of prior wakefulness from 2 to 40 hours (10–12) and can be quantified with an exponential saturating function, and the observation that both humans and rats are less easily aroused when the EEG is dominated by high amplitude slow waves, lends credence to the notion that compensation for loss of non-REM sleep may be effected by changes in its intensity.

Selected suppression of slow waves by acoustic stimulation in the first part of the sleep episode, without inducing wakefulness, results in a rebound of SWA in the second undisturbed part of the sleep episode (13). These findings indicate that the decline of SWA as observed in the course of a sleep episode is not simply related to the time elapsed since sleep onset but is related to the presence of slow waves in the sleep EEG. This implies that a process closely associated with slow waves is responsible for the decline of slow-wave propensity and indicates that SWA is a solid marker of non-REM sleep homeostasis. Actually, the behavior of this parameter during baseline sleep, recovery sleep from sleep deprivation, and extended sleep can be predicted in considerable detail under the sole assumption that it is under homeostatic control (14).

Neurophysiologic Mechanism Underlying Slow Waves and Sleep Spindles

Both sleep spindles and slow waves have been main variables of interest in research on the homeostatic regulation of non-REM sleep, especially with the advent of computer-aided quantitative analyses of the EEG. Although the EEG has been used in early studies in order to characterize the sleep process and changes in sleep induced by variations of the duration of wakefulness preceding sleep, it was not until recently that the neurophysiologic basis of slow waves and sleep spindles was identified. These developments allow for the first time investigation of the neurophysiologic basis of the profound changes exhibited by both slow waves and sleep spindles across the sleep episode and the non-REM–REM sleep cycle, as well as the response to variations in the history of sleep and wakefulness and hence the neurophysiologic correlates of processes involved in the homeostatic regulation of sleep.

Under normal conditions, sleep spindles and slow waves are absent during wakefulness and REM sleep. During these two vigilance states, firing patterns of thalamocortical neurons are characterized by a single spike firing mode. The transition from wakefulness or REM sleep to non-REM sleep is accompanied by hyperpolarization of thalamocortical neurons (15,16). The hyperpolarization switches these neurons from the single spike firing mode to the burst/pause firing mode. The nucleus reticularis is thought to play a major role in the genesis of sleep spindles, and ablation of this nucleus results in loss of sleep spindle activity. Although slow waves can be observed in isolated cortical slabs, thalamocortical neurons are thought to play an important role in the genesis of slow waves in the intact animal (17).

The transition of sleep spindle dominated EEG patterns (which can be observed at the very beginning of non-REM sleep episodes) to slow wave–dominated EEG patterns is associated with a further hyperpolarization of thalamocortical neurons, which then exhibit oscillations of their membrane potential with a period in the range of slow waves (18). These slow oscillations consist of a low threshold calcium spike crowned with a burst of action potentials (19). Slow waves and sleep spindles appear in the macroscopic EEG when thalamocortical and cortical neurons are synchronized and putative mechanisms for this synchronization have been described (17,20). The hyperpolarization of neurons in these circuits is assumed to be related to a reduced activating input from a variety of nuclei located in the upper brain stem, posterior hypothalamus, and basal forebrain. Acetylcholine, norepinephrine, serotonin, histamine and glutamate are among the neurotransmitters implicated in the effects of these activating ascending systems on thalamic and cortical neurons (21).

The modulation of SWA and sleep spindle activity by variations in the duration of prior wakefulness and sleep are thought to be mediated by a common process such as hyperpolarization of neurons in thalamocortical and cortical circuits. Thus, the more rapid increase of both slow-wave and sleep spindle activity in the very beginning of recovery sleep from sleep deprivation in both humans (3) and cats (22) could be associated with a more rapid hyperpolarization and synchronization of thalamocortical neurons. Conversely, the global changes in SWA and sleep spindle activity across the sleep episode could be associated with a global reduction in the level of hyperpolarization in non-REM sleep. These sleep-wake–dependent changes in the EEG may be mediated by neuromodulators such as adenosine. Adenosine has been shown to inhibit firing rates of cholinergic neurons in mesopontine nuclei and the nucleus basalis (23). Furthermore, adenosine may facilitate slow oscillations of thalamocortical and neocortical neurons by increasing the K^+ conductance and thereby augment membrane hyperpolarization of these neurons. It has been demonstrated that the effects of sleep deprivation on the EEG can be mimicked by adenosine agonists in the rat (24). Caffeine, which acts as an antagonist at A1 and A2 adenosine receptors, suppresses low-frequency activity and enhances activity in the frequency range of sleep spindles in humans (25). It is unlikely that adenosine is the only neuromodulator involved in mediating effects of sleep deprivation and sleep on the sleep EEG. Krueger and Obál recently suggested that the local activation of neuronal groups during wakefulness could result in local changes in sleep propensity and EEG synchronization, mediated by the release of a variety of molecules (26). These hypotheses link the concept of sleep homeostasis, as indexed by SWA, to specific neurophysiologic processes and are therefore very attractive. Whether these neurophysiologic processes are affected by outputs from the endogenous circadian pacemaker has not been investigated extensively.

CIRCADIAN PHYSIOLOGY

The recognition that an endogenous pacemaker drives circadian rhythmicity in many physiologic and behavioral variables, including sleep propensity and sleep structure led sleep researchers to adapt their concept concerning the timing of sleep which either stated that sleep was a passive process or that sleep was actively initiated by specific brain structures. The former concept implies that the sleep–wake cycle can be considered an oscillation generated by the unspecified physiologic consequences of wakefulness, which eventually result in sleep initiation, followed by reversal of these consequences during sleep. The notion that sleep is an active process, initiated by specific brain structures located in the brain stem or preoptic area, ultimately implies that these specific brain structures have intrinsic self-sustaining oscillatory properties. In both concepts the role of the circadian pacemaker in the timing of sleep and wakefulness and the regulation of sleep structure was not defined. It is now recognized that for an understanding of the alternation between sleep and wakefulness the role of the endogenous circadian pacemaker needs to be considered.

Suprachiasmatic Nuclei

The identification of the locus of the mammalian circadian pacemaker has spurred much research on the mechanisms by which this pacemaker is synchronized to the 24-hour day and research on the machinery of this biologic clock. The neuroanatomic substrate of the mammalian circadian pacemaker driving the circadian rhythms of a variety of variables including sleep–wake propensity, cortisol, melatonin, and core body temperature is generally believed to be the suprachiasmatic nuclei (SCN) of the anterior hypothalamus. The evidence supporting a pacemaker function of these two small nuclei is overwhelming and has been reviewed elsewhere (27,28). Key evidence includes the abolition of circadian rhythmicity by lesion of the SCN (29,30), demonstration of persistent circadian rhythmicity of electrical activity in individual SCN neurons (31), and restoration of circadian rhythmicity by transplantation of fetal SCN tissue to animals previously rendered arrhythmic by SCN lesions (32). In the latter experiments it could be demonstrated, by using hamsters homozygous for the so-called tau mutant—which shortens the period of the wheel-running rhythm from approximately 24.1 to 20.2 hours—that the period of the free-running rhythm is determined by the genotype of the donor. The latter finding is important because it demonstrates that SCN tissue can impose the donor's circadian period upon the host without any apparent contribution of the genotype of the host to this parameter, although the host and donor pacemaker interact at the level of the centers controlling expression of locomotor behavior (33).

Evidence supporting a pacemaker function for the human SCN region has been derived from neuropathologic studies in brain tissue of patients with a clinically documented disruption of circadian behavior (34,35) and a brain imaging study (36). In the latter study, lesion of the SCN resulted in severe disruption of the consolidation of the sleep–wake cycle with an apparent inability to sustain sleep and wakefulness for normal periods.

Neuroanatomic and histologic studies have established that in mammals other than humans, the SCN is composed of a collection of small and densely packed parvocellular neurons, located in the anterior hypothalamus just above the optic chiasm, lateral to the third ventricle. Based on cytoarchitecture and cytochemical studies, two major subdivisions—a ventrolateral and dorsomedial part—can be distinguished in the rodent SCN. Neuroactive substances that have been shown to be present in neurons of the dorsomedial SCN of the rat include arginine-vasopressin, thyrotropin-releasing hormone, gamma-aminobutyric acid, and neurophysin angiotensin II. In the ventrolateral subdivision neurons containing vasoactive intestinal polypeptide, somatostatin, gastrin-releasing peptide, corticotropin releasing hormone, and neurotensin have been identified. A number of these substances also have been identified in the human SCN in which five subdivisions have been distinguished based on their chemoarchitecture (37, 38). However, the human SCN is quite diffuse, which makes it difficult to quantify changes assumed to be associated with aging and pathologic conditions.

Inputs to the SCN

Major afferents of the SCN in mammals including humans are the monosynaptic retinohypothalamic tractus originating in basal ganglion cells of the retina and the genicohypothalamic tractus, which originates in the intergeniculate leaflet of the thalamus. Both of these visual pathways terminate in the ventrolateral region of the SCN. It is generally accepted that light information reaches the SCN via the retinohypothalamic tract (RHT), which also has been demonstrated in humans (39), and via the retina geniculate-hypothalamic tractus (GHT). Light pulses induce long-lasting increments or decrements in firing rates of specialized neurons in the SCN (40) and increase the expression of immediate early genes like c-*fos* in a phase-dependent way (41,42).

Neuropeptide Y is the neurotransmitter of the GHT, but a role for GABA also has been suggested (43). Glutamate and N-acetylaspartyl-glutamate are presently thought to be the most likely candidates for mediating signal transmission of the RHT (44–46) because application of these excitatory amino acids can mimic the effects of light in considerable detail. Early findings indicated that acetylcholine (47) and GABA (48,49) were key factors in transducing light information via the RHT. A third major afferent of the ventrolateral region of the SCN originates in the dorsal raphe nuclei and is serotonergic. In addition, both the nucleus basalis, which has been implicated in the modulation of EEG activation, and the laterodorsal tegmental and pedunculopontine tegmental nuclei, which are involved in REM sleep regulation and EEG activation (50), project to the SCN (51). This cholinergic input to the SCN provides a substrate for potential feedback effects of vigilance state on SCN function.

In addition to these major afferents, binding studies have revealed high-affinity binding sites for a number of substances that may reach the SCN tissue via non-neural pathways. In the human SCN, high-affinity binding sites are present for melatonin (52), which is produced primarily by the pineal but to a lesser extent also by the retina.

Outputs of the SCN

The neural efferents of the SCN have been studied with a variety of techniques and have been reviewed (53). The largest number of efferents of the SCN project to the adjacent subparaventricular zone, which is considered to be an important relay station for transmitting circadian information to the rest of the brain. From the subparaventricular zone, projections to the bed nucleus of the stria terminalis, lateral septal nucleus, paraventricular nucleus of the thalamus, preoptic area, retrochiasmatic area, ventral and dorsomedial nuclei of the hypothalamus, posterior hypothalamic area, and periaqueductal gray have been described. All these areas also receive direct input from the SCN, which in addition projects to the intergeniculate leaflet. These efferent connections have been considered rather limited, and it has been concluded that "the projection pattern of the SCN is remarkably deficient in terms of providing a neuroanatomic substrate to explain how the circadian generator may impart rhythmicity to motivated behaviors or to homeostatic mechanisms" (53). One important pathway that has received considerable evidence is the SCN–pineal SCN loop. The SCN drives the rhythm of melatonin synthesis by a pathway that involves the paraventricular nucleus (PVT) of the hypothalamus, and the supracervical ganglion from which sympathetic fibers innervate the pineal and stimulate the rate-limiting enzyme of pineal synthesis, i.e., N-acetyltransferase. Because melatonin receptors have been identified in the SCN and melatonin has been shown to modulate circadian parameters in rodents, this pathway has been hypothesized to play a role in stabilization of entrainment. Furthermore, melatonin administration results in sleepiness and changes the EEG during sleep and wakefulness (54–56). These hypnotic properties of melatonin are especially pronounced when endogenous levels of melatonin are low. Melatonin also has been shown to lower body temperature, and it has been hypothesized that the endogenous rhythm of melatonin plays a key role in the generation of the daily body temperature cycle.

Entrainment of the Endogenous Circadian Pacemaker by Environmental Cycles

In the absence of environmental 24-hour cycles, mammals including humans exhibit free-running rest–activity rhythms with a period different from 24 hours. Because in the natural environment rest–activity cycles are synchronized to the solar day, the question arises by which environmental 24 hour cycle(s) the endogenous circadian pacemaker is synchronized to the solar day. It is well established that the 24-hour light–dark cycle is the most important synchronizer in mammals (57,58). Synchronization of the non–24-h endogenous circadian pacemaker is achieved by a phase-dependent sensitivity of this pacemaker to light. In both diurnal and nocturnal animals, light pulses given early in the subjective night (i.e., at the beginning of the major activity period of nocturnal animals and at the beginning of the major rest period in diurnal animals) induce phase delays of endogenous circadian rhythms. Conversely, light pulses given at the end of the subjective night induce phase advances. Light pulses applied in the middle of the subjective night induce either no phase shifts or, when the light stimulus is of sufficient strength, large phase shifts, the direction of which may be unpredictable. During the subjective day, the circadian pacemaker is far less sensitive to light, and this phase of reduced sensitivity is referred to as the "dead zone" of the phase response curve. Phase response curves, i.e., a plot of phase shifts against endogenous circadian phase of light administration, have proven to be a powerful tool in understanding period and phase control of endogenous circadian pacemakers. Furthermore, naturalistic experiments in which animals have been exposed to complete 24-hour light–dark cycles in which the ratio of the duration of the light episode and dark episode have been varied [i.e., animals were exposed to different seasons (photoperiods)] demonstrated that the duration of the subjective night (i.e., the period during which the pacemaker is sensitive to light) varies as a function of photoperiod. This memory for day length has been demonstrated to be present at the level of light-induced c-*fos* expression in the SCN (59). This remarkable feature allows the SCN not only to function as a daily clock, but allows the SCN to internalize time of year and transmit this information to the rest of the central nervous system and body.

Evidence in favor of a role for light in the synchronization of circadian rhythms in humans was published as early as 1969 (60,61). Two years later, Aschoff published a paper (62) entitled "Human circadian rhythms in continuous darkness: entrainment by social cues," in which he stated that ". . . human circadian rhythms can be entrained to 24 hours by social cues from the environment" and. . . that light—at least artificial light—is a rather weak Zeitgeber for man. . . ." These conclusions were based on six subjects who were living in constant darkness for only 4 days, during which no free run of the body temperature rhythm and the rhythms of the urinary excretion of catecholamines, 17-hydroxycorticosteroids, and sodium was observed. Because in the absence of light the endogenous circadian period is close to 24 hours, 4 days was too short to discriminate between entrainment and free run. Czeisler et al. (63) reinvestigated the role of the light–dark cycle and presented evidence that a 24-hour 150 lux light–dark cycle was sufficient to entrain human circadian rhythms. Subsequently they and others (64–74) demonstrated that human circadian rhythms can be phase shifted by scheduled exposure to bright light and that this effect of light is not mediated by the sleep–wake cycle, as was originally postulated (75). Initially it was thought that light intensity needed to exceed 1,000 lux before any effect on the circadian pacemaker could be observed (76). Recently the dose-response relationship between light intensity and phase shift of the endogenous circadian system has been established. The phase-shifting effect of light appears to be proportional to the cube root of light intensity (77). Furthermore, these experiments demonstrated conclusively that even light intensity as low as 180 lux, which is close to ordinary room light, significantly affect the human circadian system.

Kronauer (78,79) developed a mathematical model to account for the phase resetting by light in humans. Besides describing the phase delays and phase advances when light exposure is scheduled shortly before and after the minimum of the core body temperature rhythms, this model predicts that a single light pulse centered around the minimum of the core body temperature (CBT) rhythm, even though it does not affect the phase of the pacemaker, does change the amplitude of the oscillator. This reduction of the amplitude then renders the pacemaker more sensitive to subsequent light pulses, which then can induce large phase shifts. The predicted reduction of the amplitude after one or two light pulses centered at the minimum of the core body temperature rhythm was subsequently verified (80). An implication of these findings and this model is that, besides phase, amplitude is an important parameter of the circadian system. Furthermore, the model makes possible the prediction of phase and amplitude, even if the light–dark schedule to which subjects are exposed is complex. This latter aspect is important to the clinical application of bright light because in real-life situations humans are exposed to complex light–dark cycles, not just single bright light pulses.

An important characteristic of the human phase response curve to light is that during entrainment the larger part of the most light-sensitive phase coincides with the nocturnal sleep episode. This implies that to shift the human circadian pacemaker efficiently, sleep needs to be displaced. In humans the effects of photoperiod have been investigated either by monitoring changes in circadian organization across season or by artificially exposing human subjects to long nights (81–83). The results of these experiments have been conflicting, demonstrating evidence for an influence of photoperiod in some experiments, whereas in other experiments no major effect of photoperiod on circadian organization could be demonstrated. These conflicting results may be related in part to the fact that in urban people, the seasonal variation in light exposure is greatly reduced due to the availability of artificial light, which even at low intensities may be sufficient to affect the circadian system. Among the results obtained in some photoperiods are the observation that phase relationships between different variables such as the sleep–wake cycle and the core body temperature change across seasons and that the duration of the interval during which melatonin is present in plasma increases during long nights. In addition, postmortem analyses of human SCN tissue has suggested changes in vasopressin neuron populations across the seasons (37). Although presently these data are not easily understood in terms of models of the human circadian pacemaker, they highlight the complexity of the human circadian system even though this system can be considered a one-pacemaker system.

The one-pacemaker concept has received substantial support from studies in which subjects were exposed to light in order to induce phase shifts of the circadian system, and the phase relationship of multiple variables was assessed before and after the phase shift. Despite the fact that these variables ranged from body temperature to plasma melatonin to subjective alertness to cognitive performance, no evidence of internal dissociation between these variables was observed (66,71,84).

The effect of scheduled bright light exposure on sleep and sleep structure has been investigated in a number of experiments. Major findings of these studies are that the rhythm of sleep propensity can be shifted by light exposure and that these (small) shifts of the circadian system as indexed by body temperature and plasma melatonin, do not affect sleep structure. Thus, in one early study (70,71), repeated exposure to bright light in the morning has been shown to phase advance the rhythm of body temperature and the evening increase of plasma melatonin. In addition the propensity to wake up from sleep was phase advanced by an amount roughly identical to the phase advance of the body temperature and plasma melatonin rhythm. This phase advance affected neither REM sleep nor the EEG during non-REM sleep. These results have been confirmed and extended in subsequent studies in both young (85) and older subjects (74). In the latter experiment it was demonstrated that inducing a phase delay of the body temperature rhythm in older subjects greatly improved sleep efficiency.

Exposure to single light pulses in the evening result in an immediate delay in the nocturnal decline in body temperature, which persists for approximately 4 hours

(86). This direct effect of light on body temperature may be mediated by the light-induced suppression of melatonin. Concurrent with this change in body temperature, a lengthening of the latency to sleep onset has been observed. Despite this profound change in the time course of temperature, the effects on the time course of SWA were minimal (87). These data and other experiments demonstrate the efficacy of bright light in phase shifting of endogenous circadian rhythm of sleep propensity and demonstrate that light does not affect SWA in the EEG in non-REM sleep. These findings also imply that bright light treatment holds promise for the treatment of sleep disorders and disturbances related to the circadian system.

It has been demonstrated recently that in the rat c-*fos* induction in the SCN and phase resetting of activity rhythms can be induced by air puffs when these air puffs have previously been paired with light pulses that induce phase shifts (88). From this experiment it thus appears that phase resetting can be conditioned. Although it is presently not known whether such a conditioning occurs under naturalistic conditions in rodents and whether it can be induced in humans, the data point to the potential complexity of phase resetting and may suggest that other stimuli could be used to reset the human circadian pacemaker.

It is only in the past decade that strong evidence for effects of nonphotic stimuli on the circadian pacemaker has accumulated, especially in rodents (89,90). These nonphotic stimuli include exposure to a novel environment and running-wheel activity. Although these (feedback) effects can be understood in light of the multitude of afferents to the SCN, their functional significance remains unclear. In at least two experiments it has been attempted to demonstrate effects of activity on circadian parameters in humans (91,92). It has been reported that scheduled vigorous activity may induce some changes in hormonal and body temperature patterns, but it has not been demonstrated that these changes are persistent and reflect a change in the phase of the endogenous circadian pacemaker.

The most compelling evidence for the existence of nonphotic zeitgebers stems from the study of blind subjects. Many completely blind subjects fail to entrain to the 24-hour day, even though many of them schedule their sleep–wake cycle to the 24-hour day (93–97). This is in accordance with the notion that light is also the most important zeitgeber in humans. Some blind subjects appear to be entrained to the 24-hour day, and at first glance this is strong evidence for the existence of nonphotic zeitgebers in humans. However, in some of these subjects a neuroendocrine response to light that is thought to be mediated by the SCN, i.e., suppression of melatonin, is intact in these subjects (98). Thus, the efficacy of nonphotic zeitgebers in humans awaits further substantiation.

EARLY CIRCADIAN STUDIES

It has been recognized early on that for a better understanding of the mechanisms underlying the timing of the sleep–wake cycle a distinction should be made between internal and environmental factors that both contribute to variations in the propensity to initiate and terminate sleep. A decade before the identification of the SCN as the locus of the endogenous circadian pacemaker, Aschoff and Wever described the timing of rest and activity in nine human subjects who were isolated from the 24-hour cycles of light, temperature, etc., and had no clocks available for the duration (on average 14 days) of the experiment (99). The main findings reported in this and a subsequent article (100) were that humans maintain a monophasic sleep–wake cycle and that the sleep–wake ratio remains approximately 1:3. The sleep–wake cycle that remained synchronized with the core body temperature rhythm exhibited a free-running period close to 25 hours. These and other data (101) demonstrated the endogenous origin of the monophasic sleep–wake cycle in the adult human. The serial correlation between the duration of subsequent sleep–wake cycles and the correlation between the duration of activity and subsequent rest both turned negative (102). This implies that a self-sustaining oscillator, and not a stochastic process or renewal process, underlies the observed rhythmicity. Further evidence for the involvement of an endogenous oscillator in the generation of the sleep–wake cycle was derived from the observed dependency of the phase angle difference between the light–dark cycle and the sleep–wake cycle on the period of the artificial light–dark cycle (60). These early data were in accordance with animal studies and supported the hypothesis that, also in humans, a single circadian pacemaker underlies circadian rhythmicity in a variety of variables. The analyses further indicated that the sleep–wake cycle is only loosely coupled to the circadian pacemaker. This was convincingly demonstrated by Aschoff, in 1967, when he reported that the human sleep–wake cycle could spontaneously desynchronize from the core body temperature cycle, which kept oscillating with a period close to 25 hours (103). Sleep–wake cycles with periods outside the circadian range, with simultaneous core body temperature cycles of 25 hours, have subsequently been reported by various researchers. The phenomenon of internal desynchronization in which two variables (i.e., the core body temperature rhythm and the sleep–wake cycle) oscillate with different periods is seemingly at variance with the hypothesis that a single circadian pacemaker directly drives both variables and has led to models in which two oscillatory processes govern the sleep–wake cycle. Because during internal desynchronization sleep is initiated at various phases of the core body temperature cycle, it allowed for an analysis of the dependency of sleep duration and sleep structure on circadian phase and thereby contributed considerably to our knowledge about the circadian regulation of sleep.

SPONTANEOUS INTERNAL DESYNCHRONIZATION

During spontaneous internal desynchronization, the period of the sleep–wake cycle becomes either substantially shorter or substantially longer than the period of the body temperature cycle, which attains a period of 24.3–25.0 hours. It should be kept in mind that in the majority of these experiments the light–dark cycle was self-selected and that light intensity during the wake episode was probably at normal indoor lighting levels. Computer simulations have recently shown that under these conditions the observed period is longer than the true intrinsic period (79). Although the period of the body temperature remains stable during spontaneous desynchronization, the period of the sleep–wake cycle is more labile. Within a subject it may vary from being close to the period of the body temperature rhythm to close to twice the period of the body temperature. Furthermore, the ratio of sleep to wakefulness varies markedly from one sleep–wake cycle to the next. Despite this variability, comprehensive analyses of the interaction of the sleep–wake cycle with the core body temperature rhythms have shown some remarkable regularities. From the analyses of spontaneous desynchrony data it appears that the duration of sleep is primarily dependent on the phase of the core body temperature rhythm at which sleep is initiated. This is to say that when prior wakefulness is of sufficient duration, sleep episodes are very long when they are initiated close to the maximum of the core body temperature rhythm, whereas they are very short when initiated on the early part of the rising limb of the core body temperature rhythm (104,105). Most sleep terminations are located on the rising limb of the temperature rhythm. In one analysis, no significant contribution of prior wake duration to sleep length could be observed, and it was concluded that the circadian contribution to the regulation of sleep duration greatly exceeds the homeostatic contribution (106). Other key observations in spontaneous desynchrony protocol have been that sleep is rarely initiated on the latter part of the rising limb of the core body temperature rhythm. This window has been called a wake maintenance zone (107). Furthermore, analyses of sleep structure as a function of circadian phase have shown that the crest of the rhythm of REM sleep is located at or shortly after the minimum of the core body temperature rhythm. Although these analyses have established the prominent influence of the circadian pacemaker on sleep duration and sleep structure, they have not addressed the role of the circadian pacemaker in sleep timing under entrained conditions. In addition, these analyses did not allow for a quantitative analysis of the relative contribution of the circadian pacemaker and the sleep homeostat to sleep propensity and sleep structure because of the confounding of variations in the duration of prior wakefulness and sleep and circadian phase at which sleep occurred.

FORCED DESYNCHRONIZATION

The forced desynchrony protocol, pioneered by Kleitman (108), allows for an analysis of the interaction of sleep-dependent and circadian aspects of the regulation of alertness during wakefulness (109) and the interaction of sleep-dependent and circadian aspects of sleep (110,111). In this protocol subjects live in the laboratory for a prolonged period of time, i.e., 1 month or longer. After an initial assessment of the phase of the endogenous circadian pacemaker during entrainment, subjects are scheduled to a non–24-hour sleep–wake cycle, with a period length (e.g., 28 hours) that is outside the range of entrainment. When light intensity during the scheduled waking episodes is kept at low levels (i.e., 10–15 lux), it is reasonable to assume that the pacemaker freeruns with a near stable period (79). As a consequence, scheduled sleep and wake episodes occur at virtually all circadian phases (Fig. 1). Because subjects are scheduled to stay in bed in darkness, i.e., a sleep conducive condition, the variation in wakefulness preceding sleep episode is minimized. Results of this protocol have confirmed the results of spontaneous desynchrony protocols and the results of studies in which the circadian regulation of sleep was studied in so-called 90-minute days or 3-hour days (111). Key findings of these protocol are that the maximum circadian drive for sleep, as indexed by sleep latency and wakefulness within scheduled sleep episodes, is located close to the minimum of the core body temperature rhythm, in accordance with previous results (Fig. 2). Paradoxically, this maximum circadian drive for sleep is under entrained conditions thus located close to habitual wake time because the CBT minimum occurs 1–2 hours before habitual wake time. The minimum of the circadian drive for sleep, as indexed by sleep latency and wakefulness in a scheduled sleep episode, occurs approximately 8 hours before the temperature minimum (Fig. 2). Thus, under entrained conditions the circadian pacemaker opposes sleep initiation most strongly shortly before habitual bedtime. Analyses of the interaction of circadian and sleep-dependent components of the propensity to wake up, demonstrated nonlinear components, which are such that the circadian influences became progressively stronger when the homeostatic drive for sleep subsided. These data strongly suggest that under entrained conditions the circadian pacemaker promotes the consolidation of sleep and wakefulness by opposing during the habitual waking day the progressive increase in sleep propensity associated with sustained wakefulness. During the habitual sleep episode the circadian pacemaker promoted sleep consolidation by opposing the progressive decline in the homeostatic drive for sleep associated with sustained sleep.

Actually, analyses of the interaction of sleep-dependent and circadian components demonstrated that high sleep efficiency can be maintained only when sleep is initiated close to the minimum of the circadian drive for sleep (110). These analyses thus demonstrate that besides circadian aspects—which were highlighted in spontaneous desynchrony protocols—sleep-dependent aspects play a key-role in the regulation of sleep propensity.

Analysis of REM sleep regulation in this forced desynchrony protocol demonstrated that apart from the well-known circadian regulation of this sleep state, a sleep-dependent disinhibition of REM sleep contributes to the high levels of REM sleep, which are observed at the end of the sleep episode, under entrained conditions. The application of spectral analysis in the forced desynchrony protocol has allowed for an assessment of the contribution of the circadian pacemaker to the spectral composition of the EEG during sleep, whereas the confounding influence of variations in the duration of wakefulness preceding sleep was minimized. In accordance with previous data, SWA was shown to be primarily dependent on the time elapsed since sleep onset and to be largely independent of

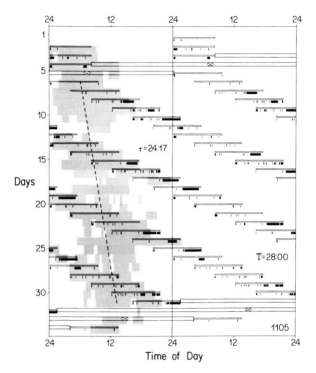

FIG. 1. Double plot of the forced desynchrony protocol. Successive days are plotted both next to and beneath each other. Scheduled sleep episodes (*open narrow bars*), polysomnographically determined wakefulness within each sleep episode (*black tick marks below narrow open bars*), and intervals during which core body temperature was below the mean (stippled areas) are indicated. An intrinsic temperature cycle period of 24.3 hours was estimated by a nonparametric spectral analysis of the core body temperature data during the forced desynchrony part of the protocol. The time of the minimum of the circadian temperature rhythm as estimated by this nonparametric spectral analysis is indicated by the broken line. The minimum of the endogenous circadian rhythm of core body temperature as unmasked by a 40-hour constant routine protocol is indicated by an encircled X. Reprinted with permission (110).

circadian phase (Figs. 3 and 4). Surprisingly, the crest of the low-amplitude circadian modulation of SWA coincided with the minimum of the circadian sleep propensity rhythm. Thus, the circadian rhythm in SWA did not parallel the circadian rhythm in sleep propensity. In contrast to slow waves, sleep spindle activity exhibited both a marked sleep-dependent and a marked circadian component. The interaction of the sleep-dependent and circadian components is such that when the second half of the sleep episode coincides with the minimum of the core body temperature rhythm, sleep spindles are abundant. In contrast, when the second half of the sleep episode coincides with the rising limb of the core body temperature rhythm, sleep spindle activity is at low levels. These data indicate that the circadian and homeostatic contribution to slow waves and sleep

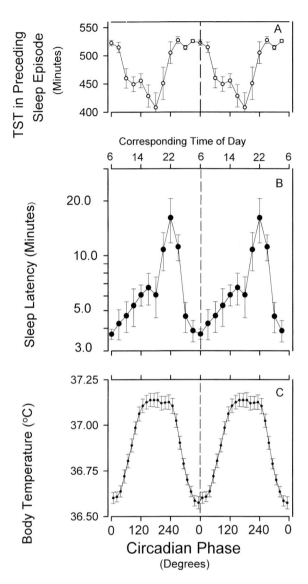

FIG. 2. Circadian variation of the latency to sleep onset (**B**), the educed wave-form of core body temperature (**C**), and total sleep time in sleep episodes preceding the assessment of sleep latency (**A**). Sleep latency data (i.e., the duration of the interval between lights-off and the first occurrence of stage 1 or any other sleep stage) were first log transformed and then for each subject averaged per 30° bin (i.e., 2 circadian hours). Next, the retransformed data were averaged per 30° bin over subjects. The data are plotted at the mid-point of the bins and double plotted. Note the logarithmic scale on the ordinate. Temperature data were first for each subject folded at the endogenous circadian period as assessed by nonparametric spectral analysis and then averaged per 15° (i.e., 1 circadian hour). Next the data were averaged per 15° over subjects. The estimated minimum of the educed wave-form (9) of core body temperature was arbitrarily assigned circadian phase 0. Vertical bars correspond to ±1 SEM. To facilitate interpretation of the data, the clock time that would correspond to the circadian phase of the core body temperature rhythm in young subjects under normal entrained conditions (12) is indicated on the upper abscissa of panel B. Total sleep times (TST) in the sleep episodes preceding the assessment of sleep latency for each bin were first averaged per subject and next averaged over subjects. The TST data are plotted at the circadian phase at which sleep latency was assessed. Reprinted with permission (110).

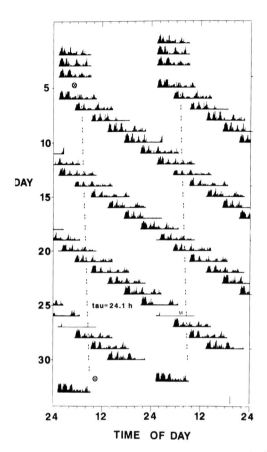

FIG. 3. Double plot of the time course of SWA during sleep episodes in the forced desynchrony protocol (subject 1136). Artifacts during sleep and wakefulness within the scheduled sleep episodes were removed. One-minute averaged values are plotted for SWA. The time of the minimum of the circadian temperature rhythm, estimated by nonparametric spectral analysis, is indicated by the broken line. Successive days are plotted both next to and beneath each other. The minimum of the endogenous circadian rhythm of core body temperature as assessed in the initial and final constant routine is indicated by an encircled X. M indicates missing data. The data were plotted with respect to clock time. The vertical line in the right hand lower corner corresponds to 200 $\mu V^2/Hz$. Reprinted with permission (111).

spindle activity are quantitatively different and challenge the notion that their reciprocal relationship depends on one common process.

PATIENT CARE IMPLICATIONS

The study of the effects of light on human circadian physiology, the establishment of the importance of homeostatic mechanism in the regulation of sleep, the progress in the understanding of the neurophysiologic basis of slow waves

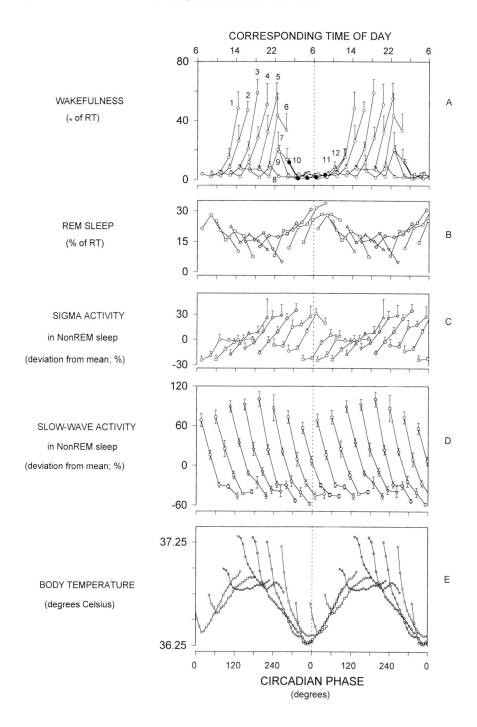

and sleep spindles, and the new insights in the role of the circadian pacemaker in the regulation of sleep provide key components for an integrative approach to the study of human sleep and its disorders. An emerging consensus from these approaches and animal studies (112,113) is that sleep propensity and sleep structure result from a complex interaction of circadian and homeostatic processes. Under entrained conditions the phase relationship between the sleep–wake cycle and the endogenous circadian rhythm of sleep propensity and REM sleep propensity is such that the consolidation of sleep and wakefulness, as well as the transition between these vigilance states, is facilitated. Light exposure may be used to shift the circadian component and normalize the phase relationship between the sleep–wake cycle and circadian rhythm of sleep propensity in conditions in which this ideal phase relationship is not maintained, although it may not be effective in those dysregulations that may be more related to changes in the homeostatic aspects of sleep regulation.

An integrative approach, inspired by concepts (114,115) and pioneering experiments (116) developed and carried out in the early 1980s, may lead to new experimental protocols and eventually result in new and more effective therapies for sleep disorders and disturbances in the blind, shift workers, and older people.

ACKNOWLEDGMENTS

Part of the research reported in this chapter was supported by U.S. Public Health Service National Institutes of Health Awards NIA-1-P01-AG09975, NCRR-GCRC-M01-RR02635, and NIMH-1-R01-MH45130 to Dr. Charles A. Czeisler and by a grant from Philips Lighting to Dr. D-J Dijk. I also wish to thank Drs. Alexander A. Borbély and Charles Czeisler for support and inspiration.

FIG. 4. Sleep-dependent changes as a function of circadian phase at start of sleep episodes. **A:** Sleep episodes were assigned to 12 30° bins of the core body temperature rhythm, based on the circadian phase at lights out. **B–E:** Sleep episode were assigned to eight 45° bins. ○, −22.5–22.5°; ●, 22.5–67.5°; ▽, 76.5–112.5°; ▼, 112.5–157.5°; □, 157.5–202.5°; ■, 202.5–247.5°; △, 247.5–292.5°; ▲, 292.5–337.5°. **A:** Wakefulness in scheduled sleep episodes, expressed as a percentage of recording time. ●, sleep episodes initiated between 255° and 285° (23:01 hours), which corresponds to the habitual timing of sleep during entrained conditions. The numbers in the graph identify bin number: 1, −15–15°; 2, 15–45°; 3, 45–75°; 4, 75–105°; 5, 105–135°; 6, 135–165°; 7, 165–195°; 8, 195–225°; 9, 225–255°; 10, 255–285°; 11, 285–315°; 12, 315–345°. **B:** REM sleep, expressed as a percentage of recording time. **C:** Sigma activity in non-REM sleep, expressed as a deviation from each individual's mean value. **D:** SWA in non-REM sleep, expressed as a deviation from each individual's mean value. **E:** Core body temperature. Note that the first value of each temperature curve represents the average core body temperature during the last 30 minutes before lights out. Reprinted with permission (111).

REFERENCES

1. Dijk DJ, Brunner DP, Borbély AA. Time course of EEG power density during long sleep in humans. *Am J Physiol* 1990;258:R650–R661.
2. Aeschbach D, Borbély AA. All-night dynamics of the human sleep EEG. *J Sleep Res* 1993;2:70–81.
3. Dijk DJ, Hayes B, Czeisler CA. Dynamics of electroencephalographic sleep spindles and slow wave activity in men: effect of sleep deprivation. *Brain Res* 1993;626:190–199.
4. Borbély AA, Baumann F, Brandeis D, Strauch I, Lehmann D. Sleep deprivation: effect on sleep stages and EEG power density in man. *Electroencephalogr Clin Neurophysiol* 1981;51:483–493.
5. Dijk D-J, Wieser HG. Intracranial recording of SWA in man. In: Horne J, ed. *Sleep '90. Proceedings of the 10th congress of the European Sleep Research Society.* Bochum. Germany: Pontenagel;1990: 3–7.
6. Lancel M, Van Riezen H, Glatt A. Enhanced slow-wave activity within NREM sleep in the cortical and subcortical EEG of the cat after sleep deprivation. *Sleep* 1992;15:102–118.
7. Borbély AA. Sleep homeostasis and models of sleep regulation. In: Kryger MH, Roth T, Dement WC, eds. *Principles and practice of sleep medicine.* 2nd ed. Philadelphia: WB Saunders; 1994: 309–320.
8. Rosenthal L, Roehrs TA, Rosen A, Roth T. Levels of sleepiness and total sleep time following various time in bed conditions. *Sleep* 1993;16:226–232.
9. Carskadon MA, Dement WC. Effect of total sleep loss on sleep tendency. *Percept Motor Skills* 1979; 48:495–506.
10. Dijk DJ, Beersma DGM, Daan S. EEG power density during nap sleep: reflection of an hourglass measuring the duration of prior wakefulness. *J Biol Rhythms* 1987;2:207–219.
11. Dijk DJ, Brunner DP, Beersma DGM, Borbély AA. EEG power density and slow wave sleep as a function of prior wakefulness and circadian phase. *Sleep* 1990;13:430–440.
12. Brunner DP, Dijk D-J, Tobler I, Borbély AA. Effect of partial sleep deprivation on sleep stages and EEG power spectra: evidence for non-REM and REM sleep homeostasis. *Electroencephalogr Clin Neurophysiol* 1990;75:492–499.
13. Dijk D-J, Beersma DGM, Daan S, Bloem GM, Van den Hoofdakker RH. Quantitative analysis of the effects of slow wave sleep deprivation during the first 3 h of sleep on subsequent EEG power density. *Eur Arch Psychiatr Neurol Sci* 1987;236:323–328.
14. Achermann P, Dijk DJ, Brunner DP, Borbély AA. A model of human sleep homeostasis based on EEG slow-wave activity: quantitative comparison of data and simulations. *Brain Res Bull* 1993;31: 97–113.
15. Hirsch JC, Fourment A, Marc ME. Sleep-related variations of membrane potential in the lateral geniculate body relay neurons of the cat. *Brain Res* 1983;259:308–312.
16. Steriade M, McCormick DA, Sejnowski TJ. Thalamocortical oscillations in the sleeping and aroused brain. *Science* 1993;262:679–685.
17. Steriade M, Curró Dossi R, Nuñez A. Network modulation of a slow intrinsic oscillation of cat thalamocortical neurons implicated in sleep delta waves: cortically induced synchronization and brainstem cholinergic suppression. *J Neurosci* 1991;11:3200–3217.
18. Curró Dossi R, Nuñez A, Steriade M. Electrophysiology of a slow (0.5–4 Hz) intrinsic oscillation of cat thalamocortical neurones in vivo. *J Physiol* 1992;447:215–234.
19. Steriade M, Contreras D, Amzica F. Synchronized sleep oscillations and their paroxysmal developments. *Trends Neurosci* 1994;17:199–208.
20. Soltesz I, Crunelli V. A role for low-frequency, rhythmic synaptic potentials in the synchronization of cat thalamocortical cells. *J Physiol* 1992;457:257–276.
21. McCormick DA. Neurotransmitter actions in the thalamus and cerebral cortex. *J Clin Neurophysiol* 1992;9:212–223.
22. Lancel M, Van Riezen H, Glatt A. The time course of sigma activity and slow wave activity during NREMS in cortical and thalamic EEG of the cat during baseline and after 12 hours of wakefulness. *Brain Res* 1992;596:285–295.
23. Rainnie DG, Grunze HCR, McCarley RW, Greene RW. Adenosine inhibition of mesopontine cholinergic neurons: implications for EEG arousal. *Science* 1994;263:689–692.
24. Benington JH, Kodali SK, Heller HC. Stimulation of A1 adenosine receptors mimics the electroencephalographic effects of sleep deprivation. *Brain Res* 1995;692:79–85.
25. Landolt HP, Werth E, Borbély AA, Dijk D-J. Caffeine intake (200 mg) in the morning affects human sleep and EEG power spectra at night. *Brain Res* 1995;675:67–74.
26. Krueger JM, Obál F. A neuronal group theory of sleep function. *J Sleep Res* 1993;2:63–69.

27. Meijer JH, Rietveld WJ. Neurophysiology of the suprachiasmatic circadian pacemaker in rodents. *Physiol Rev* 1989;69:671–707.
28. Klein DC, Moore RY, Reppert SM, eds. *Suprachiasmatic nucleus: the mind's clock*. New York: Oxford University Press, 1991.
29. Stephan FK, Zucker I. Circadian rhythms in drinking behavior and locomotor activity of rats are eliminated by hypothalamic lesion. *Proc Natl Acad Sci U S A* 1972;69:1583–1586.
30. Moore RY, Eichler VB. Loss of circadian adrenal corticosterone rhythm following suprachiasmatic nucleus lesions in the rat. *Brain Res* 1972;42:201–206.
31. Welsh DK, Logothetis DE, Meister M, Reppert SM. Individual neurons dissociated from rat suprachiasmatic nucleus express independently phase circadian firing rhythms. *Neuron* 1995;14:697–706.
32. Ralph MR, Foster RG, Davis FC, Menaker M. Transplanted suprachiasmatic nucleus determines circadian period. *Science* 1990;247:975–978.
33. Vogelbaum M, Menaker M. Temporal chimeras produced by hypothalamic transplants. *J Neurosci* 1992;12:3619–3627.
34. Fulton JF, Bailey B. Tumors in the region of the third ventricle: their diagnosis and relation to pathological sleep. *J Nerv Ment Dis* 1929;69:1–23,145–164,261–277.
35. Schwartz WJ, Busis NA, Hedley-White ET. A discrete lesion of ventral hypothalamus and optic chiasm that disturbed the daily temperature rhythm. *J Neurol* 1986;233:1–4.
36. Cohen RA, Albers HE. Disruption of human circadian and cognitive regulation following a discrete hypothalamic lesion: a case study. *Neurology* 1991;41:726–729.
37. Hofman MA, Purba JS, Swaab DF. Annual variations in the vasopressin neuron population of the human suprachiasmatic nucleus. *Neuroscience* 1993;53:1103–1112.
38. Mai JK, Kedziora O, Teckhaus L, Sofroniew MV. Evidence for subdivisions in the human suprachiasmatic nucleus. *J Comp Neurol* 1991;305:508–525.
39. Sadun AA, Schaechter JD, Smith LEH. A retinohypothalamic pathway in man: light mediation of circadian rhythms. *Brain Res* 1984;302:371–377.
40. Groos GA, Meijer JH. Effects of illumination on suprachiasmatic nucleus electrical discharge. *Ann N Y Acad Sci* 1985;153:134–146.
41. Rusak B, Robertson HA, Wisden W, Hunt SP. Light pulses that shift rhythms induce gene expression in the suprachiasmatic nucleus. *Science* 1990;248:1237–1240.
42. Kornhauser JM, Nelson DE, Mayo KE, Takahashi JS. Photic and circadian regulation of c-fos gene expression in the hamster suprachiasmatic nucleus. *Neuron* 1990;5:127–134.
43. Card JP, Moore RY. The organization of visual circuits influencing the circadian activity of the suprachiasmatic nucleus. In: Klein DC, Moore RY, Reppert SM, eds. *Suprachiasmatic nucleus: the mind's clock*. New York: Oxford University Press; 1991:51–76.
44. Meijer JH, Van der Zee EA, Diets M. Glutamate phase shifts circadian activity rhythms in hamsters. *Neurosci Lett* 1988:86:177–183.
45. Vindlacheruvu RR, Ebling FJP, Maywood ES, Hastings MH. Blockade of glutaminergic neurotransmission in the suprachiasmatic nucleus prevents cellular and behavioural responses of the circadian system to light. *Eur J Neurosci* 1992;4:673–679.
46. Ding JM, Chen D, Weber ET, Faiman LE, Rea M, Gillette MU. Resetting the biological clock: mediation of nocturnal circadian shifts by glutamate and NO. *Science* 1994;266:1713–1717.
47. Earnest DJ, Turek FW. Neurochemical basis for the photic control of circadian rhythms and seasonal reproductive cycles: role for acetylcholine. *Proc Natl Acad Sci U S A* 1985;82:4277–4281.
48. Ralph MR, Menaker M. Bicuculline blocks circadian phase delays but not advances. *Brain Res* 1985;325:362–365.
49. Ralph MR, Menaker M. Effects of diazepam on circadian phase advances and delays. *Brain Res* 1986;372:405–408.
50. McCarley RW, Greene RW, Rainnie D, Portas CM. Brainstem neuromodulation and REM sleep. *Semin Neurosci* 1995;7:341–354.
51. Bina KG, Rusak B, Semba K. Localization of cholinergic neurons in the forebrain and brainstem that project to the suprachiasmatic nucleus of the hypothalamus in rat. *J Comp Neurol* 1993;335:295–307.
52. Reppert SM, Weaver DR, Rivkess SA, Stopa EG. Putative melatonin receptors in a human biological clock. *Science* 1982;42:78–81.
53. Watts AG. The efferent projections of the suprachiasmatic nucleus: anatomical insights into the control of circadian rhythms. In: Klein DC, Moore RY, Reppert SM, eds. *Suprachiasmatic nucleus: the mind's clock*. New York: Oxford University Press; 1991:77–106.

54. Dollins AB, Zhdanova IV, Wurtman RJ, Lynch HJ, Deng MH. Effect of inducing nocturnal serum melatonin concentrations in daytime sleep, mood, body temperature and performance. *Proc Natl Acad Sci U S A* 1994;91:199–209.

55. Dijk D-J, Roth C, Landolt HP, et al. Melatonin effect on daytime sleep in men: suppression of EEG low-frequency activity and enhancement of spindle frequency activity. *Neurosci Lett* 1995;201: 13–16.

56. Cajochen C, Krauchi K, Von Arx MA, Mori D, Graw P, Wirz-Justice A. Daytime melatonin administration enhances sleepiness and theta/alpha activity in the waking EEG. *Neurosci Lett* 1996;207:209–213.

57. Czeisler CA. The effect of light on the human circadian pacemaker. In: *Circadian clocks and their adjustments.* Ciba Foundation Symposium 183. Chichester, England: Wiley; 1995:254–302.

58. Dijk D-J, Boulos Z, Eastman CI, Lewy AJ, Campbell SS, Terman M. Light treatment for sleep disorders: consensus report II. Basic properties of circadian physiology and sleep regulation. *J Biol Rhythms* 1995;10:113–125

59. Sumova A, Travnickova Z, Peters R, Schwartz WJ, Illnerova H. The rat suprachiasmatic nucleus is a clock for all seasons. *Proc Natl Acad Sci U S A* 1995;92:7754–7758.

60. Aschoff J, Pöppel E, Wever R. Circadiane Periodik des Menschens unter dem Einfluss von Lich-Dunkel-Wechseln unterschiedlicher Periode. *Pflugers Arch* 1969;306:58–70.

61. Wever R. Autonome circadiane Periodik des Menschen unter dem Einfluss verschiedener Beleuchtungs-Bedingen. *Pflugers Arch* 1969;306:71–91.

62. Aschoff J, Fatranska M, Giedke H, Doerr P, Stamm D, Wisser H. Human circadian rhythms in continuous darkness: entrainment by social cues. *Science* 1971;171:213–215.

63. Czeisler CA, Richardson GS, Zimmerman JC, Moore-Ede MC, Weitzman ED. Entrainment of human circadian rhythms by light-dark cycles: a reassessment. *Photobiol Photochem* 1981;34: 239–247.

64. Czeisler CA, Allan JS, Strogatz SH, et al. Bright light resets the human circadian pacemaker independent of the timing of the sleep-wake cycle. *Science* 1986;233:667–671.

65. Czeisler CA, Kronauer RE, Allan JS, et al. Bright light induction of strong (type 0) resetting of the human circadian pacemaker. *Science* 1989;244:1328–1333.

66. Czeisler CA, Johnson MP, Duffy JF, Brown EN, Ronda JM. Exposure to bright light and darkness to treat physiologic maladaptation to night-work. *N Engl J Med* 1990;322:1253–1259.

67. Lewy AJ, Sack RL, Singer CM. Imediate and delayed effects of bright light on human melatonin production: shifting "dawn" and "dusk" shifts the dim light melatonin onset (DLMO). *Ann N Y Acad Sci* 1985;453:253–259.

68. Lewy A, Sack R, Miller L, Hoban T. Antidepressant and circadian phase-shifting effects of light. *Science* 1987;235:352–354.

69. Wever RA, Polasek J, Wildgruber CM. Bright light affects human circadian rhythms. *Pflugers Arch* 1983;396:85–87.

70. Dijk DJ, Visscher CA, Bloem GM, Beersma DGM, Daan S. Reduction of human sleep duration after bright light exposure in the morning. *Neurosci Lett* 1987;73:181–186.

71. Dijk DJ, Beersma DGM, Daan S, Lewy AJ. Bright morning light advances the human circadian system without affecting NREM sleep homeostasis. *Am J Physiol* 1989;256:R106–R111.

72. Drennan M, Kripke DF, Gillin JC. Bright light can delay human temperature rhythm independent of sleep. *Am J Physiol* 1989;257:R136–R141.

73. Rosenthal NE, Joseph-VanderPool JR, Levendosky AA. Phase shifting effects of bright morning light as treatment for delayed sleep phase syndrome. *Sleep* 1990;13:354–361.

74. Campbell S, Dawson D, Anderson M. Alleviation of sleep maintenance insomnia with timed exposure to bright light. *J Am Geriatr Soc* 1993;41:829–836.

75. Kronauer RE, Czeisler CA, Pilato SF, Moore-Ede MC, Weitzmann ED. Mathematical model of the human circadian system with two interacting oscillators. *Am J Physiol* 1982;242:R3–R17.

76. Lewy AJ, Wehr TA, Goodwin FK, Newsome DA, Markey SP. Light suppresses melatonin secretion in humans. *Science* 1980;210:267–269.

77. Boivin DB, Duffy JF, Kronauer RE, Czeisler CA. Dose-response relationships for resetting of human circadian clock by light. *Nature* 1996;379:540–542.

78. Kronauer RE. A quantitative model for the effects of light on the amplitude and phase of the deep circadian pacemaker, based on human data. In: Horne J, ed. *Sleep '90.* Bochum, Germany: Pontenagel; 1990:306–309.

79. Klerman EB, Dijk D-J, Kronauer RE, Czeisler CA. Simulations of light effects on the human circadian pacemaker: implications for assessment of intrinsic period. *Am J Physiol* 1996;270: R271–R282.
80. Jewett ME, Kronauer RE, Czeisler CA. Light induced suppression of endogenous circadian amplitude in humans. *Nature* 1991;350:59–62.
81. Illnerova H, Zvolsky P, Vanecek J. The circadian rhythm in plasma melatonin concentration of the urbanized man: the effect of winter and summer. *Brain Res* 1985;328:186–189.
82. Wehr TA. The durations of human melatonin secretion and sleep respond to changes in day length (photoperiod). *J Clin Endocrinol Metab* 1991;73:1276–1280.
83. Honma K, Honma S, Kohsaka M, Fukuda N. Seasonal variation in the human circadian rhythm: dissociation between sleep and temperature rhythm. *Am J Physiol* 1992;262:R885–R891.
84. Shanahan TL, Czeisler CA. Light exposure induces equivalent phase shifts of the endogenous circadian rhythms of circulating plasma melatonin and core body temperature in men. *J Clin Endocrinol Metab* 1991;73:227–235.
85. Carrier J, Dumont M. Sleep propensity and sleep architecture after bright light exposure at three different times of day. *J Sleep Res* 1995;4:202–211.
86. Dijk D-J, Cajochen C, Borbély AA. Effect of a single 3-h exposure to bright light on core body temperature and sleep in humans. *Neurosci Lett* 1991;121:59–62.
87. Cajochen C, Dijk D-J, Borbély AA. Dynamics of EEG slow-wave activity and core body temperature in human sleep after exposure to bright light. *Sleep* 1992;15:337–343.
88. Amir S, Stewart J. Resetting of the circadian clock by a conditioned stimulus. *Nature* 1996;379:542–545.
89. Van Reeth O, Turek FW. Stimulated activity mediates phase shifts in the hamster circadian clock induced by dark pulses or benzodiazepines. *Nature* 1989;339:49–51.
90. Mrosovsky N, Salmon PA. A behavioral method for accelerating re-entrainment of rhythms to new light-dark cycles. *Nature* 1987;330:372–373.
91. Van Reeth O, Sturis J, Byrne MM, et al. Nocturnal exercise phase delays circadian rhythms of melatonin and thyrotropin secretion in normal men. *Am J Physiol* 1994;266:E964–E974.
92. Eastman CI, Hoese EK, Youngstedt SD, Liu Liwen. Phase-shifting human circadian rhythms with exercise during the night shift. *Physiol Behav* 1995;58:1287–1291.
93. Miles LEM, Wilson MA. High incidence of cyclic sleep/wake disorders in the blind. *Sleep Res* 1977;6:192.
94. Lewy AJ, Newsome DA. Different types of melatonin circadian secretory rhythms in some blind subjects. *J Clin Endocrinol Metab* 1983;56:1103–1107.
95. Sack RL, Lewy AJ, Blood ML, Keith D, Nakagawa H. Circadian rhythm abnormalities in totally blind people: incidence and clinical significance. *J Clin Endocrinol Metab* 1992;75:127–134.
96. Nakagawa H, Sack RL, Lewy AJ. Sleep propensity free-runs with the temperature, melatonin and cortisol rhythms in a totally blind person. *Sleep* 1992;15:330–336.
97. Klein T, Martens H, Dijk DJ, Kronauer RE, Seely EW, Czeisler CA. Circadian sleep regulation in the absence of light perception: chronic non-24-hour circadian rhythm sleep disorder in a blind man with a regular 24-hour sleep-wake schedule. *Sleep* 1993;16:333–343.
98. Czeisler CA, Shanahan TL, Klerman EB, et al. Suppression of melatonin secretion in some blind patients by exposure to bright light. *N Engl J Med* 1995;332:6–11.
99. Aschoff J, Wever R. Spontanperiodik des Menschen bei Ausschlus aller Zeitgeber. *Die Naturwissenschaften* 1962;49:337–342.
100. Aschoff J, Circadian rhythms in man. *Science* 1965;148:1427–1432.
101. Wever RA. *The circadian system of man.* New York: Springer Verlag; 1979.
102. Wever RA. Properties of human sleep-wake cycles: parameters of internally synchronized freerunning rhythms. *Sleep* 1984;7:27–51.
103. Aschoff J, Gerecke U, Wever R. Desynchronization of human circadian rhythms. *Jpn J Physiol* 1967;17:450–457.
104. Czeisler CA, Weitzman ED, Moore-Ede MC, Zimmerman JC, Knauer RS. Human sleep: its duration and organization depend on its circadian phase. *Science* 1980;210:1264–1267.
105. Zulley J, Wever R, Aschoff J. The dependence of onset and duration of sleep on the circadian rhythm of rectal temperature. *Pflugers Arch* 1981;391:314–318.
106. Strogatz SH, Kronauer RE, Czeisler CA. Circadian regulation dominates homeostatic control of sleep length and prior wake length in humans. *Sleep* 1986;9:353–364.

107. Strogatz SH, Kronauer RE, Czeisler CA. Circadian pacemaker interferes with sleep onset at specific times each day: role in insomnia. *Am J Physiol* 1987;253:R172–R178.
108. Kleitman N. *Sleep and wakefulness.* Chicago: University of Chicago Press; 1939.
109. Dijk D-J, Duffy JF, Czeisler CA. Circadian and sleep-wake dependent aspects of subjective alertness and cognitive performance. *J Sleep Res* 1992;1:112–117.
110. Dijk D-J, Czeisler CA. Paradoxical timing of the circadian rhythm of sleep propensity serves to consolidate sleep and wakefulness in humans. *Neurosci Lett* 1994;166:63–68.
111. Dijk D-J, Czeisler CA. Contribution of the circadian pacemaker and the sleep homeostat to sleep propensity, sleep structure and electroencephalographic slow waves and sleep spindle activity in humans. *J Neurosci* 1995;15:3526–3538.
112. Czeisler CA, Dijk D-J, Duffy JF. Entrained phase of the circadian pacemaker serves to stabilizes alertness and performance throughout the habitual waking day. In: Ogilvie RD, Harsh JR, eds. *Sleep onset normal and abnormal processes.* Washington, DC: American Psychological Association; 1995:89–110.
113. Edgar DM, Dement WC, Fuller CA. Effect of SCN-lesions on sleep in squirrel monkeys: evidence for opponent processes in sleep-wake regulation. *J Neurosci* 1993;13:1065–1079.
114. Borbély AA. A two-process model of sleep regulation. *Hum Neurobiol* 1982;1:195–204.
115. Daan S, Beersma DGM, Borbély AA. Timing of human sleep:recovery process gated by a circadian pacemaker. *Am J Physiol* 1984;246:R161–R178.
116. Åkerstedt T, Gillberg M. The circadian variation of experimentally displaced sleep. *Sleep* 1981;4: 159–169.

Physiology, Stress, and Malnutrition: Functional Correlates, Nutritional Intervention, edited by J.M. Kinney and H.N. Tucker. Lippincott–Raven Publishers © 1997.

Disordered Rhythms: Strategies for Treatment and Their Relation to Pancreatic and Metabolic Function

Josephine Arendt, Stephen J. Deacon, Linda M. Morgan, Shelagh M. Hampton, *Simon Folkard, *Deborah S. Owens, and David C. O. Ribeiro

*School of Biological Sciences, University of Surrey, Guildford, Surrey GU2 5XH, United Kingdom, and *Medical Research Council Body Rhythms and Shiftwork Centre, Department of Psychology, University of Wales Swansea, Singleton Park, Swansea SA2 8PP, United Kingdom*

BIOLOGIC RHYTHMS

Biologic rhythms of various periodicity occur in all eukaryotic organisms. The frequency displayed varies from fractions of a second (e.g., the firing of neurones) to years (e.g., population variations). Rhythms with a periodicity of less than a day are known as ultradian (e.g., pulse rate, pulsatile secretion of hormones), and of more than a day, infradian (e.g., the estrous cycle). Rhythms corresponding to major periodicities in the external environment (daily, lunar, annual) are the most prominent, and by far the most information is available concerning daily rhythms. These are of particular interest with regard to human physiology and pathology.

Rhythms are externally imposed, internally generated, or more frequently a combination of the two. Internally generated rhythms are known as circadian (approximately a 24-hour period, from the Latin for "about a day"), circannual (about a year), circalunar, circatidal, etc. Circadian rhythms serve to temporally program the daily sequence of metabolic and behavioral changes (1). They also may serve as reference points for annual changes.

A rhythm displaying its endogenous period (tau or t) in the absence of time cues is said to be free running and is desynchronized from environmental periodicity. The manifested endogenous period depends on species, individuals, experimental conditions, and previous history. It is an inheritable characteristic. The environmental factors that entrain or synchronize a rhythm to a given periodicity are referred to as zeitgebers (time givers). Some species, e.g., humans, show free-running circadian rhythms that are usually longer than 24 hours (average 24.2 hours), whereas others have an endogenous periodicity shorter than 24 hours (1,2).

Endogenous rhythms are driven by a pacemaker (oscillator, biologic clock). The major biologic clock in higher vertebrates is situated within the suprachiasmatic nucleus (SCN) of the hypothalamus (3), whereas in some birds and lower vertebrates the pineal gland is the principal rhythm generator. Zeitgebers that effect entrainment or synchronization to the environment include light–dark, temperature, social cues, rhythmic feeding, and knowledge of clock time. Zeitgebers with a period T force endogenous cycles to run with a period T. This means that in each cycle the zeitgeber changes the intrinsic period (tau) by t − T. If the endogenous period of a circadian rhythm is greater than 24 hours, synchronization requires a phase advance of the pacemaker each day by this amount. If tau is less than 24 hours, the pacemaker must be phase delayed each day.

The general structure of the circadian system has three components: a pacemaker, an input pathway for entrainment of the pacemaker, and an output pathway for the expression of overt rhythms (Fig. 1). This scheme is well represented by the mammalian melatonin rhythm generating and entraining system. The pacemaker is the SCN, the input is the retina-retino-hypothalamic tract, and the output is along neuronal connections to the pineal gland. In all other amniote species, circadian rhythms are synchronized to the light–dark cycle via photoreceptors in the pineal gland, parapineal structures, and deep diencephalic photoreceptors in addition to the retinal pathway.

The light–dark cycle is the major synchronizer of circadian (and seasonal) rhythms (4) and the circadian activity–rest cycle is the most easily measured overt rhythm in small animals and in humans. Hence, an enormous amount of information has accrued on the formal properties of circadian rhythms using

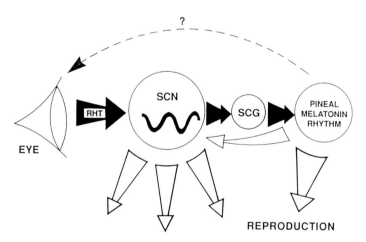

FIG. 1. Basic concepts of the circadian system: inputs and outputs of the central rhythm generating system in the suprachiasmatic nucleus (SCN). RHT, retino-hypothalamic tract; SCG, superior cervical ganglion. Melatonin can feed back at the level of the SCN and probably the retina.

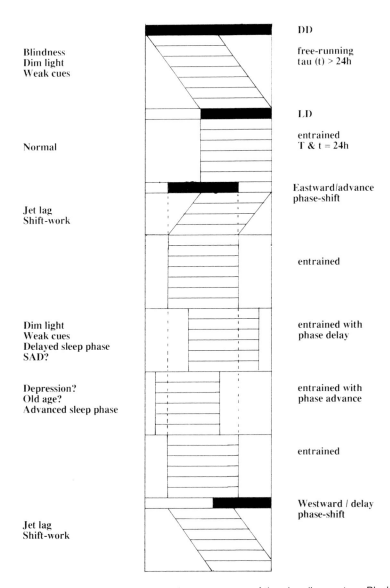

FIG. 2. Diagrammatic representation of various responses of the circadian system. Black bars represent darkness. Each thin horizontal bar represents an endogenous clock component, for example sleep in consecutive days. Free run with a period tau (t) >24h in continuous darkness (DD), entrainment by a light-dark cycle (T) of 12 hours light and 12 hours darkness (LD), advancing transients following a 6h phase advance of the light-dark cycle, entrainment with a negative and then with a positive phase angle difference, delaying transients following a phase delay of the light-dark cycle. Note that during adaptation to a new light dark cycle the endogenous biological clock is out of phase with the ambient time cues (in this case light-dark).

these variables. It has been assumed that information derived from rest activity can be extrapolated to all circadian rhythms. This may be true in ideal conditions with no "masking." When external factors significantly modify an endogenous rhythm in addition to synchronizing it, the rhythm is said to be masked. Examples of masking of circadian rhythms include the suppression of melatonin secretion by light (5), the rapid increase in body temperature at night with bright light (6), and the stress-induced increase of cortisol secretion. Human studies in particular suggest that in an uncontrolled environment, e.g., in shift workers, and in artificially disturbed rhythms in environmental isolation, different circadian rhythms behave quite differently from the rest activity cycle.

In continuous darkness or in dim light below a particular intensity and in the absence of other major time cues, mammalian rhythms free run (1). In constant light, disruption of the activity rest cycle is often but not always present. In the presence of weak zeitgebers, rhythms may be synchronized to the appropriate periodicity but with an abnormal phase relationship to the driving zeitgebers. In a species such as humans with a free-running tau greater than 24 hours, this implies an abnormal phase delay relative to the zeitgeber. When the light–dark cycle (standard laboratory lighting) is artificially advanced or delayed, the circadian system adapts slowly to the new phase position passing through intermediate phases known as transients (Fig. 2). The time taken to adapt depends on the size of the phase shift, the zeitgeber strength (e.g., photoperiod), and the light intensity, but often approximates to 1 hour of adaptive shift per day. During the process of adaptation, endogenous rhythms are out of phase with the external environment (external desynchronization). They also may be out phase with each other, i.e., assume a transitory abnormal phase relationship (internal desynchronization). These situations occur regularly in shift workers and in jet-lagged travelers and are considered to be responsible for many health and performance problems encountered by these groups (7).

DISORDERED RHYTHMS

Common conditions in which circadian rhythms are known to be disturbed include shift work, rapid time zone change, blindness (in the absence of the light–dark time cue), certain types of insomnia, and old age.

The most frequently reported problem in such conditions is poor sleep. However, gastrointestinal problems are also common in shift workers. This population has an incidence of cardiovascular disease higher than that found in day workers together with evidence of lipid intolerance. Because shift workers comprise approximately 20% of the population in developed countries, such health problems are of economic and industrial importance (7–10).

Endogenous circadian rhythms such as melatonin do not adapt to rapidly rotating shifts. Depending on a number of factors such as amount and timing of natural light exposure, usually only partial adaptation is seen in slow rotations or permanent night shift work (7,8,11–13). This means that during the night shift subjects are attempting to work during the peak of their melatonin rhythm and the nadir of their core body temperature, alertness, and performance rhythms. However, with rapid rotations, only the night shift is compromised in this way. Exceptionally, complete adaptation is seen in unusual situations such as shift work in Antarctica (14). Here, during winter, without conflicting natural light, complete adaptation (assessed by melatonin secretion profiles) is seen within 7 days to a 12-hour shift. Subjects sleep better on the night shift than on the day shift and have more problems readapting to the normal daytime schedule. Abrupt changes of time zone have many features in common with shift work, but in this case ambient time cues act to reinforce adaptation rather than to conflict with it.

In addition to behavioral problems, a much neglected aspect of abrupt phase shift is the metabolic and pancreatic response to meals taken during the night shift. Gastrointestinal complaints are common in this population, and investigations are warranted. There is evidence that both insulin and glucose show diurnal variations that are to some extent endogenous.

Glucose tolerance decreases during the day in normal individuals (15). Studies have shown that postprandial plasma glucose levels after oral glucose, intravenous glucose, and test meal are markedly increase in the latter part of the day compared with the morning (15,16). The persistence of a diurnal variation of glucose tolerance in the absence of sleep and in constant environmental conditions, continuously low levels of activity, and constant caloric intake strongly suggest that this diurnal variation must be at least partially controlled by signals originating from the body clock (17). Recent studies into the effect of time of day on meal tolerance have shown that glucose and insulin responses are modulated by circadian rhythmicity and are inversely correlated with the circadian rhythm of cortisol secretion (18). The mechanisms involved in time-dependent changes of glucose tolerance are unknown, but both diminished insulin sensitivity and decreased insulin secretion have been implicated (15,17,19). When nutrients are given orally, rates of gastric emptying and intestinal motility may influence postprandial hormone and metabolic responses. Diurnal variation also has been reported in a number of gastrointestinal hormones, including glucose-dependent insulinotropic polypeptide (GIP), gastrin, and motilin, hormones that influence insulin secretion and gut motility (20,21).

Numerous factors influence postprandial circulating lipid levels. The rates of gastric emptying, intestinal triacylglycerol (TAG) hydrolysis, and intestinal motility all contribute to the rate of entry of TAG into the circulation (22). The enzyme lipoprotein lipase (LPL), whose activity is influenced by both insulin and GIP, plays a key regulatory role in postprandial TAG clearance (23). Nonesterified fatty acids (NEFA) have been reported to exhibit a diurnal rhythm with higher postprandial levels seen after a standard meal in the morning than the evening (24). Insulin also influences circulating NEFA levels via its inhibitory action on hormone-sensitive lipase. In rats there is recent evidence for a circadian rhythm in hepatic low-density lipoprotein (LDL)-receptor expression and plasma LDL levels (25).

Recently we found both sleep-related and endogenous circadian components to the variations of plasma triacylglycerol and insulin in constant routine conditions (unpublished observations).

COUNTERMEASURES

A number of strategies can be envisaged to counter such problems. Short pulses of very high intensity light or longer pulses of lower intensity light predictably advance or delay circadian rhythms according to a phase-response curve (26). Bright light during the entire night shift suppresses melatonin and hastens adaptation of endogenous rhythms of hormones and behavior (27). Melatonin itself acutely lowers body temperature and alertness and shifts the endogenous clock according to a phase-response curve that is opposite to that of light (28–30). It also can be used to hasten phase shift of circadian rhythms and improve daytime sleep. Combinations of suitably timed melatonin and light may well prove to be advantageous. Inappropriately timed exposure to natural light, or theoretically to melatonin, can delay adaptation.

There is substantial published evidence that in field studies and one simulation study, suitably timed melatonin can alleviate subjective jet lag, primarily due to improvement of night-time sleep and daytime alertness, and hasten the objectively measured rate of re-synchronization of the endogenous circadian system. In two small field studies on 7-day rotating shift workers, melatonin likewise had beneficial effects on daytime sleep and night shift alertness and shifted the internal clock such that it was more appropriate to daytime sleep and night-time work. A simulation study comparing the use of timed bright light and melatonin found improvement of sleep with both countermeasures, but only light treatment improved performance (31–33).

Field studies on shift workers and time zone travelers are expensive and difficult to control. The use of constant routines that eliminate masking factors (such as sleep, meals, exercise, posture, and bright light exposure) has substantial constraints, and subjects can be studied only during selected windows. We have therefore established a technique for simulating rapid phase shifts with exposure to ambient time cues during adaptation, with continuous assessment of hormonal and behavioral variables. Using timed combinations of bright light (1,200 lux, 9 hours) and imposed darkness (8 hours), with the remaining time in a normal environment, it is possible to generate a synchronized phase advance or delay of 9 hours in 5 days. Subjects are then released into their normal environments, and readaptation can be studied in detail with exposure to normal time cues (34,35).

Using this technique we have investigated the effects of melatonin on adaptation of hormonal and behavioral rhythms to a simulated abrupt phase shift, together with combinations of melatonin and conflicting bright light (34,35).

Furthermore, we have investigated the metabolic and pancreatic response to a test meal (preceded by a set breakfast and a 6-hour fast) at the same clock time (13:30 h) before and immediately after an abrupt 9-hour phase delay, without countermeasures (36,37).

AN EXPERIMENTAL MODEL FOR SHIFT WORK AND JET LAG

Using an average light intensity of 1,200 lux (full-spectrum light) specifically timed for periods of 9 hours per day, it is possible to nudge the circadian system to later and later or earlier and earlier times. A maximum advance or delay of 9 hours has been accomplished to date. Apart from the periods of light treatment subjects are required to stay in total darkness for specific periods of 8 hours per day. The rest of the time they live in normal ambient light but avoid intense natural light exposure by wearing sunglasses outside. The schedules used to advance and delay are shown in Figs. 3 and 4. Circadian status is evaluated by continuous recording of rectal temperature and continuous sequential urine collections for the

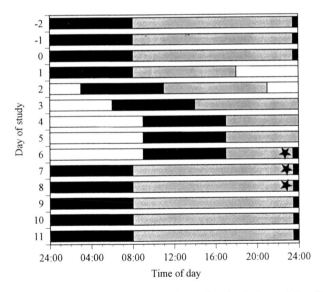

FIG. 3. Diagrammatic representation of a forced, synchronized phase delay, followed by an abrupt phase advance. The black bars are periods of imposed darkness-sleep, the white bars periods of wake and light exposure (average 1,200 lux), and the gray bars periods of normal activity in ambient light (<500 lux, sunglasses are worn when outdoors). This treatment reliably induces a 9-hour delay in the marker rhythms of core body temperature and 6-sulphatoxymelatonin, with no important detrimental effects on sleep, mood or performance. The abrupt phase advance on days 6–7 represents an eastward time zone flight of 9 hours or a change in work shift. During readaptation to the ambient light–dark cycle, melatonin or placebo treatment (*) is given at 23:30 h on days 6, 7, and 8. Reprinted with permission (34).

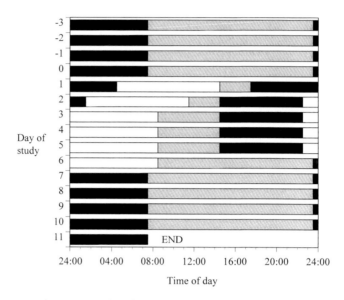

FIG. 4. Diagrammatic representation of a forced, synchronized phase advance, followed by an abrupt phase delay. The black bars are periods of imposed darkness-sleep, the white bars periods of wake and light exposure (average 1,200 lux), and the gray bars periods of normal activity in ambient light (<500 lux, sunglasses are worn when outdoors). This treatment reliably induces a 9-hour advance in the marker rhythms of core body temperature and 6-sulphatoxymelatonin, with only transient detrimental effects on sleep, mood, or performance during days 1–2. The abrupt phase delay on days 6–7 represents a westward time zone flight of 9 hours or a change in work shift. For evaluation of pancreatic and metabolic responses, a pre–meal is given at 07:30h and a test meal at 13:30h on day 0 and on day 6, with appropriate blood sampling. Adapted with permission (34).

measurement of the major melatonin metabolite 6-sulphatoxymelatonin. Sleep is quantified by logs (latency, number of night awakenings, duration of night awakenings, quality-visual analogue scale), and in some experiments by actigraphy and polysomnography. Subjects perform low- and high-memory load tests at intervals, usually every 2 hours when awake, and record mood (alertness, cheerfulness, calmness) on visual analogue scales every 2 hours. At the end of a 5-day treatment period, subjects are fully shifted by 9 hours as assessed by the marker rhythms of core temperature and melatonin. During a period of forced delay shift, there are no important deleterious effects on sleep, mood, or performance. In contrast, during a forced 9-hour advance, sleep deteriorates but only during the first 1–2 days. Thus, the endogenous circadian clock is positioned 9 hours ahead or behind local time. At this point subjects are required to assume the initial baseline sleep–wake and light–dark cycle (Figs. 3 and 4), thereby undergoing either an abrupt 9 hour advance or delay identical to the experience of, e.g., arriving in Paris from Los Angeles or vice versa. It is then possible to study their adaptation in a normal but controlled environment using different strategies to hasten adaptation.

Using this approach we have investigated the ability of timed low-dose melatonin to hasten adaptation to an abrupt 9-hour advance shift (after a synchronized 9-hour delay) together with the effects of conflicting bright light treatment, i.e., timed to counter the predicted phase shifting ability of melatonin. In addition, we have observed the pancreatic and metabolic response to a standard test meal taken at 13:30 h in the initial baseline environment and immediately after an abrupt 9-hour delay (after a synchronized 9-hour advance) with no concomitant countermeasures.

MELATONIN HASTENS ADAPTATION TO AN ABRUPT 9-HOUR ADVANCE PHASE SHIFT

Melatonin, timed to phase advance, abolished the decrements in sleep, alertness, and performance seen under placebo treatment on the first and subsequent nights after the shift (Fig. 5). The effects were manifested during the first 24 hours and subsequent days after the abrupt shift, well before complete circadian adaptation was seen. During treatment by exogenous melatonin, it is not possible to assess circadian phase using the endogenous rhythm as a marker. Phase can only be assessed when treatment has ceased and the exogenously derived metabolite has cleared. This late assessment of phase nevertheless showed more rapid circadian adaptation with melatonin. Thus, it is likely that the acute sleepiness-inducing and body temperature–lowering effects of melatonin combine to enhance sleep already during the first night of treatment and to improve alertness and performance during the first and subsequent days. The more rapid adaptation of the internal clock probably represents a combination of acute and cumulative effects of melatonin acting in concert with ambient time cues. The phase-shifting effects of bright light (2,000 lux) timed to phase delay (i.e., counter to the most desirable direction of re-entrainment) were attenuated by melatonin treatment (35). These results extend field observations on the use of melatonin to treat jet lag and shift work (33). They show clearly in a placebo-controlled randomized crossover study in the presence of ambient zeitgebers that melatonin does indeed alleviate many aspects of the jet lag phenomenon and that this is accompanied by faster circadian adaptation.

ABNORMAL PANCREATIC AND METABOLIC RESPONSES AFTER AN ABRUPT 9-HOUR DELAY

Both the postprandial glucose and insulin levels were approximately 25% higher and delayed after phase shifting subjects notably 2–6 hours after the meal (Figs. 6 and 7). The differences in glucose levels were similar to those found by other workers when test meals were given at different times of the day (15,16), although not all previous studies have demonstrated increased

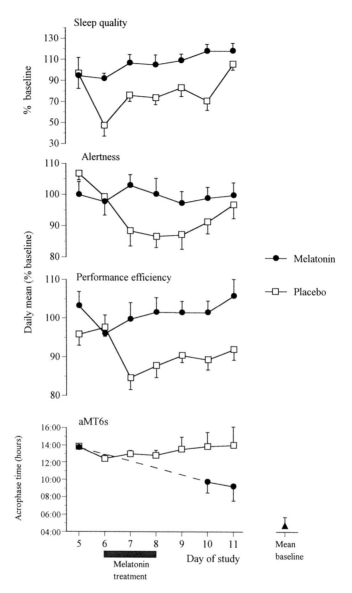

FIG. 5. Effects of melatonin treatment (5 mg fast release) or placebo at 23:00 h (see Fig. 3) on self-recorded sleep quality (VAS), alertness (VAS), performance efficiency [5 target letter cancellation (SAM-5) task] and readaptation of the 6-sulphatoxymelatonin rhythm, expressed as calculated peak time (acrophase) after an abrupt 9-hour phase advance (n = 7) on day 6. The behavioral parameters are expressed as difference from mean baseline levels (see Fig. 3), and all data are means ±1 SEM. Note the deleterious effects of abrupt phase shift on sleep, mood, and performance, which are immediately countered by melatonin administration. 6-sulpha-toxymelatonin has not returned to the baseline phase position (*lowest panel on the right*) by day 11, but faster resynchronization is seen with melatonin treatment (ANOVA, raw data). Diagram reproduced from (43) by permission.

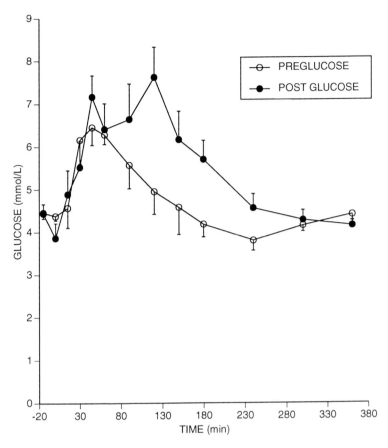

FIG. 6. Plasma glucose response before and immediately after a synchronized phase advance (see Fig. 4). The test meal was consumed at 13:30 h clock time on both occasions, but after forced phase shift (as assessed by 6-sulphatoxymelatonin and core temperature), the test meal was consumed at 22:30 h body clock time. A significant increase in glucose (AUC 2–6 hours after the meal) was found after the phase shift (closed symbols; n = 6). The response is comparable with that found to a test meal during the late evening. Diagram courtesy of Hampton et al. (unpublished), with some data from (37).

postprandial insulin levels in the evening relative to the morning (16,18). Insulin sensitivity appears to be reduced after phase shift. Reduced sensitivity of the peripheral tissues to insulin in the evening compared with the morning has been reported (38), and a separate study has demonstrated relatively impaired insulin secretion in response to intravenous glucose (39). The findings of the present study are consistent with decreased insulin sensitivity together with a degree of impaired insulin secretion after phase shift: further studies, using a euglycemic insulin clamp or similar technique are required to demonstrate this conclusively.

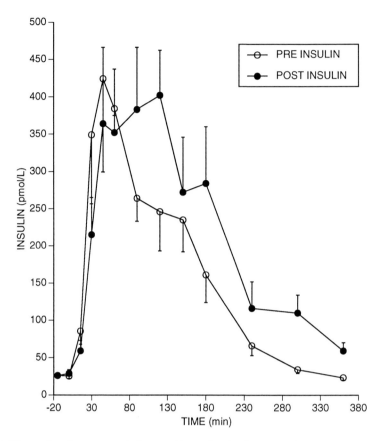

FIG. 7. Plasma insulin response before and immediately after a synchronized phase advance (see Fig. 4). The test meal was taken at 13:30h clock time on both occasions, but after forced phase shift body clock time (as assessed by 6-sulphatoxymelatonin and core temperature) was 22:30 h at the time of the test meal. A significant increase in insulin (AUC 2–6 hours after the meal) was found after the phase shift (closed symbols). Diagram courtesy of Hampton et al. (unpublished), with some data from (37).

Postprandial lipid levels were also affected by the phase shift. Plasma TAG levels peaked after 5 hours in the first test meal, in contrast to the post–phase shift meal, where they were still increasing at the end of the study period. This pattern is suggestive of impaired chylomicron TAG clearance, a risk factor for cardiovascular disease (40). Elevation of both plasma TAG and plasma cholesterol levels has been reported in some shift workers (10,41), consistent with our present findings. Plasma NEFA levels decreased immediately after food consumption both pre– and post–phase shift. Their return to basal levels was significantly delayed post–phase shift. This was probably due to the higher circulating insulin levels that occurred in the latter part of the study post–phase shift, inhibiting the action of hormone-sensitive lipase and consequent release of

NEFA from the hydrolysis of TAG. This pattern is consistent with Gibson's observation of a diurnal variation in postprandial NEFA levels (24).

Insulin resistance is considered to be a risk factor for coronary heart disease: shift workers are reported to have significantly more heart disease than age-matched day workers. An increase in plasma triacylglycerol and total and low-density lipoprotein-cholesterol is one of the few major metabolic effects reported in night shift workers (42). This is also associated with cardiovascular problems. Whereas in field conditions these observations could be attributed to dietary factors, these are eliminated (in the short term) in our experiments.

Thus, after an abrupt phase shift, metabolic and pancreatic responses are abnormal. We do not yet know how long these abnormalities persist, or to what extent they are influenced by the nutritional content of the meal preceding the test meal. However, if repeated at each shift change, such abnormalities could have cumulative effects leading to major health problems. It is clear that a forced synchronized phase shift such as we have described here is able to shift pancreatic and metabolic responses such that characteristic night-time responses are found during the day. This suggests that bright light during the night shift hastens adaptation of the enteroinsular axis as well as rhythms of sleep, mood, performance and hormones. Whether such forced adaptation at frequent intervals is desirable remains a matter for debate.

SUMMARY

The 24-hour society of developed countries leads to major conflicts between our biologic rhythms and work schedules. In addition to poor performance and sleep, night shift workers have a high incidence of major health problems. The extent to which rhythm disturbance contributes to such problems is only beginning to be investigated. The influence of phase shifting strategies such as bright light and melatonin on these responses is of obvious interest. In the future, both dietary advice and phase-shifting strategies should improve the quality of life of shift workers and decrease their use of national health resources in the short- and long-term.

ACKNOWLEDGMENTS

These studies were supported by the MRC and Stockgrand Ltd.

REFERENCES

1. Wever R A. *The circadian system of man. Results of experiments under temporal isolation.* New York: Springer Verlag; 1979.
2. Middleton B, Arendt J, Stone B. Human circadian rhythms in constant dim light (8 lux) with knowledge of clock time. *J Sleep Res* 1996;5:69–76.

3. Klein DC, Moore RY, Reppert SM, eds. *Suprachiasmatic nucleus. The minds clock.* New York: Oxford University Press; 1991:197–219.
4. Wetterberg L, ed. *Light and biological rhythms in man.* Wenner-Gren International Series, Vol. 63. Oxford, England: Pergamon; 1993.
5. Lewy AJ, Wehr TA, Goodwin FK, Newsome DA, Markey SP. Light suppresses melatonin secretion in humans. *Science* 1980;210:1267.
6. Strassman RJ, Qualls CR, Lisansky EJ, Peake GT. Elevated rectal temperature produced by all night bright light is reversed by melatonin infusion in man. *J Appl Physiol* 1991;71:2178–2181.
7. Akerstedt T. Adjustment of physiological circadian rhythms and the sleep wake cycle to shift work. In: Folkard S, Monk TH, eds. *Hours of work: temporal factors in work scheduling.* New York: Wiley; 1985:185–198.
8. Rosa RR, Bonnet MH, Bootzin RR, et al. Intervention factors for promoting adjustment to nightwork and shiftwork. *Occup Med* 1990;5:391–415.
9. Knutsson A. Shift work and coronary heart disease. *Scand J Sociol Med Suppl* 1989;44:1–36.
10. Romon M, Nuttens M-C, Fievet C. et al. Increased triglyceride levels in shift-workers. *Am J Med* 1992;93:259–262.
11. Hall R, English J, Wood P, Arendt J. Assessment of 6-sulphatoxymelatonin rhythms in fast rotating shift workers [Abstr]. Presented at the *European Pineal Society Conference,* Sitges, Spain, March 28–31, 1996.
12. Koller M, Harma M, Laitinen JT, et al. Different patterns of light exposure in relation to melatonin and cortisol rhythms and sleep of night workers. *J Pineal Res* 1994;16:127–135.
13. Sack R, Blood M, Lewy A. Melatonin rhythms in night-shift workers. *Sleep* 1992;15,5:434–441.
14. Ross JK, Arendt J, Horne J, Haston W. Night-shift work during Antarctic winter: sleep characteristics and adaptation with bright light treatment. *Physiol Behav* 1995;57:1169–1174.
15. Carroll KF, Nestel PJ. Diurnal variation in glucose tolerance and in insulin secretion in man. *Diabetes* 1973;22:333–348.
16. Service FJ, Hall LD, Westland RE, et al. Effect of size, time of day and sequence of meal ingestion on carbohydrate tolerance in normal subjects. *Diabetologia* 1983;25:316–321.
17. Van Cauter E, Desir D, Decoster C, Fery F, et al. Nocturnal decrease of glucose tolerance during constant glucose infusion. *J Clin Endocrinol Metab* 1989;69:604–611.
18. Van Cauter E, Shapiro ET, Tillil H, Polonsky KS. Circadian modulation of glucose and insulin response to meals: relationship to cortisol. *Am J Physiol* 1992;262:E467–475.
19. Van Cauter E, Blackman JD, Roland D, et al. Modulation of glucose regulation and insulin secretion by circadian rhythmicity and sleep. *J Clin Invest* 1991;88:934–942.
20. Minors DS, Waterhouse JM. *Circadian rhythms and the human.* Bristol, England: Wright; 1981.
21. Amland PF, Jorde R K, Burhol PG. Diurnal GIP, PP and insulin levels in morbid obesity before and after stapled partitioning with gastric-gastrostomy. *Int J Obesity* 1984;8:117–122.
22. Cohn J, McNamara J, Krasinski S, et al. Role of triglyceride-rich lipoproteins from the liver and intestines in the aetiology of postprandial peaks in plasma triglycerides. *Metabolism* 1989;38: 484–490.
23. Knapper JME, Puddicombe SM, Morgan LM, Fletcher JM. Enteroinsular hormones glucose-dependent insulinotropic polypeptide and glucagon-like peptide-1 (7-36)amide; effects on lipoprotein lipase activity in explants of rat adipose tissue. *J Nutr* 1995;125:183–188.
24. Gibson T, Stimmler L, Jarrett RJ, et al. Diurnal variation in the effect of insulin on blood glucose, plasma non-esterified fatty acids and growth hormone. *Diabetologia* 1975;11:83–89.
25. Balasubramaniam S, Szanto A, Roach P. Circadian rhythm in hepatic low-density-lipoprotein (LDL)-receptor expression and plasma LDL levels. *Biochem J* 1994;298:39–43.
26. Minors D, Waterhouse J, Wirz-Justice A. A human phase-response curve to light. *Neurosci Lett* 1991;133:36–40.
27. Czeisler CA, Johnson PJ, Duffy JF, et al. Exposure to bright light and darkness to treat physiologica maladaption to night work. *N Engl J Med* 1990;322:1253–1259.
28. Arendt J, Bojkowski C, Folkard S, et al. Some effects of melatonin and the control of its secretion in man. *Ciba Found Symp* 1985;117:266–283.
29. Deacon S, Arendt J. Melatonin-induced temperature suppression and its acute phase shifting effects correlate in a dose-dependent manner in humans. *Brain Res* 1995;688:77–85.
30. Lewy A, Saeeduddin A, Latham Jackson J, Sack R. Melatonin shifts human circadian rhythms according to a phase-response curve. *Chronobiol Int* 1992;9:380–392.
31. Arendt J, Aldhous M, Marks M, et al. Some effects of jet-lag and their treatment by melatonin. *Ergonomics* 1987;30:1379–1393.

32. Folkard S, Arendt J, Clarke M. Can melatonin improve shiftworkers tolerance of the night shift? Some preliminary findings. *Chronobiol Int* 1993;10:315–320.
33. Arendt J, Deacon S, English J, et al. In: Melatonin and adjustment to phase shift. Work hours, sleepiness and accidents. Proceedings of the International Workshop, Karolinska Institute, Stockholm, September 1994. *J Sleep Res* 1995;(suppl 2):74–79.
34. Deacon S, Arendt J. Adapting to phase-shifts. I. An experimental model for jet lag and shift work. *Physiol Behav* 1995;59:665–673.
35. Deacon S, Arendt J. Adapting to phase-shifts. II. Effects of melatonin and conflicting light treatment. *Physiol Behav* 1995;59:675–682.
36. Hampton S, Morgan L, Lawrence N, et al. Pancreatic function in simulated shift work. 14th Joint Meeting of British Endocrine Societies. *J Endocrinol* 1995;144(suppl):P217.
37. Hampton SM, Morgan LM, Lawrence N, et al. Postprandial hormone and metabolic responses in simulated shift work. *J Endocrinol* 1996;151:259–267.
38. Verrillo UA, DeTeresa A, Martino C, DiChiara G, Pinto M, Verrillo L, Torello F, Gattoni A. Differential roles of splanchic and peripheral tissues in determining diurnal fluctuation of glucose tolerance. *Amer J Physiol* 1989;257:E459–E465.
39. Shapiro T, Tillil H, Polonsky KS, et al. Oscillations in insulin secretion during constant glucose infusion in normal man: relationship to changes in plasma glucose. *J Clin Endocrinol Metab* 1988;67:307–314.
40. Sethi S, Gibney M, Williams CM. Postprandial lipoprotein metabolism. *Nutr Res Rev* 1993;6:161–183.
41. De Backer M, Kornitzer M, Dramix M, Peeters H, Kittel F. Irregular working hours and lipid levels in men. In: Schlierf G, Morl H, eds. *Expanding horizons in atherosclerosis research*. Berlin: Springer-Verlag; 1987:217–224.
42. Lennernas MA-C. *Nutrition and shift work. The effect of work hours on dietary intake, meal patterns and nutritional status parameters* [Thesis]. Uppsala, Sweden: University of Uppsala, 1995.
43. Arendt J, Deacon S. Treatment of circadian rhythm disorders: melatonin. *Chronobial Internat* 1997; in press.

Physiology, Stress, and Malnutrition: Functional Correlates, Nutritional Intervention,
edited by J.M. Kinney and H.N. Tucker.
Lippincott–Raven Publishers © 1997.

Surgical Stress: Pain, Sleep, and Convalescence

Henrik Kehlet and Jacob Rosenberg

*Department of Surgical Gastroenterology, Hvidovre University Hospital,
DK-2650 Hvidovre, Denmark*

Postoperative outcome has shown a steady improvement during recent decades because of developments within anesthesiology and surgical care as well as in surgical techniques to minimize surgical trauma (minimally invasive surgery). Despite these improvements, a common feature of most surgical patients is pain, fatigue, alterations in sleep, and a prolonged convalescence period with inability to work, etc. In addition, trauma-induced alterations in various endocrine glands, leukocytes, and other cascade systems (surgical stress response) may influence body organ functions. These alterations are pathogenic factors of common postoperative complications such as cardiopulmonary, thromboembolic, cerebral, and infectious complications.

We review in this chapter the role of pain, sleep disturbances, surgical stress (catabolism), and nutritional factors for the development of postoperative fatigue and convalescence. Finally, these recovery-related physiologic changes are brought together in a unifying concept for early postoperative rehabilitation. References are given to original work unless the topic has been reviewed within the past 2–3 years.

THE SURGICAL STRESS RESPONSE: A MAJOR DETERMINANT OF POSTOPERATIVE OUTCOME

Surgical injury leads to a multi-component response characterized by pronounced endocrine metabolic changes with increased secretion of catabolic acting hormones and decreased secretion and/or effect of anabolic hormones (1,2). Metabolic changes include hyperglycemia, lipolysis and negative protein economy. In addition to the classical hormonal stress response, injury leads to activation of several humoral cascade systems such as the arachidonic acid cascade, complement activation, cytokines, etc. (3). The catabolic response to surgery may have profound consequences for the later postoperative period and convalescence, due to major changes in body composition with loss of weight and muscle mass. Thus, after a major operation, loss of skeletal muscle may be as high as 1–2 kg (4). These changes together with alterations in the peripheral and central nervous system (pain, sleep disturbances) may have additive or synergistic effects on postoperative recovery by delaying gastrointestinal motility, oral intake, and mobilization. These may add to postoperative fatigue and impairment in muscle function.

The main release mechanism of the stress response in elective procedures is the afferent neurogenic pathway that activates various endocrine systems (2). Humoral mediators become more important when infectious complications occur during major trauma and multiple organ failure (3). Consequently, interventions against the undesirable functional sequelae of the surgical stress response have been pain relief by various techniques, including neural blockade, nutritional support (5), and reduction of trauma by minimally invasive surgery. Of these, minimally invasive surgery has been most effective in reducing the inflammatory response [C-reactive protein and interleukin-6 (IL-6)], as well as a reduced immunomodulatory response, and with improvement in pulmonary function and hypoxemia (6). Early responses in classical endocrine metabolic parameters (cortisol, glucose, and catecholamines) may be slightly inhibited when compared with a similar open operation. Protein economy also seems to be somewhat better preserved in patients undergoing laparoscopic surgery (6).

Neural blockade with epidural or spinal anesthesia is effective in reducing the classical hormonal responses such as the increase in cortisol, aldosterone, catecholamines, growth hormone, and renin (2,7). The effect is most pronounced in lower body procedures with lumbar epidural analgesia with local anesthetics. Epidural analgesia with opioids provides a more selective nociceptive blockade and thereby less inhibition of the surgical stress response. Neural blockade has no important effect on inflammatory responses (acute phase proteins, IL-6, etc.) and most immunologic changes (2). However, due to the reduction in the classical catabolic hormonal response to surgery, postoperative nitrogen economy is improved by epidural analgesia and has been demonstrated in more than ten studies (2,7). Nitrogen balance is improved with less postoperative changes in muscle amino acid composition in most of these studies (2,7). A single dose block has no important effect on nitrogen economy in contrast to a block continued beyond 24 hours (2).

Nutritional support with the parenteral or enteral route has been demonstrated to reduce, but not normalize, postoperative changes in body composition and function (5).

The effects of neural blockade and other pain-relieving techniques, nutrition, and minimal invasive surgery on postoperative pain, sleep disturbances, and fatigue are discussed below.

POSTOPERATIVE PAIN

Postoperative pain is uncomfortable and serves no useful purpose with its usual intensity, which instead may amplify unwarranted autonomic and somatic reflex and endocrine responses, making the patient unable to breathe, cough, or move. Much effort has therefore been directed toward treating postoperative pain effectively (8,9) in the hope that various aspects of the surgical stress response could be abated and recovery enhanced by earlier mobilization and restoration of oral intake. In recent years there has been a tremendous increase in our understanding of the physiology of acute (postoperative) pain, development of new analgesics and techniques for their delivery, and introduction of "acute pain services."

After injury there is development of hyperalgesia, both in the periphery and centrally at the spinal cord level (10,11). These neuroplastic changes, mediated in the periphery by bradykinin, arachidonic cascade metabolites, substance P, and various cytokines (11) and centrally by excitatory amino acids, nitric oxide, etc. (10), are assumed to result in an increased intensity and duration of postoperative pain and a risk of transition into a chronic postoperative pain state (10). Considering the advances within acute pain physiology other therapeutic approaches have focused on preemptive analgesia (10,12,13) (i.e., treatment before the injury to "prevent" the neuroplastic changes and thereby the intensity and duration of postoperative pain). Although rational, clinical controlled studies comparing identical analgesic treatment given before versus after the surgical injury have not demonstrated a substantial improvement in the postoperative pain status (12,13). Furthermore, improvement of the technique of preemptive analgesia with more intense and prolonged afferent neural blockade or specific modification of spinal cord neuroplasticity (NMDA-receptor blockade, inhibition of nitric oxide synthesis, etc.) is warranted. The hitherto most effective technique to treat postoperative pain is based on the concept of "balanced" or "multimodal" analgesia (14). Different analgesics with additive or synergistic effects are combined, thereby improving pain relief and at the same time reducing side effects because of differences in adverse effect profiles. This concept has proven valid for the combination of nonsteroidal anti-inflammatory drugs (NSAIDs) and opioids and to some extent the combination of NSAIDs with neural blockade techniques (14). The most effective pain treatment in major operations is continuous epidural analgesia with a combination of epidural local anesthetics and opioids. This approach results in improved pain relief during cough and mobilization and a reduction in side effects (14,15). Most importantly, the central neural blockade techniques with local anesthetics are more effective on movement-related pain than any opioid technique available. Addition of alpha-2 agonists (clonidine, etc.) also improves pain relief after epidural or systemic application, although this has to be weighed against the risk of hypotension (14). The peripheral approach in the treatment of acute pain is rational, but unfortunately the local anesthetic techniques with presently available agents have only an effect lasting only 6–16 hours. The development of new, slow-release preparations may offer a future optimization of postoperative pain relief. The recent demonstration of a postinflammatory increase in opioid receptors on the peripheral nerve terminals (16) has offered a new possibility for peripheral opioid treatment (16). Up to this point, however, peripheral opioid treatment has been demonstrated to be effective only in arthroscopic procedures (16).

The peripheral approach for management of postoperative pain seems to be promising, especially with the use of future long-acting local anesthetic agents together with modifiers of the inflammatory response, including substance P antagonists, peripheral opioids, lipoxygenase inhibitors, etc. (17).

The effect of the various pain alleviation techniques (Fig. 1) on the surgical stress response was recently reviewed (2,7,8). These can be summarized by the following statements. NSAIDs have little effect on the classical hormonal responses or protein economy, and opioids given systemically in conventional intermittent doses or by the patient controlled analgesia (PCA) technique are not effective in reducing catabolism. The use of epidural opioids may reduce the catabolic hormonal responses slightly, but with minimal effects on protein economy. Clonidine has only a slight inhibitory effect on the stress response. In contrast, a central neuraxial blocking technique with local anesthetics may have a profound inhibitory effect on the stress responses (especially in lower body procedures) and may improve postoperative protein economy. Simultaneously, continuous epidural analgesia with local anesthetics has positive effects on pulmonary function (2) and postoperative ileus is reduced (2,15), thereby offering the possibility for early oral nutrition with further improvement of protein economy. Also, these techniques may offer the most pronounced relief of pain due to movement allowing early mobilization and avoidance of immobilization-induced detrimental effects on muscle and pulmonary function (hypoxemia).

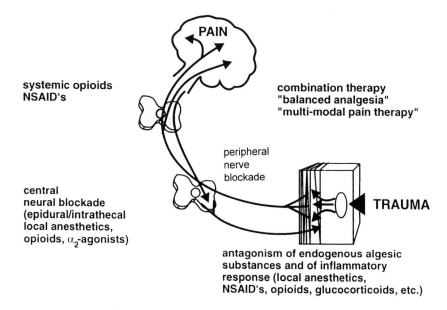

FIG. 1. Measures to provide postoperative pain relief.

Reduction of trauma by the use of laparoscopically assisted surgery also reduces postoperative pain (18), which may be one of the factors allowing early restoration of function when compared with conventional open techniques (6).

Effective postoperative pain relief allowing early mobilization and restoration of oral intake is a prerequisite to early recovery of postoperative organ functions and a primary component of the multimodal approach in "accelerated stay" programs.

POSTOPERATIVE SLEEP DISTURBANCES

It is well known that anesthesia and surgery may be followed by delirium or other acute confusional states. Specific risk factors are old age, self-reported alcohol abuse, poor preoperative cognitive and functional status, and abnormal preoperative electrolytes (19). Furthermore, postoperative use of psychoactive medication such as opioids and benzodiazepines (20), as well as hypoxemia (21), may contribute to postoperative delirium. In addition, cerebral functional changes may include pronounced alterations in sleep pattern during the postoperative period, as reviewed recently (22), which may contribute to changes in mental function, episodic hypoxemia, and hemodynamic instability.

Although the exact function of sleep is largely unknown, it is essential for preservation of normal cerebral function. Thus, deprivation of sleep, being either rapid eye movement (REM) sleep or slow-wave sleep (SWS) in volunteers leads to confusion, anxiety, irritability, impaired concentration, and impaired performance on psychometric tests (23). Also, sleep deprivation results in a rebound response when the inhibition is removed, which may have detrimental effects into the postoperative period.

The normal sleep pattern is divided into REM and non-REM sleep based on their electrophysiologic characteristics. Of particular interest for the postoperative patient is the REM sleep phase, which may be associated with marked variations in arterial pressure and heart rate, rate and depth of breathing, and metabolic rate. Changes in sleep pattern also may be important for airway patency that is maintained by the muscles surrounding the oropharynx and pharyngopharynx. During different sleep stages, and especially during REM sleep, atonia of these muscles may predispose to instability of the airway leading to obstructive apnea episodes and thereby progressive hypoxia, bradycardia, and hypercapnia. This may result in sympathetic stimulation and increased oxygen demands at a time when myocardial hypoxia and hypertension are marked and cardiac ischemic injury may become likely (22).

The physiologic effects of the different sleep stages are well described in nonsurgical patients and may be coupled to an increased risk of myocardial ischemia and infarction as well as cerebral hypoperfusion and stroke, especially in the early morning hours. In the postsurgical stage, pronounced changes in sleep pattern take place (22). These changes may be unfortunate. At this time the body is influenced by the surgical stress response and increased metabolic demands setting up the potential for an unfavorable ratio between oxygen demands and oxygen supply. Although relatively little information is available on postoperative sleep disturbances, the observation that most of the unexplained postoperative deaths take place during the night (24) calls for further attention on postoperative sleep changes.

Postoperative Sleep Pattern

Postoperative changes in sleep have been studied either with electroencephalographic (EEG) recordings or by sleep interviews. Relatively little information is available derived from the optimal EEG technique. Only seven studies have been performed in noncardiac surgery, including 35 patients after major abdominal surgery (25–28), 10 patients after laparoscopic cholecystectomy (29), 18 patients after herniorrhaphy (26,30), and 46 patients after minor undefined surgery (31) (Table 1). The results of these studies have demonstrated abdominal surgery to lead to a highly fragmented sleep during the first 1 to 2 nights, with pronounced reduction of total sleep time, including REM and SWS. REM sleep is usually almost absent for the first and sometimes the second and third postoperative nights, with a subsequent reappearance with increased density and duration. During REM rebound, there is an increased total REM sleep time as well as increased REM density (27). The increase in REM activity is often associated with nightmares (27). The amount of SWS decreases significantly in the postoperative period and in fact was absent in all 10 patients on the first and second night after major abdominal surgery (28).

TABLE 1. *Summary of clinical studies with EEG-measured sleep after noncardiac surgery*

	Type of surgery	Postoperative nights	Total sleep time	Duration of REM sleep	Duration of SWS	No. of patients
Aurell and Elmqvist (25)	Major noncardiac surgery	1–4	↓	↓	↓	9
Ellis and Dudley (26)	Inguinal hernia repair	1,2	↓	↓	↓	8
	Upper abdominal surgery	1,2	↓	↓	↓	4
Knill et al. (27)	Cholecystectomy	1,2,(3)	—	↓	↓	6
		(3),4,5,6	—	↑	↓	
	Gastroplasty	1,2,(3)	—	↓	↓	6
		(3),4,5	—	↑	↓	
Rosenberg et al. (28)	Major abdominal surgery	1,(2)	—	↓	↓	
		(2),3	—	↑	↓	10
Rosenberg-Adamsen et al. (29)	Laparoscopic cholecystectomy	1	—	—	↓	10
Kavey and Altshuler (30)	Herniorrhaphy	1,2	↓	↓	↓	10
		3,4	—	↑	↓	
Lehmkuhl et al. (31)	Minor surgery	1	—	↓	↓	46

↑, increased; ↓, decreased; —, unchanged.

Corresponding to the rebound of REM sleep, there also may be a rebound of SWS in the later postoperative period (28).

The duration of the postoperative sleep abnormalities is poorly described because no EEG study has monitored beyond the 6th postoperative night. It appears that the sleep disturbances may gradually change toward normal values within the first postoperative week, although in no study did all patients show normal sleep pattern within this period.

In sleep interview studies the subjective recall has been that sleep quality is markedly deteriorated during the first postoperative night with gradual normalization before discharge (22). However, some studies have shown that about 25% of the patients have reduced sleep quality for more than 2 weeks after discharge (32). Because postoperative sleep disturbances may have an important influence on postoperative convalescence—mental performance, feeling of fatigue, etc.— there is a need for more detailed descriptive studies using the EEG technique into the later postoperative period. Additionally, further information is needed on pathogenic factors of postoperative sleep disturbances.

Pathogenesis of Postoperative Sleep Disturbances

Figure 2 describes some of the factors responsible for the postoperative sleep disturbances. The changes in postoperative sleep pattern may be related to the magnitude of surgery (Table 1). Of particular interest is our recent demonstration that no significant changes in REM sleep occur and that there is less change in SWS after laparoscopic cholecystectomy (29) when compared with open laparotomy (28). Also, questionnaire studies have demonstrated that the greatest changes in sleep pattern take place after the more major procedures (22). These studies may therefore suggest that factors related to the surgical stress response may be of importance for the precipitation of sleep abnormalities. Unfortunately, existing studies with stress reduction by regional anesthesia versus surgery performed during general anesthesia have not shown differences in postoperative sleep pattern (30,31). However, these studies have used a single-dose regional anesthetic technique, a technique that has no endocrine metabolic effects into the later postoperative period (2). It can therefore only be concluded that postoperative sleep disturbances are not a result of general anesthesia per se (22) because these disturbances were avoided by using the regional anesthetic technique.

On the various components in the endocrine metabolic surgical stress response, several factors may potentially influence postoperative sleep pattern. Thus, cortisol may cause reduction in REM sleep and increase in non-REM sleep after administration to healthy volunteers (33,34). The conventional increase in postoperative sympathetic activity may be important also because high levels of noradrenergic activity may maintain wakefulness (35). Postoperative changes in cytokine activity may be another pathogenic factor. Experimental studies have shown IL-1 administration to result in hyperthermia and increase

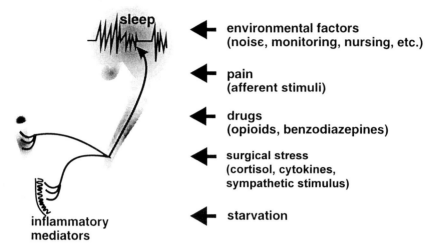

FIG. 2. Pathogenic factors leading to postoperative sleep disturbances.

in non-REM sleep and suppressions of REM sleep resembling the postoperative situation (36). Pretreatment with an IL-1 receptor antagonist prevented the IL-1–induced sleep disturbances (36). Similarly, intracerebroventricular injection of tumor necrosis factor in rabbits caused deprivation of REM sleep and an increase in non-REM sleep (37). Finally, endotoxin administration to healthy volunteers, which may release the classical catabolic hormones as well as various cytokines, also leads to deprivation of REM sleep and increase in non-REM sleep (38). Thus, several of the classical parameters of the surgical stress response may in themselves have an effect on sleep patterns. However, a noncausal relationship cannot be excluded. Rather than being caused by specific mediators of the surgical stress response, the postoperative sleep disturbances may represent only a global excitatory effect of the entire surgical stress (afferent stimulation) on the brain.

Postoperative pain may be another important cause of postoperative sleep disturbances (22). Unfortunately, no information is available on sleep patterns with optimal multimodal postoperative analgesia. Opioids are one of the most commonly used analgesics in the postoperative period and may have significant effects on postoperative sleep pattern. Morphine 0.1 and 0.2 mg/kg led to a disrupted sleep in a dose-dependent manner in healthy volunteers. The smaller dose reduced SWS and the larger dose reduced both REM sleep and SWS (39). The importance of opioids for postoperative sleep pattern (39,40) needs further evaluation in postoperative patients with different opioid techniques (PCA, epidural low-dose combinations, etc.), as well as with different opioid agonists. The use of NSAIDs for postoperative pain relief may have an advantageous effect on postoperative sleep disturbances because of their opioid-sparing effect. Thus, preliminary studies have shown improved subjective feeling of sleep quality with NSAID-induced opioid sparing (41). Monitoring procedures as well as the noise level in the surgical ward may disturb sleep during the first postoperative night, as mentioned in patient reported studies (22). Finally, starvation, which often occurs after major operations, may in itself be associated with a decreased SWS, as demonstrated in volunteers (42).

Clinical Implications of Postoperative Sleep Disturbances

The postoperative rebound of REM sleep may be of importance for the development of breathing abnormalities during sleep (apnea) and nocturnal hypoxemia (28,43). Thus, episodic hypoxemia is more frequent during periods of REM rebound than during other sleep stages in the postoperative period (28). Because REM sleep is normally associated with profound sympathetic activation and hemodynamic instability, the pronounced REM rebound in the middle of the first postoperative week may contribute to cardiac complications. REM sleep induced sympathetic stimulation with tachycardia and hypertension, and time-related episodic hypoxemia may be an important pathogenic factor for postoperative myocardial ischemia and infarction, although this hypothesis obviously needs further documentation. However, this hypothesis is supported by the finding of a majority of unexpected postoperative deaths to occur at night (24).

Postoperative mental deterioration occurs in about 5–10% of elderly patients and may be related to postoperative sleep disturbances. Studies in nonsurgical patients with sleep deprivation have shown similar changes in mental function (22). However, so far no study has directly related the occurrence of postoperative sleep disturbances with postoperative cerebral dysfunction. Efforts to prevent or normalize postoperative sleep disturbances have not been correlated with cerebral performance. Finally, postoperative sleep disturbances may be linked with the development of early postoperative fatigue, although this has not been studied.

Prevention and Treatment of Postoperative Sleep Disturbances

The principal strategies to reduce postoperative sleep disturbances are a reduction of the trauma by minimally invasive surgery techniques, by efficient stress-reducing neural blockade techniques, and by avoidance of opioids in the perioperative analgesic regimens. Also, a reduction of noise and unnecessary monitoring and the early use of nutrition may be of importance. Pharmacologic issues involve the use of newer hypnotic agents that have no important influence on sleep architecture, such as zopiclone and zolpidem (22). The effect of melatonin administration needs consideration. Except for a preliminary study in opioid-free laparoscopic cholecystectomy surgery that showed less sleep disturbance (29), to date none of these methods has been adequately studied with specific attention to postoperative sleep patterns.

In summary, the postoperative sleep disturbance is a rather neglected surgical stress response. However, because of the pronounced abnormalities in the sleep cycle and the fact that sleep represents a vital parameter for preservation of cerebral function, intervention studies with the reduction or prevention of postoperative sleep disturbances are urgently needed. Finally, the potential detrimental effects of sleep disruption on cerebral and cardiac function and postoperative recovery need to established.

POSTOPERATIVE FATIGUE AND CONVALESCENCE

Even though fatigue has been recognized as a common complaint in most patients after surgical procedures, there was little information available on this undesirable sequelae of otherwise successful operations until a fatigue analog scale was described in 1982 (44). Subsequently, an increasing number of studies have described the phenomenon and time course of postoperative fatigue as well as pathogenic mechanisms and intervention techniques (45,46). There is now a general agreement that the subjective feeling of postoperative fatigue after major procedures (assessed as the ability to cope with daily working demands and need of sleep) increases to a peak on days 7–10. A subsequent normalization appears within the next 3–4 weeks, and a slight improvement follows 3 months postoperatively when compared with preoperative fatigue scores (45–47). The most important pathogenic mechanisms leading to postoperative fatigue are shown in Fig. 3.

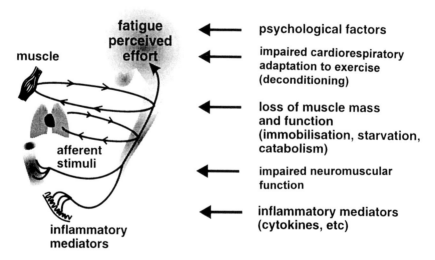

FIG. 3. Pathogenic factors leading to postoperative fatigue.

Influence of Preoperative Factors on Postoperative Fatigue

In relatively fit patients, preoperative age, sex, fatigue score, and nutritional status parameters (body weight, triceps skinfold caliber, arm muscle circumference) did not predict postoperative fatigue (45,46). However, in a group including malnourished patients, preoperative fatigue as well as weight, weight loss, total body protein, grip strength, and age correlated slightly with development of postoperative fatigue (48). Preoperative level of anxiety is not a predictor of postoperative fatigue (45,46,48).

Influence of Intra- and Postoperative Factors on Postoperative Fatigue

The magnitude of surgical trauma is of obvious importance for development of postoperative fatigue. Minor surgery (such as middle ear surgery) does not lead to postoperative fatigue despite a duration of surgery of about 3 hours (46). Reduction of the inflammatory response by the minimal surgical technique (6) results in reduced fatigue scores after cholecystectomy (49,50) and colectomy (51). This occurred despite an unaltered early increase in plasma glucose and cortisol (50). The choice of anesthesia is probably not important, and general anesthesia is not an important pathogenic factor per se for the development of postoperative fatigue (52). The effect of intraoperative, single-dose regional anesthesia on development of postoperative fatigue has not been evaluated but is probably negligible because its effect on the surgical stress response is transient (2).

The effect of various analgesic techniques per se on postoperative fatigue is probably relatively small. Effective postoperative pain relief with multimodal epidural analgesia and NSAIDs did not reduce fatigue after open cholecystectomy. This was true for patients who were pain free during mobilization (53) and even when pain relief was continued for up to 4 days. Similarly, a low-dose epidural local anesthetic–opioid regimen had no effect on early and late postoperative fatigue scores after major abdominal surgery (54). Neither epidural opioids alone (55) nor intrapleural local anesthetics (56) had any influence on postoperative fatigue. In contrast, a single bolus of preoperative high-dose glucocorticoid combined with epidural analgesia and NSAID reduced fatigue scores and the deterioration of pulmonary function after open cholecystectomy and colonic resection (57,58). At the same time, the IL-6 and hyperthermic responses were reduced compared with surgery using general anesthesia with systemic opioids for postoperative pain treatment. This suggests that these responses must be controlled in order to reduce postoperative fatigue.

Postoperative changes in psychologic function (anxiety and depression scores, etc.) do not play an important role in the development of postoperative fatigue (46,48).

In contrast, changes in nutritional parameters may be of importance for the development of postoperative fatigue. Postoperative weight loss correlated with

increase in fatigue as well as with loss of triceps skinfold thickness (46). However, no correlation was found between postoperative reduction of arm muscle
circumference and fatigue (46). Although fatigue increases and total body protein decreases postoperatively, no clear relationships between these parameters
have been demonstrated (47,48). The catabolic response to surgery is also characterized by profound changes in muscle amino acid composition and muscle
protein synthesis. However, despite these changes that persist 3 to 4 weeks postoperatively, no relationship between muscle amino acid composition and development of fatigue could be demonstrated (59). In another study, late postoperative depression of protein synthesis was demonstrated by a decreased number
of ribosomes in muscle biopsies and with a simultaneous increase in fatigue
(60). Unfortunately, no correlation analysis between changes in fatigue and protein synthesis was performed (60). In summary, changes in nutritional parameters may therefore be only one of several pathogenic factors of postoperative
fatigue.

The relationship between muscle function as assessed by exercise performance (daily work, walking stairs, etc.) and development of postoperative
fatigue has been investigated. Voluntary maximum muscle force of elbow flex-
ors decreased 5–10% postoperatively and endurance during a sustained contraction decreased about 30% (61). There was a correlation of both muscle function
parameters and the development of postoperative fatigue (59). However, other
studies have not been able to demonstrate a clear relationship between changes
in postoperative hand grip strength and development of postoperative fatigue
(47,53) despite the fact that grip strength decreased after operation and fatigue
increased (47). Objective assessment of muscle function by induction of adductor pollicis muscle contraction with ulnar nerve stimulation showed no significant decrease in muscle function postoperatively despite an increase in postoperative fatigue (47,62). However, in both studies there was a slight (5–10%) but
insignificant decrease in muscle function on days 7–10 (47,62).

Other studies have demonstrated an increase in mean amplitude during elec-
tromyographic monitoring under sustained contractions and a correlation with
development of fatigue (61). These results may suggest that postoperative
fatigue is partly explained as muscle fatigue of peripheral origin. In studies of
postoperative changes in muscle fiber characteristics, the decrease in slow
twitch fibers did correlate with loss of body weight, but not with increase in
postoperative fatigue (63). The relative distribution of fiber types was
unchanged 21 days after surgery and without any relation to postoperative
fatigue (63). However, the number of patients studied were limited, and because
no other information is available in the literature, final conclusions are hindered.

In studies during pre- and postoperative bicycle exercise, there was no correlation between development of postoperative fatigue and changes in various
muscle enzymes and substrates (64). Neither could any correlation be found
between the exercise-induced development of postoperative fatigue and the
responses in various stress hormones and serum lactate (65).

In contrast, several studies have shown a correlation between the increase in postoperative fatigue and impaired cardiovascular adaptation (i.e., increase in heart rate) to orthostatic stress or exercise (44,64,65). Zeiderman et al. (62) measured energy expenditure from oxygen consumption and carbon dioxide production and muscular efficiency as defined by the ratio of the net change in work rate divided by the net change in energy expenditure during exercise on a thread mill. At identical work loads 3 days after surgery, the muscular efficiency was 12% lower than preoperatively and was accompanied by a 19% increase in net energy expenditure (62). In all patients there was an increase in postoperative fatigue, but unfortunately a direct correlation analysis between cardiorespiratory responses to exercise and development of postoperative fatigue was not performed (62).

The available studies suggest a relationship between loss of muscle mass and amplified cardiorespiratory responses to a given exercise and development of fatigue. Studies of skeletal muscle function as a result of direct stimulation have not established a direct relationship with the development of postoperative fatigue. However, the overall increase in perceived effort to perform an exercise does seem to correlate with the development of fatigue (47), probably due to physiologic changes on several levels (Fig. 3). Intervention studies aimed at reducing or preventing development of postoperative fatigue should therefore consist of several modalities. These should include avoidance of immobilization and semistarvation, both of which may have detrimental effects on muscle function and may contribute to fatigue.

Interventional Studies on Postoperative Fatigue

Relatively few intervention studies to demonstrate a reduction of postoperative fatigue have been performed. As mentioned above, conventional techniques for postoperative pain relief per se have not been able to decrease postoperative fatigue (53–56). The use of enteral nutrition as a single modality treatment had well-known positive effects on body weight and wound collagen accumulation (66). However, no significant effects were obtained on body composition or muscle function assessed by the ulnar nerve stimulation test. Additionally, the development of postoperative fatigue was not influenced (66). Similarly, short-term (3 days) glutamine supplementation prevented postoperative reduction of protein synthesis as assessed by ribosome changes in skeletal muscle but had no effect on fatigue (67). These studies therefore suggest that, in accordance with its multifactorial pathogenesis, unimodal intervention may not result in reduction of postoperative fatigue (Fig. 3). In contrast, the use of minimally invasive surgery, which reduces the all-over stress response to surgery (6), including catabolism and inflammatory response, pain, and sleep disturbances, seems to be effective in reducing postoperative fatigue (49–51). Of most interest, a multimodal intervention with laparoscopic surgery, epidural local anesthetics to enhance restoration of postoperative ileus, avoidance of opioids, and immediate enteral nutrition did prevent development of postoperative fatigue after colonic resection in high-risk patients (51). These results suggest that sufficient stress reduction by minimal invasive surgery or sufficient neural blockade techniques, avoidance of opioids with their delaying effects on recovery, as well as effective pain relief with early institution of enforced mobilization and oral nutrition may be effective. Unfortunately, no controlled studies are available, but uncontrolled observations in 17 patients undergoing open colectomy with effective epidural analgesia, early oral nutrition, and enforced mobilization demonstrated less postoperative fatigue (68) than usually observed (46,47). Perioperative administration of growth hormone to promote anabolism also may reduce postoperative fatigue (69).

In conclusion, development of postoperative fatigue is a nonpsychologic but somatically precipitated event of multifactorial origin. Important pathogenic factors are postoperative deconditioning of muscle function, catabolism, impaired cardiorespiratory adaptation to exercise, immobilization, and semistarvation. Although definitive studies describing the relative role of each of these predisposing factors are still warranted, existing data suggest that single-parameter intervention has no important effects on postoperative fatigue. A multimodal approach with stress reduction, effective pain relief, early mobilization, and oral nutrition may be effective in reducing or preventing fatigue.

A MULTIMODAL APPROACH TO IMPROVE POSTOPERATIVE REHABILITATION AND CONVALESCENCE

Recent advances in perioperative care have included optimization of pain relief, nutrition, fluid management, anesthetic and surgical technique, antithrombotic prophylaxis, and antimicrobial prophylaxis, all adding to a continuous decrease in hospital stay and postoperative morbidity. Nevertheless, major procedures are still beset with a clinically important risk of organ dysfunction (pulmonary, cardiac, thromboembolic, and cerebral complications) as well as postoperative fatigue and lengthy convalescence. This is complicated increasingly with the admission of more elderly patients and more patients with severe pre-existing disease. In this chapter the interactions of the surgical stress response, postoperative pain, postoperative sleep disturbance, and fatigue have been discussed. Considering unimodal intervention studies, it appears that the pathogenesis of these "unspecific" postoperative sequelae is multifactorial. Experiences with the minimally invasive surgical techniques suggest that reduction of trauma and thereby the inflammatory, humorally mediated responses may be of major importance to reduce the surgical convalescence period, including changes in sleep patterns and fatigue. Other mechanisms include the detrimental effects of immobilization and semistarvation, which often unintentionally takes place in the traditional surgical care programs. An additional pathogenic factor may be

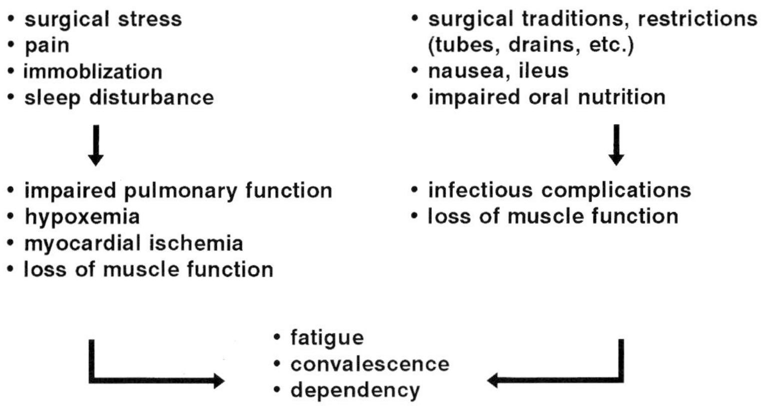

- surgical stress
- pain
- immoblization
- sleep disturbance

↓

- impaired pulmonary function
- hypoxemia
- myocardial ischemia
- loss of muscle function

- surgical traditions, restrictions (tubes, drains, etc.)
- nausea, ileus
- impaired oral nutrition

↓

- infectious complications
- loss of muscle function

- fatigue
- convalescence
- dependency

FIG. 4. The postoperative cascade to dependency.

opioids, which may have detrimental effects such as sleep disruption, nausea, gastrointestinal paralysis, and sedation, thereby retarding recovery (70).

Subsequently, a rational strategy to reduce perioperative morbidity and shorten convalescence must be multimodal to counteract all pathogenic mechanisms, leading to the "postoperative cascade to dependency" (Fig. 4) (71). Such efforts include an intensified preoperative information, stress reduction with neural blockade or humoral mediator modification, and sufficient pain relief allowing early mobilization facilitating recovery of gastrointestinal function and thereby early restoration of oral intake. Normalization of postinjury gastrointestinal function may be a key factor in early recovery because this may reduce the general trauma response (72) and the risk of infectious complications (73). Although the relative role of these factors to enhance recovery remains to be established, single-modality treatment seems to be outdated. Efforts should be directed toward reducing harmful aspects of the stress response in combination with an enhancement of positive effects through the use of biologic response modifiers, nutritional support, and growth factors.

REFERENCES

1. Bessey PQ. Metabolic response to critical illness. In: Wilmore DW, Cheung LY, Harken AH, Holcroft JW, Meakins JL, eds. *Scientific American surgery.* New York: Scientific American Inc.; 1995:1–31.
2. Kehlet H. Modification of responses to surgery by neural blockade. Clinical implications. In: Cousins MJ, Bridenbaugh PO, eds. *Neural blockade in clinical anesthesia and management of pain.* Philadelphia: JB Lippincott; 1997.
3. Beal AL, Cerra FB. Multiple organ failure syndrome in the 1990s. *JAMA* 1994;271:226–233.
4. Hill G, Douglas RG, Schroeder, D. Metabolic basis for the management of patients undergoing major surgery. *World J Surg* 1993;17:146–153.
5. Hill GL. Impact of nutritional support on the clinical outcome of the surgical patient. *Clin Nutr* 1994;13:331–340.

6. Kehlet H, Nielsen HJ. Impact of laparoscopic surgery on stress responses, immunofunction and risk of infectious complications—a review. *J Am Coll Surg* 1997.
7. Kehlet H. Effect of neural blockade in the acute catabolic stage. In: Revhaug A, ed. *Acute catabolic stage. Update in intensive care and emergency medicine.* Vol. 21. Berlin: Springer-Verlag; 1996:207–215.
8. Kehlet H. Postoperative pain. In: Wilmore DW, Cheung LY, Harken AH, Holcroft JW, Meakins JL, eds. *Scientific American surgery.* New York: Scientific American Inc.; 1995:1–12.
9. Kehlet H. Postoperative pain—what is the issue? *Br J Anaesth* 1994;72:375–378.
10. Woolf CJ. Somatic pain—pathogenesis and prevention. *Br J Anaesth* 1995;75:169–175.
11. Treede R-D, Meyer RA, Raja SN, Campbell JN. Peripheral and central mechanism of cutaneous hyperalgesia. *Prog Neurobiol* 1992;38:397–421.
12. Woolf CS, Chong M-S. Preemptive analgesia—treating postoperative pain by preventing the establishment of central sensitisation. *Anesth Analg* 1993;77:362–379.
13. Kehlet H, Dahl JB. Preemptive analgesia—is it effective in clinical pain states? In: Gebhart GF, ed. *Visceral pain.* Seattle: IASP Press; 1995:489–504.
14. Kehlet H, Dahl JB. The value of multi-modal or balanced analgesia on post operative pain relief. *Anesth Analg* 1993;77:1048–1056.
15. Liu SS, Carpenter RL, Mackey DC, et al. Effects of perioperative analgesic technique on rate of recovery after colon surgery. *Anesthesiology* 1995;83:757–765.
16. Stein C. The control of pain in peripheral tissues by opioids. *N Engl J Med* 1995;332:1685–1690.
17. Dray A. Inflammatory mediators of pain. *Br J Anaesth* 1995;75:125–131.
18. McMahon AJ, Russell IT, Ramsey G, et al. Laparoscopic and mini-laparotomy cholecystectomy: a randomized trial comparing postoperative pain and pulmonary function. *Surgery* 1994;115:533–539.
19. Marcantonio ER, Goldman L, Mangione CM, et al. A clinical prediction rule for delirium after elective non-cardiac surgery. *JAMA* 1994;271:134–139.
20. Marcantonio ER, Juaraz G, Goldman L, et al. The relationship of postoperative delirium with psychoactive medications. *JAMA* 1994;272:1518–1522.
21. Rosenberg J, Kehlet H. Postoperative mental confusion—association with postoperative hypoxemia. *Surgery* 1993;114:76–81.
22. Rosenberg-Adamsen S, Kehlet H, Dodds C, Rosenberg J. Postoperative sleep disturbances: mechanisms and clinical implications. *Br J Anaesth* 1996;76:552–559.
23. Gilberg M, Åkerstedt T. Sleep restriction and SWS-suppression: effects on day time alertness and night-time recovery. *J Sleep Res* 1994;3:144–151.
24. Rosenberg J, Pedersen NH, Ramsing T, Kehlet H. Circadian variation in unexpected postoperative death. *Br J Surg* 1992;7:1300–1302.
25. Aurell J, Elmqvist D. Sleep in the surgical intensive care unit: continuous polygraphic recording of sleep in nine patients reveiving postoperative care. *Br Med J* 1985;290:1029–1032.
26. Ellis BW, Dudley HAF. Some aspects of sleep research in surgical stress. *J Psychosom Res* 1976;20: 303–308.
27. Knill RL, Moote CA, Skinner MI, Rose EA. Anesthesia with abdominal surgery leads to intense REM sleep during the first postoperative week. *Anesthesiology* 1990;73:52–61.
28. Rosenberg J, Wildschiødtz G, Pedersen MH, et al. Late postoperative nocturnal episodic hypoxaemia and associated sleep pattern. *Br J Anaesth* 1994;72:145–150.
29. Rosenberg-Adamsen S, Skarbye M, Wildschiødtz G, et al. Sleep after laparoscopic cholecystectomy. *Br J Anaesth* 1996;76:552–556.
30. Kavey NB, Altshuler KZ. Sleep in herniorrhaphy patients. *Am J Surg* 1979;138:682–687.
31. Lehmkuhl P, Prass D, Pichlmayr I. General anaesthesia and postnarcotic sleep disorders. *Neuropsychobiology* 1987;18:37–42.
32. Beydon L, Rauss A, Lofasso F, et al. Assessment of quality of perioperative sleep: study of the factors favouring insomnia. *Ann Fr Anesth Reanim* 1994;13:669–674.
33. Fehm HL, Benkowitsch R, Kern W, et al. Influences of corticosteroids, dexamethasone and hydrocortisone on sleep in humans. *Neuropsychology* 1986;16:198–204.
34. Friess E, von Bardeleben U, Wiedemann K, et al. Effects of pulsatile cortisol infusion on sleep-EEG and nocturnal growth hormone release in healthy men. *J Sleep Res* 1994;3:73–79.
35. Hilakivi I. Biogenic amines in the regulation of wakefulness and sleep. *Med Biol* 1987;65:97–104.
36. Opp MR, Krueger JM. Interleukin 1-receptor antagonist blocks interleukin 1-induced sleep and fever. *Am J Physiol* 1991;260:R453–R457.
37. Kapas L, Hong L, Cady AB, et al. Somnogenic, pyrogenic and anorectic activities of tumor necrosis factor-alpha and TNF-alpha fragments. *Am J Physiol* 1992;263:R708–R715.

38. Trachsel L, Schreiber W, Holsboer F, Poilmächer T. Endotoxin enhances EEG alpha and beta power in human sleep. *Sleep* 1994;17:132–139.
39. Moote CA, Knill RL, Skinner MI, Rose EA. Morphine disrupts nocturnal sleep in a dose-dependent fashion. *Anesth Analg* 1989;68:S200.
40. Kay DC, Eisenstein RB, Jersinsky DR. Morphine effects on human REM sleep stage, waking stage, and NREM sleep. *Psychopharmacologia* 1969;14:404–416.
41. Parker RK, Holtmann B, Smith I, White PF. Use of ketorolac after lower abdominal surgery. *Anesthesiology* 1994;80:6–12.
42. MacFayden UM, Oswald I, Lewis SA. Starvation and human slow wave sleep. *J Appl Physiol* 1973; 35:391–394.
43. Knill RL, Moote CA, Rose EA, Skinner MI. Marked hypoxemia after gastroplasty due to disorders of breathing in REM sleep. *Anesthesiology* 1987;67:3A.
44. Christensen T, Bendix T, Kehlet H. Fatigue and cardiorespiratory function following abdominal surgery. *Br J Surg* 1982;69:417–419.
45. Christensen T, Kehlet H. Postoperative fatigue. *World J Surg* 1993;17:220–225.
46. Christensen T. Postoperative fatigue. *Dan Med Bull* 1995;42:314–322.
47. Schroeder D, Hill G. Postoperative fatigue: a prospective physiological study of patients undergoing major abdominal surgery. *Aust NZ J Surg* 1991;61:774–779.
48. Schroeder D, Hill GL. Predicting postoperative fatigue: importance of preoperative factors. *World J Surg* 1993;17:226–231.
49. Delaunay L, Bonnet F, Cherqui D, et al. Laparoscopic cholecystectomy minimally impairs postoperative cardio-respiratory and muscle performance. *Br J Surg* 1995;82:373–376.
50. Hill AG, Finn P, Schroeder D. Postoperative fatigue after laparoscopic surgery. *Aust NZ J Surg* 1993;63:946–951.
51. Bardram L, Funch-Jensen P, Jensen P, et al. Recovery after laparoscopic colonic surgery with epidural analgesia, and early oral nutrition and mobilization. *Lancet* 1995;345:763–764.
52. Christensen T, Hougård F, Kehlet H. Influence of pre- and intra-operative factors on the occurrence of postoperative fatigue. *Br J Surg* 1985;72:63–65.
53. Schulze S, Roikjær O, Hasselstrøm L, et al. Epidural bupivacaine and morphine plus systemic indomethacin eliminates pain but not the systemic response and convalescence after cholecystectomy. *Surgery* 1988;103:321–327.
54. Hjortsø N-C, Andersen T, Frøsig F, et al. A controlled study of the effect of epidural analgesia with local anaesthetics and morphine on morbidity after abdominal surgery. *Acta Anaesthesiol Scand* 1985;29:790–796.
55. Zeiderman MR, Welchew EA, Clark RG. Influence of epidural analgesia upon postoperative fatigue. *Br J Surg* 1991;78:1457–1460.
56. Schroeder D. Baker P. Interpleural catheter for analgesia after cholecystectomy: the surgical perspective. *Aust NZ J Surg* 1990;60:689–694.
57. Schulze S, Møller IW, Bang U, et al. Effect of combined prednisolone, epidural analgesia and indomethacin on pain, systemic response and convalescence after cholecystectomy. *Acta Chir Scand* 1990;156:203–209.
58. Schulze S, Sommer P, Bigler D, et al. Effect of epidural analgesia, indomethacin and methylprednisolone on pain, cytokines, acute phase and pulmonary response to colonic surgery. *Arch Surg* 1992;127:325–331.
59. Christensen T, Kehlet H, Vesterberg K, Vinnars E. Fatigue and muscle amino acids during surgical convalescence. *Acta Chir Scand* 1987;153:567–570.
60. Petersson B, Wernerman J, Waller S-O, et al. Elective abdominal surgery depresses muscle protein synthesis and increases subjective fatigue: effects lasting more than 30 days. *Br J Surg* 1990;77: 796–800.
61. Christensen T, Wulff C, Fuglsang-Frederiksen A, Kehlet H. Electrical activity and arm muscle force in postoperative fatigue. *Acta Chir Scand* 1985;151:1–5.
62. Zeiderman MR, Welchew EA, Clark RG. Changes in cardiorespiratory and muscle function associated with the development of postoperative fatigue. *Br J Surg* 1990;77:576–580.
63. Christensen T, Nygaard E, Kehlet H. Skeletal muscle fiber composition, nutritional status and subjective feeling of fatigue during surgical convalescence. *Acta Chir Scand* 1988;154:335–338.
64. Christensen T, Nygaard E, Stage JG, Kehlet H. Skeletal muscle enzyme activities and metabolic substrates during exercise after abdominal surgery. *Br J Surg* 1990;77:312–315.
65. Christensen T, Stage JG, Galbo H, et al. Fatigue and cardiac and endocrine metabolic response to exercise after abdominal surgery. *Surgery* 1989;105;46–50.

66. Schroeder D, Gillanders L, Mahr K, Hill GL. Effects of immediate postoperative enteral nutrition on body composition, muscle function and wound healing. *J Parenter Enter Nutr* 1991;15:376–383.
67. Petersson B, von der Decken A, Vinnars E, Wernerman J. Long-term effects of postoperative total parenteral nutrition supplemented with glycylglutamine on subjective fatigue and muscle protein synthesis. *Br J Surg* 1994;81:1520–1523.
68. Møiniche S, Bülow S, Hesselfeldt P, et al. Convalescence and hospital stay after colonic surgery with balanced analgesia, early oral feeding and enforced mobilization. *Eur J Surg* 1995;161;283–288.
69. Vara-Thorbeck R, Guerrero JA, Ruiz-Requena E, Garcia-Carriazo M. Can the use of growth hormone reduce the postoperative fatigue syndrome? *World J Surg* 1996;20:81–87.
70. Kehlet H, Rung GW, Callesen T. Postoperative opioid analgesia—time for a reconsideration? *J Clin Anesth* 1996;8:441–445.
71. Kehlet H. Multimodal approach to control postoperative pathophysiology and rehabilitation. *Br J Anaesth* 1997 (May, in press).
72. Fong Y, Marano MA, Barber A, et al. Total parenteral nutrition and bowel rest modify the metabolic response to endotoxin in humans. *Ann Surg* 1989;210:449–457.
73. Moore FA, Feliciano V, Andrassy RJ, et al. Early enteral feeding, compared with parenteral, reduces postoperative complications. *Ann Surg* 1992;216:172–183.

Physiology, Stress, and Malnutrition: Functional Correlates, Nutritional Intervention,
edited by J.M. Kinney and H.N. Tucker.
Lippincott–Raven Publishers © 1997.

Stress, Brain, and Behavior: Life-Long Effects upon Health and Disease

Bruce S. McEwen

Laboratory of Neuroendocrinology, Rockefeller University, New York, New York 10021

Stress is a widely misunderstood human experience that is often blamed as a cause of disease. A stressful stimulus represents a challenge to an organism's physiologic systems (1), and the degree of the perceived or real threat determines the magnitude of the stress response (2). Yet, stressors are heterogeneous, and health professionals are often baffled as to how to respond to patients' complaints that they are "stressed." There are physical stressors, such as exertion, heat, cold, trauma, infection, and inflammation, as well as psychological stressors, such as fear and anxiety, social defeat and humiliation, disappointment and sometimes even intense joy. The physiologic responses to such stressors are variable, and there are individual differences both physiologically and behaviorally in how a person perceives a challenge (3). Nevertheless, it is important to take stress seriously even though it is an individual experience and only one factor in the etiology of disease, because there are very real physiologic and pathophysiologic consequences in at least some individuals who experience stress.

Individual differences in responding to challenge are a product of genetics, developmental influences, and experience. Genetic predisposition is an important factor, but genetics alone does not explain individual differences. The 40–60% concordances of identical twins for diseases such as atherosclerosis (4) and type I diabetes (5), and only 19% for asthma (6), emphasizes the importance of environmental as well as genetic factors.

In particular, it is necessary to re-evaluate what it is about stress that contributes to disease processes. The environment and experiences that individuals have are translated into responses of the central nervous system, endocrine system, and autonomic nervous system. Responses to acute stress often synergize with the actions of chronic stress, as in cardiovascular disease (7,8). Chronic stress places a strain on physiologic systems that maintain homeostasis and it leads to chronic wear and tear and changes the operating range of physiologic systems. Therefore, one goal is to understand what factors come together acutely to precipitate a myocardial infarction or to exacerbate a viral infection or potentiate the metastasis of a tumor. Another task is to understand the long-term (sometimes life-long) antecedents and predisposing factors that lead to acute pathology. For example, diet and metabolism, influenced in part by personality factors and intrinsic neurochemistry, can increase progression toward atherosclerosis (8–11).

This article summarizes recent information pointing to chronic and acute aspects of the stress response that contribute to disease processes. First, there is a summary of the connections between stress and a number of pathophysiologic conditions, based largely on correlational studies. Second, we redefine the role of the hormonal stress response in adaptation and coping with experiences and, as a substitute for "chronic stress," we introduce the notion of "allostatic load" or chronic wear and tear produced by excessive activity of adaptive systems. Third, we note the importance of the social environment in regulating activity of stress hormone systems and then discuss the role of the brain and behavior in determining whether an event is stressful to an individual. Finally, we consider the role of the brain itself as a target of allostatic load as well as the master controller and intepreter of what is stressful.

EVIDENCE FOR EFFECTS OF STRESS ON HEALTH

The evidence for effects of stress on health involves what is largely a correlational analysis of stress with occurrence of disorders based on autonomic, cardiovascular, gastrointestinal, and immune system pathophysiology. For each system, there is evidence that acute or chronic stress contributes significantly as a risk factor to the expression of disease.

Atherosclerosis and Myocardial Infarction

Myocardial infarction (MI) is the best-known example of an acute health crisis that is often precipitated by recent physical or psychological stress (12) and which also involves long-term antecedents, particularly how stress accelerates atherosclerosis (8). The interactions between diet and stress lead to a chronic, long-term condition that promotes endocrine imbalances that alter metabolism and body fat distribution and increase atherosclerosis (13).

Diabetes

Although diabetes is a heterogeneous disease, there is evidence that stressful experience is a significant risk factor in both animal studies and in humans (14,15). The linkage is somewhat stronger for the effects of stress on type II diabetes (14). However, stressful experiences are also risk factors for exacerbation of type I diabetes in an animal model (16) as well as in humans (15), and for the onset of type I diabetes in children (17).

Gastrointestinal Disorders

Stress-induced ulceration of the gastrointestinal tract is well-recognized in human beings and well-studied in experimental animals (1). Ulcerative colitis is a disease in which the symptoms come and go in relation to factors such as the continuity of the doctor–patient relationship and whether the patient is optimistic or helpless in dealing with life events (1). For various forms of inflammatory bowel disease, major stressful life events were the most significant indicators of disease activity, even though only 7% of the variance was uniquely attributable to stress (18).

Asthma

Asthma is an example of an acute effect of stress on health. The role of emotional stress as an important stimulus has emerged after recognition that asthma involves both intrinsic and extrinsic pathways. The intrinsic pathway, involving autonomic nervous system effects on the airway passages, is susceptible to acute effects of emotional stressors (6). Long-term antecedents of the asthmatic condition are not understood, but they must exist because concordances among identical twins for asthma are on the order of 19% (6).

Cancer, Viral Infections, and Autoimmunity

The immune system is responsive to behavioral influences and to stress, with both positive and negative outcomes. Stress enhances the delayed-type hypersensitivity response, which is good for fighting infections and tumors but is deleterious when the response is an allergic one (19). Moreover, also on the positive side is the report that supportive group therapy doubled the survival time for patients with metastatic breast cancer after the end of intervention (20). On a more negative side is the report that psychological stress increased susceptibility to the common cold, elevating infection rates from 74% to 90% and clinical colds from 27% to 47% (21). Earlier studies had shown increased incidence of mononucleosis with examination stress in medical students (22).

There is less information available regarding long-term stress effects on diseases related to the immune system. However, a study of type I diabetes in children found that stressful life events stemming from actual or threatened losses within the family during ages 5–9 years significantly increased the relative risk for the disease, and this was true after the investigators had standardized for possible confounding factors such as age, sex, and family socioeconomic status (17). Newly diagnosed Graves' disease in adults also has been associated with an increased frequency of negative life events (23). Moreover, psychosocial influences on rheumatoid arthritis, another autoimmune disease, are strongly suggestive, but are confounded, as in the case of asthma (6), by the heterogeneity of the disease (24). Personality features such as the ability to express anger and irritation and stressful life events have been implicated as risk factors in women with rheumatoid arthritis in whom there was not a family history of this disease (24).

IMPORTANCE OF THE STRESS HORMONE AXIS FOR ADAPTATION AND COPING

The stress hormone axis is frequently called upon by the organism in response to challenge, and stress hormone actions play an important role in adaptation and coping, as well as contributing to certain diseases. One way of defining a stressful event is that it activates secretion of hormones such as adrenalin, adrenocorticotrophic hormone (ACTH) and glucocorticoids. It is well known that, without these hormones, the organism would not survive many stressors, and their role in adaptation and coping is well-recognized. One example is the ability of stress hormones to enhance the cellular immune response to a pathogen through delayed-type hypersensitivity (19). Another aspect of glucocorticoid action in the aftermath of stress is to counteract and contain other stress responses, such as inflammation (25) or the release of catecholamines (26), thus keeping the primary responses to stressors under some negative feedback control (27).

One important feature of successful coping with stress is that physiologic systems are not only turned on efficiently by the stressor but that they are turned off again after the stress has ceased (28–33). Dominant baboons, for example, turn on their stress response rapidly and efficiently, whereas the opposite is true of subordinates (34). Likewise, successful air controllers show precise control of their cortisol stress responses, whereas unsuccessful controllers do not (28–30). Boys who are at risk for substance abuse show poor cortisol responses to laboratory challenge of an anticipated stressor (35), and individuals who are clinically anxious show lesser catecholamine responses to acute stressors (33). A subgroup of what appear to be the most stressed subordinate rats in a chronic psychosocial stress situation showed a failure to mount a glucocorticoid stress response to a restraint stress paradigm (36).

The bottom line is that a successful organism must mobilize the physiologic stress response when needed and then turn it off in order to minimize the overall exposure to stress hormones and use them only when needed. In fact, repeated stress has the effect of enhancing or at least maintaining a high level of stress responsiveness to novel stressors (37–40) while at the same time leading to adaptation or habituation to repetitions of the same stressor (33,40–43). Depending on the intensity and modality of the chronic stressor, it is also possible to sometimes see sensitization to presentation of the same stressor (44–46).

When they are not shut off properly, stress hormones exacerbate pathologic processes. This is true of elevated blood pressure in relation to atherosclerosis (8,47) and glucocorticoid, insulin, and catecholamine production in relation to abdominal obesity (13,48). Stress-responsive systems such as catecholamines and glucocorticoids, which are involved in adaptation of the organisms, operate within a range that has been referred to as allostasis, maintaining stability through change (49). In the process of maintaining allostasis, physiologic systems sometimes work for periods of time at higher or lower levels than average, and the increased activity of these systems can accelerate pathologic processes if the elevation occurs chronically over long periods. This is because the products of the elevated activity produce various effects on tissue of the body, and we have termed this "allostatic load" (50).

Allostatic load is the wear-and-tear on the body and brain resulting from chronic overactivity of physiologic systems that are normally involved in adaptation to environmental challenge. Although it is true that physiologic parameters like blood oxygen and pH are maintained in a narrow range (homeostasis), the cardiovascular system, metabolic machinery, immune system, and central nervous system all show a large range of activity as a function of the time of day and in response to external and internal demands (allostasis). These systems are involved in coping and adaptation, and, as a general rule, they are most useful when they can be rapidly mobilized and then turned down in their activity again when not needed. It is when they are not turned off or turned down that these systems become dangerous for health (Table 1). Mediators involved in modulating these adaptive systems consist of hormones (principally, but not confined to, adrenalin and noradrenalin, ACTH and glucocorticoids, insulin and glucagon) and cytokines (produced not only by immune cells but also by the liver and brain).

An important aspect of allostasis and allostatic load is the notion of anticipation. Although originally introduced by Sterling and Eyer (49) in relation to explaining the reflex that prevents us from blacking out when we get out of bed

TABLE 1. Interacting adaptive systems of the body

System	Acute response to challenge	Problems associated with chronic activity
Cardiovascular	Maintaining erect posture (avoiding "black-out") Physical exertion	Hypertension, potential for stroke, MI
Metabolic	Activating and maintaining energy reserves, including energy supply to the brain	Obesity, diabetes, atherosclerosis
Immune	Response to pathogens Surveillance for tumors	Inflammatory, autoimmune disorders Immunosuppression
Brain, CNS	Learning, memory Neuroendocrine and autonomic regulation	Neuronal atrophy, death of nerve cells

Mediators involved in modulating these adapative systems consist of hormones (principally, but not confined to, adrenalin and noradrenalin, ACTH and glucocorticoids, insulin and glucagon) and cytokines (produced not only by immune cells but also by the liver and brain).

in the morning, anticipation also implies psychological states such as worry and anxiety as well as cognitive preparation for a coming event (51). Because anticipation can drive the output of mediators (particularly true of hormones such as ACTH, cortisol, and adrenalin), it is likely that states of prolonged anxiety and anticipation can result in allostatic load. However, this is one of many notions that need experimental testing.

STUDIES OF STRESS AND THE SOCIAL ENVIRONMENT

The social environment plays an important role in determining the level of stress hormone secretion. Poor social support, isolation, and conflict lead to elevated stress hormone production (52). In this context it is important to note that studies of health across socioeconomic status have shown gradients not only of mortality but also of indices of morbidity such as blood pressure and abdominal obesity (53–56). Because we have noted that these indices of morbidity are sensitive to excessive activity of stress hormones, it is tempting to suggest that socioeconomic status reflects differences in the social environment that are accompanied by different levels of allostatic load, leading individuals at lower levels of socioeconomic status to express diseases more rapidly.

Although the causes of these gradients are undoubtedly complex, and the individual differences within socioeconomic strata are considerable, it is important that these conditions be investigated because our future as a species is more and more dependent on understanding how our behavior and social organization affects our mental and physical health. In particular, the health consequences of job loss and social instability need to be investigated, along with interventions that may help to alleviate the allostatic load and its impact on physical and mental health. Recent dramatic evidence of increased mortality and morbidity in Eastern Europe, especially in Russia, since the fall of communism (54) also imply connections between the social environment and health.

ROLE OF BEHAVIOR IN DETERMINING THE STRESS RESPONSE AND ALLOSTATIC LOAD

Events that are stressful to one individual may not be stressful to another person, and a primary role is performed by the brain and by behavioral responses in interpreting and responding to events in ways that make them more or less stressful. To help understand the behavioral and physiologic significance of allostasis and allostatic load, Fig. 1 diagrams the multiple factors operating and the general sequence of events that occur under conditions of stress.

On the behavioral side (Fig. 1A), what is important is how the individual interprets and reacts to a challenge, as is explained in the following sequence:

1. The reaction to potentially stressful physical and psychological stimuli is determined in part by the social context in which they occur. The social status

of the individual (e.g., dominant or submissive) undoubtedly plays a significant role.

2. The effect of the potentially stressful stimulus on the individual's "information processor"—the nervous system—is determined in part by the genetic makeup, stage of biologic development, and gender, as well as by past learning and social history. The hippocampus and amygdala are two brain regions that are involved, respectively, in the processing and recall of recent events and the processing of emotionally laden memories (57–59).

3. When processed, the stimulus is perceived as a threat, or not as a threat. If it is a threat, the source of the threat is either known or not known; if not known, the individual becomes highly vigilant and remains physiologically aroused until the decision can be made that it is, or is not, a threat (*dotted arrow in Fig. 1*). If the source is known, then the next question is whether there is a coping response available. If no response is available, then helplessness or hopelessness may result, with altered physiologic responses. If a response is available, it may be a low-cost response and therefore not stressful; or it may be a high-cost response such as aggression or some kind of thrill-seeking or risk-taking behavior, like driving recklessly, that can lead to its own physically or psychologically serious consequences. Smoking or drinking behavior are also high-cost responses. Alternatively, the available response can be blocked or thwarted, leading either to helplessness, frustration, displaced aggression, and some of the same types of high-cost responses. Perceptions of threat and selection of response are also key aspects of the assessment of risk; they are also aspects involved in choosing health-damaging and health-promoting behaviors, including compliance or noncompliance with medical treatments (60,61).

The biologic side of the stress response (Fig. 1B) can be divided into three components: mediators, effectors and disease outcomes, which have already been discussed above in some detail. There are wide individual variations in both behavioral and biologic reactions to stressful situations, depending on genetic factors, gender, developmental stage, and past physiologic and psychological history. Some individuals are highly resilient and cope with stress easily; others are highly vulnerable (62). Much remains to be learned about exactly why there are these individual differences and how they may be recognized. Determining physiologic correlates of the resilient state is especially important as a goal of future investigation.

THE BRAIN AS A TARGET OF STRESS AND STRESS HORMONES

As noted in Fig. 1, the brain interprets what is stressful as well as deciding on a response. Moreover, the brain is a target for the actions of stress and stress hormones, and many of these actions are mediated by the effects of stress hormones to modify gene expression via intracellular stress hormone receptors

(63). According to modern cell and molecular biology, genes are regulated by environmental signals, and this regulation goes on for the entire lifespan. It is a common pattern in development that genes are made available, or unavailable, in different tissues for regulation by hormonal or other inter- and intracellular messengers at a later time.

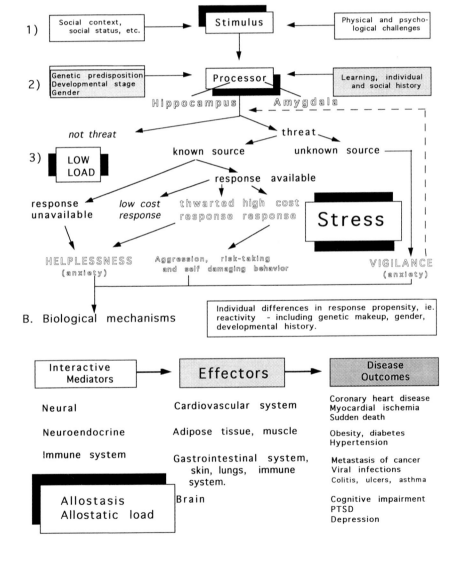

There is an additional constraint in the brain related to the fact that nerve cells for the most part are born early in life and then are not replaced during the rest of the lifespan. Moreover, neural circuits and nerve cell structures have been assumed for many years to be largely static in adult life. Only during development has the brain been regarded as plastic. However, this idea is changing because recent studies have shown in certain adult brain regions the occurrence of cyclic synaptogenesis, atrophy, and elongation of dendrites after stress and hibernation, as well as regulated neurogenesis. Moreover, the adult brain's plastic response to its environment is shaped by events that occur early in brain development, and hormones of the gonads, adrenals, and thyroid gland play an important role in the developmental programming of adult responses.

Developmental Events

Individual differences in brain function and behavior are shaped, in part, by the effects of early experience and by hormones. Sexual differentiation of the brain is an example of a hormonally directed event in which the presence or absence of testosterone during fetal and neonatal life causes brain development to diverge in

---

FIG. 1. Conceptual model of biology and behavior in which responses that are stressful result from the interpretation of, and behavioral and physiologic responses to, environmental challenges that may be stressful to some individuals and less or not stressful to others. **A:** 1. Physical and psychological challenges operate within a social context that includes individual social status. 2. The processing of this information by the nervous system is biased by such factors as genetic predisposition that are operated upon by developmental history, learning, and socioeconomic status; developmental age and gender are also important factors. 3. Interpretation of a stimulus as threatening results in behavioral responses that vary in degree and cost to the individual and are therefore stressful to varying degrees. Nonthreatening situations and low cost responses are not considered stressful because they do not elevate physiologic responses. STRESS refers to responses that are costly in terms of arousal of physiologic systems and elicitation of behaviors that are harmful. Thwarted responses may lead to aggression or result in helplessness that is similar to a response being unavailable. High-cost responses, which may include aggression, are ones that consume energy and further increase risk to further challenge. All of these responses, including vigilance and helplessness, have biologic counterparts, and they feed back to influence further stimulation and processing of that stimulation. **B:** Behavioral responses are accompanied by neural, neuroendocrine, and immune system responses that act on effectors, such as the immune and cardiovascular systems and adipose tissue and muscle, as well as the brain. As noted in the text, chronic or repeated stimulation of these effectors may be due to thwarted or high-cost responses or to anxiety associated with vigilance or helplessness and may lead to allostatic load that, over time, increases risk for pathology and disease. Acute stress more readily precipitates disease when chronic stress has laid a pathophysiologic foundation. Modified with permission (50). Steve Manuck, University of Pittsburgh, deserves major credit for proposing the essential features of this model at the first of two MacArthur Foundation Health and Behavior Network meetings on stress. Participants at these meetings were C. Blanchard, D. Brindley, M. Dallman, J. Kagan, C. Kuhn, D. Kupfer, S. Leibowitz, J. Liebeskind, S. Maier, S. Manuck, K. Matthews, B. McEwen, M. Meaney, J. Muller, M. Rebuffe-Scrive, J. Rodin, R. Rose, R. Sapolsky, A. Selwyn, E. Stellar, J. Weiss, R. Williams, D. York, and M. Zigmond.

two directions: male or female. As a result, male and female brains differ in subtle ways, both in terms of structure and connectivity as well as different responses to hormonal signals (64–67). In other words, besides differences in numbers and distributions of synaptic connections and cell densities within groups of neurons, male and female brains differ in that they use the same hormonal signals—androgens, estrogens, and progestins—to achieve somewhat different consequences in various brain regions. For example, estrogens induce progestin receptors in female brain cells to a greater extent than in the same cells in males, and estrogens induce new synapses to form in female hypothalamus and hippocampus and do not have the same effect in these regions of the male brain (65). Androgens regulate synaptic and dendritic plasticity of specific regions of the male nervous system that are not present in the female, such as the spinal nucleus that innervates muscles of the penis (68).

Likewise, effects of prenatal stressful experiences, or the opposite effects of postnatal handling, appear to involve adrenal and thyroid hormone actions, respectively, that program the brain to have either higher or lower reactivity to novel experiences later in life (69–71). According to this model, once the reactivity of the adrenocortical system is established by events early in life, it is the subsequent actions of the hypothalamo-pituitary-adrenal (HPA) axis in adult life that play a major role in determining the rate of brain and body aging. Increased HPA activity is associated with increased brain aging, whereas the opposite is true of animals with reduced HPA reactivity to novel situations.

The hippocampal formation of the brain turns out to be one of the most vulnerable and plastic of brain regions and one in which many of these processes can be studied, and recent studies have shown that rats that show high levels of stress hormone reactivity show earlier decline of cognitive function as they age (71), whereas rats with a lower stress hormone reactivity have a slower rate of cognitive aging and a reduced loss of hippocampal neurons and function (69,70).

Plasticity of the Adult Brain

The hippocampus is an important brain structure for working and spatial memory in animals and humans, and in episodic memory as well as memory for "context" in which positive and negative experiences have taken place (72,73). The hippocampus is also a vulnerable as well as plastic brain structure in terms of sensitivity to epilepsy, ischemia, head trauma, stress, and aging (31). The hippocampus is also a target brain area for the actions of hormones of the steroid/thyroid hormone family (63,74), which traditionally have been thought to work by regulating gene expression (75). Genomic actions of steroid hormones involve intracellular receptors, whereas nongenomic effects of steroids involve putative cell surface receptors (76). Although this distinction is valid, it does not go far enough in addressing the variety of mechanisms that steroid hormones use to produce their effects on cells. This is because cell surface receptors may signal changes in gene expression, whereas genomic actions sometimes affect neuronal excitability, often doing so quite rapidly (77).

Moreover, steroid hormones and neurotransmitters may operate together to produce effects, and sometimes these effects involve collaborations between groups of neurons. For example, a number of steroid actions in the hippocampus involve the coparticipation of excitatory amino acids (63,74). These interactions are evident for the regulation of synaptogenesis by estradiol in the CA1 pyramidal neurons of the hippocampus (74,78) and for the induction of dendritic atrophy of CA3 neurons by repeated stress as well as by glucocorticoid injections (63,79). Estrogen-regulated synaptogenesis is a cyclic event in the 4- to 5-day estrous cycle of the female rat, whereas stress-induced atrophy of dendrites is slower, taking almost 3 weeks to occur. However, atrophy of dendrites of CA3 pyramidal neurons has been reported as a result of hibernation in squirrels and hamsters, and the reversal of this atrophy has been found 1–2 hours after waking the animals (80; Magarinos and Pevet, unpublished observations). In addition to synaptic and dendritic plasticity, neurogenesis in the adult and developing dentate gyrus is "contained" by adrenal steroids as well as by excitatory amino acids, and these events may play a role in long-term, e.g., seasonal changes in the size and functional capacity of the hippocampus, at least in small mammals (81,82).

In each of these three examples of plasticity in the rat hippocampus, we have found that NMDA receptors are involved (63,74,83). This finding means that the process of neurotransmission interacts with the endocrine system to regulate the structure and function of both developing and adult brain cells. One of the implications of this interaction is that experiences which cause hormone secretion and alter neural activity can govern brain structural and functional changes and they do so synergistically.

THE IMPLICATIONS OF THE PLASTICITY AND VULNERABILITY OF THE BRAIN FOR HEALTH AND DISEASE

Importance of the Brain for Coping with the Environment

The brain, particularly the limbic system including the hippocampus and amygdala (Fig. 1), plays a pivotal role in processing of psychosocial experiences and in determining behavioral responses. Important functions of the hippocampus and amygdala involve episodic memory and memory of emotionally laden events, respectively, and of the context in which they have occurred (57,58). As a result, the health and functional capacity of the brain is an essential factor in human behavior and health because if the brain fails to perform its memory functions adequately or is programmed to over-react to certain stimuli, as in posttraumatic stress disorder, then aberrant or inappropriate behavior is likely to result. One outcome of such failure is captured in the popular adage, "Stress makes you stupid."

Homeostasis, Allostasis, and Allostatic Load

Some of this translates into how the brain processes events and determines if they will trigger a neuroendocrine and neural stress response. We have noted that what is stressful to one individual is not necessarily stressful to another, and prior experience plays an important role (2,50). We hypothesize that allostatic load, meaning wear and tear from chronically elevated activity of physiologic systems involved in adaptation, leads certain individuals down a pathway toward various diseases. Allostatic load is a better description for the sometimes subtle long-term influences that can compromise health than is the term "chronic stress," which evokes images of more dramatic physiologic changes than are actually needed to accelerate disease processes. Some examples of allostatic load can be illustrated by the metabolic system (leading to obesity, diabetes, and atherosclerosis) and by the brain (chronic effects of stress that impair cognition). Here the challenge is to find measures to assess these long-term load factors and their relevance to the progression of pathologic states.

Examples of allostatic load include fat deposition and progression toward diabetes and atherosclerosis, each of which is accelerated by dietary factors and by stressful events (50). Likewise, as noted above, long-term actions of stress hormones cause hippocampal damage and cognitive impairment, and there is evidence for more rapid brain aging in rats that are intrinsically more reactive to novelty by showing greater stress hormone responses (71). In contrast, rats that are less reactive to novelty show evidence of slower brain aging (70). There is now new evidence in humans for allostatic load on human cognitive function with increasing age (84,85). In each of these examples, early experience, as well as the process of sexual differentiation, all play a role in determining an individual's susceptibility.

Importance of Gender Differences

Sex differences in brain structures and mechanisms occur in other brain regions besides the hypothalamus, such as the hippocampus, and they appear to be involved in aspects of cognitive function and other processes that go beyond the reproductive process itself (86), such as the higher incidence of depression in women and of substance abuse in men (87). There are also sex differences in the severity of brain damage resulting from transient ischemia (88) and sex differences in the response of the brain to lesions (89) and to severe, chronic stress (90,91).

Psychosocial Determinants of Health

Psychosocial interactions and social hierarchies appear to be powerful determinants of allostatic load, not only in animal societies but also in human societies, where, as we have noted, there are reported gradients of health and disease across the entire spectrum of socioeconomic status (53). We have noted that psychosocial interactions regulate neuroendocrine function, and social support is related to lower levels of adrenocortical activity (52). The repeated psychosocial stress of being subordinate has been reported in tree shrews to cause dendritic atrophy in the hippocampus and in vervet monkeys to cause actual loss of hippocampal neurons (90,92). Psychosocial stress produces an allostatic load in cynomolgus monkeys that increases atherosclerosis in dominant males in unstable social hierarchies (8) and in subordinate females (93). These are some examples of what further investigation may show is a wide range of psychosocial and environmental influences that create allostatic load and alter the progression toward disease.

Genetic Traits as Risk Factors for Allostatic Load

So far we have only briefly mentioned genotype as a factor involved in determining individual differences. There is no question that the genetic traits are important in this regard, and genes that underlie diabetes, atherosclerosis, obesity, susceptibility to depressive illness, schizophrenia, and Alzheimer's disease increase the risk that experiences and other aspects of the life-long environment will ultimately produce disease. In other words, genetic traits contribute to allostatic load by making it more potent in certain individuals. The example of stress-induced increases in the incidence of type I diabetes in the BB rat is one example of the impact of allostatic load on disease in a genetically susceptible genotype (16). Therefore, it is not sufficient simply to find and describe the genes responsible for diseases, but rather it is necessary to understand how these genes are involved in the pathophysiology of disease and, in particular, how they are regulated.

The life-long interplay between genes and the environment is instrumental in shaping the structure and function of the body, and this now includes the brain as a plastic and ever-changing organ of the body. Key brain areas such as the hippocampus are vital to the processing of information that affect how each individual adapts to and responds to life events, and the response of the brain through its control of endocrine and autonomic function in turn determines the degree of allostatic load that an individual will experience, and this allostatic load in turn works with the intrinsic genetic susceptibility to determine the progression toward declining health.

ACKNOWLEDGMENTS

Research support in the author's laboratory for work described in this article was provided by the National Institutes of Health (R01 Grants MH41256 and NS07080) and from the Health Foundation (New York) and Servier (France). Besides my many laboratory colleagues, past and present, I thank my colleagues at the MacArthur Foundation Health Program and the Socioeconomic Status and Health Planning Initiative (Nancy Adler, Chair; Grace Castellazzo, Administrator; Ralph Horwitz; Karen Matthews; Michael Marmot, Burt Singer) for their contributions to many of the topics covered in this article dealing with health. I also thank Dr. Robert Rose, Director of the MacArthur Foundation Health Program, and Dr. Teresa Seeman of the Andrus Gerontology Center, USC, for their colleagueship and many stimulating discussions. Finally, this article is dedicated to the memory of Eliot Stellar, with whom I wrote the first paper defining allostatic load (50).

REFERENCES

1. Weiner H. *Perturbing the organism: the biology of stressful experiences.* Chicago: University of Chicago Press; 1992.
2. Lazarus RS, Folkman S. *Stress, appraisal and coping.* New York: Springer-Verlag; 1984.
3. Mason JW. Hormones and metabolism: psychological influences on the pituitary-adrenal cortical system. *Recent Prog Hormone Res* 1959;15:345–389.
4. Berg K. Genetics of coronary heart disease. *Prog Med Genet* 1983;5:35–90.
5. Barnett AH, Eff C, Leslie R, Pyke D. Diabetes in identical twins: a study of 200 pairs. *Diabetologia* 1981;20:87–93.
6. Mrazek DA, Klinnert M. In: Ader R, Felten DL, Cohen N, eds. Asthma: psychoneuroimmunologic consideration. *Psychoneuroimmunology* 1991;1013–1033.
7. Muller JE, Tofler G, Stone P. Circadian variation and triggers of onset of acute cardiovascular disease. *Circulation* 1989;79:733–743.
8. Manuck SB, Kaplan JR, Adams MR, Clarkson TB. Studies of psychosocial influences on coronary artery atherosclerosis in cynomologus monkeys. *Health Psychol* 1995;7:113–124.
9. Muldoon M, Kaplan J, Manuck S, Mann J. Effects of a low-fat diet on brain serotonergic responsivity in cynomologus monkey. *Biol Psychol* 1992;31:739–742.
10. Muldoon MF, Manuck SB, Matthews KA. Lowering cholesterol concentrations and mortality: a quantitative review of primary prevention trials. *Br Med J* 1990;301:309–314.
11. Williams RB, Chesney MA. Psychosocial factors and prognosis in established coronary artery disease. The need for research on interventions. *JAMA* 1993;270:1860–1861.
12. Muller JE, Tofler GH. A symposium: triggering and circadian variation of onset of acute cardiovascular disease. *Am J Cardiol* 1990;66:1–70.
13. Brindley DN, Rolland Y. Possible connections between stress, diabetes, obesity, hypertension and altered lipoprotein metabolism that may result in atherosclerosis. *Clin Sci* 1989;77:453–461.
14. Surwit RS, Ross SL, Feinglos MN. In: McCabe P, Schneidermann N, Field TM, Skylar JS, eds. Stress, behavior, and glucose control in diabetes mellitus. *Stress Coping Dis* 1991;97–117.
15. Cox DJ, Gonder-Frederick LA. In: McCabe P, Schneidermann N, Field TM, Skylar JS, eds. The role of stress in diabetes mellitus. *Stress Coping Dis* 1991;118–134.
16. Lehman C, Rodin J, McEwen BS, Brinton R. Impact of environmental stress on the expression of insulin-dependent diabetes mellitus. *Behav Neurosci* 1991;105:241–245.
17. Hagglof B, Bloom L, Dahlquist G, Lonnberg G, Sahlin B. The Swedish childhood diabetes study: indications of severe psychological stress as a risk factor for type I (insulin-dependent) diabetes mellitus in childhood. *Diabetologia* 1991;34:579–583.
18. Duffy LC, Zielezny MA, Marshall JR, et al. Relevance of major stress events as an indicator of disease activity prevalence in inflammatory bowel disease. *Behav Med* 1991;17:101–110.
19. Dhabhar F, McEwen BS. Stress-induced enhancement of antigen-specific cell-mediated immunity. *J Immunol* 1996;156:2608–2615.
20. Spiegel D, Bloom JR, Kraemer HC, Gottheil E. Effect of psychosocial treatment on survival of patients with metastatic breast cancer. *Lancet* 1989;2:888–891.
21. Cohen S, Tyrrell DAJ, Smith AP. Psychological stress and susceptibility to the common cold. *N Engl J Med* 1991;325:606–612.

22. Kiecolt-Glaser JK, Glaser R. Stress and immune function in humans. *Psychoneuroimmunology* 1991;849–865.
23. Winsa B, Adami HO, Bergstrom R, et al. Stressful life events and Graves' disease. *Lancet* 1991; 338:1475–1479.
24. Weiner H. Social and psychobiological factos in autoimmune disease. In: Arder R, Felten OL, Cohen N, eds. *Psychoneuroimmunology.* New York: Academic; 1991:995–1011.
25. Munck A, Guyre PM, Holbrook NJ. Physiological functions of glucocorticoids in stress and their relation to pharmacological actions. *Endocr Rev* 1984;5:25–43.
26. Kvetnansky R, Fukuhara K, Pacak K, Cizza G, Goldstein DS, Kopin IJ. Endogenous glucocorticoids restrain catecholamine synthesis and release at rest and during immobilization stress in rats. *Endocrinology* 1993;133:1411–1419.
27. McEwen BS, Angulo J, Cameron H, et al. Paradoxical effects of adrenal steroids on the brain: protection versus degeneration. *Biol Psychol* 1992;31:177–179.
28. Rose R, Jenkins C, Hurst M, Livingston L, Hall R. Endocrine activity in air traffic controllers at work. I. Characterization of cortisol and growth hormone levels during the day. *Psychoneuroendocrinology* 1982;7:101–111.
29. Rose R, Jenkins C, Hurst M, Herd J, Hall R. Endocrine activity in air traffic controllers at work. II. Biological, psychological and work correlates. *Psychoneuroendocrinology* 1982;7:113–123.
30. Rose R, Jenkins C, Hurst M, Kreger B, Barrett J, Hall R. Endocrine activity in air traffic controllers at work. III. Relationship to physical and psychiatric morbidity. *Psychoneuroendocrinology* 1982; 7:125–134.
31. Sapolsky R. *Stress, the aging brain and the mechanisms of neuron death.* Cambridge, MA: MIT Press; 1992:1–423.
32. Sapolsky R. Stress in the wild. *Sci Am* 1990;262:116–123.
33. Dienstbier R. Arousal and physiological toughness: implications for mental and physical health. *Psychol Rev* 1989;96:84–100.
34. Sapolsky RM. Endorinology al fresco: psychoneuroendocrinology of wild baboons. *Res Prog Horm Res* 1991;48:437–467.
35. Moss HB, Vanyukov MM, Martin CS. Salivary cortisol responses and the risk for substance abuse in prepubertal boys. *Biol Psychiatry* 1995;38:547–555.
36. McKittrick CR, Blanchard DC, Blanchard RJ, McEwen BS, Sakai RR. Serotonin receptor binding in a colony model of chronic social stress. *Biol Psychiatry* 1995;37:383–393.
37. Armario A, Hidalgo J, Giralt M. Evidence that the pituitary-adrenal axis does not cross-adapt to stressors: comparison to other physiological variable. *Neuroendocrinology* 1988;47:162–167.
38. Armario A, Restrepo C, Castellanos JM, Balasch J. Dissociation between adrenocorticotropin and corticosterone responses to restraint after previous exposure to stress. *Life Sci* 1985;36:2085–2092.
39. Kant GJ, Anderson SM, Dhillon GS, Moughey EH. Neuroendocrine correlates of sustained stress: the activity-stress paradigm. *Brain Res Bull* 1996;20:407–414.
40. Watanabe Y, Stone E, McEwen BS. Induction and habituation of c-FOS and ZIF/268 by acute and repeated stressors. *NeuroReport* 1994;5:1321–1324.
41. Watanabe Y, Gould E, McEwen BS. Stress induces atrophy of apical dendrites of hippocampal CA3 neurons. *Brain Res* 1992;588:341–345.
42. Nisenbaum LK, Zigmond MJ, Sved AF, Abercrombie ED. Prior exposure to chronic stress results in enhanced synthesis and release of hippocampla norepinephrine in response to a novel stressor. *J Neurosci* 1995;11:1478–1484.
43. Yehuda R, Resnick H, Kahana B, Giller E. Long-lasting hormonal alterations to extreme stress in humans: normative or maladaptive? *Psychosomat Med* 1993;55:274–286.
44. Brady LS, Smith MA, Gold PW, Herkenham M. Altered expression of hypothalamic neuropeptide mRNAs in food-restricted and food-deprived rats. *Neuroendocrinology* 1990;52:441–447.
45. Pitman DL, Ottenweller JE, Natelson BH. Plasma corticosterone levels during repeated presentation of two intensities of restraint stress: chronic stress and habituation. *Physiol Behav* 1988;43: 47–55.
46. Pitman DL, Ottenweller JE, Natelson BH. Effect of stressor intensity on habituation and sensitization of glucocorticoid responses in rats. *Behav Neurosci* 1990;104:28–36.
47. Kaplan JR, Pettersson K, Manuck SB, Olsson G. Role of sympathoadrenal medullary activation in the initiation and progression of atherosclerosis. *Circulation* 1991;84(suppl 6):VI23–VI32.
48. Marin P, Darin N, Amemiya T, Andersson B, Jern S, Bjorntorp P. Cortisol secretion in relation to body fat distribution in obese premenopausal women. *Metabolism* 1992;41:882–886.

49. Sterling P, Eyer J. Allostasis: a new paradigm to explain arousal pathology. In: Fisher S, Reason J, eds. *Handbook of life stress, cognition and health.* New York: Wiley; 1988:631–651.
50. McEwen BS, Stellar E. Stress and the indvividual: mechanisms leading to disease. *Arch Intern Med* 1993;153:2093–2101.
51. Schulkin J, McEwen BS, Gold PW. Allostasis, amygdala, and anticipatory angst. *Neurosci Biobehav Rev* 1994;18:385–396.
52. Seeman TE, McEwen BS. The impact of social environment characteristics on neuroendocrine regulation. *Psychosomat Med* 1996;58:459–471.
53. Adler N, Boyce WT, Chesney M, Folkman S, Syme L. Socioeconomic inequalities in health: no easy solution. *JAMA* 1993;269:3140–3145.
54. Bobak M, Marmot M. East-West mortality divide and its potential explanations: proposed research agenda. *Br Med J* 1996;312:421–425.
55. Larsson B, Seidell J, Svardsudd K, et al. Obesity, adipose tissue distribution and health in men—the study of men born in 1913. *Appetite* 1989;13:37–44.
56. Lapidus L, Bengtsson C, Hallstrom T, Bjorntorp P. Obesity, adipose tissue distribution and health in women—results from a population study in Gothenburg, Sweden. *Appetite* 1989;12:25–35.
57. Phillips RG, LeDoux JE. Differential contribution of amygdala and hippocampus to cued and contextual fear conditioning. *Behav Neurosci* 1992;106:274–285.
58. Cahill L, Prins B, Weber M, McGaugh JL. Beta-Adrenergic activation and memory for emotional events. *Nature* 1994;371:702–704.
59. Eichenbaum H, Otto T, Cohen NJ. Two functional components of the hippocampal memory system. *Behav Brain Sci* 1994;17:449–518.
60. Redelmeier DA, Rozin P, Kahneman D. Understanding patients' decisions cognitive and emotional perspectives. *JAMA* 1993;270:72–76.
61. Horwitz RJ, Horwitz SM. Adherence to treatment and health outcomes. *Arch Intern Med* 1993;133: 1863–1868.
62. Rutter M. Resilience in the face of adversity. *Br J Psychiatry* 1985;147:598–611.
63. McEwen BS, Albeck D, Cameron H, et al. Stress and the brain: a paradoxical role for adrenal steroids. In: Litwack GD, ed. *Vitamins and hormones.* San Diego: Academic; 1995:371–402.
64. Witelson S. Hand and sex differences in the isthmus and genu of the human corpus callosum. *Brain* 1989;112:799–835.
65. McEwen BS. Our changing ideas about steroid effects on an ever-changing brain. *Semin Neurosci* 1991;3:497–507.
66. Kimura D. Sex differences in the brain. *Sci Am* 1992;267:119–125.
67. Witelson SF, Glezer II, Kigar DL. Women have greater density of neurons in posterior temporal cortex. *J Neurosci* 1995;15:3418–3428.
68. Forger NG, Breedlove SM. Steroid influences on a mammalian neuromuscular system. *Semin Neurosci* 1991;3:459–468.
69. Catalani A, Marinelli M, Scaccianoce S, et al. Progeny of mothers drinking corticosterone during lactation has lower stress-induced corticosterone secretion and better cognitive performance. *Brain Res* 1993;624:209–215.
70. Meaney MJ, Tannenbaum B, Francis D, et al. Early environmental programming hypothalamic-pituitary-adrenal responses to stress. *Semin Neurosci* 1994;6:247–259.
71. Dellu F, Mayo W, Vallee M, LeMoal M, Simon H. Reactivity to novelty during youth as a predictive factor of cognitive impairment in the elderly: a longitudinal study in rats. *Brain Res* 1994;653:51–56.
72. LeDoux JE. In search of an emotional system in the brain: leaping from fear to emotion and consciousness. In: Gazzaniga M, ed. *The cognitive neurosciences.* Cambridge, MA: MIT Press; 1995: 1049–1061.
73. Eichenbaum H, Otto T. The hippocampus—what does it do? *Behav Neural Biol* 1992;57:2–36.
74. McEwen BS, Gould E, Orchinik M, Weiland NG, Woolley CS. Oestrogens and the structural and functional plasticity of neurons: implications for memory, ageing and neurodegenerative processes. *Ciba Found Symp* 1995;191:52–73.
75. Miner JN, Yamamoto KR. Regulatory crosstalk at composite response elements. *Trends Biochem Sci* 1991;16:423–426.
76. McEwen BS. Steroids affect neural activity by acting on the membrane and the genome. *TIPS* 1991;12:141–147.
77. Orchinik M, McEwen BS. Rapid actions in the brain: a critique of genomic and non-genomic mechanisms. In: *Genomic and non-genomic effects of aldosterone.* Boca Raton, FL: CRC Press; 1995: 77–108.

78. Woolley C, McEwen BS. Estradiol regulates hippocampal dendritic spine density via an N-methyl-D-aspartate receptor dependent mechanism. *J Neurosci* 1994;14:7680–7687.
79. Magarinos AM, McEwen BS. Stress-induced atrophy of apical dendrites of hippocampal CA3c neurons: involvement of glucocorticoid secretion and excitatory amino acid receptors. *Neuroscience* 1995;69:89–98.
80. Popov VI, Bocharova LS, Bragin AG. Repeated changes of dendritic morphology in the hippocampus of ground squirrels in the course of hibernation. *Neuroscience* 1992;48:45–51.
81. Gould E, McEwen BS. Neuronal birth and death. *Curr Opin Neurobiol* 1993;3:676–682.
82. Cameron HA, McEwen BS, Gould E. Regulation of adult neurogenesis by excitatory input and NMDA receptor activation in the dentate gyrus. *J Neurosci* 1995;15:4687–4692.
83. Gould E, Cameron HA. The regulation of neuronal birth, migration and death in the rat dentate gyrus. *Dev Neurosci* 1996;18:1–31.
84. Lupien S, Lecours AR, Lussier I, Schwartz G, Nair NPV, Meaney MJ. Basal cortisol levels and cognitive deficits in human aging. *J Neurosci* 1994;14:2893–2903.
85. McEwen BS, Sapolsky RM. Stress and cognitive function. *Curr Opin Neurobiol* 1995;5:205–216.
86. McEwen BS. In: Berg G, Hammer M, eds. Ovarian steroids have diverse effects on brain structure and function. *Mod Management Menopause.* New York: Parthenon; 1994;269–278.
87. Regier DA, Boyd JH, Burke JD, et al. One-month prevalence of mental disorders in the U.S. *Arch Gen Psychiatry* 1988;45:977–986.
88. Hall ED, Pazara KE, Linseman KL. Sex differences in postischemic neuronal necrosis in gerbils. *J Cereb Blood Flow Metabolism* 1991;11:292–298.
89. Morse JK, Dekosky ST, Scheff SW. Neurotrophic effects of steroids on lesion-induced growth in the hippocampus. *Exp Neurol* 1992;118:47–52.
90. Uno H, Ross T, Else J, Suleman M, Sapolsky R. Hippocampal damage associated with prolonged and fatal stress in primates. *J Neurosci* 1989;9:1705–1711.
91. Mizoguchi K, Kunishita T, Chui DH, Tabira T. Stress induces neuronal death in the hippocampus of castrated rats. *Neurosci Lett* 1992;138:157–160.
92. Fuchs E, Uno H, Flugge G. Chronic psychosocial stress induces morphological alterations in hippocampal pyramidal neurons of the tree shrew. *Brain Res* 1995;673:275–282.
93. Shively CA, Clarkson TB. Social status incongruity and coronary artery athersclerosis in female monkeys. *Arteriosclerosis Thrombosis* 1994;14:721–726.

Physiology, Stress, and Malnutrition: Functional
Correlates, Nutritional Intervention,
edited by J.M. Kinney and H.N. Tucker.
Lippincott–Raven Publishers © 1997.

Overview of Brain Metabolism, Sleep, and Stress

Torbjörn Åkerstedt

Department of Public Health Sciences, Karolinska Institute, S-171 77 Stockholm, Sweden.

The emphasis of this part of the text is on sleep: its regulation and function, which to a great extent involves metabolism. The section is composed of six chapters. In the first chapter, Dinges and Chugh's view of sleep as a boost to immune defense and brain restitution (in addition to energy conservation) was discussed. McGinty's chapter focused in detail on the latter and presents sleep as a means of energy conservation and body temperature as a regulator of sleep. Dijk described how sleep and alertness are precisely regulated by circadian and homeostatic factors—both probably linked to metabolism—and introduced light as the circadian phase regulator. Arendt et al. described the detailed role of pineal melatonin in the circadian regulation of the body, as well as the place of food in this regulation. They also described the applied aspects of shift work and time zone travel and how phase adjustment may counteract the associated problems. Kehlet et al. introduced the role of stress as an influence on sleep. McEwen took the stress issue further and integrated it with the psychosocial environment.

Before discussing the chapters in detail, it may be necessary to summarize some basic facts about sleep. All species of homeotherms studied (n = 100) exhibit sleep (1). Human sleep is mainly described through the electroencephalogram (EEG) and contains five different stages (2). Stages 1–4 are merely steps on a frequency/amplitude continuum, with stage 1 being the entrance sleep stage showing 4–7 Hz activity and being superficial in terms of arousability. After a few minutes stage 2 appears, with a lowered frequency and phasic events such as occasional K complexes (high amplitude), single waves, and rapid sleep spindles (14–16 Hz). Stage 2 usually makes up 50% of normal sleep and has markedly decreased arousability. Stages 3 and 4 constitute slow-wave sleep (SWS), characterized by a preponderance of slow (<2 Hz) waves with high amplitude (>75 µV). SWS makes up about 15% of normal sleep, but more if preceded by sleep loss. The progression from stages 1 to 4 is characterized by a gradual decrease in heart rate, blood pressure, respiration, body temperature, metabolic rate, etc. Stages 1–4 make up non–rapid eye movement (non-REM) sleep. The remaining sleep stage is REM sleep, characterized by stage 1–like

131

EEG patterns, rapid eye movements, and markedly reduced muscle tension in the neck, back, and legs. Dream experience is common on awakenings from REM sleep but rare on awakening from non-REM sleep. Today spectral analysis of the EEG expressed as μV^2 is partly replacing the classical sleep stages, yielding the measure "spectral power density" (μV^2) for different frequency bands. SWS corresponds, for example, to spectral power density in the low-frequency delta band (0.5–2.5 Hz).

Across a sleep episode stages 1–4 usually occur in sequence, followed by REM, thus producing a sleep cycle that is repeated every 80–100 minutes. That is, each sleep usually contains five to six sleep cycles. SWS is abundant in the first sleep cycle, somewhat less in the second, and almost absent in the third. Cycles 5 and 6 only rarely contain any SWS at all. Using spectral analysis, the pattern across sleep cycles is one of exponential decrease of spectral density in the slow frequencies (0–4 Hz).

With respect to neural organization, wakefulness seems to be maintained by a number of structures in the reticular activating system (RAS) (3), projecting to the thalamus and neocortex. Input of acetylcholine, serotonin, histamine, and noradrenaline maintain wakefulness and an activated (desynchronized) EEG. Withdrawal of these activating inputs leads to thalamic neuronal hyperpolarization and a synchronized EEG.

The hyperpolarization of thalamic and cortical neurons deinactivates a slow depolarizing calcium current (I_t), leading to spike bursts and a slow potassium-mediated after-hyperpolarizaton (4,5). Thalamocorticothalamic circuits are important for these slow oscillations (6), showing oscillations of their membrane potential (7). EEG slow waves appear when thalamocortical and cortical neurons are synchronized (6,8). The effects of prior wakefulness may occur through hyperpolarization of neurons in thalamocortical and cortical circuits, sleep loss causing more rapid hyperpolarization and synchronization of thalamocorical neurons (9,10). Within sleep, hyperpolarization gradually decreases.

The non-REM–promoting systems include the lower brain stem (11), dorsomedial (DM) thalamus (12), and preoptic–anterior hypothalamic (POAH) area (13). Putative endogenous sleep factors include prostaglandin D2 (PGD2) (14), interleukin-1 (IL-1) and other cytokines (15), uridine (16), and adenosine (17). The latter facilitates slow oscillations of thalamocortical and neocortical neurons by increasing the K^+ conductance, increasing membrane hyperpolarization. Adenosine agonists cause sleep deprivation (SD) like that induced by EEG and caffeine (18), and adenosine A1 and A2 antagonists suppress low-frequency activity and enhance spindle activity (19).

PHYSIOLOGIC CORRELATES OF SLEEP DEPRIVATION

The first chapter of this volume (Dinges and Chugh) focused on total sleep deprivation (TSD) as one means of investigating the function of sleep. Of particular interest is mortality, neurobehavior, neuroendocrinology, immunology, and metabolism. However, starting with areas not responding to SD, we find that one such area is physical performance capacity, although endurance is reduced (20–22). Nor is there any effect on energy substrates (23,24), but glucose tolerance may be decreased (25). Neither do monoamines seem to react to SD (26), although immediate cellular and molecular changes may occur in brain tissue in response to SD in rats (27–29). Remarkably, considering the common-sense notion of SD as stressful, the glucocorticoid stress hormones of the hypothalamic-pituitary-adrenal axis do not seem to show any effects of SD (25,30–36). Thus, SD cannot really be considered a stressor in the classical sense (see chapter by McEwen in this section).

In contrast, the most obvious and well-established effects of SD is found on neurobehavioral variables. Thus, subjective alertness and all types of psychomotor or cognitive performance decrease dramatically across 3 days of sleep loss (20,37–40). On the third day, most tasks are beyond the capacity of the sleep-deprived individual, and sleep onset is always close. Similar effects, although more drawn out, occur in connection with partial SD (41). Other neurobehavioral effects of SD include the improvement of mood in depression (42,43), improvement of motor function in Parkinson's disease (44), and reduction of seizure threshold in patients (45).

The neurophysiologic effects involve increased alpha and theta activity in the wake EEG, reduced amplitude of evoked potentials (46), slowed eye movements (47), decreased sleep latency (48), and reduced glucose metabolism in the prefrontal cortex, thalamus, basal ganglia, limbic system, and brain stem (49,50). The thalamus in particular seems to show reduced metabolism (51). Recovery after SD in humans show markedly increased SWS (52–54), whereas rats show REM increases in recovery (34,55,56). In both cases one night of recovery reverses all changes incurred during SD. Most of the sleep loss induced changes in neurophysiologic parameters have close connections to the corresponding changes in sleepiness and performance discussed above.

If neurobehavior/neurophysiology show clear and dramatic effects of sleep loss, such effects are still reversible. However, prolonged SD also appears to be lethal. This was demonstrated in early studies (57) but was questioned on grounds of methodology (control for deprivation method). However, the recent series of studies by the Rechtschaffen group have supported such claims (58) and extended them in a series of studies with disk-over-water and yoked controls (32). Total sleep deprivation led to death within 2–3 weeks, whereas partial deprivation took twice as long. No specific biochemical or functional change was responsible for death (59), but it was correlated with disturbances of metabolism, thermogenesis, and immunity. The progressive syndrome of TSD includes debilitated appearance, decreased core body temperature, heat-seeking behavior, hyperphagia, weight loss, increased metabolic rate, elevated plasma norepinephrine, decreased plasma thyroxine, and increase in enzymes mediating thermogenesis of brown adipose tissue. Importantly, animals that are permitted to sleep after many days of SD and development of syndrome recover, provided hypothermia has not gone too far (33,34,55).

A second set of evidence for the lethality of SD derives from the (rare) inherited prion protein disease termed "fatal familial insomnia" (12). Insomnia occurs in middle age in the form of gradually decreasing nocturnal sleep. Wakefulness starts to include dreamlike states, reduced environmental contact, sweating, elevated heart rate and blood pressure, slightly increased body temperature, increased norepinephrine, increased adrenocorticotrophic hormone (ACTH; no increase in plasma cortisol), mild brain atrophy, but profound reduction of thalamic metabolism. Further on, ataxia, motor abnormalities, and inability to stand and walk develop. Death occurs after 7–9 months when acute and after 25–30 months when chronic (60), and postmortem brain studies confirm the loss of neurons and reactive astrogliosis in the anteroventral and dorsomedial thalamic nuclei. Some of the effects of this disease are similar to what is seen in sleep-deprived rats.

One key effect of prolonged SD clearly is impaired temperature regulation and failure to conserve energy. This issue is discussed in more detail below in connection with the chapter by McGinty. Another important related observation is diet; malnutrition secondary to heightened catabolism might be the lethal mechanism of SD in rats (33,61), and the state has been compared with that of critically ill patients (61). Rats fed a protein-rich diet during SD had accelerated weight loss, developed skin lesions sooner, and had markedly reduced life spans compared with rats on a fat-rich diet (61). Furthermore, the protein-fed rats maintained a steady food intake, whereas it increased by 250% in the fat-diet group. The latter showed no weight gain or abnormal lipid or glucose levels. Calorie intake during the first 14 days was significantly correlated with the length of survival ($r = 0.84$), whereas protein intake or carbohydrate intake did not. Thus, dietary fat and calorie augmentation was beneficial but did not prevent death, whereas a single night of sleep did (33). However, far less is known about diet and sleep loss in humans.

Among neuroendocrinologic variables, the glucocorticoids did not show any reaction to sleep loss, but thyroid hormones decrease in rats (33,36) (possibly related to energy conservation) and seem to increase in humans (62–64) (who are exposed to a much shorter wake span). Interestingly, administration of thyroxine to sleep-deprived rats increased metabolic rates, elevated body temperature, reduced warming behavior, but reduced life span by 37% (65). Norepinephrine is increased in rats (35) but not in humans (66–69). Again, human SD has normally been short.

Immune function has not shown a clear-cut response to SD (70–72). Bacteremia and septicemia is found in terminal TSD rats (73), although antibiotic treatment does not seem to reverse these conditions (Bergman et al., in press). Increased levels of leukocytes, granulocytes, and monocytes are often found in humans (31,74,75), but markers of infection or illness do not seem to react (31,75).

THERMOREGULATORY CONTROL OF NON-REM SLEEP

McGinty's chapter addresses the energy conservation and temperature regulation of sleep, and reduced body temperature, metabolic rate, and heat loss during sleep are major arguments. Lower body temperature during sleep reduces the use of cellular energy and thus conserves energy. This is similar to what occurs during both torpor (mild temperature reduction) and hibernation, which both occur as extensions of SWS (76). Fasting in pigeons increases non-REM, and the temperature decrease in sleep and the effects are similar in humans (increased SWS) (76).

The lethal effects seen in the previously cited studies of SD in rats (33) seem to involve a dysregulation of temperature control and/or energy exchange. Thus, sleep-deprived rats lose fat, become mildly hypothermic, double their food intake, and prefer very hot environments (77). This is amplified by the observation that hyperthyroid animals die faster (33), that high-calorie diets prolong survival (61), jejunal mitosis is reduced, serum albumin is reduced, and cerebral metabolic rate is reduced.

A supporting argument for the importance of sleep to energy conservation derives from the observation that across mammalian species there is a significant negative relationship between body mass and sleep length (1). This would save energy in small animals, which, while awake, lose more mass-specific heat through the skin due to their low mass/surface ratio. Ectothermic animals sleep but show no (temperature-reducing) SWS (78). They also go in and out of sleep or torpor slowly, whereas the homeotherms do this rapidly and show SWS-like sleep. SWS then would be one way to help mammals and birds compensate for the increased mass-specific metabolic rate required to maintain body temperature.

It should be emphasized that, despite the arguments above, one major explanatory problem for the hypothesis of energy conservation as a reason for sleep is that metabolic rate during sleep is reduced by only 20% in humans (120 Kcal—a slice of bread). This energy saving does not in itself seem to justify such a dramatic behavioral state as sleep (although one may speculate that the downregulation of body temperature serves to help maintain the functioning of regulatory system).

The author suggests that the control of sleep by thermoregulation occurs around the preoptic anterior hypothalamus (POAH) such that when local hypothalamic temperature exceeds the set point, sleep is signaled, the size of the effect being proportional to size of the error signal. The set point is regulated by, for example, the biologic clock situated in the suprachiasmatic nucleus (SCN) (79,80), by sleep onset (81,82), or by a number of other factors. The SCN may trigger night sleep by reducing the set point, causing an error signal signaling sleep (causing a further reduction of set point and a steady reduction of body temperature). The increasing set point after the circadian trough would then reverse this trend. Several experiments of POAH local warming and cooling have shown the expected effects on sleep (83,84) and SWS (85), as well as on the activity of POAH warm- and cold-sensitive neurons. Heating, for example, increases non-REM in rats (86) and humans (87,88) and reduces discharge in posterior hypothalamus (PH) arousal-related neurons (89). Selective activation of POAH warm-sensitive neurons and/or deactivation of cold-sensitive neurons by local POAH warming (2°) facilitates non-REM and delta wave sleep and inhibits wake-promoting PH neurons. Selective deactivation/activation suppresses sleep. The same relationship holds true for spontaneous sleep (90,91).

With respect to the circadian (SCN) regulation of sleep (92,93), the author suggests that it reflects the thermoregulatory hypnogenic control of sleep. Activation of POAH warm-sensitive neurons could mediate both the circadian decrease in body temperature and the onset of sleep later in the evening, perhaps through SCN modulation of the activity or excitability of POAH thermosensitive neurons. The thermoregulatory control of sleep has been turned into a sleep regulatory model using as components the interaction between T_{hypo} and T_{set}. A circadian X oscillator (and a Y for the afternoon dip) affecting T_{hypo} is combined with a homeostatic component representing heat load since awakening. The output would be sleepiness, a large excess of body heat (relative to set point) being associated with increased sleepiness. Although intriguing, the model clearly requires further verification.

LIGHT, CIRCADIAN RHYTHMS, AND THE HOMEOSTATIC REGULATION

Dijk's chapter introduced a detailed discussion of the homeostatic and circadian regulation of sleep. Sleep homeostasis is reflected in the compensation during sleep for variations in prior time awake or prior sleep intensity (94). However, the time lost is never fully recovered (94,95). Instead, recovery occurs through increased amounts of SWS (96–98) and decreased latency (99). Selected deprivation of SWS causes a rebound of SWS.

The effects of prior wakefulness may occur through hyperpolarization of neurons in thalamocortical and cortical circuits, sleep loss causing more rapid hyperpolarization and synchronization of thalamocortical neurons (9,10). Within sleep, hyperpolarization gradually decreases. As discussed in the introduction, one interesting neuromodulator that may be involved is adenosine, which facilitates slow oscillations of thalamocortical and neocortical neurons by increasing the K^+ conductance, increasing membrane hyperpolarization. Adenosine agonists cause SD like that induced by EEG and caffeine (18), and adenosine A1 and A2 antagonists suppress low-frequency activity and enhance spindle activity (19).

The pacemaker function that drives so much of our physiology (including body temperature, cortisol, melatonin, and sleep propensity) is generally believed to be the SCN of the anterior hypothalamus (100–103). The SCN receives light information via the retinohypothalamic tract (RHT) and the geniculate-hypothalamic tract (GHT) (103,104). The SCN also contains high-affinity binding sites (e.g., for melatonin) (105). With respect to output there are yet fewer efferent paths identified than what may be expected from the impact of the SCN on the circadian physiology (105). The pineal hormone melatonin has been identified as having hypnotic effects (106–108) and been shown to lower body temperature.

The synchronization of the circadian system to the solar day occurs through the light/dark cycle (109,110) through phase-dependent sensitivity of the pacemaker. Light at the start of subjective night delays circadian rhythms, and light at the end phase advances the rhythms (111–114), whereas light centered on the circadian temperature trough actually could abolish the rhythm (reduce the amplitude) (115–117). The size of the phase shift is proportional to the cube root of light intensity (118). Exposure to single light pulses in the evening results in an immediate delay in the nocturnal decline in body temperature (119), possibly mediated by the light-induced suppression of melatonin, but not affecting SWS (120).

The regulation of sleep was by some first thought to be mainly due to circadian influences because studies of sleep during isolation showed a roughly 25-hour period (121,122) with a negative serial correlation of sleep length (123). Studies that exploited the phenomenon of spontaneous internal desynchronization (different periods of the body temperature and sleep/wake rhythms) supported this circadian influence (93,124–126), also demonstrating that sleep initiated close to the maximum core temperature rhythm would be long and that initiated on the early rising phase would be short. Sleep initiation was particularly facilitated shortly before the minimum and terminated shortly before the maximum. Homeostatic regulation did not seem to be of any importance, probably because prior time awake and the prior length of sleep were strongly confounded with the circadian phase of sleep.

With the advent of the forced desynchrony protocol (which induced a sleep/wake period too long or short for circadian entrainment, e.g., 28 hours), prior sleep length or time awake could be better controlled and the circadian regulation of sleep was confirmed (92,127–129). It was also found that the maximum circadian drive for sleep (sleep latency) was located close to the minimum of the core body temperature and the minimum drive 8 hours before. That is, normal bedtime occurs close to minimum sleep propensity. It was also observed that the rising phase of the temperature rhythm compensated for the homeostatic fall of alertness which started at awakening.

HORMONES, FOOD, AND SLEEP

There are several important applications of the regulatory mechanisms discussed by Dijk: shift work, jet lag, and other types of disturbed rhythmicity (130,131). The two former are more directly addressed by Arendt, with a particular emphasis on light and melatonin as countermeasures. With respect to sleep, night shift work is associated with 2–4 hours shorter sleep, mainly through reduced stage 2 sleep and stage REM sleep (dream sleep) (132–137). Sleepiness in connection with night shift work is markedly increased with intrusions of patterns of sleep in the EEG (135,138,139). The increased sleepiness has been thought to be related to the higher accident risk in connection with night work (140–142). Shift work is also associated with increased risks of cardiovascular and gastrointestinal disease (143).

The sleep wake disturbances are likely caused by demands for work at the circadian nadir and demands for sleep at the peak (130). Cardiovascular and gastrointestinal problems may have a similar origin. Thus, phase shifts of the circadian rhythm would be one obvious countermeasure. The use of light for phase shifting was discussed by Dijk in his chapter. Arendt introduced the pineal hormone melatonin for the same purpose (144). Melatonin is almost totally suppressed by bright light (113,145) and is phase shifted (146). Melatonin acutely lowers body temperature and alertness and shifts the endogenous clock according to a phase response curve opposite that of light (147–149). It has been used successfully to counteract jet lag (150) and shift work insomnia (151). In the laboratory, melatonin and light may cancel each other out or enforce each other's effect, depending on phase of application (152,153).

Another point brought up by Arendt is the metabolic and pancreatic responses to meals taken during night work. Several studies indicate a circadian variation in glucose tolerance (154–156). The mechanism may be diminished insulin sensitivity and decreased insulin secretion. Diurnal variation in insulinotropic polypeptide, gastrin, and motilin also have been observed (157,158). Interestingly, postprandial glucose and insulin levels were higher and delayed after phase shifting subjects (153). The results indicate that shifted rhythms in night workers may involve metabolic parameters, which may have a bearing on cardiovascular and gastrointestinal disease in shift workers. However, this has yet to be proven.

SURGICAL STRESS: PAIN, SLEEP, AND CONVALESCENCE

The chapter by Kehlet and Rosenberg switches to the effects of acute surgical stress on sleep and recovery. Apart from the pain, disturbed sleep and fatigue are common features of most surgical patients. Surgical injury leads to, among other changes, pronounced endocrine metabolic changes with increased secretion of catabolic hormones and decreased secretion of anabolic hormones (159,160), as well as loss of skeletal muscle (161). The mechanism is partly revealed in the effects of pain reduction, including epidural analgesia (162–164) and minimization of invasive size (165,166), which seem to reduce much of the classical stress reactions.

The profound metabolic and psychologic changes are also likely to disturb sleep and interfere with recovery from surgery. Thus, postsurgery sleep is highly fragmented, with decreased REM and SWS (167–169), and a gradual normalization (170). The pattern of results seems to suggest that the postoperative disturbances are caused by the size of the surgery, pain, surgical stress, and starvation. The clinical implications of postoperative sleep disturbances include sleep-related breathing abnormalities (168,171), as well as increase in death during sleep (172), postoperative mental deterioration (170), and fatigue. The authors suggest that postoperative sleep disturbances are reduced by minimizing invasive surgery techniques, by using stress-reducing neural blockade techniques, and by avoiding opioids in perioperative analgesia. Noise and unnecessary monitoring also should be reduced, and proper nutrition should be instituted earlier than what is common practice. However, long-term studies on the effects of such counter-measures on postoperative complications seem to be lacking.

A related outcome of surgical stress is the profound postoperative fatigue, often related to increased need for sleep, reaching a peak after a week and remaining for several weeks postsurgery (173–175). The mechanism is not clear, but Kehlet et al. argued that the factors involved are postoperative deconditioning of muscle function, catabolism, impaired cardiorespiratory adaptation to exer-cise, immobilization, and semistarvation. The countermeasures would, accord-ingly, include stress reduction, pain relief, early mobilization, and early oral nutrition.

STRESS, BRAIN, AND BEHAVIOR: LIFE-LONG EFFECTS ON HEALTH AND DISEASE

In the last chapter of this section, by McEwen, more general aspects of stress are introduced. The author sees stress as a challenge to an organism's physiologic systems (176) and involves physical (cold, trauma, infection, inflammation, exertion, heat) and psychologic stressors (fear, social defeat, humiliation, disap-pointment, joy). The effects may be pathophysiologic through the translation of experience into responses of the central nervous system, the endocrine system, and the autonomic nervous system. Responses to acute stress often are in syn-ergy with the actions of chronic stress (177,178), and chronic stress involves a long-term strain on homeostatic systems, leading to wear and tear and changes in their operating range.

A number of (correlative) studies have found that stress has a role in myocar-dial infarction (179), atherosclerosis (178), diabetes (180–182), gastrointestinal ulceration (176), inflammatory bowel disease (183), asthma (184), immune system delayed-type hypersensitvity response (185), cancer (group therapy increasing survival time) (186), and common cold infection rate (50% increase) (187). Psychosocial stress increases atherosclerosis in dominant males in unstable social hierarchies (178) and in subordinate females (188).

The key system in the stress response is the hypothalamus-pituitary-adrenal axis with ACTH, glucocorticoids, catecholamines, etc. Increased activity in this system enhances immune system activity (185) but also counteracts inflammation (189). The ability to turn off the stress response is also important, as found in suc-cessful air traffic controllers (190–192). On the other hand, dampened stress responses are seen in boys at risk for substance abuse (193), in the clinically anx-ious (194), and in subordinate rats (195). Also, repeated stress enhances stress responsiveness to novel stressors (196–198) but reduces it to repetition of the same stressor (194,198–200).

The authors also bring up the new concept of allostasis, that is, long-term changes in stress system activity in order to maintain stability through change (201,202). Such allostatic load (chronic stress) involves long-term wear and tear leading to disease. One important contributor to allostatic load is anticipation, which can drive the stress system (203) for long periods.

The social environment (support, conflict, submissive role, etc.) plays an important role in modifying the stress responses (204–206). The effect of the perceived challenge on the nervous system is modified by genetics, biologic development, gender, past learning, etc., and the hippocampus and amygdala in particular are involved in the processing of prior emotional learning (207,208). In the next step a perceived threat causes extreme arousal if the source is not known. If the source is known but no coping mechanism is available, then helplessness and its physiologic changes may follow. If coping is possible, it may involve negative behaviors such as drug intake, violence, etc. The biologic responses involve the physiologic and pathophysiologic changes discussed above.

It is important to remember that the brain is a target for stress hormones (209). Early in fetal or neonatal life, testosterone and estrogen can cause subtle changes in brain development (210–212). Also pre- or neonatal stress may affect the reactivity to novel experiences in later life (213,214), and increased hypothalamic, pituitary-adrenal activity later in life accelerates brain aging in rats and humans (213–215). The hippocampus may be particularly implicated and is a target area for steroid/thyroid hormones (209), and has demonstrated dendritic atrophy in tree shrews and loss of hippocampal neurons in monkeys (216,217).

SUMMARY

This section has addressed several key points concerning sleep, perhaps the most important being that we still do not understand exactly why we sleep. This remains one of the major questions to resolve in biology. On the other hand, it is obvious that sleep is essential for long-term survival and for short-term functioning. The links, as delineated in this section, suggest energy conservation as one central function of sleep, perhaps also build-up of central nervous system cell energy levels, whereas the immune system responses to sleep loss, although often dramatic, are difficult to interpret. Energy conservation or strengthening of the regulatory system for temperature is also implied by the poikilothermic state during REM sleep.

The central role of sleep is also suggested by its remarkably elegant regulation by a combination of circadian and homeostatic regulation, presumably to assure that the organism obtains an optimal balance of sleep and waking, with consideration of our ecologic niche, that is, our unsuitability for life in the darkness of the night. Logically, the circadian phasing of our physiology and psychology is influenced by lighting, and melatonin and body temperature appear to function as key mediators of circadian influence. It is also suggested that one key parameter in both circadian and homeostatic regulation is the difference between hypothalamic temperature and the temperature set point, excessive body heat requiring sleep for efficient return to set point.

The applied aspects of sleep regulation and function are particularly obvious in individuals on an abnormal sleep/wake schedule, such as shift workers and time zone travelers; sleep and alertness are often grossly impaired due to the conflict between the required time of activity and the setting of circadian phase and homeostasis. Some of the countermeasures may be strategic use of light or melatonin in order to rephase rhythms. Use of both may either enhance adjustment or prevent it, depending on their relative phase. Possibly, the circadian phasing is of importance also with respect to the metabolic response to nutritional substances. Abnormally timed food intake in night workers or jet travelers may thus have unwanted metabolic consequences, possibly related to cardiovascular and gastrointestinal disturbances.

One important source of disturbed sleep is surgical stress. Direct stress effects and pain affect sleep, and disturbed sleep in turn may be related to the outcome of the surgical procedure. Immobility, starvation, and environmental disturbances also may be involved. Finally, stress of a physical or psychosocial nature profoundly affects our physiology and as a consequence interferes with sleep. Long-term stress may lead to chronic upregulation (allostasis) of the stress response axis, presumably leading to several of the stress-related pathologies (cardiovascular diseases, asthma, etc.).

REFERENCES

1. Zepelin H. Mammalian sleep. In: Kryger M, Roth T, Dement W, eds. *Principles and practice of sleep medicine*. Philadelphia: WB Saunders; 1994:69–80.
2. Rechtschaffen A, Kales A, eds. *A manual of standardized terminology, techniques and scoring system for sleep stages of human subjects*. Bethesda: US Department of Health, Education and Welfare, Public Health Service; 1968.
3. Morruzzi G, Magoun HW. Brain stem reticular formation and activation of the EEG. *Electroencephalogr Clin Neurophysiol* 1949;1:445–473.
4. Hirsch J, Fourment A, Marc M. Sleep-related variations of membrane potential in the lateral geniculate body relay neurons of the cat. *Brain Res* 1983;259:308–312.
5. Steriade M, McCormick DA, Sejnowski TJ. Thalamocortical oscillations in the sleeping and aroused brain. *Science* 1993;262:679–685.
6. Steriade M, Curro Dossi R, Nunez A. Network modulation of a slow intrinsic oscillation of cat thalamocortical neurons implicated in sleep delta waves: cortically induced synchronization and brainstem cholinergic suppression. *J Neurosci* 1991;11:3200–3217.
7. Curro Dossi R, Nunez A, Steriade M. Electrophysiology of a slow (0.5–4 Hz) intrinsic oscillation of cat thalamocortical neurones in vivo. *J Physiol* 1992;447:215–234.
8. Soltesz I, Crunelli V. A role for low-frequency, rhythmic synaptic potentials in the synchronization of cat thalomocortical cells. *J Physiol* 1992;457:257–276.
9. Dijk D-J, Hayes B, Czeisler CA. Dynamics of electroencephalographic sleep spindles and slow wave activity in men: effect of sleep deprivation. *Brain Res* 1993;626:190–199.
10. Lancel M, Van Riezen H, Glatt A. The time course of sigma activity and slow wave activity during non-REMS in cortical and thalamic EEG of the cat during baseline and after 12 hour of wakefulness. *Brain Res* 1992;596:285–295.
11. Jones B. Basic mechanisms of sleep-wake states. In: Kryger M, Roth T, Dement W, eds. *Principles and practice of sleep medicine*. Philadelphia: WB Saunders; 1994:145–162.

12. Lugaresi E, Medori R, Baruzzi A, et al. Fatal familial insomnia and dysautonomia with selective degeneration of thalamic nuclei. *N Engl J Med* 1986;315:997–1003.
13. McGinty D, Szymusiak R. Keeping cool: a hypothesis about the mechanisms and functions of slow wave sleep. *Trends Neurosci* 1990;13:480–487.
14. Matsumura HNT, Osaka T. Prostaglandin D2-sensitive, sleep-promoting zone defined in the ventral surface of the rostral basal forebrain. *Proc Natl Acad Sci USA* 1994;91:11998–12002.
15. Kreuger J, Opp M, Toth L, Johannsen L, Cady A. Somnogenic cytokines and models concerning their effects on sleep. *Yale J Biol Med* 1990;63:157–172.
16. Ticho S, Radulovacki M. Role of adenosine in sleep and temperature regulation in the preoptic area of rats. *Pharmacol Biochem Behav* 1991;40:33–40.
17. Kimura-Takeuchi M, Inoue S. Lateral preoptic lesions void slow-wave sleep enhanced by uridine but not by muramyl dipeptide in rats. *Neurosci Lett* 1993;157:17–20.
18. Benington J, Kodali S, Heller H. Stimulation of A1 adenosine receptors mimics the electroencephalographic effects of sleep deprivation. *Brain Res* 1995;692:79–85.
19. Landolt H-P, Werth E, Borbély A, Dijk D-J. Caffeine intake (200 mg) in the morning affects human sleep and EEG power spectra at night. *Brain Res* 1995;675:67–74.
20. Horne J, eds. *Why we sleep—the functions of sleep in humans and other mammals.* Oxford, England: University Press; 1988.
21. Rodgers C, Paterson D, Cunningham D. Sleep deprivation: effects on work capacity, self-paced walking, contractile properties and perceived exertion. *Sleep* 1995;18:30–38.
22. Angus RG, Heslegrave RJ, Myles WS. Effects of prolonged sleep deprivation, with and without chronic physical exercise, on mood and performance. *Psychophysiology* 1985;22:276–282.
23. Symons JD, Vanhelder T, Myles WS. Physical performance and physiological responses following 60 hours of sleep deprivation. *Med Sci Sports Exerc* 1988;20:374–380.
24. Martin B, Bender B, Chen H. Stress hormonal response to exercise after sleep loss. *Eur J Appl Physiol* 1986;55:210–214.
25. VanHelder T, Radomski M. Sleep deprivation and the effect on exercise performance. *Sports Med* 1989;7:235–247.
26. Bergmann B, Seidan L, Landis C. Sleep deprivation in the rat. XVIII. Regional brain levels of monoamines and their metabolites. *Sleep* 1994;17:583–589.
27. Feng P, Bergmann B, Rechtschaffen A. Effect of total sleep deprivation on neuronal ultrastructure in the rat. *Sleep Res* 1996;25:466.
28. O'Hara B, Young K, Watson F. Immediate early gene expression in brain during sleep deprivation: preliminary observations. *Sleep* 1993;16:1–7.
29. Neuner-Jehle M, Rhyner T, Borbély A. Sleep deprivation differentially alters the mRNA and protein levels of neurogranin in rat brain. *Brain Res* 1995;685:143–153.
30. Kollar EJ, Slater GR, Palmer JO, Docter RF, Mandell AJ. Stress in subjects undergoing sleep deprivation. *Psychosom Med* 1966;28:101–113.
31. Dinges D, Douglas S, Zaugg L. Leukocytosis and natural killer cell function parallel neurobehavioral fatigue induced by 64 hours of sleep deprivation. *J Clin Invest* 1994;93:1930–1939.
32. Rechtschaffen A, Gilliland BM, Winter JB. Physiological correlates of prolonged sleep deprivation in rats. *Science* 1983;221:182–184.
33. Rechtschaffen A, Bergmann BM. Sleep deprivation in the rat by the disk-over-water method. *Behav Brain Res* 1995;65:55–63.
34. Everson CA, Gilliland MA, Kushida CA. Sleep deprivation in the rat. IX. Recovery. *Sleep* 1989;12:60–67.
35. Bergmann B, Everson C, Kushida C. Sleep deprivation in the rat. V. Energy use and mediation. *Sleep* 1989;12:31–41.
36. Everson C, Reed H. Pituitary and peripheral thyroid hormone responses to thyrotropin-releasing hormone during sustained sleep deprivation in freely moving rats. *Endocrinology* 1995;136:1426–1434.
37. Dinges D, Kribbs N. Performing while sleepy: effects of experimentally induced sleepiness. In: Monk T, ed. *Sleep, sleepiness and performance.* Chichester, England: Wiley; 1991:97–128.
38. Johnson LC. Sleep deprivation and performance. In: Webb WB, eds. *Biological rhythms, sleep and performance.* Chichester, England: Wiley; 1982:111–141.
39. Dinges DF. Probing the limits of functional capability: the effects of sleep loss on short-duration tasks. In: Broughton RJ, Ogilvie RD, eds. *Sleep, arousal, and performance.* Boston: Birkhauser; 1992:176–188.

40. Bonnet MH. Sleep deprivation. In: Kryger M, Roth T, Dement W, eds. *Principles and practice of sleep medicine.* Philadelphia: WB Saunders; 1994:50–67.
41. Carskadon MA, Roth T. Sleep restriction. In: Monk T, ed. *Sleep, sleepiness and performance.* New York: Wiley; 1991:155–167.
42. Ebert D, Kaschka WP, Loew T, Beck G. Cortisol and beta-endorphin responses to sleep deprivation in major depression—the hyperarousal theories of sleep deprivation. *Neuropsychobiology* 1994;29: 64–68.
43. Wehr TA. Effects of sleep and wakefulness on depression and mania. In: Montplaisir J, Godbout R, eds. *Sleep and biological rhythms.* London: Oxford Press; 1991.
44. Riest C, Sokolski KN, Chen C. The effect of sleep deprivation on motor impairment and retinal adaptation in Parkinson's disease. *Prog Neuropsychopharmacol Biol Psychiatry* 1995;19:445–454.
45. Tartara A, Moglia A, Manni R, Corbellini C. EEG findings and sleep deprivation. *Eur Neurol* 1980;19:330–334.
46. Schlesinger A, Dahl R, Redfern MJR. Sleep deprivation impairs the control of postural balance while performing a cognitive task. *Sleep Res* 1996;25:477.
47. Naitoh P. Sleep deprivation in human subjects: a reappraisal. *Waking Sleeping* 1976;1:53–60.
48. Carskadon M, Dement W. Daytime sleepiness: quatification of a behavioral state. *Neurosci Biobehav Review* 1987;11:307–317.
49. Wu J, Gillin J, Buchsbaum M. The effect of sleep deprivation on cerebral glucose metabolic rate in normal humans assessed with positron emission tomography. *Sleep* 1991;14:155–162.
50. Thomas M, Sing H, Belenky G. Cerebral glucose utilization during task performance and prolonged sleep loss. *J Cereb Blood Flow Metab* 1993;13:5531.
51. Thakkar M, Mallick B. Rapid eye movement sleep-deprivation–induced changes in glucose metabolic enzymes in rat brain. *Sleep* 1993;16:691–694.
52. Dinges DF. Differential effects of prior wakefulness and circadian phase on nap sleep. *Electroencephalogr Clin Neurophysiol* 1986;64:224–227.
53. Borbély AA, Baumann F, Brandeis D, Strauch I, Lehmann D. Sleep deprivation: effects on sleep stages and EEG power density in man. *Electroencephalogr Clin Neurophysiol* 1981;51:483–493.
54. Achermann P, Dijk D, Brunner D, Borbély A. A model of human sleep homeostasis based on EEG slow-wave activity: quantitative comparison of data and simulations. *Brain Res Bull* 1993;31: 97–113.
55. Tsai L, Bergmann BM, Rechschaffen A. Sleep deprivation in the rat. XVI. Effects in a light-dark cycle. *Sleep* 1992;15:537–544.
56. Feinberg I, March J. Observations on delta homeostasis, the one-stimulus models of non-REM-REM alernation and the nuerobiologic implications of experimental dream studies. *Behav Brain Res* 1995; 69:97–108.
57. Kleitman N, eds. *Sleep and wakefulness.* Chicago: University of Chicago Press; 1963.
58. Montagna P, Cortelli P, Tinuper P. Fatal familial insomnia: a disease that emphasizes the role of the thalamus in regulation of sleep and vegetative functions. In: Guilleminault C, Lugaresi E, Montagna P, Gambetti P, eds. *Fatal familial insomnia: inherited prion diseases, sleep, and the thalamus.* New York: Raven; 1994:1–14.
59. Gilliland MA, Wold L, Wollmann R. Pathology in sleep deprived rats is not reflected in histologic abnormalities. *Sleep Res* 1984;13:190.
60. Montagna P, Cortelli P, Gambetti P, Lugaresi ER. Fatal familial insomnia: sleep, neuroendocrine and vegetative alterations. *Adv Neuroimmunol* 1995;5:13–21.
61. Everson C, Wehr T. Nutritional and metabolic adaptations to prolonged slepp deprivation in the rat. *Am J Physiol* 1993;264:R376–R387.
62. Parker D, Rossman L, Pekary A, Hershman J. Effect of 64-hour sleep deprivation on the circadian waveform of thyrotropin (YSH): further evidence of sleep-related inhibition of THS release. *J Clin Endocrinol Metab* 1987;64:157–161.
63. Allan J, Czeisler C. Persistence of the circadian thyrotropin rhythm under constant conditions and after light-induced shifts of circadian phase. *J Clin Endocrinol Metab* 1994;79:508–512.
64. Gary K, Winokur A, Douglas S. Total sleep deprivation and the thyroid axis: effects of sleep and waking activity. *Aviat Space Environ Med* 1996;67:189–203.
65. Bergmann B, Gilliland M, Balzano S. Sleep deprivation in the rat: XIX. effects of thyroxine administration. *Sleep* 1995;18:317–324.
66. Palmblad J, Åkerstedt T, Fröberg J, Melander A, von Schenk H. Thyroid and adrenomedullary reactions during sleep deprivation. *Acta Endocrinol* 1979;90:233–239.

67. Fröberg JE, Karlsson C-G, Levi L, Lidberg L. Circadian rhythms of catecholamine excretion, shooting range performance and self-ratings of fatigue during sleep deprivation. *Biol Psychol* 1975;2: 175–188.
68. Åkerstedt T, Fröberg J. Sleep, stress and sleep deprivation in relation to circadian rhythms in catecholamine excretion. *Biol Psychol* 1979;8:69–80.
69. Candito M, Pringuey D, Jacomet Y. Circadian rhythm in plasma noradrenaline of healthy sleep-deprived subjects. *Chronobiol Int* 1992;9:444–447.
70. Toth L, Opp M, Mao L. Somnogenic effects of sleep deprivation and Escherichia coli inoculation in rabbits. *J Sleep Res* 1995;4:30–40.
71. Brown R, Pang G, Husband A. Sleep deprivation and the immune response to pathogenic and non-pathogenic antigens. In: Husband A, eds. *Behaviour and immunity*. Boca Raton, FL: CRC Press; 1992:127–133.
72. Brown R, Price R, King M, Husband A. Interleukin-1β and muramyl dipeptide can prevent decreased antibody response associated with sleep deprivation. *Brain Behav Immun* 1989;3: 320–330.
73. Everson C. Sustained sleep deprivation impairs host defense. *Am J Physiol* 1993;265:R1148–R1154.
74. Kuhn E, Brodan V, Brodanova M, Rysanek K. Metabolic reflection of sleep deprivation. *Activitas Nervosa Superior* 1969;11:165–174.
75. Dinges D, Douglas S, Hamarman S. Sleep deprivation and human immune function. *Adv Neuroimmunol* 1995;5:97–110.
76. Berger R, Phillips N. Energy conservation and sleep. *Behav Brain Res* 1995;69:65–73.
77. Prete FR, Bergmann BM, Holtzman P, Obermeyer W, Rechtschaffen A. Sleep deprivation in the rat. XII. Effect on ambient temperature choice. *Sleep* 1991;14:109–115.
78. McGinty D. Amphibians. In: Carskadon M, Rechtschaffen A, Richardson G, Roth T, Siegel J, eds. *Encyclopedia of sleep and dreaming*. New York: MacMillan; 1993:34–35.
79. Edgar D, Dement W, Fuller C. Effect of SCN lesions on sleep in squirrel monkeys: evidence for opponent processes in sleep-wake regulation. *J Neurosci* 1993;13:1065–1079.
80. Ibuka N, Kawamura H. Loss of circadian rhythm in sleep-wakefulness cycle in the rat by suprachiasmatic nucleus lesions. *Brain Res* 1975;96:76–81.
81. Glotzbach S, Heller H. Central nervous regulation of body temperature during sleep. *Science* 1976;194:537–539.
82. Parmeggiani P, Franzini C, Lenzi P, Zamboni G. Threshold of respiratory responses to preoptic heating during sleep in freely moving cats. *Brain Res* 1973;52:189–201.
83. Glotzbach S, Heller H. Temperature regulation. In: Kryger MH, Roth T, Dement WC, eds. *Principles and practice of sleep medicine*. Philadelphia: WB Saunders; 1994:260–276.
84. Proppe D, Gale C. Endocrine thermoregulatory responses to local hypothalamic warming in unanesthetized baboons. *Am J Physiol* 1970;219:202–207.
85. McGinty D, Szymusiak R, Thomson D. Preoptic/anterior hypothalamic warming increases EEG delta frequency activity within non-rapid eye movement sleep. *Brain Res* 1994;667:273–277.
86. Morairty S, Szymusiak RDT, McGinty D. Selective increases in nonrapid eye movement sleep following whole body heating in rats. *Brain Res* 1993;617:10–16.
87. Horne JA, Reid AJ. Night-time sleep EEG changes following body heating in a warm bath. *Electroencephalogr Clin Neurophysiol* 1985;60:154–157.
88. Jordan J, Montgomery I, Trinder J. The effect of afternoon body heating on body temperature and slow wave sleep. *Psychophysiology* 1990;27:560–566.
89. Krilowicz B, Szymusiak R, McGinty D. Regulation of posterior lateral hypothalamic arousal related neuronal discharge by preoptic anterior hypothalamic warming. *Brain Res* 1995;668:30–38.
90. Alam MN, McGinty DS R. Neuronal discharge of preoptic/anterior hypothalamic neurons: relation to non-REM sleep. *Am J Physiol* 1995;269:R1240–R1249.
91. Alam MN, Szymusiak R, Steininger T, McGinty D. Discharge during wakefulness and sleep of rat preoptic/anterior hypothalamic (POAH) neurons. *Soc Neurol Abstr* 1995;21:955.
92. Dijk D-J, Czeisler CA. Contribution of the circadian pacemaker and the sleep homeostat to sleep propensity, sleep structure, electroencephalographic slow waves, and sleep spindle activity in humans. *J Neurosci* 1995;15:3526–3538.
93. Czeisler CA, Weitzman ED, Moore-Ede MC, Zimmerman JC, Knauer RS. Human sleep: its duration and organization depend on its circadian phase. *Science* 1980;210:1264–1267.
94. Borbély A. Sleep homeostasis and models of sleep regulation. In: Kryger M, Roth T, Dement W, eds. *Principles and practice of sleep medicine*. Philadelphia: WB Saunders; 1994:309–320.
95. Rosenthal L, Roehrs TA, Rosen A, Roth T. Level of sleepiness and total sleep time following various time in bed conditions. *Sleep* 1993;16:226–232.

96. Dijk DJ, Beersma DGM, Daan S. EEG power density during nap sleep: reflection of an hourglass measuring the duration of prior wakefulness. *J Biol Rhythms* 1987;3:207–219.

97. Dijk DJ, Brunner DP, Beersma DGM, Borbély AA. Electroencephalogram power density and slow wave sleep as a function of prior waking and circadian phase. *Sleep* 1990;13:430–440.

98. Brunner DP, Dijk D-J, Tobler I, Borbély AA. Effect of partial sleep deprivation on sleep stages and EEG power spectra: evidence for non-REM and REM sleep homeostasis. *Electroencephalogr Clin Neurophysiol* 1990;75:492–499.

99. Carskadon MA, Dement WC. Effects of total sleep loss on sleep tendency. *Percept Motor Skills* 1979;48:495–506.

100. Klein DC, Morre RY, Reppert SM, eds. *Suprachiasmatic nucleus: the mind's clock.* New York: Oxford University Press; 1991.

101 Moore R, Eichler V. Loss of circadian adrenal corticosterone rhythm following suprachiasmatic nucleus lesions in the rat. *Brain Res* 1972;42:201–206.

102. Welsh D, Logothetis D, Meister M, Reppert S. Individual neurons dissociated from rat suprachiasmatic nucleus express independently phase circadian firing rhythms,. *Neuron* 1995;14:697–706.

103. Groos G, Meijer J. Effects of illumination on suprachiasmatic nucleus electrical discharge. *Ann N Y Acad Sci* 1985;153:134–146.

104. Sadun A, Schaechter J, Smith L. A retinohypothalamic pathway in man: light mediation of circadian rhtyhms. *Brain Res* 1984;302:371–377.

105. Reppert S, Weaver D, Rivkess S, Stopa E. Putative melatonin receptors in a human biological clock. *Science* 1982;42:78–81.

106. Dollins A, Zhdahova IV, Wurtman R, Lynch H, Denmg M. Effect of inducing nocturnal serum melatonin concentration in daytime sleep, mood, body temperature and performance. *Proc Natl Acad Sci U S A* 1994;91:199–209.

107. Dijk D-J, Roth C, Laandolt H, et al. Melatonin effect on daytime sleep in men: suppression of EEG low-frequency activity and an hancement of spindle frequency activity. *Neurosci Lett* 1995;201:13–16.

108. Cajochen C, Krauchi K, Von Arx M, Mori DGP, Wirz-Justice A. Daytime melatonin administration enhances sleepiness and theta/alpha activity in the waking EEG. *Neurosci Lett* 1996;207:209–213.

109. Czeisler CA. The effect of light on the human circadian pacemaker. In: Chadwick DJ, Ackrill K, eds. *Circadian clocks and their adjustment.* Chichester: Ciba/Foundation. 1995;254–302.

110. Dijk D-J, Boulos Z, Eastman C, Lewy A, Campbell S, Terman M. Light treatment for sleep disorders: consensus report. II: Basic properties of circadian physiology and sleep regulation. *J Biol Rhythms* 1995;10:113–125.

111. Czeisler CA, Allan JS, Strogatz SH, et al. Bright light resets the human circadian pacemaker independent of the timing of the sleep-wake cycle. *Science* 1986;233:667–671.

112. Czeisler CA, Kronauer RE, Allan JS, et al. Bright light induction of strong (type 0) resetting of the human circadian pacemaker. *Science* 1989;244:1328–1333.

113. Lewy A, Sack R, Singer C. Immediate and delayed effects of bright light on human melatonin production: shifting "dawn" and "dusk" shifts the dim light melatonin onset (DLMO). *Ann N Y Acad Sci* 1985;453:253–259.

114. Rosenthal NE, Joseph-Vanderpool JR, Levendosky AA, et al. Phase-shifting effects of bright morning light as treatment for delayed sleep phase syndrome. *Sleep* 1990;13:354–361.

115. Jewett E, Kronauer RE, Czeisler CA. Light-induced suppression of endogenous circadian amplitude in humans. *Nature* 1991;350:59–62.

116. Kronauer RE. A quantitative model for the effects of light on the amplitude and phase of the deep circadian pacemaker, based on human data. In: Horne J, eds. *Sleep '90.* Bochum: Pontenagel Press;1990:306–309.

117. Klerman E, Dijk D-J, Kronauer R, Czeisler C. Simulations of light effects on the human circadian pacemaker: implications for assessment of intrinsic period. *Am J Physiol* 1996; 270:R271–R282.

118. Boivin D, Duffy J, Kronauer R, Czeisler C. Dose-response relationships for resetting of human circadian clock by light. *Nature* 1996;379:540–542.

119. Dijk D-J, Cajochen C, Borbély A. Effect of a single 3-h exposure to bright light on core body temperature and sleep in humans. *Neurosci Lett* 1991;121:59–62.

120. Cajochen C, Dijk D-J, Borbély A. Dynamics of EEG slow-wave activity and core body temperature in human sleep after exposure to bright light. *Sleep* 1992;15:337–343.

121. Aschoff J, Wever R. Spontanperiodik des Menschen bei Ausschlus aller Zeitgeber. *Die Naturwissenschaften* 1962;49:337–342.

122. Aschoff J. Circadian rhythms in man. *Science* 1965;148:1427–1432.

123. Wever RA. Properties of human sleep-wake cycles: parameters of internally synchronized free-running rhythms. *Sleep* 1984;7:27–51.
124. Aschoff J, Gerecke U, Wever R. Desynchronization of human circadian rhythms. *Jpn J Physiol* 1967;17:450–457.
125. Zulley J, Wever R, Aschoff J. The dependence of onset and duration of sleep on the circadian rhythm of rectal temperature. *Pflugers Arch* 1981;391:314–318.
126. Strogatz SH, Kronauer RE, Czeisler CA. Circadian regulation dominates homeostatic control of sleep length and prior wake length in humans. *Sleep* 1986;9:353–364.
127. Dijk DJ, Duffy JF, Czeisler CA. Circadian and sleep-wake dependent aspects of subjective alertness and cognitive performance. *J Sleep Res* 1992;1:112–117.
128. Dijk DJ, Czeisler CA. Paradoxical timing of the circadian rhythm of sleep propensity serves to consolidate sleep and wakefulness in humans. *Neurosci Lett* 1994;166:63–68.
129. Czeisler C, Dijk D-J, Duffy J. Entrained phase of the circadian pacemaker serves to stabilizes alewrtness and performance throughout the habitual waking day. In: Ogilvie R, Harsh J, eds. *Sleep onset normal and abnormal processes.* Washington, DC: American Psychological Association; 1995:89–110.
130. Åkerstedt T. Work hours, sleepiness and the mechanism. *J Sleep Res* 1995;4(suppl 2):15–22.
131. Samel A, Wegmann HM, Vejvoda M. Jet lag and sleepiness in aircrew. *J Sleep Res* 1995;4(suppl 2):30–36.
132. Foret J, Benoit O. Shiftwork: the level of adjustment to schdule reversal assessed by a sleep study. *Waking Sleeping* 1978;2:107–112.
133. Torsvall L, Åkerstedt T, Gillberg M. Age, sleep and irregular work hours: a field study with EEG recording, catecholamine excretion, and self-ratings. *Scand J Work Environ Health* 1981;7:196–203.
134. Tilley AJ, Wilkinson RT, Drud M. Night and day shifts compared in terms of the quality and quantity of sleep recorded in the home and performance measured at work: a pilot study. In: Reinberg A, Vieux N, Andlauer P, eds. *Night and shift work. Biological and social aspects.* Oxford: Pergamon; 1981:187–196.
135. Torsvall L, Åkerstedt T, Gillander K, Knutsson A. Sleep on the night shift: 24-hour EEG monitoring of spontaneous sleep/wake behavior. *Psychophysiology* 1989;26:352–358.
136. Åkerstedt T, Arnetz BB, Anderzén I. Physicians during and following night call duty—36 hour ambulatory recording of sleep. *Electroencephalogr Clin Neurophysiol* 1990;76:193–196.
137. Åkerstedt T, Kecklund G, Knutsson A. Spectral analysis of sleep electroencephalography in rotating three-shift work. *Scand J Work Environ Health* 1991;17:330–336.
138. Torsvall L, Åkerstedt T. Sleepiness on the job: continuously measured EEG changes in train drivers. *Electroencephalogr Clin Neurophysiol* 1987;66:502–511.
139. Kecklund G, Åkerstedt T. Sleepiness in long distance truck driving: an ambulatory EEG study of night driving. *Ergonomics* 1993;36:1007–1017.
140. Smith L, Folkard S, Poole CJM. Increased injuries on night shift. *Lancet* 1994;344:1137–39.
141. Horne JA, Reyner LA. Sleep related vehicle accidents. *Br Med J* 1995;310:565–567.
142. Mitler MM, Carskadon MA, Czeisler CA, Dement WC, Dinges DF, Graeber RC. Catastrophes, sleep and public policy. Concensus report. *Sleep* 1988;11:100–109.
143. Costa G. Effects on health and well-being. In: Colquhoun WP, Costa G, Folkard S, Knauth P, eds. *Shiftwork, problems and solutions.* Frankfurt: Peter Lang GmbH; 1996:113–139.
144. Arendt J, Deacon S, English J, Hampton S, Morgan L. Melatonin and adjustment to phase shift. *J Sleep Res* 1995;4(suppl 2):74–79.
145. Czeisler CA, Shanahan T, Klerman EB, et al. Suppression of melatonin secretion in some blind patients by exposure to bright light. *N Engl J Med* 1995;332:6–11.
146. Czeisler CA, Johnson MP, Duffy JF, Brown EN, Ronda JM, Kronauer RE. Exposure to bright light and darkness to treat physiologic maladaptation to night work. *N Engl J Med* 1990;322:1253–1259.
147. Arendt J, Bojkowski C, Folkard S, Franey C. Some effects of melatonin and the control of its secretion in man. *Ciba Found Symp* 1985;117:266–283.
148. Deacon S, Arendt J. Melatonin-induced temperature suppression and its acute phase shifting effects correlate in a dose-dependent manner in humans. *Brain Res* 1995;688:77–85.
149. Lewy A, Saeeduddin A, Latham Jackson J, Sack R. Melatonin shifts human circadian rhythms according to a phase-response curve. *Chronobiol Int* 1992;9:380–392.
150. Arendt J, Aldhous M, English J, et al. Some effects of jet lag and their alleviation by melatonin. *Ergonomics* 1987;30:1379–1393.
151. Folkard S, Arendt J, Clarke M. Can melatonin improve shiftworkers tolerance of the night shift? Some preliminary findings. *Chronobiol Int* 1993;10:315–320.

152. Deacon S, Arendt J. Adapting to phase-shifts. I. An experimental model for jet lag and shift work. *Physiol Behav* 1995;59:665–673.
153. Deacon S, Arendt J. Adapting to phase-shifts. II. Effects of melatonin and conflicting light treatment. *Physiol Behav* 1995;59:675–682.
154. Carroll K, Nestel P. Diurnal variation in glucose tolerance and in insulin secretion in man. *Diabetes* 1973;22:333–348.
155. Service F, Hall L, Westland R, O'Brian P. Effect of size, time of day and sequence of meal ingestion on carbohydrate tolerance in normal subjects. *Diabetologia* 1983;25:316–321.
156. Van Cauter E, Desir D, Decoster C, Fery F. Nocturnal decrease of glucose tolerance during constant glucose infusion. *J Clin Endocrinol Metab* 1989;69:604–611.
157. Minors DS, Waterhouse JM, eds. *Circadian rhythms and the human*. Bristol, England: John Wright & Sons; 1981.
158. Amland P, Jorde R, Burhol P. Diurnla GIP, PP and insulin levels in morbid obesity before and after stapled partitioning with gastric-gastrostomy. *Int Obesity* 1984;8:117–122.
159. Bessey P. Metabolic response to critical illness. In: Wilmore D, Cheung L, Harken A, Holcroft J, Meakins J, eds. *Scientific American surgery*. New York: Scientific American Inc.; 1995:1–31.
160. Kehlet H. Modification of responses to surgery by neural blockade. Clinical implications. In: Cousins M, Bridenbaugh P, eds. *Neural blockade in clinical anesthesia and management of pain*. Philadelphia: JB Lippincott; 1996 (in press).
161. Hill G, Douglas R, Schroeder D. Metabolic basis for the management of patients undergoing major surgery. *World J Surg* 1993;17:146–153.
162. Hill G. Impact of nutritional support on the clinical outcome of the surgical patient. *Clin Nutr* 1994;13:331–340.
163. Kehlet H. Effect of neural blockade in the acute catabolic stage. In: Revhaug A, eds. *Acute catabolic stage. Update in intensive care and emergency medicine*. Berlin: Springer-Verlag; 1996:207–215.
164. Dray A. Inflammatory mediators of pain. *Br J Anaesth* 1995;75:125–131.
165 Kehlet H, Nielsen H. Impact of laparoscopic surgery on stress responses, immunofunction and risk of infectious complications—a review. *J Am Coll Surg* 1996 (in press).
166 McMahon A, Russell I, Ramsey G. Laparoscopic and mini-laparotomy cholecystectomy: a randomized trial comparing postoperative pain and pulmonary function. *Surgery* 1994;115:533–539.
167. Ellis B, Dudley H. Some aspects of sleep research in surgical stress. *J Psochosomat Res* 1976;20: 303–308.
168. Rosenberg J, Wildschiødtz G, Pedersen M. Late postoperative nocturnal episodic hypoxaemia and associated sleep pattern. *Br J Anaesth* 1994;72:145–150.
169. Kavey N, Altshuler K. Sleep in herniorrhaphy patients. *Am J Surg* 1979;138:682–687.
170. Rosenberg-Adamsen S, Kehlet H, Dodds C, Roseberg J. Postoperative sleep disturbances: mechanisms and clinical implications. *Br J Anaesth* 1996;76:552–559.
171. Knill R, Moote C, Rose E, Skinner M. Marked hypoxhemia after gastroplasty due to disorders of breathing in REM sleep. *Anesthesiology* 1987;67:3A.
172. Rosenberg J, Pedersen N, Ramsing T, Kehlet H. Circadian variation in unexpected postoperative death. *Br J Surg* 1992;7:1300–1302.
173. Christensen T, Kehlet H. Postoperative fatigue. *World J Surgery* 1993;17:220–225.
174. Christensen T. Postoperative fatigue. *Dan Med Bull* 1995;42:314–322.
175. Schroeder D, Hill G. Postoperative fatigue: a prospective physiological study of patients undergoing major abdominal surgery. *Aust N Z J Surg* 1991;61:774–779.
176. Weiner H, eds. *Perturbing the organism: the biology of stressful experiences*. Chicago: University of Chicago Press; 1992.
177. Muller J, Tofler G, Stone P. Circadian variation and triggers of onset of acute cardiovascular disease. *Circulation* 1989;79:733–743.
178. Manuck S, Kaplan J, Adams M, Clarkson T. Studies of psychosocial influences on coronary artery atherosclerosis in cynomolgus monkeys. *Health Psychol* 1995;7:113–124.
179. Muller J, Tofler G. Triggering and circadian variation of onset of acute cardiovascular disease. (A symposium). *Am J Cardiol* 1990;66:1–70.
180. Surwit R, Ross S, Feinglos M. Stress, behavior, and glucose control in diabetes mellitus. *Stress Coping Dis* 1991;97:117.
181. Cox D, Gonder-Frederick L. The role of stress in diabetes mellitus. *Stress Coping Dis* 1991;97:118–134.
182. Lehman C, Rodin J, McEwen B, Brinton R. Impact of environmental stress on the expression of insulin-dependent diabetes mellitus. *Behav Neurosci* 1991;105:241–245.

183. Duffy L, Zielezny M, Marshall J, et al. Relevance of major stress events as an indicator of disease activity prevalence in inflammatory bowewl disease. *Behav Med* 1991;17:101–110.
184. Mrazek D, Klinnert M. Asthma: psychoneuroimmunologic consideration. *Psychoneuroimmunology* 1991;1013–1033.
185. Dhabhar F, McEwen B. Stress-induced enhancement of antigen-specific cell-mediated immunity. *J Immunol* 1996;156:2608–2615.
186. Spiegel D, Bloom J, Kraemer H, Gottheil E. Effect of psychosocial treatment on survival of patients with metastatic breast cancer. *Lancet* 1989;2:888–891.
187. Cohen S, Tyrrell D, Smith A. Psychological stress and susceptibility to the common cold. *N Engl J Med* 1991;325:606–612.
188. Shively C, Clarkson T. Social status incongruity and coronary artery athersclerosis in female monkeys. *Arteriosclerosis Thrombosis* 1994;14:721–726.
189. Munck A, Guyre P, Holbrook N. Physiological functions of glucocorticoids in stress and their relation to pharmacological actions. *Endocr Rev* 1984;5:25–43.
190. Rose R, Jenkins C, Hurst M, Livingston L, Hall R. Endocrine activity in air traffic controllers at work. I. Characterization of cortisol and growth hormone levels during the day. *Psychoneuroendocrinology* 1982;7:101–111.
191. Rose R, Jenkins C, Hurst M, Herd J, Hall R. Endocrine activity in air traffic controllers at work. II. Biological, psychological and work correlates. *Psychoneuroendocrinology* 1982;7:113–123.
192. Rose R, Jenkins C, Hurst M, Kreger B, Barrett J, Hall R. Endocrine activity in air traffic con trollers at work. III. Relationship to physical and psychiatric morbidity. *Psychoneuroendocrinology* 1982;7:125–134.
193. Moss H, Vanyukov M, Martin C. Salivary cortisol responses and the risk for substance abuse in prepubertal boys. *Biol Psychol* 1995;38:547–555.
194. Dienstbier R. Arousal and physiological toughness: implications for mental and physical health. *Psychol Rev* 1989;96:84–100.
195. McKittrick C, Blanchard D, Blanchard R, McEwen B, Sakai R. Serotonin receptor binding in a colony model of chronic social stress. *Biol Psychiatry* 1995;37:383–393.
196. Armario A, Hidalgo J, Giralt M. Evidence that the pituitary-adrenal axis does not cross-adapt to stressors: comparison to other physiological variable. *Neurendo* 1988;47:162–167.
197. Kant G, Anderson S, Dhillon G, Moughey E. Neuroendocrine correlates of sustained stress: the activity-stress paradigm. *Brain Res Bull* 1996;20:407–414.
198. Watanabe Y, Stone E, McEwen B. Induction and habituation of C-FOS and ZIF/268 by acute and repeated stressors. *NeuroReport* 1994;5:1321–1324.
199. Nisenbaum L, Zigmond M, Sved A, Abercrombie E. Prior exposure to chronic stress results in enhanced synthesis and release of hippocampla norepinephrine in response to a novel stressor. *J Neurosci* 1995;11:1478–1484.
200. Yehuda R, Resnick H, Kahana B, Giller E. Long-lasting hormonal alterations to extreme stress in humans: normative or maladaptive? *Psychosom Med* 1993;55:274–286.
201. Sterling P, Eyer J. Allostasis: a new paradigm to explain arousal pathology. In: Fisher S, Reason J, eds. *Handbook of life stress, cognition and health*. New York: Wiley; 1988:631–651.
202. McEwen B, Stellar E. Stress and the individual: mechanisms leading to disease. *Arch Intern Med* 1993;153:2093–2101.
203. Schulkin J, McEwen B, Gold P. Allostasos, amygdala, and anticipatory angst. *Neurosci Biobehav Rev* 1994;18:385–396.
204. Seeman T, McEwen B. The impact of social environment characteristics on neuroendocrine regulation. *Psychosom Med* 1996;58:459–471.
205. Bobak M, Marmot M. East-west mortality divide and its potential explanations: proposed research agenda. *Br Med J* 1996;312:421–425.
206. Larsson B, Seidell J, Svardsudd K, et al. Obesity, adipose tissue distribution and health in men—the study of men born in 1913. *Appetite* 1989;13:37–44.
207. Phillips R, LeDoux J. Differential contribution of amygdala and hippocampus to cued and contextual fear conditioning. *Behav Neurosci* 1992;106:274–285.
208. Cahill L, Prins B, Weber M, McGaugh J. Beta-adrenergic activation and memory for emotional events. *Nature* 1994;371:702–704.
209. McEwen B, Albeck D, Cameron H, et al. Stress and the brain: a paradoxical role for adrenal steroids. In: Litwack G, eds. *Vitamins and hormones*. San Diego: Academic; 1995:371–402.
210. Witelson S. Hand and sex differences in the isthmus and genu of the human corpus callosum. *Brain* 1989;112:799–835.

211. McEwen B. Our changing ideas about steroid effects on an ever-changing brain. *Semin Neurosci* 1991;3:497–507.
212. Witelson S, Gleze II, Kigar D. Women have greater density of neurons in posterior temporal cortex. *J Neurosci* 1995;15:3418–3428.
213. Catalani A, Marinelli M, Scaccianoce S, et al. Progeny of mothers drinking corticosterone during lactation has lower stress-induced corticosterone secretion and better cognitive performance. *Brain Res* 1993;624:209–215.
214. Dellu F, Mayo W, Vallee M, LeMoal M, Simon H. Reactivity to novelty during youth as a predictive factor of cognitive impairment in the elderly: a longitudinal study in rats. *Brain Res* 1994;653:51–56.
215. McEwen B, Sapolsky R. Stress and cognitive function. *Curr Opin Neurobiol* 1995;5:205–216.
216. Uno H, Ross T, Else J, Suleman M, Sapolsky R. Hippocampal damage associated with prolonged and fatal stress in primates. *J Neurosci* 1989;9:1705–1711.
217. Fuchs E, Uno H, Flugge G. Chronic psychosocial stress induces morphological alterations in hippocampal pyramidal neurons of the tree shrew. *Brain Res* 1995;673:275–282.

Physiology, Stress, and Malnutrition: Functional Correlates, Nutritional Intervention,
edited by J.M. Kinney and H.N. Tucker.
Lippincott–Raven Publishers © 1997.

Anorexia: A Neglected Clinical Problem

Susan A. Jebb

Medical Research Council Dunn Clinical Nutrition Centre, Cambridge CB2 2DH, United Kingdom

Pathologic processes in humans are frequently accompanied by anorexia. In the acute situation when the organism requires energy to mount an acute-phase response, it seems inconsistent that food intake should be suppressed, but there may be good teleologic reasons for this to occur. Certainly overfeeding during infective periods can increase morbidity and mortality (1–3) and can exacerbate respiratory difficulties (4). However, diseases associated with prolonged anorexia, are likely to lead to cachexia and frank malnutrition, with deleterious consequences.

Chronic anorexia leading to cachexia has been observed in a wide range of chronic diseases, including cancer (5), human immunodeficiency virus (HIV) infection (6), bacterial and parasitic diseases (7), chronic inflammatory bowel disease (8), Crohn's disease (9), chronic liver disease, chronic obstructive pulmonary disease (10), rheumatoid arthritis (11), and many more.

In 1974 malnutrition in hospitalized patients was condemned as "the skeleton in the hospital closet" (12). This was quickly followed by a succession of articles confirming the high prevalence of malnutrition in medical and surgical inpatients (13–16). For example, in the study of Bistrian et al. (13), 50% of patients had evidence of protein-energy malnutrition and a third of patients were classified as severely depleted.

In 1979, Weinsier et al. (16) showed an increase in the incidence of malnutrition during a patient's hospital stay. Encouragingly, a follow-up study in the US (17) showed that this trend had been reversed. This improvement was attributed to the increase in nutrition education among health professionals and the existence of a multi-disciplinary nutrition support service. However, there was still a significant margin of error; 39% of patients who may have benefited from nutritional support were still not referred.

Unfortunately, the situation in the United Kingdom is still bleak. Figure 1 shows data from a comprehensive survey of patients admitted to a teaching hospital in Scotland (18), compared with population estimates (19). Of 500 patients, 187 (38%) had a body mass index (BMI) of less than 20 kg/m^2, yet only 96 had any nutritional information documented in the notes. Among 112 patients reassessed

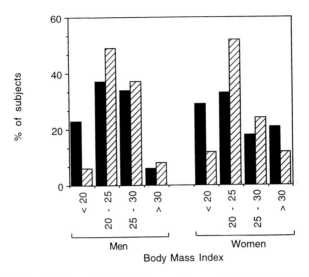

FIG. 1. Distribution of BMI in patients 16–64 years of age admitted to hospital (18) compared with population estimates (19). Solid bars represent patients and hatched bars represent controls.

at discharge, only 18% of undernourished patients had been referred for nutritional support, and of these 70% gained weight, whereas 80% of undernourished patients not referred lost weight. This lack of attention to nutritional status resulted in a further decrease in body weight during hospitalization.

This negligence occurs even though the deleterious effect of undernutrition is well recognized. In initially healthy volunteers, experimental semi-starvation with a 25% loss of body weight was associated with apathy, depression, and fatigue, which were reversible with refeeding (20). In patients with coexisting injury or disease, there are additional effects on morbidity and mortality, which recently were reviewed in a report from the British Association of Parenteral and Enteral Nutrition (21). Malnutrition delays recovery, increases the incidence of serious complications, and increases treatment costs. A recent study in patients admitted to an intensive care unit has shown a significant increase in the incidence of complications and number of patients not discharged from the hospital in malnourished compared with well-nourished patients (22). Numerous other examples of the detrimental effects of malnutrition are given elsewhere in this symposium.

The extent of undernutrition among patients with disease or injury and its negative consequences are clear. Its correction should be a priority for health professionals and managers alike, yet it remains a neglected area of medicine. A plausible hypothesis is that progress is hindered by a lack of understanding of the causes of malnutrition and the efficacy of intervention strategies. This chapter reviews each of these areas in an attempt to replace some of the anecdotal information with objective data.

CAUSES OF WEIGHT LOSS

Subjective reports of anorexia as a primary symptom are unreliable and correlate poorly with objective measures of weight loss (23). The depletion of body protein and fat reserves only occurs if the patient is in a state of net negative energy balance, so in many cases conclusions regarding the etiology of weight loss are made from studies of energy expenditure.

Reports of increased basal or resting energy requirements have encouraged the claim that excessive energy requirements rather than inadequate intake is the cause of weight loss in sick patients. However, our current understanding of energy metabolism in disease suggests that the elevation may be less than previously believed (24). In many cases the increase in resting energy expenditure (REE) is more than counterbalanced by decreases in physical activity, such that total energy expenditure (TEE) is rarely increased. Figure 2 shows measurements of TEE in a variety of patients in comparison with data collated by Black et al. (25) for age- and sex-matched controls. The lower energy expenditure of the patient groups suggests that the principal factor influencing weight loss must be decreases in energy intake of greater magnitude than the decrease in energy expenditure. In healthy volunteers energy intake is matched to energy expenditure across a wide range of energy requirements. Moreover, at a population level in affluent societies there is a net imbalance toward positive energy balance (26). Yet in patients with

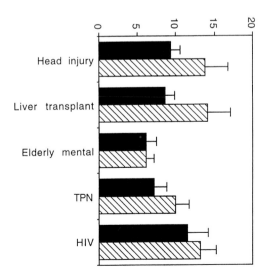

FIG. 2. Total energy expenditure in sick patients (29,37,91,178,179) compared with age- and sex-matched controls (25). Solid bars represent patients and hatched bars represent controls.

disease there is commonly a breakdown of energy homeostasis and a failure to consume sufficient energy to meet the body's requirement.

In many cases there is a clear indication of the cause of the decrease in food intake. These include many physical symptoms (e.g., nausea, vomiting, or pain); social causes (e.g., isolation or economic hardship); and behavioral or psychiatric causes, (e.g., anxiety or depression). These have been reviewed elsewhere (27).

Inadequate Food Supply

It is clear that weight loss in some patients, frequently the elderly, is caused by an inadequate or inappropriate food supply (28). Retrospective data from a single ward in a geriatric mental hospital showed that 15 of 18 patients had lost weight over a 2-year period since their admission, of which four had lost more than 30% of their initial body weight (29). In 14 patients, a detailed study of energy balance was performed. All patients had a history of weight loss, and the average BMI was only 19 ± 2 kg/m^2.

Basal metabolic rate was close to predicted values, and the energy expended on physical activity was highly correlated with a subjective activity score made by the dietitian ($r = 0.81$, $p < 0.001$). TEE was 6.1 ± 1.4 MJ/day, with a ratio of basal metabolic rate (BMR) to TEE averaging 1.5, which is similar to or less than that observed in other studies (25). These data provide no support for the hypothesis that these patients are hypermetabolic. Patients were in energy balance and weight stable at the time of the measurements, supporting the notion that weight loss in these patients is episodic. However, because it is inconceivable that the habitual energy expenditure of these patients coincidentally matched their food intake, it may be assumed that subjects have adapted their energy expenditure to achieve energy balance. This may have occurred either by a suppression of activity or a loss of body mass until energy equilibrium is achieved. This implies that supplementation of the available food supply with additional energy would lead to a desirable increase in body weight.

Numerous other studies, particularly in the elderly, suggest that a poor food supply is the cause of weight loss. A study in Swedish nursing homes recorded that patients who were dependent on their caregiver for food received only 6–10 minutes of attention per meal by 15–20 different personnel each week (30). Van Ort and Phillips (31) characterized the interactions between caregivers and demented patients using videotapes. They discerned no clear organizational pattern or consistency in the feeding arrangements and formulated strategies that they felt would improve feeding in these patients. Unfortunately, no follow-up data are yet available to indicate the efficacy of this approach. However, it seems logical that these basic failures in the food supply to patients, particularly in hospitals or other institutions, should be addressed before more complex interventions are considered.

Physical Limitations to Food Intake

In many cases adequate intake is difficult to achieve due to physical handicaps [e.g., patients who are dysphagic after a stroke (32) or patients with motor neuron disease (33)]. Malabsorption may also reduce energy intake, both as a consequence of gastrointestinal losses and an apparent diminution of intake (34). Reductions in gastric emptying have been observed in animal models of disease (35), and recently this also has been observed in patients with head injuries (36). In this study, enteral feeding was restricted due to a twofold reduction in gastric emptying compared with controls ($p < 0.001$) and significant regurgitation of food into the mouth. As a consequence, energy intake was only 3.56 ± 2.05 MJ/day, compared with their measured expenditure of 9.32 ± 1.20 MJ/day.

Anorexia of Disease

Only if energy intake remains inadequate, despite the availability of food and the ability to digest and absorb nutrients, is it reasonable to attribute the weight loss to the anorexia of disease. This phenomena has been comprehensively studied in patients with HIV infection (37). Figure 3 shows data from 52 men with HIV infection. Measurements of total energy expenditure by doubly labeled water showed no evidence of hypermetabolism; indeed, TEE was significantly lower in patients who were losing weight. Despite this decrease, patients lost weight since weighed diet records show that their energy intake had dropped even lower. Patients were consuming as little as 1.8 MJ/day despite free access to food, nutritional supplements, and dietetic counseling. Longitudinal studies of weight change in this population suggest that patients experience episodic periods of weight loss, frequently associated with acute opportunistic infections during which appetite is suppressed. However, after successful treatment of the infection, appetite returns and weight is spontaneously regained (6).

This phenomena is all too familiar to health professionals. Many patients recognize the consequences of their failure to eat, yet despite their motivation they are still unable to overcome their anorexia. However, successful treatment of their underlying disease results in a rebound of appetite and regain of body weight. This nebulous condition is the anorexia of disease.

CONTROL OF FOOD INTAKE

Sensory Influences

Under experimental conditions the sensory influences on food intake have been qualitatively identified (38). However, there has been almost no quantification of the effects of these sensory influences on day-to-day food choices and net intake.

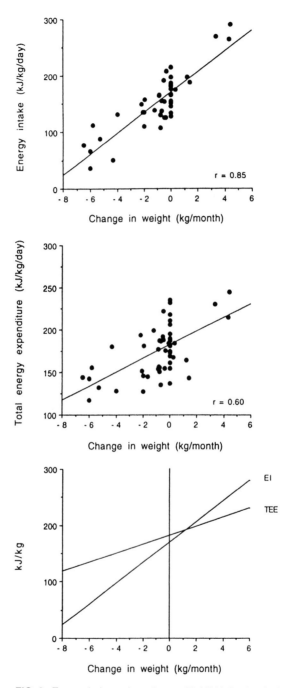

FIG. 3. Energy balance in patients with HIV infection (37).

Changes in sensory preferences in patients with cancer have been widely reported, particularly in relation to taste changes. Approximately one third of patients are reported to have an elevated sweet threshold and one sixth a lower threshold for the bitter taste. These changes have been correlated with reduced energy intake and disease status (39).

Gastrointestinal Factors

Gastrointestinal mechanisms influence both the initiation of a meal and its termination (40). Through a variety of postprandial signals they may also affect the intermeal interval.

Gastric distention appears to provide a physical limitation to food intake. In humans, inflating a balloon in the stomach is a recognized technique to reduce food intake in obese people (41). However, this is reported to give an uncomfortable feeling of fullness rather than the satisfaction associated with post-meal satiety. Furthermore, satiety usually lasts for a few hours after a meal, whereas gastric distention is short lived. This has led to the suggestion that it is the rate of emptying of nutrients into the small intestine that is primarily responsible for postmeal satiety. These effects appear to be mediated in a number of ways, including vagal nerve stimulation and chemoreceptors. If lipid is infused into the small intestine at the same time that the stomach is inflated with a balloon, the normal satiety response can be elicited (42).

Gastrointestinal hormones, including cholecystokinin (CCK), bombesin, gastric-inhibitory protein, insulinotrophic peptide, and pancreatic glucagon, are believed to play an important role in the control of food intake. Perhaps the greatest body of evidence relates to CCK, a peptide in the duodenal epithelium that is released by luminal lipid and peptides. Although intravenous infusions of CCK reduce food intake and enhance satiety (43,44), more recent studies have failed to show an effect of CCK-A receptor antagonists in humans (45,46). There is a poor correlation between CCK concentrations and sensations of hunger or fullness in human volunteers after a meal (47). Although this diminishes the likelihood that CCK is a direct hunger or satiety hormone, it does not eliminate the possibility that it may act as a paracrine agent or neurotransmitter. Alternatively, it may interact with other neuroendocrine mediators. For example, the level of insulin in the brain influences the sensitivity of the central nervous system (CNS) to the effects of CCK (48).

Studies of the effect of disease or injury on the gastrointestinal appetite regulation are limited. However, the common symptom of fullness or early satiety reported by anorectic patients would support the possibility of inhibitory signals from the gastrointestinal tract on subsequent food intake. Decreases in gastric emptying (36) and atrophic changes in intestinal integrity may delay the digestion and assimilation of nutrients (39). Numerous studies have reported changes in many of the peptides purported to induce satiety or decrease hunger.

Oxidative Fuel Supply

During periods of undernutrition uncomplicated by disease or injury, there is a progressive switch from the oxidation of carbohydrate to fatty acids (49). This reduces the breakdown of lean tissue mass to provide gluconeogenic precursors. Plasma insulin levels decrease, leading to increased lipolysis and ß-oxidation, which inhibits pyruvate dehydrogenase, thus decreasing carbohydrate oxidation (50). However, in the presence of infection or inflammation, this adaptive mechanism is disrupted. At a clinical level this is manifest as a failure to decrease protein oxidation in response to the energy deficit and hence sustained negative nitrogen balance. Evidence from animal studies suggests that this may be due either to a failure to inhibit pyruvate oxidation (51) or to develop an appropriate ketosis (52).

Studies in healthy volunteers suggest that the oxidation of carbohydrate generates a strong satiety signal, which exerts a powerful negative feedback on appetite, whereas fat oxidation is associated with a only a weak satiety effect and therefore has a more permissive influence on subsequent food intake (53). This would explain the powerful hunger drive in starving individuals, who are predominately oxidizing fat. In contrast, in patients with blunted fat oxidation and continued carbohydrate oxidation consequent to lean body mass catabolism, the hunger drive is suppressed. Although theoretically plausible, there is little direct experimental evidence to support this model. Indeed studies in healthy, lean volunteers show no tendency to increase voluntary food intake in response to carbohydrate deprivation and low carbohydrate oxidation rates (54,55).

Neuroendocrine Mediators

Numerous mediators have been proposed whose effects on food intake are believed to operate through a central regulatory system (56). The dual-center hypothesis proposes that the ventromedial hypothalamic nucleus acts as a satiety center that inhibits the activity of the lateral hypothalamic area, believed to be a feeding center. This concept was originally based on studies in animals involving the destruction of each of these centers, but more recently it has been possible to reproduce these effects using specific neuropeptides. Table 1 lists some substances, acting via the CNS, that have been proposed to have either appetite-stimulating or appetite-suppressing properties.

There has been a recent stimulus to work in this area with the sequencing of the gene responsible for obesity in the ob/ob mouse, coding for a protein now named leptin (57). Low circulating levels of leptin have been linked to the hyperphagia seen in these animals. Injection of leptin increases plasma concentrations and reduces food intake. In humans, the concentration of circulating leptin in obese individuals is higher than in lean controls, suggesting that obesity is a consequence of a relative leptin resistance (58). The production of leptin is regulated by insulin and glucocorticosteriods, and it is suppressed by feeding and enhanced by starva-

TABLE 1. *Neuroendocrine mediators of feeding*

Appetite stimulating	Appetite suppressing
Neuropeptide Y	Leptin
Galanin	Serotonin
Opiates	Dopamine
Growth hormone–releasing factor	Corticotrophin-releasing factor
Norepinephrine	Insulin
	Glucagon
	Glucagon-like-peptide 1
	Enterostatin
	Calcitonin
	Amylin
	Bombesin
	Somatostatin
	Thyroid releasing hormone

tion. It seems probable that leptin controls energy intake through the balance of activity of the neurotransmitters neuropeptide-Y (NPY; appetite-stimulating) and glucagonlike peptide 1 (GLP-1; appetite-suppressing) (59).

To date there has been little work on NPY and GLP-1 in disease states, and it is unclear whether these neurotransmitters are important contributors to the anorexia of disease. The concentration of NPY in patients with sepsis has been shown to be increased (60), although it is decreased in patients with Alzheimer's disease (61). Neither study has correlated NPY to changes in food intake. However, it is apparent that anorexigenic molecules liberated during the disease process may reset the body's appetite regulation via effects on this central regulatory system (62).

Cytokines

A considerable body of literature has suggested that the release of cytokines from activated cells during pathologic processes is associated with the anorectic response to injury and disease (63,64). Peripheral administration of cytokines suppresses food intake, as does the administration of factors, such as endotoxin, known to provoke endogenous cytokine release (65). These responses can be blocked by cytokine antagonists. The mechanism of their action is not clear, but effects have been reported at the molecular, cellular, neurologic, and behavioral level.

However, not all cytokines are equivalent in their anorectic effects. The most potent seems to be interleukin-1β (IL-1β), which suppresses both short- and long-term feeding patterns (66). It decreases meal size, predominantly through a reduction in eating rate. At higher doses it also may decrease meal frequency. Interferon seems to affect only short-term eating, leading to decreases in meal size and duration without affecting meal frequency (67), whereas IL-8 and tumor necrosis factor (TNF) reduce meal size without significantly affecting meal duration or feeding frequency (68).

Psychological Influences

Anxiety, depression, and other psychological effects of disease may all contribute to anorexia (69). Depression is the most common cause of weight loss in most elderly nursing home residents (70). Learned aversions to food are commonly reported in patients with cancer (71). Anorexia may be the somatic consequence of the patient's beliefs and attitudes toward his or her illness. Overcoming these influences may be an important component of restoring normal appetite control.

Because there is clearly a large component of cognitive control in normal feeding processes, it has been suggested that the internal stimuli tending to promote anorexia and reduce food intake can be overcome by a high degree of motivation and/or cognitive control (72). Anecdotal evidence is not encouraging because even the most enthusiastic approach is often insufficient to overcome the anorexia of disease, but further research is warranted.

Integration of Food Intake Regulation in Disease

It seems probable that the normal control of feeding behavior is achieved through a hierarchy of strategies operating over different time frames. A hypothetical model is shown in Fig. 4 (40). The sensory properties may determine what and how much is eaten within any eating episode. Gastrointestinal factors seem to regulate how much food is consumed at a given meal and perhaps the timing of the next meal. Metabolic signals such as the composition of fuels oxidized and hormonal or neuroendocrine mediators may operate over the course of a day or more to set the overall energy budget.

Unfortunately, the effect of disease, perhaps operating through cytokines or other inflammatory mediators, seems to exert its effect above all the normal appetite control mechanisms, which limits food intake and cannot easily be overridden. However, adapting foods to optimize their sensory properties to an individual's food choice, manipulating the macronutrient composition, and suppressing the anorectic environment created by the acute phase response are all possible methods to overcome the anorexia of disease.

STRATEGIES FOR THE MANAGEMENT OF ANOREXIA

The efficacy of strategies for the management of anorexia is most usually assessed by monitoring the restoration of body weight and composition and the resumption of normal energy intake, rather than by direct measures of the anorexia itself. This is a reflection of the difficulties of reliably quantifying anorexia both within and between individuals. Clearly the most fundamental method to reverse the anorexia of disease is to successfully treat the underlying condition. In patients in whom the etiology of anorexia is apparent, appropriate strategies can usually be devised to resolve or attenuate the problem, e.g., increasing the quantity of food

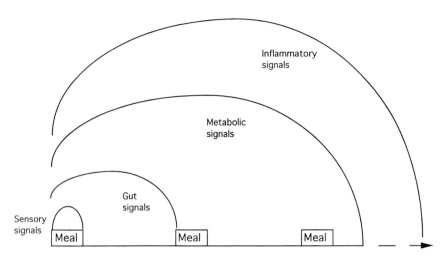

FIG. 4. A putative model of food intake regulation in disease. Adapted from (40).

available, modifying the form or texture, or providing intravenous nutrition to overcome gastrointestinal losses. In other cases, more empirical options must be explored.

Nutritional Strategies

Dietary Advice

Nutritional advice is often the first attempt to restore normal food intake in an anorexic patient (73). The process is often derided simply as "common sense," and evidence of its efficacy remains the most anecdotal of all intervention strategies.

Many studies in this area are merely retrospective audits of clinical care: they lack a control group, follow-up data on many patients are incomplete, and little or no data are offered to examine the functional consequences of the apparent improvements in nutrient intake. Recently a number of studies have been conducted in patients with HIV infection. Schwenk et al. (74) showed a small mean weight gain (1.4 ± 6.2%) in 40 of 75 patients, including 15 who gained more than 5% of body weight following dietary advice alone. However, due to the wide variety of patients and assorted symptoms, it was not possible to clearly identify factors predictive of a positive response. In the study of Murphy et al. (75) there were highly significant increases in energy intake over 16 weeks of dietetic counseling from 8.1 to 11.4 MJ/day. This was associated with a mean increase in body weight of 5.1 kg. Dowling et al. (76) achieved a significant increase in total energy intake and of a wide range of micronutrients in 12 weeks of dietetic counseling. Among the symptomatic patients, body weight and mid-arm circumference increased significantly, although there was less impact in the asymptomatic patients. Other studies also have demonstrated the efficacy of dietary advice to improve the quality of the diet. In a group of patients with Crohn's disease, there were significant improvements in the nutrient density of the diet with respect to most micronutrients in those who received monthly diet counselling for 6 months compared with a control group (77).

Some experimental evidence taken from laboratory-based studies, usually in healthy volunteers, supports specific components of dietary advice given to anorectic patients. Three such examples will be considered.

Energy Density

Dietary advice to increase the energy density of the diet usually focuses on the addition of energy-dense items to habitual components of the diet. For example, adding additional butter or cream to mashed potatoes or scrambled eggs, or putting sugar on breakfast cereals or fruit.

Numerous metabolic studies in healthy volunteers have shown that such energy-dense diets result in hyperphagia, and a number of mechanisms have been proposed to explain this phenomena. Under conditions of normal food intake, energy density is closely correlated to the fat content of the food, and it is difficult to dissociate the relative effects of the fat content of the food and its energy density (78). Because fat contains more than twice the energy per unit weight of carbohydrate or protein, high-fat meals are smaller in volume than their isoenergetic high-protein or high-carbohydrate equivalents. Eating a similar volume of food or eating for a similar period of time therefore tends to produce the greatest energy intake on a high-fat diet. Studies also show that fat is less satiating than carbohydrate (79–81). This may be a reflection of the decreased bulk of the food, which minimizes satiety signals from gastric stretch receptors or decreases the rate of gastric emptying. It also may exert its effect as a consequence of a low oxidative feedback mechanism because the consumption of fat does not produce the autoregulatory increase in its own oxidation, which is seen after the ingestion of other macronutrients (82–84). Finally, it may be that fat simply serves to enhance the sensory properties of a meal (85,86). The addition of fat to food heightens the flavor and increases the subjective palatability of the food, thus stimulating consumption.

However, evidence that it is the energy density of the food and not fat per se that invokes the hyperphagic response comes from a number of sources. In rats fed diets of similar energy density, differing only in their macronutrient content, there was no high-fat hyperphagia. However, when energy density was fixed, the weight of food consumed was unchanged, and net energy intake was directly proportional to the energy density of the diet (87). In humans consuming liquid diets over 14 days, energy intake was unchanged on diets of 24% or 47% fat, with constant energy density (88). In the studies of Stubbs et al. (89,90), depicted in Fig. 5, the hyperphagia seen on 60% fat relative to 20% fat diets was abolished when the energy density of the diets was equalized.

Most of this work has been conducted within the context of the etiology of obesity. However, it is probable that similar mechanisms operate even in disease, such that energy intake is maximized on energy-dense diets. Figure 6 shows data from two studies in which neutral energy supplements were added to increase the energy density of food provided to patients with cancer. Parkinson et al. (91) achieved a significant increase in energy (+1.74 MJ/day) and protein (+28 g/day) intake over a single supplemented day compared with a control day. This suggests that the increased energy density of the diet was not counterbalanced by a decrease in the volume of food consumed. Unfortunately, this study did not assess whether the increase in energy density could be achieved by patients at home or sustained over a clinically significant period. A similar increase in energy intake (+1.04 MJ/day) was reported in a study of 12 geriatric patients receiving hospital meals supplemented with a glucose polymer (92). In a further study patients with HIV infection randomized to a standard-energy or increased-energy density sip feed consumed less of the high-energy feed, but not enough to counteract the benefits of the increased energy density (93).

Other strategies to increase the energy density of the diet could include greater use of high-fat foodstuffs. In clinical practice there has been some caution about promoting high-fat, energy-dense foods for weight regain because of concerns about fat intolerance and the apparent contradiction with established healthy

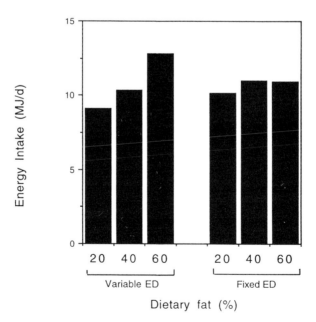

FIG. 5. Effect of high fat diets on energy intake under conditions of variable or fixed energy density (89,90).

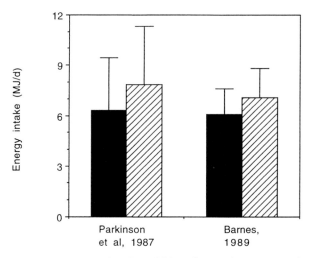

FIG. 6. Increase in energy intake after the addition of neutral energy supplements to food (91,92). Solid bars represent unsupplemented intake and hatched bars represent supplemented intake.

eating practices. Clearly, some patients are unable to absorb fat, but this should not be a justification for putting all patients on low-fat diets, which may deprive many of an important energy source. Finally, there is some evidence that liquid foods may cause earlier satiety than solids (94). The textural properties of liquid-based formulations mean that drinks with an energy content of greater than 8 kJ/ml are difficult to achieve, whereas for solid foods energy densities in excess of 16 kJ/g are commonplace. For example, even commercial milkshakes have an energy density of only 4 kJ/ml compared with 19 kJ/g for digestive biscuits and 24 kJ/g for peanuts.

Meal Frequency

It is common practice to recommend that anorectic patients, particularly those reporting early satiety, should consume frequent small meals to maximize energy intake. Community-based studies show a direct relationship between feeding frequency and energy intake in healthy volunteers (95,96). Figure 7 shows data from 7,147 individuals as part of the National Health and Nutrition Examination Survey. Total energy was significantly lower ($p < 0.05$) in those eating less than twice per day to those eating on more than seven occasions, increasing from 6.08 to 11.74 MJ/day in men and 4.10 to 7.69 MJ/day in women. However, such data must be treated with caution in view of the clear evidence of under-reporting in at least a proportion of participants.

Once again there is no direct evidence of the effect of meal frequency on energy intake in sick patients. In children recovering from malnutrition, but with

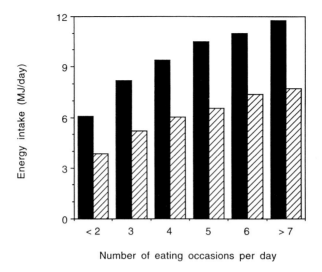

FIG. 7. Effect of feeding frequency on energy intake (96). Solid bars represent men and hatched bars represent women.

no specific organic disorder, increasing the number of meals from three to four per day increased energy intake by 16% and a further 7% when the frequency was increased from four to five meals (97). This study also demonstrated an increased energy intake with increased energy density of the feed.

Alcohol

The use of small quantities of alcohol as an appetite stimulant has received much anecdotal support, although currently there is no experimental evidence in anorectic patients. After fat, alcohol is the most energy-dense of the macronutrients (29 kJ/g) and is 98% absorbed. One possible mechanism for its appetite-stimulant effects is that it suppresses gluconeogenesis and the oxidation of fat (98). Community-based studies suggest that total energy intake increases when alcohol is added to the diet (99–102) and that drinkers consume more energy on days when they have alcohol than on alcohol-free days (102). However, these findings cannot be easily extrapolated to patients because alcohol consumption in a free-living environment is often also linked to social events that may independently promote hyperphagia (103).

When alcohol is added to the diet under experimental conditions (2.4 or 4.6 MJ/day), there was a net increase in total energy intake (104). However, this effect was similar in magnitude to that resulting from the addition of carbohydrate, suggesting that there is no specific appetite-stimulant effect of alcohol. A recent study of the so-called "aperitif effect" of alcohol showed similar results (104a). Subjects were given a drink of water, 0.72 MJ carbohydrate, or 0.91 MJ

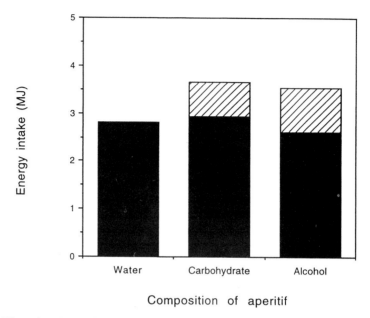

FIG. 8. Effect of an "aperatif" on energy intake at the subsequent meal. Solid bars represent energy intake of the meal and hatched bars represent the energy content of the aperatif.

alcohol. Energy intake at a subsequent meal was similar regardless of the nature of the "aperatif" (Fig. 8). These data suggest that subjects simply fail to compensate for a preload of energy rather than a specific appetite-stimulant effect of alcohol. This is perhaps demonstrating the phenomenon of increased energy intake associated with a small, frequent meals.

Sip Feeds

In contrast to the paucity of data on the efficacy of dietary advice, numerous controlled clinical trials have considered the use of sip feeds. Their findings have been mixed, but to some extent this can perhaps be attributed to a failure to accurately separate compliance to the prescribed regimen from the observed efficacy.

Palatability of the supplement is a key issue. Although taste panels typically produce good palatability ratings, there is less evidence of long-term acceptability. Indeed, the phenomenon of flavor fatigue is well described (105). In a comprehensive study, Bolton et al. (106) found that 18 of 52 patients with cancer declined a range of sip feeds because they were considered to be unpalatable, and a further 10 patients discontinued the supplements due to flavor fatigue, a total of 54% of the sample. Only 10% of patients continued taking the sip feeds for 90 days or more. Moreover, palatability does not always assure consumption. Ovesen (107) found high palatability scores for two different liquid diets with only a small nonsignificant decrease in the taste rating after 8 days, yet patients consumed only half the prescribed intake.

Differences in compliance may explain some of the discrepancies in the reported efficacy of sip feeds. In a study of patients with head and neck cancer, Arnold and Richter (108) showed that none of the 23 patients in the intervention group consumed all of a 4 MJ/day oral supplement. The average intake was 67% in men and 56% in women, with only 30% of patients consuming at least 80% of the prescribed volume. Williams et al. (109) analyzed the results of an intervention trial in elderly orthopedic patients by comparing those in whom successful supplementation was achieved with noncompliant patients. Noncompliant patients experienced a significant decline in triceps skinfold thickness and mid-arm muscle circumference, similar in magnitude to that of the unsupplemented group, whereas there were no significant changes in patients with "fair or good" intakes of the supplement (mean supplement intake = 1.68 MJ/day). However, most studies have been analyzed on an "intention to treat" basis, and this may confound the outcome measures.

The net effect of supplementation programs depends not only on the compliance to the prescribed supplement regimen, but the concomitant effects on voluntary food intake. Relatively few studies have documented the extent of substitution or supplementation of net energy intake. In the study of Elmstahl et al. in patients with head and neck cancer, a sip feed increased net energy intake, although 43% of the energy content of the supplement substituted for the habitual diet (110). In geriatric patients, 15–50% of a sip feed replaced the hospital diet (108). In the latter study the highest daily energy intake and least suppression of habitual food intake was seen in patients receiving the most energy-dense supplement, apparently confirming the lower satiety value of foods with a higher energy density. However, in a more recent study (107) a group of geriatric patients showed a greater suppression of their hospital food intake while consuming an energy-dense (6.3 kJ/ml) supplement than did patients taking the lower energy density (4.2 kJ/ml) supplement, although total energy intakes were similar in the two groups. Although not statistically significant, patients consuming the 4.2 kJ/ml supplement showed an increase in their habitual energy intake of the order of approximately 1.2 MJ/day. This is particularly important because it implies that rather than simply addressing the weight loss, supplements may in fact be reversing the anorexia of disease. Confirmation of this phenomenon can be found in the study of Rana et al. (111) (Fig. 9). A group of 40 postoperative patients received a mean of 1.97 MJ/day from a sip feed. Mean energy intake from the hospital diet averaged 1.05 MJ/day greater than an unsupplemented control group, resulting in a highly significant increase in net energy intake.

A number of studies have not measured net energy intake, but used body weight or other measures of nutritional status to assess the efficacy of the

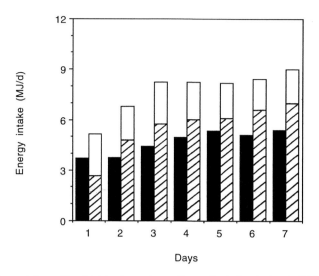

FIG. 9. Supplementation of food intake in postoperative patients by sip feeds (111). Solid bars represent the energy intake of control patients, hatched bars the energy intake from food in the intervention group and open bars the energy intake from the sip feed.

intervention. Sip feeds have been shown to increase body weight or attenuate weight loss (111–115), increase skinfold thickness and mid-arm muscle circumference (109,112,113,115–117), or increase grip strength (111,118). Unosson et al. (119) reported significant improvements in physical activity in supplemented geriatric patients receiving long-term care.

Other studies have shown improvements in micronutrient status, independent of changes in energy intake, presumably reflecting the superior nutrient density of sip feeds relative to everyday foods (76,116–118). Improvements in micronutrient status may be related to the disinhibition of appetite seen in some studies because there is some evidence that the correction of even moderate deficiencies of micronutrients may enhance appetite. Deficiencies of zinc in particular have been related to anorexia (120).

Enteral and Parenteral Feeding

Enteral and parenteral feeding are predominantly used as techniques to overcome the consequences of anorexia (i.e., weight loss) rather than a treatment of the symptom itself. There are numerous reports of the benefits of artificial nutrition in terms of morbidity and even mortality (21). In the context of anorexia, understanding the consequences of artificial nutritional support on voluntary food intake is essential if these therapies are to be used optimally in the period during which oral feeding is recommenced. Because clinicians are reluctant to withdraw artificial nutritional support until voluntary oral intake is established, it is important to define the regimens associated with minimal suppression of appetite. Conversely, in cases in which nutritional support is provided to obviate the need for oral nutrition (e.g., in patients receiving total parenteral nutrition for bowel rest), it may be advantageous to use a regimen associated with maximum satiety. Furthermore, by studying the consequences of enteral and parenteral nutrition on voluntary food intake, it may be possible to elucidate some of the mechanisms of appetite control and hence the nature of its dysregulation in disease states.

Only a limited number of studies are available that have considered the effects of artificial nutritional support on appetite and food intake in animals or humans. However, already some interesting hypotheses have arisen that require further attention.

Disinhibition of Appetite by Feeding

There are reports from patients receiving enteral nutrition that a threshold of energy intake is required to reinvigorate the body's own appetite mechanisms. This may be analogous to the stimulation of appetite associated with sip feeds (111). The mechanism of this effect is not at all clear, but the phenomenon has been reported both as a single case history (28) and within the context of a study of nocturnal enteral feeding (121). In the latter, 10 patients who were unable to consume sufficient nutrition to meet their energy needs began a period of nocturnal enteral feeding that provided 7.53 MJ in 1 L. On average, patients doubled their voluntary oral intake.

Timing of Feeds

Evidence from diverse sources suggests that the timing of nutritional supplements may determine the effects on voluntary energy intake. A night-time intragastric feed of 8.37 MJ/day in healthy lean men was not associated with any significant change in habitual energy intake (122) and led to significant weight gain. However, consuming 4.18 MJ/day orally in the late evening reduced habitual energy intake by 1.95 MJ/day, thus attenuating although not abolishing the weight gain (123). Even modest energy preloads given in the early part of the day are followed by accurate energetic compensation at the next meal (124). Clearly a definitive analysis of this effect requires a systematic evaluation within a single study, but already the theory that nocturnal feeding produces less suppression of voluntary intake than daytime feeding has widespread anecdotal support. In patients the success of a sip feed supplementation trial in which there was no decrease in habitual intake has been attributed to giving the supplement in the late evening (125).

Route of Feeding

There has been considerable interest in the extent to which bypassing all or part of the gut by the artificial delivery of nutrients undermines appetite control. Patients receiving parenteral feeding may complain of hunger, yet when offered food they are quickly satiated (126). Such patients are not ideal for experimental studies because the effects of total parenteral nutrition are complicated by changes in their clinical status that may have independent effects on appetite.

Short-term studies in which gastrointestinal cues may be expected to dominate the appetite control system seem to show that enteral nutrients satiate while parenteral nutrients do not. In the rat, intragastric feeding inhibits food intake to precisely counterbalance the infused energy (127), whereas intravenous infusions of lipid had no effect on eating behavior (128). In healthy male volunteers the infusion of lipid into the small intestine leads to enhanced satiety and decreased food intake, yet no such effects are seen when the same lipid emulsion is infused into a peripheral vein (129). Shide et al. (130) have made a series of studies to investigate the effect of fat and carbohydrate given intragastrically or intravenously on the feeding response within a single day. Figure 10 illustrates that no compensation was observed at meals 1 hour (lunch) or 6.5 hours (dinner) after the end of 3.5-hour parenteral infusions leading to a net increase in energy

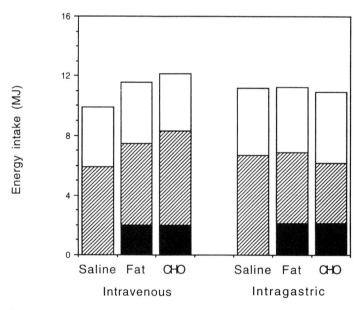

FIG. 10. Compensation for intragastric or intravenous energy infusions in healthy volunteers (130). Solid bars represent the energy content of the preload, hatched bars the energy intake at lunch, and open bars the energy intake at dinner.

intake. After 15-minute intragastric infusions there was a significant suppression of energy intake at a meal (lunch) 15 minutes later, although no further effect at a second meal (dinner) 6.5 hours later. Here the infusion produced no net increase in energy intake over the 24-hour period.

Unfortunately, data from prolonged studies complicates this simplistic assessment. Infusions of a mixed nutrient solution, providing 85% of basal energy requirements for 5 days, led to a decrease in daily voluntary food intake by the last 2 days that compensated for $103 \pm 19\%$ of the infused energy (131), suggesting the presence of a postabsorptive control mechanism sensitive to the circulating supply of fuels.

It is evident that the presence of nutrients in the gut plays at least a part in appetite regulation, but there is as yet no clear view of its relative importance in integrative models of appetite control. Food consumed orally may exert a satiating influence via cognitive, gastrointestinal, or metabolic (oxidative or neuroendocrine) mechanisms. Intragastric nutrients bypass cognitive control, and parenteral nutrients can only be equally satiating if metabolic factors are the dominant mechanism of satiation. It would seem logical that the least satiating route would be parenteral, followed by intragastric and lastly oral because each step bypasses an additional level of appetite control, but definitive evidence is as yet absent.

Macronutrient Composition

The oral ingestion of macronutrients may have differential effects on satiety and subsequent food intake (53). This observation has led to an interest in the role of these nutrients in artificial nutrition to modulate anorexia. In the short-term studies described above assessing the feeding response to fat or carbohydrate within a 24-hour period (130), there was no significant difference between the two macronutrients. However, results of the 5-day studies of Gil et al. (131) suggest that glucose alone infused intravenously to provide 68% of basal energy requirements decreased oral intake by 78% of the infused energy, whereas when isoenergetic amounts of fat were infused the compensation in voluntary intake was only 29%.

A range of studies are currently underway in our unit to address each of these effects on long-term voluntary oral intake in healthy volunteers and weight-losing patients (M. Elia et al., unpublished observations). This may shed some light on the mechanisms of appetite control but will also provide practical guidelines for effective nutritional support. Until we begin to understand the mechanisms underlying the anorexia of disease, our nutritional interventions will remain largely empirical.

Specific Nutritional Substrates

Recent research has shown the dramatic effect that dietary factors may have on the cytokine response. Because cytokine effects on appetite may be an important contributor to the anorexia of disease, it is a plausible strategy to use anticytokine agents as therapeutic modalities. Supplementation of the diet with n-3 fatty acids decreases the production of IL-1, TNF, and interferon by peripheral blood mononuclear cells in vitro (132), and feeding with fish oil diminishes the anorectic effect of IL-1 (133) and TNF (134).

Appetite-stimulant effects have been attributed to ornithine oxo-glutarate (OXG). In a randomized, placebo-controlled trial (135), OXG led to a significant increase in reported appetite and greater body weight gain compared with placebo in a group of 185 elderly subjects. The mechanism of this effect is not clearly defined, although other studies have suggested that glutamine and its precursor OXG may have mood-enhancing properties (136).

Non-Nutritional Interventions

Cytokine Inhibitors

Cytokine action also may be inhibited by specific anticytokine monoclonal antibodies and receptor antagonists (137). Corticosteroids inhibit the transcription of IL-1, TNF, and other cytokines. Other agents, known as cytokine-suppressing anti-inflammatory drugs, seem to act by binding a mitogen-activating protein kinase that is required for the translation of messenger RNAs.

The anorectic effects of IL-1 can be blocked by ibuprofen, a cyclooxygenase inhibitor, which is presumed to operate in a manner analogous to that of fish oil (66). Experimental studies have shown that an IL-1 receptor antagonist can block the behavioral, cellular, and molecular action of this cytokine (63), but no clinical study has yet demonstrated that this approach can be exploited therapeutically to combat IL-1 induced anorexia. It has been suggested that the drug pentoxifylline, a nonspecific inhibitor of TNF in vitro, may be useful in the management of HIV-associated wasting (138), and a number of clinical trials are underway.

Neuropeptide inhibitors also seem to exert their action by modulating cytokine activity. Melanocyte-stimulating hormone inhibits IL-1 induced anorexia (139) and other biologic effects of cytokines, including fever (140).

Steroidal Agents

Corticosteroids have long been used to boost appetite, although their effect may be short term. In a randomized double-blind trial of dexamethasone treatment in patients with gastrointestinal cancer, Moertel et al. (141) showed significant symptomatic improvement in appetite after 2 weeks of treatment with the active drug, although the effect had disappeared by 4 weeks. Likewise, Willcox et al. (142) achieved subjective improvements in appetite and well-being using prednisolone. However, the failure to elicit an increase in body weight suggests that these findings may be a consequence of the mood-enhancing properties of steroids (143) and not necessarily a specific effect on appetite leading to increased intake. In a 14-day, randomized, double-blind study in patients with cancer (144), 32 mg/day of methylprednisolone led to improvements in appetite and food intake in approximately two thirds of patients. However, in a 20-day follow-up open phase of the trial, these nutritional parameters had returned to baseline levels. Moreover, the toxicity of prolonged treatment with corticosteroids preclude its use in many patients.

Chemical derivatives with more specific effects such as megesterol acetate and medroxyprogesterone acetate have frequently been shown to increase food intake and body weight and to enhance quality of life in patients with cancer and HIV infection (145–151). Although the results appear promising in terms of weight gain, the change in body composition is less clear and may include significant amounts of water or fat rather than lean tissue mass (152). The doses necessary to achieve its appetite-stimulant properties range from 400–800 mg/day, which is expensive and a significant burden to patients already taking numerous medications. Side effects are not uncommon and include nausea, vomiting, and edema. Again the mechanism is not fully elucidated, although recent evidence has implicated neuropeptide-Y (153).

If the principal mechanism of the effect of steroidal agents is through improvements in quality of life, other nonpharmacologic methods may achieve a similar effect on appetite. We are currently investigating this relationship in a longitudinal study of patients with lung cancer, focusing on appetite, nutritional status, functional well-being, and quality of life (J. Kramer et al., unpublished observations).

Other Pharmacologic Agents

A number of other pharmacologic agents have received intermittent attention as potential strategies to reverse the anorexia of disease, particularly in relation to cancer and HIV infection. However, none have yet become standard therapy.

Serotinergic Drugs

Evidence from experimental animals suggests that the injection of serotonin into the brain in pharmacologic doses decreases food intake. Systemic administration of its dietary precursor, tryptophan, increases brain serotonin levels and decreases food intake. In humans the appetite suppressant dexfenfluramine is a highly specific serotonin agonist that acts by both stimulating serotonin release and inhibiting reuptake and has been shown to produce significant weight loss in overweight individuals (154). These observations have led to the suggestion that cyproheptadine, a serotonin receptor blocker, may promote food intake.

Early studies in humans showed that it could increase appetite and food intake in healthy but underweight adults (155), patients with anorexia nervosa

(156), and patients with pulmonary tuberculosis (157). However, in the largest clinical trial to date, in which 295 patients with advanced cancer were randomized in a double-blind manner to receive oral cyproheptadine or placebo, the effects on appetite and food intake were extremely modest and did not ameliorate the progressive weight loss (158).

Hydrazine Sulfate

Hydrazine sulfate is a metabolic inhibitor that blocks the gluconeogenic enzyme phosphoenolpyruvate carboxykinase. In patients with lung cancer, it decreased hepatic glucose production (159) and resulted in a significant reduction in amino acid flux (160). The results of clinical trials of hydrazine sulfate have been mixed (161) but sufficiently encouraging to instigate two large multicenter studies to examine its effect on appetite, weight, nutritional status, quality of life, and survival. The results of these studies are not yet known.

Growth Hormone

Growth hormone has the potential to reverse some of the metabolic abnormalities of the cachexic syndrome. Cachexia is characterized by inappropriately large losses of protein associated with the oxidation of glucose and amino acids. Growth hormone increases lipolysis in the adipocyte and exerts a carbohydrate- and protein-sparing effect (162,163). However, there is no evidence that it exerts an anti-anorectic effect.

Growth hormone has been used therapeutically in a number of diseases in addition to growth hormone deficiency, including injury (164), surgery (162), critical illness (165), burns (164,166,167), and HIV infection (168). In each case protein conservation has been maintained throughout treatment in the presence of adequate or hyperenergetic feeding. Furthermore, Manson et al. (169) have demonstrated positive nitrogen balance in healthy male subjects in the presence of hypoenergetic feeding. Numerous studies are currently underway to investigate optimal treatment strategies, often in combination with nutritional support and exercise. The principal limiting factor in this form of therapy is the cost.

Cannabinoids

Weight gain is a well-recognized feature associated with the use of marijuana and its derivatives (161). Like corticosteroids, it is difficult to distinguish any specific appetite-inducing effects from the more generic mood enhancement effects. Dronabinol capsules (the principal psychoactive substance in *Cannabis sativa L.*) are approved by the U.S. Food and Drug Administration for the treatment of the anorexia induced by acquired immunodeficiency syndrome, for which they have been shown to enhance appetite and promote weight gain

(170,171). However, preliminary clinical data are not particularly encouraging. In the study of Struwe et al. (172), two of 12 patients withdrew because of drug intolerance. Only five patients completed the 5-week treatment period, and the increase in body weight and appetite was small and not significant.

CONCLUSIONS

Anorexia is a poorly defined, under-recognized and inadequately treated symptom of disease. All too often, appropriate nutritional support is not provided to patients at times when food intake is compromised. In some cases this is a consequence of the lack of training of health professionals about the importance of nutrition or a failure of communication between physicians, nurses, dietitians, and caterers. The beneficial effect of nutrition teams in raising the profile of nutrition and coordinating interventions has now been clearly documented (173,174). Not only do such teams lead to an improvement in the quality of care but ultimately also to cost savings. To date, nutrition teams have tended to focus on enteral and parenteral nutrition. If they are to achieve the maximum benefit to the greatest number of patients, they must widen their perspective to include the whole spectrum of nutritional and non-nutritional interventions to alleviate anorexia and not just use artificial nutrition to override the anorexia of disease.

However, resolving anorexia is not an end in itself. Cachexia is frequently characterized by a disproportionate loss of body cell mass. Therapies that simply overcome anorexia do not consistently restore an appropriate body composition (175,176). It has been suggested that the chronic production and release of proinflammatory cytokines may inhibit the normal anabolic processes essential for nutritional repletion. This would imply that nutritional strategies targeted at the diminution of the inflammatory response may be of the greatest benefit because they may improve nutrient use in addition to reversing the anorexia of disease (177). Alternatively, increases in food intake (achieved by nutritional or pharmacologic approaches) may have to be accompanied by mechanisms to modulate the metabolic response. The success of such strategies should be measured not by a reversal of the symptom of anorexia, or even by increases in body weight or composition, but by changes in the functional capacity of patients and decreases in morbidity and mortality.

Until we begin to understand the mechanisms underlying the anorexia of disease, nutritional interventions will remain largely empirical. At this stage the least we can do is to rigorously evaluate these interventions to achieve optimum results. A clearer understanding of the efficacy of current interventions may in itself shed some light on the mechanisms causing the anorexia of disease.

ACKNOWLEDGMENT

I thank Beckie Moore for collating the literature on sip feeds.

REFERENCES

1. Murray MJ, Murray AB. Anorexia of infection as a mechanism of host defense. *Am J Clin Nutr* 1979;32:593–596.
2. Yamazaki K, Maiz A, Moldawer LL, Bistrian BR, Blackburn GL. Complications associated with overfeeding of infected animals. *J Surg Res* 1986;40:152–158.
3. Alexander JW, Gonce ST, Miskell PW, Peck MD, Sax H. A new model for studying nutrition in peritonitis. *Ann Surg* 1989;209:338–340.
4. Askanazi J, Nordenstrom J, Rosenbaum H, et al. Nutrition for the patient with respiratory failure. *Anaesthesiology* 1981;54:373–377.
5. Dewys WD, Begg L, Larin PT, et al. Prognostic effect of weight loss prior to chemotherapy in cancer patients. *Am J Med* 1980;69:491–497.
6. Macallan DC, Noble C, Baldwin C, Foskett M, McManus T, Griffin GE. Prospective analysis of patterns of weight change in stage IV human immunodeficiency virus infection. *Am J Clin Nutr* 1993;58:417–424.
7. Hart BL. Behavioral adaptations to pathogens and parasites: five strategies. *Neurosci Biobehav Rev* 1990;14:274.
8. Hodges P, Thomson ABR. Nutritional status of patients with Crohn's disease. *J Can Diet Assoc* 1982;43:100.
9. Rigaud D, Angel LA, Cerf M, et al. Mechanisms of decreased food intake during weight loss in adult Crohn's disease patients without obvious malabsorption. *Am J Clin Nutr* 1994;60:775–781.
10. Difrancia M, Barbier D, Mege JL, Orehek J. Tumor necrosis factor alpha levels and weight loss in chronic obstructive pulmonary disease. *J Respir Crit Care Med* 1994;150–155:1453.
11. Roubenhoff R, Rall L. Humoral mediation of changing body composition during aging and chronic inflammation. *Nutr Rev* 1993;51:1–6.
12. Butterworth CE. The skeleton in the hospital closet. *Nutr Today* 1974;9:4–8.
13. Bistrian BR, Blackburn GL, Hallowell E, Heddle R. Protein status of general surgical patients. *JAMA* 1974;230:858–860.
14. Bistrian BR, Blackburn GL, Vitale J, Cochran D, Naylor J. Prevalence of malnutrition in general medical patients. *JAMA* 1976;253:1567–70.
15. Hill GL, Pickford I, Young GA et al. Malnutrition in surgical patients: an unrecognised problem. *Lancet* 1977;1:689–692.
16. Weinsier RL, Hunker EM, Krumdieck CL, Butterworth CE. Hospital malnutrition: a prospective evaluation of general medical patients during the course of hospitalisation. Am J Clin Nutr 1979;32:418–426.
17. Coats KG, Morgan SL, Bartolucci AA, Weinsier RL. Hospital associated malnutrition: a reevaluation 12 years later. *J Am Diet Assoc* 1993;93:27–33.
18. McWhirter JP, Pennington CR. Incidence and recognition of malnutrition in hospital. *Br Med J* 1994;308:945–948.
19. Gregory J, Foster K, Tyler H, Wiseman M. The dietary and nutritional survey of British adults. London: Her Majesty's Stationery Office; 1990.
20. Keys AJ, Brozek J, Henschel O, Michelson O, Taylor HL. In: *The biology of human starvation.* Minneapolis: University of Minnesota Press; 1950:140–60.
21. British Association for Parenteral and Enteral Nutrition. Enteral and parenteral nutrition in the community. Maidenhead, British Association for Parenteral and Enteral Nutrition; 1994.
22. Giner M, Laviano A, Meguid M, Gleason J. In 1995 a correlation between malnutrition and poor outcome in critically ill patients still exists. *Nutrition* 1996;12:23–29.
23. Moore R, Kramer JA, Elia M, Jebb SA. Screening for malnutrition in oncology patients. *Proc Nutr Soc* 1996;55:181a.
24. Elia M, Jebb SA. Changing concepts of energy requirements of critically ill patients. *Clin Nutr* 1992;1:35–37.
25. Black AE, Coward WA, Cole TJ, Prentice AM. Human energy expenditure in affluent societies: an analysis of 574 doubly-labelled water measurements. *Eur J Clin Nutr* 1996;50:72–92.
26. Prentice AM, Jebb SA. Obesity in Britain: gluttony or sloth. *Br Med J* 1995;311:437–439.
27. Reife CM. Involuntary weight loss. *Med Clin North Am* 1995;79:299–312.
28. Allison SP. Cost-effectiveness of nutritional support in the elderly. *Proc Nutr Soc* 1995;54:693–699.

29. Prentice AM, Leavesley K, Murgatroyd PR, et al. Is severe wasting in elderly mental patients caused by an excessive energy requirement? *Age Ageing* 1989;18:158–167.
30. Sandman PO, Adolfsson R, Nygren C, Hallmans G, Winblad B. Nutritional status and dietary intake in institutionalised patients with Alzheimer's disease and multi-infarct dementia. *J Am Geriatr Soc* 1987;35:31–38.
31. Van Ort S, Phillips L. Feeding nursing home residents with Alzheimers Disease. *Geriatr Nursing* 1992;13:249–253.
32. Norton B, McKaig B, Booth S, Gornall C, Long R, Holmes G. A randomised comparison of percutaneous endoscopic gastrostomy feeding and nasogastric tube feeding following acute dysphagic stroke. *Proc Nutr Soc* 1996;55:147a.
33. Gazis A, Rawlings J, Allison S, Jefferson D. A prospective study of nutritional changes and gastrostomy feeding in motor neurone disease. *Proc Nutr Soc* 1996 (in press).
34. Kotler D, Tierney A, Brenner S, Couture S, Wang J, Pierson R. Preservation of short-term energy balance in clinically stable patients with AIDS. *Am J Clin Nutr* 1990;51:7–13.
35. Jennings G, Lunn P, Elia M. Effect of endotoxin on gastrointestinal transit time and intestinal permeability. *Clin Nutr* 1995;14:35–41.
36. Weekes E, Elia M. Observations on the patterns of 24 hour energy expenditure, changes in body composition and gastric emptying in head-injured patients receiving nasogastric tube feeding. *J Parenter Enter Nutr* 1995;20:31–37.
37. Macallan DC, Noble C, Baldwin C, et al. Energy expenditure and wasting in human immunodeficiency virus infection. *N Engl J Med* 1994;333:83–88.
38. Booth DA. Sensory influences on food intake. *Nutr Rev* 1990;48:71–77.
39. DeWys WD. Anorexia as a general effect of cancer. *Am Cancer Soc* 1979;43:2013–2019.
40. Read N, French S, Cunningham K. The role of the gut in regulating food intake in man. *Nutr Rev* 1994;52:1–10.
41. Pasquali R, Besteghi L, Casimirri F et al. Mechanisms of the action of the intragastric balloon in obesity: effects on hunger and satiety. *Appetite* 1990;15: 3–11.
42. Khan MI, Read NW. The effect of duodenal lipid infusions upon gastric pressure and sensory responses to balloon distension. *Gastroenterology* 1992;102:467.
43. Kissileff HR, Pi-Sunyer XF, Thornton J, Smith GP. C-terminal octapeptide of cholecystokinin decreases food intake in man. Am J Clin Nutr 1981;34:154–160.
44. Stacher G, Steinringer H, Schmierer G, et al. Cholecystokinin octapeptide decreases intake of solid food in man. *Peptides* 1982;3:133–136.
45. Wolkowitz OM, Gertz B, Weingartner H, Beccaria L, Thompson K, Liddle RA. Hunger in humans induced by MK-329 a specific peripheral-type cholecystokinin receptor antagonist. *Biol Psychol* 1990;28:169–173.
46. Drewe J, Gadien A, Rovati LC, Begliner C. Role of circulating cholecystokinin in control of fat-induced inhibition of food intake in humans. *Gastroenterology* 1992;102:1654–1659.
47. French SJ, Murray B, Rumsey RDE, Sepple CP, Read NW. Is cholecystokinin a satiety hormone? Correlations of plasma cholecystokinin with hunger, satiety and gastric emptying in normal volunteers. *Appetite* 1993;21:95–104.
48. Schwartz M, Figlewicz D, Baskin D, Woods S, Porte D. Insulin in the brain: a hormonal regulator of energy balance. *Endocr Rev* 1992;13:387–414.
49. Langhans W, Scharrer E. Metabolic control of eating. In: Simopoulous AP, ed. *Energy expenditure and the bioenergetics of obesity. World review of nutrition and dietetics.* Basel, Switzerland: Karger; 1992:1–67.
50. Cahill G. Starvation in man. *Clin Endocrinol Metabolism* 1976;5:397–415.
51. Vary TC, Siegel JM, Nakatani T, et al. Effect of sepsis on activity of pyruvate dehydrogenase complex in skeletal muscle and liver. *Am J Physiol* 1986;250:E634–E640.
52. Williamson DH, Farrell R, Kerr A, et al. Muscle protein catabolism after injury in man, as measured by urinary excretion of 3-methylhistidine. *Clin Sci* 1977;52:527–533.
53. Stubbs RJ. Macronutrient effects on appetite. *Int J Obesity* 1995;19:511–519.
54. Stubbs R, Goldberg G, Murgatroyd P, Prentice AM. Carbohydrate balance and day to day food intake in man. *Am J Clin Nutr* 1993;57:897–903.
55. Shetty PS, Prentice AM, Goldberg GR, et al. Alterations in fuel selection and voluntary food intake in response to isoenergetic manipulation of glycogen stores in man. *Am J Clin Nutr* 1994;60:534–543.
56. Rohner-Jeanrenaud F. A neuroendocrine reappraisal of the dual-centre hypothesis: its implications for obesity and insulin resistance. *Int J Obesity* 1995;19:517–534.

57. Zhang Y, Proenca R, Maffei M, et al. Positional cloning of the mouse obese gene and its human homologue. *Nature* 1994;372:425–432.
58. Lonnquist F, Arner P, Nordfos L, Schalling M. Overexpression of the obese (ob) gene in adipose tissue of human obese subjects. *Nature Med* 1995;1:950–953.
59. Scott J. New chapter for the fat controller. *Nature* 1996;379:113–114.
60. Arnalich F, Sanchez JF, Martinez M, et al. Changes in plasma concentrations of vasoactive neuropeptides in patients with sepsis and septic shock. *Life Sci* 1994;56:75–81.
61. Koide S, Onishi H, Hashimoto H, Kai T, Yamagami S. Plasma neuropeptide-Y is reduced in patients with Alzheimers disease. *Neurosci Lett* 1995;198:149–151.
62. Theologides A. The anorexia-cachexia syndrome: a new hypothesis. *NY Acad Sci* 1974;230:14–22.
63. Plata-Salaman CR. Cytokines and feeding suppression: an integrative view from neurologic to molecular levels. *Nutrition* 1995;11:674–677.
64. Dinarello C. The interleukin-1 family: 10 years of discovery. *FASEB J* 1994;8:1314.
65. Plata-Salaman C. Cytokines and injestive behaviour: methods and overview. *Methods Neurosci* 1993;17:151.
66. Plata-Salaman CR. Meal patterns in response to the intracerebroventricular administration of interleukin-1B in rats. *Physiol Behav* 1994;55:727.
67. Plata-Salaman CR. Interferons and central regulation of feeding. *Am J Physiol* 1992;263:R1222.
68. Plata-Salaman CR, Borkoski JP. Centrally administered bacterial lipopolysaccharide depresses feeding in rats. *Pharmacol Biochem Behav* 1993;46:787.
69. Schmale AH. Psychological aspects of anorexia. *Cancer* 1979;43:2087–2092.
70. Morley JE, Kraenzle D. Causes of weight loss in a community nursing home. *J Am Geriatr Soc* 1994;42:583–585.
71. Bernstein I, Webster M. Learned taste aversions in humans. *Physiol Behav* 1980;25:363–366.
72. Dewys WD. Anorexia in cancer patients. *Cancer Res* 1977;37:2354–2358.
73. Barrocas A, Craig LD, Foltz MB. Nutrition support, supplementation and replacement. *Nutr Old Age* 1994;21:149–173.
74. Schwenk A, Burger B, Ollenschlager G, et al. Evaluation of nutritional counselling in HIV associated malnutrition. *Clin Nutr* 1994;13:212–220.
75. Murphy J, Cameron DW, Garber G, Conway B, Denomme N. Dietary counselling and nutritional supplementation in HIV infection. *J Can Diet Assoc* 1992;53:205–208.
76. Dowling S, Mulcahy F, Gibney MJ. Nutrition in the management of HIV antibody positive patients: a longitudinal study of dietetic out-patient advice. *Eur J Clin Nutr* 1990;44:823–829.
77. Imes S, Pinchbeck BR, Thompson ABR. Diet counselling modifies nutrient intake of patients with Crohn's disease. *J Am Diet Assoc* 1987;87:456–463.
78. Poppitt SD. Energy density of diets and obesity. *Int J Obesity* 1995;19:520–526.
79. Hill AJ, Blundell JE. Macronutrients and satiety: the effects of a high-protein or high-carbohydrate meal on subjective motivation to eat and food preferences. *Nutr Behav* 1986;3:133–144.
80. DeCastro JM. Macronutrient relationships with meal patterns and mood in the spontaneous feeding behaviour of humans. *Physiol Behav* 1987;39:561–569.
81. Cotton JR, Burley VJ, Westrate JA, Blundell JE. Dietary fat and appetite: similarities and differences in the satiating effect of meals supplemented with either fat or carbohydrate. *J Hum Nutr Diet* 1994;7:11–24.
82. Flatt JP, Ravussin E, Acheson HJ, Jequier E. Effects of dietary fat on postprandial substrate oxidation and on carbohydrate and fat balances. *J Clin Invest* 1985;76:1019–1024.
83. Abbot WGH, Howard BV, Christin L, et al. Short-term energy balance: relationship with protein, carbohydrate and fat balances. *Am J Physiol* 1988;255:E322–E337.
84. Schutz Y, Flatt JP, Jequier E. Failure of dietary fat to promote fat oxidation: a factor favouring the development of obesity. *Am J Clin Nutr* 1989;50:307–314.
85. Drewnowski A, Riskey D, Desor JA. Feeling fat yet unconcerned: self-reported overweight and the restraint scale. *Appetite* 1982;3:273–279.
86. Tourila H. Preferences and attitudes related to fat containing foods. In: *Dietary fats: determinants of preference, selection and consumption.* London: Elsevier Applied Science; 1992.
87. Ramirez I, Friedman MI. Dietary hyperphagia in rats: role of fat, carbohydrate and energy content. *Physiol Behav* 1990;47:1157–1163.
88. van Stratum P, Lussenberg RN, van Wezel LA, Vergroesen AJ, Cremer HD. The effect of dietary carbohydrate:fat ratio on energy intake by adult women. *Am J Clin Nutr* 1978;31:206–212.

89. Stubbs RJ, Harbron CG, Murgatroyd PR, Prentice AM. Covert manipulation of dietary fat and energy density: effect on substrate flux and food intake in men eating ad libitum. *Am J Clin Nutr* 1995;62:316–29.

90. Stubbs RJ, Ritz P, Coward WA, Prentice AM. Covert manipulation of the ratio of dietary fat to carbohydrate and energy density: effect on food intake and energy balance in free living men, eating ad libitum. *Am J Clin Nutr* 1995;62:330–337.

91. Parkinson SA, Lewis J, Morris R, Allbright A, Plant H, Slevin MA. Oral protein and energy supplements in cancer patients. *Hum Nutr* 1987;41A:233–243.

92. Barnes E. Increasing energy intake in hospital food. *Nursing Standard* 1989;4:30–31.

93. Chlebowski RT, Beall G, Grosvenor M, et al. Long-term effects of early nutritional support with a new enterotropic peptide-based formula vs. standard enteral formula in HIV-infected patients: randomized prospective trial. *Nutrition* 1993;9:507–512.

94. Kissileff HR. Effects of physical state (liquid-solid) of foods on food intake: procedural and substantive contributions. *Am J Clin Nutr* 1985;42:956–965.

95. Edelstein SL, Barrett-Connor EL, Wingard DL, Cohn BA. Increased meal frequency associated with decreased cholesterol concentrations. *Am J Clin Nutr* 1992;55:664–669.

96. Kant AK, Schatzkin A, Graubard BI, Ballard-Barbash R. Frequency of eating occasions and weight change in the NHANES I Epidemiologic Survey. *Int J Obesity* 1995;19:466–474.

97. Brown KH, Sanchez-Grinan M, Perez F, Peerson JM, Ganoza L. Effects of dietary energy density and feeding frequency on total daily energy intakes of children recovering from malnutrition. *Am J Clin Nutr* 1995;62:13–18.

98. Shelmet JJ, Reicherd GA, Skutches CL, Hoeldtke RD, Owen OE, Bodin G. Ethanol causes acute inhibition of carbohydrate, fat and protein oxidation and insulin resistance. *J Clin Invest* 1988;81:1137–1145.

99. Bebb HT, Houser HB, Witschi JC, Littell AS, Fuller RK. Calorie and nutrient contribution of alcoholic beverages to the usual diets of 155 adults. *Am J Clin Nutr* 1971;24:1042–1052.

100. Jones BR, Barret-Conner E, Criqui MH, Holdbrook MJ. A community study of calorie and nutrient intake in drinkers and non-drinkers of alcohol. *Am J Clin Nutr* 1982;35:135–141.

101. Fisher M, Gordon T. The relationship of drinking and smoking habits to diet: the Lipid Research Clinics prevalence study. *Am J Clin Nutr* 1985;41:623–630.

102. DeCastro JM, Orozco S. Moderate alcohol intake and spontaneous eating patterns of humans: evidence of unregulated supplementation. *Am J Clin Nutr* 1990;52:246–253.

103. DeCastro JM, DeCastro ES. Spontaneous meal patterns in humans: Influence of the presence of other people. *Am J Clin Nutr* 1989;50:237–247.

104. Foltin RW, Kelly TH, Fischman MW. Ethanol as an energy source in humans: comparison with dextrose-containing beverages. *Appetite* 1993;20:95–110.

104a. Poppitt SD, Eckhardt JW, McGonagle J, et al. Short-term effects of alcohol consumption on appetite and energy intake. *Physiol Behav* 1996;60:1063–1070.

105. Soukop M, Calman KC. Nutritional support in patients with malignant disease. *J Hum Nutr* 1979;33:179–188.

106. Bolton J, Abbott R, Kiely M, et al. Comparison of three oral sip-feed supplements in patients with cancer. *J Hum Nutr Diet* 1992;5:79–84.

107. Ovesen J. The effect of a supplement which is nutrient dense compared to standard concentration on the total nutritional intake of anorectic patients. *Clin Nutr* 1992;11:154–157.

108. Arnold C, Richter MP. The effect of oral nutritional supplements on head and neck cancer. *Int J Radiat Oncol Biol Physics* 1988;16:1595–1599.

109. Williams CM, Driver LT, Older J, Dickerson WT. Controlled trial of sip-feed supplements in elderly orthopaedic patients. *Eur J Clin Nutr* 1989;43:267–274.

110. Elmstahl S, Steen B. Hospital nutrition in geriatric long-term care medicine II. Effects of dietary supplements. *Age Ageing* 1987;16:73–80.

111. Rana SK, Bray J, Menzies-Gow N, et al. Short term benefits of post-operative oral dietary supplements in surgical patients. *Clin Nutr* 1992;11:337–344.

112. McEnvoy AW, James O. The effect of a dietary supplement (build-up) on nutritional status in hospitalized elderly patients. *Hum Nutr Appl Nutr* 1982;36A:374–376.

113. Larsson J, Unosson M, Ek AC, et al. Effect of a dietary supplement on nutritional status and clinical outcome in 501 geriatric patients—a randomised study. *Clin Nutr* 1990;9:179–184.

114. Johnson LE, Dooley PA, Gleick JB. Oral nutritional supplement use in elderly nursing home patients. *J Am Geratr Soc* 1993;41:947–952.

115. Carver A, Dobson A. Effects of dietary supplementation of elderly demented hospital residents. *J Hum Nutr Diet* 1995;8:389–394.
116. Banerjee AK, Brocklehurst JC, Wainwright H, Swindell R. Nutritional status of long-stay geriatric in patients: effects of a food supplement (Complan). *Age Ageing* 1978;7:237–243.
117. Hankey CR, Summerbell J, Wynne HA. The effect of dietary supplementation in continuing-care elderly people: nutritional, anthropometric and biochemical parameters. *J Hum Nutr Diet* 1993;6: 317–322.
118. Katakity M, Webb JF, Dickerson JWT. Some effects of a food supplement in elderly hospital patients. *Hum Nutr Appl Nutr* 1983;37A:85–93.
119. Unosson M, Larsson J, Ek AC, Bjurulf P. Effects of a dietary supplement on functional condition and clinical outcome measured with a modified norton scale. *Clin Nutr* 1992;II:134–139.
120. O'Dell B, Reeves P. Zinc status and food intake. In: *Zinc in human biology.* International Life Sciences Institute; 1989:173–182.
121. Bastow D, Rawlings J, Allison SP. Overnight nasogastric tube feeding. *Clin Nutr* 1985;4:7–11.
122. Ashworth N. Effects of nightly food supplements on food intake in man. *Lancet* 1962;2:685–687.
123. Fryer JH. The effects of a late-night caloric supplement upon body weight and food intake in man. *Am J Clin Nutr* 1958;6:354–364.
124. Rolls BT, Tim-Harris S, Fischmann MW, Faltin RW, Maran TH, Stoner SA. Satiety after preloads with different amounts of fat and carbohydrate: implications for obesity. *Am J Clin Nutr* 1994;60: 476–487.
125. Delmi M, Rapin CH, Bengoa JM, Delmas PD, Vasey H, Bonjour JP. Dietary supplementation in elderly patients with fractured neck of femur. *Lancet* 1990;335:1013–1016.
126. Jordan HA, Moses H, MacFayden BV, Dudrick SJ. Hunger and satiety in humans during parenteral hyperalimentation. *Psychosomat Med* 1974;36:144–155.
127. Booth DA. Satiety and behavioral caloric compensation following intragastric glucose loads in the rat. *J Compar Physiol Psychol* 1972;78:412–432.
128. Greenberg D, Becker DC, Gibbs J, Smith GP. Intraportal administration of fat fails to elicit satiety. *Soc Neurosci* 1986;12:213.
129. Welch I, Saunders K, Read NW. Effect of ileal and intravenous infusions of fat emulsions on feeding and satiety in human volunteers. *Gastroenterology* 1985;89:1293–1297.
130. Shide DJ, Caballero B, Reidelberger R, Rolls BJ. Accurate energy compensation for intragastric and oral nutrients in lean males. *Am J Clin Nutr* 1995;61:754–764.
131. Gil KM, Skeie B, Kvetan V, Askanazi J, Friedman MI. Parenteral nutrition and oral intake: effect of glucose and fat infusions. *J Parenter Enter Nutr* 1990;15:426–432.
132. Endres S, Gharbani R, Kelley VE, et al. The effect of dietary supplementation with n-3 polyunsaturated fatty acids on the synthesis of interleukin-1 and tumor necrosis factor by mononuclear cells. *N Engl J Med* 1989;320:265–271.
133. Hellerstein MK, Meydani SN, Meydani M, Wu K, Dinarello CA. Interleukin-1–induced anorexia in the rat. Influence of prostaglandins. *J Clin Invest* 1989;84:228.
134. Mulrooney HM, Grimble RF. Influence of butter and of corn, coconut and fish oils on the effects of recombinant human tumour necrosis factor alpha in rats. *Clin Sci* 1993;84:105–107.
135. Brocker P, Vellas B, Albarede JL, Poynard T. A two-centre, randomized, double-blind trial of ornithine oxoglutarate in 194 elderly, ambulatory, convalescent subjects. *Age Ageing* 1994;23:303–306.
136. Young L, Bye N, Scheltinga M, Ziegler T, Jacobs D, Wilmore D. Patients receiving glutamine-supplemented intravenous feedings report an improvement in mood. *J Parenter Enter Nutr* 1993;17: 422–427.
137. Dinarello CA. Controlling the production of interleukin-1 and tumor necrosis factor in disease. *Nutrition* 1995;11:695–697.
138. Ambrus JL, Lillie MA. Pentoxifylline in treatment of acquired immunodeficiency syndrome? [Letter]. *Blood* 1992;79:535–536.
139. Uehara Y, Shimizu H, Sato N, et al. Carboxyl-terminal tripeptide of α-melanocyte–stimulating hormone antagonizes interleukin-1–induced anorexia. *Eur J Pharmacol* 1992;220:119.
140. Catania A, Lipton JM. α-Melanocyte stimulating hormone in the modulation of host reactions. *Endocr Rev* 1992;14:564.
141. Moertel CG, Schutt AJ, Reitemeier RJ, Hahn RG. Corticosteroid therapy of preterminal gastrointestinal cancer. *Cancer* 1974;33:1607–1609.
142. Willcox JC, Carr J, Shaw J, Richardson M, Calman KC, Drennan M. Prednisolone as an appetite stimulant in patients with cancer. *Br Med J* 1984;288:27.

143. Schell H. Adrenal corticosteroid therapy in far-advanced cancer. *Geriatrics* 1972;27:131–141.
144. Bruera E, Roca E, Cedaro L, Carraro S, Chacon R. Action of oral methylprednisolone in terminal cancer patients: a prospective randomized double-blind study. *Cancer Treat Rep* 1985;69:751–754.
145. Tchekmedyian NS, Tait N, Moody M, Aisner J. Appetite stimulation with megestrol acetate in cachectic cancer patients. *Semin Oncol* 1986;13(suppl 4):37–43.
146. Tchekmedyian NS, Tait N, Moody M, Aisner J. High-dose megestrol acetate: a possible treatment for cachexia. *JAMA* 1987;257:1195–1198.
147. Tchekmedyian NS, Hariri L, Siau J, et al. Megestrol acetate in cancer anorexia and weight loss. *Proc ASCO* 1990;9:336.
148. Aisner J, Parnes H, Tait N, Hickman M. Appetite stimulation and weight gain with megestrol acetate. *Semin Oncol* 1990;17(suppl 9):2–7.
149. Cruz JM, Muss HB, Brockschmidt JK, Evans GW. Weight changes in women with metastatic breast cancer treated with megestrol acetate: a comparison of standard versus high does therapy. *Semin Oncol* 1990;17(suppl 9):63–67.
150. Loprinzi CL, Ellison NM, Schaid DJ, et al. A controlled trial of megestrol acetate for the treatment of cancer anorexia and cachexia. *J Natl Cancer Inst* 1990;82:1127–1132.
151. Von Roenn JH, Murphy RL, Wegener N. Megestrol acetate for treatment of anorexia and cachexia associated with human immunodeficiency virus infection. *Semin Oncol* 1990;17(suppl 9):13–16.
152. Beck SA, Tisdale MJ. Effect of megestrol acetate on weight loss induced by tumor necrosis factor α and a cachexia-inducing tumor (MAC16) in NMRI mice. *Br J Cancer* 1990;62:420–424.
153. McCarthy HD, Crowder RE, Dryden S, Williams G. Megestrol acetate stimulates food and water intake in the rat: effects on regional hypothalamic neuropeptide-y concentration. *Eur J Pharmacol* 1994;265:99.
154. Guy-Grand B, Apfelbaum M, Crepaldi G, Gries A, Lefebvre P, Turner P. International trial of long term dexfenfluramine in obesity. *Lancet* 1989;2:1142–1145.
155. Noble RE. Effect of cyproheptadine on appetite and weight gain in adults. *JAMA* 1969;209:2054–2055.
156. Goldberg SC, Halmis KA, Eckert ED, Casper RC, Davies JM. Cyproheptadine in anorexia nervosa. *Br J Psychiatry* 1979;134:67–70.
157. Shah NM. A double-blind study on appetite stimulation and weight gain with cyproheptadine as an adjunct to specific therapy in pulmonary tuberculosis. *Curr Med Practice* 1968;12:861–864.
158. Kardinal CG, Loprinzi CL, Schaid DJ, et al. A controlled trial of cyproheptadine in cancer patients with anorexia and/or cachexia. *Cancer* 1990;65:2657–2662.
159. Chlebowski RJ, Heber D, Richardson B, Block JB. Influence of hydrazine sulphate on abnormal carbohydrate metabolism in cancer patients with weight loss. *Cancer Res* 1984;44:857–861.
160. Tayek JA, Chlebowski RT, Heber D. Effect of hydrazine sulphate on whole-body protein breakdown measured by C-lysine metabolism in lung cancer patients. *Lancet* 1987;240–245.
161. Bruera E. Clinical management of anorexia and cachexia in patients with advanced cancer. *Oncology* 1992;49:35–42.
162. Ward HC, Halliday D, Sin AJW. Protein and energy metabolism and biosynthetic human growth hormone after gastrointestinal surgery. *Ann Surg* 1987;206:56–61.
163. Grunfeld C, Kotler DP, Hamadeh R, et al. Hypertriglyceridemia in the acquired immunodeficiency syndrome. *Am J Med* 1989;86:27–31.
164. Belcher HJCR, Mercer D, Judkins KC, et al. Biosynthetic human growth hormone in burned patients: a pilot study. *Burns* 1989;15:99–107.
165. Ziegler TR, Young LS, Ferrari-Baliviera E, et al. Use of human growth hormone combined with nutritional support in a critical care unit. *J Parenter Enter Nutr* 1990;14:574–581.
166. Herndon DN, Barrow RE, Kunkel KR, et al. Effects of recombinant human growth hormone on donor-site healing in severely burned children. *Ann Surg* 1990;212:424–429.
167. Gore DC, Honeycutt D, Jahoor F, Wolfe RR, Herndon DN. Effect of exogenous growth hormone on whole-body and isolated-limb protein kinetics in burned patients. *Arch Surg* 1991;126:38–43.
168. Mulligan K, Grunfeld C, Hellerstein MK, Neese RA, Schambelan M. Anabolic effects of recombinant human growth hormone in patients with wasting associated with human immunodeficiency virus infection. *J Clin Endocrinol Metab* 1993;77:956–962.
169. Manson J, Wilmore DW. Positive nitrogen balance and human growth hormone and hypocaloric intravenous feeding. *Surgery* 1986;100:188–197.
170. Plasse TF, Gorter RW, Krasnow SH, et al. Recent clinical experience with dronabinol. *Pharmacol Biochem Behav* 1991;40:695–700.

171. Conant M, Roy D, Shepard KV, et al. Dronabinol enhances appetite and controls weight loss in HIV patients. *Proc ASCO* 1991;10:35.
172. Struwe M, Kaaempfer S, Geiger C, Pavia A, Plasse T, Shepard K, et al. Effect of dronabinol on nutritional status in HIV infection. *Ann Pharmacother* 1993;27:827–831.
173. Allison S. The uses and limitations of nutritional support. *Clin Nutr* 1992;11:319–330.
174. Hassel J, Games A, Shaffer B, Harkins L. Nutrition support team management of enterally fed patients in a community hospital is cost-beneficial. *J Am Diet Assoc* 1994;94:993–995.
175. Cohn S, Vartsky D, Vaswani AN, et al. Changes in body composition of cancer patients following combined nutritional support. *Nutr Cancer* 1982;4:107–119.
176. Shike M, Russell DM, Detsky AS, et al. Changes in body composition in patients with small cell lung cancer. The effect of total parenteral nutrition as an adjunct to chemotherapy. *Ann Intern Med* 1984;101:303–309.
177. Hellerstein MK, Kahn J, Mudie H, Viteri F. Current approaches to the treatment of human immunodeficiency virus-associated weight loss: pathophysiologic considerations and emerging management strategies. *Semin Oncol* 1990;17:17–33.
178. Pullicino E, Goldberg G, Elia M. Energy expenditure and substrate metabolism measured by 24h whole-body calorimetry in patients receiving cyclic and continuous total parenteral nutrition. *Clin Sci* 1991;80:571–582.
179. Pullicino E. *Aspects of energy metabolism in hospitalised patients* [PhD Thesis]. CNAA. British Lending Library No. 96679 1992.

*Physiology, Stress, and Malnutrition: Functional
Correlates, Nutritional Intervention,*
edited by J.M. Kinney and H.N. Tucker.
Lippincott–Raven Publishers © 1997.

Late Postoperative Hypoxemia

Jacob Rosenberg and Henrik Kehlet

*Department of Surgical Gastroenterology, Hvidovre University Hospital,
DK-2650 Hvidovre, Denmark*

Major surgery may be followed by complications such as myocardial infarction, wound infection, impaired wound healing, and mental disturbances, which cannot only be explained by imperfections in surgical technique but rather may be due to increased organ demands caused by the endocrine metabolic response to surgical trauma (1). One of the stress responses after operation is impaired pulmonary function with arterial hypoxemia, which may lead to decreased oxygen supply to body organs, thereby representing a pathogenic factor in the above mentioned postoperative morbidity parameters (2). Residual sedation or intraoperative mechanisms impairing pulmonary function may contribute to early postoperative hypoxemia in the recovery room, a common and well-known phenomenon (3). In the late postoperative period, however, hypoxemia may be unrecognized, severe, and sustained with constant hypoxemia lasting for 2–5 days after major abdominal surgery (4) and with superimposed episodic hypoxemia, especially during the night (5). This review addresses the mechanisms and clinical implications of hypoxemia in the late postoperative period, that is, when the patient is back in the surgical ward, and usually without routine noninvasive monitoring.

DEFINITIONS

Constant hypoxemia refers to a constantly low oxygen saturation (SpO_2) in the arterial blood, usually defined as a mean value for a study period below, e.g., 90% SpO_2 (4,6–8).

Episodic hypoxemia in the postoperative period has been defined as a decrease in SpO_2 arterial oxygen saturation of 5% (6,9) or more than 5% (7) from baseline. It is emphasized that terms such as "desaturation" (10) or "episodes of hypoxemia" (11–13), as used for a certain time spent below a certain SpO_2 value, are inaccurate definitions of episodic hypoxemia. They could merely represent physiological 1–2% oscillations around the line of the defined limit and therefore not a pathophysiologic event (presumably a ventilatory dysrhythmia) often linked to simultaneous cardiovascular changes. A definition of

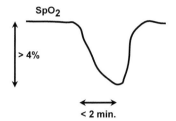

FIG. 1. Definition of episodic hypoxemia. The decrease in arterial oxygen saturation (SpO_2) should occur within 2 minutes and SpO_2 should decrease more than 4% from baseline.

episodic hypoxemia holding criteria of the magnitude of sudden desaturation (e.g., a 5% decrease in SpO_2) and of the $dSpO_2/dt$ is therefore more suitable when looking at the relationship to postoperative morbidity parameters (e.g., the decline in SpO_2 should occur within 2 minutes; Fig. 1) (9).

Another problem is methodologic differences in the reporting of hypoxemia in the literature, making extraction of incidence data difficult. For example, when using the compressed SpO_2 distribution diagram (Fig. 2) to describe oxygenation in a single patient during a study night, the incidence and severity of each hypoxemia event cannot be seen (14). The above mentioned definition of episodic hypoxemia requires that the actual SpO_2 curve is available. An international agreement on the recommendations for reporting of hypoxemia in scientific publications is warranted in order to make comparisons and extractions of data possible regarding time course and incidence.

TIME COURSE

Episodic Hypoxemia

Reeder et al. monitored nocturnal oxygen saturation during the first 5 nights after major abdominal vascular surgery and observed episodes of hypoxemia, especially on nights 3–5 after operation (15). However, the natural course of

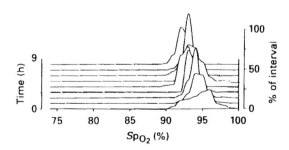

FIG. 2. Example of a compressed SpO_2 distribution diagram showing hypoxemia. Reprinted with permission (14).

postoperative hypoxemia was disturbed by the routine use of supplemental oxygen therapy in the majority of their patients for the first two postoperative nights (15). Entwistle et al. monitored patients for four nights after thoracotomy, and patients were given oxygen during the first night after operation (14). However, episodic hypoxemia was not documented specifically, only as a "pattern of unstable hypoxemia," and from their data presentation using the compressed SpO_2 distribution diagram it was not possible to derive the time course of late postoperative episodic hypoxemia. A number of studies in which patients have been monitored for up to three nights after major operation and without oxygen therapy have reported episodic hypoxemia to be most pronounced on the second or third night after surgery (5,7,9,16). Another study in patients undergoing open cholecystectomy and studied for three nights after operation and without oxygen therapy reported episodic hypoxemia to be most frequent on the first and the second nights after operation (17). Only one study reported continuous monitoring of nocturnal oxygenation for five nights after major surgery and without oxygen therapy (4). This study showed episodic hypoxemia to be most frequent on the third night after general anesthesia and abdominal surgery (Fig. 3) (4).

Constant Hypoxemia

Studies using daytime blood gas analyses have evaluated the time course of constant hypoxemia after abdominal (18–20), thoracic (21,22), thoracoabdominal

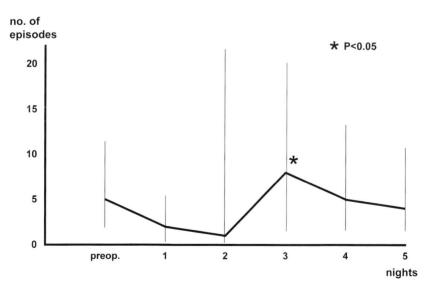

FIG. 3. Number of hypoxemic episodes (medians and quartiles) on the preoperative and first five nights after major abdominal surgery in 17 patients studied without supplementary oxygen therapy. Data from Rosenberg et al. (4).

(18,23), and hip surgery (24), and they all found lowest arterial oxygen levels on the second or third day after operation. Studies using continuous nocturnal oximetry have found comparable results, with mean SpO_2 being lowest on the second night after thoracotomy (14) or abdominal surgery (4,5,7,9,10,16,17,25).

INCIDENCE

Hypoxemia in the surgical ward has been known for many years, but the incidence in larger patient series has not been studied until recently (8). In 78 patients undergoing major abdominal surgery and studied without oxygen therapy, 41% of patients had a mean oxygen saturation during the second postoperative night of less than 90%; 38% of patients had episodes of sudden desaturation to below 80% oxygen saturation; and 23% of patients had more than 30 episodes (regardless of end-point) of sudden desaturation on the second postoperative night. Otherwise well-designed studies (26,27) have unfortunately not been able to control postoperative oxygen therapy, making them ineffective for evaluating the true incidence of hypoxemia. Other studies have ceased to monitor after the first postoperative night (6,11,12,13,28,29), thereby overlooking observations of more pronounced oxygen desaturations on the second and third postoperative nights. Incidence data from other patient categories and using different perioperative regimens (minimal invasive surgery versus conventional techniques, and with different types of anesthesia and postoperative analgesia) are not available.

MECHANISMS OF LATE POSTOPERATIVE HYPOXEMIA

Extensive reviews on the classical pathogenic factors to postoperative hypoxemia have been published recently (30,31), and the following is a short update. In summary, the mechanism leading to postoperative constant hypoxemia is primarily a pulmonary shunt caused by a reduction in functional residual capacity and is most pronounced after abdominal or thoracic operations (32), whereas postoperative episodic hypoxemia may be caused by ventilatory dysrhythmias (hypoventilation and apneas) related to analgesic administration and/or rebound of rapid eye movement (REM) sleep on the second and third nights after operation (16,30,31).

Postoperative Pulmonary Function and Ventilatory Pattern

The early postoperative phase (within the first 2 hours) is characterized by arterial hypoxemia directly related to the continuing effects of general anesthesia. This is followed by a second delayed phase in which mechanical abnormalities dominate with accompanying arterial hypoxemia (32). During anesthesia, gas exchange is impaired as a result of reduced tone in the muscles of the chest

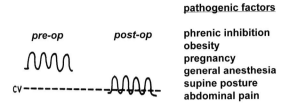

pathogenic factors

phrenic inhibition
obesity
pregnancy
general anesthesia
supine posture
abdominal pain

FIG. 4. Relationship of closing volume (CV) to functional residual capacity (basis of the curve showing ventilation). Preoperatively and in young healthy patients, FRC normally is larger than CV (left). If FRC decreases (right), as seen during and after operation, small airway closure may occur during normal breathing. Adapted with permission (32).

wall, and probably alterations in bronchomotor and vascular tone, and the resulting changes may persist somewhat into the postoperative period, contributing to early postoperative constant hypoxemia (30). The most important mechanisms contributing to hypoxemia in the first hours after operation are diffusion hypoxia, compression atelectases in dependent areas of the lungs, and posthyperventilation hypoventilation (32).

The maximum decrease in lung volume occurs approximately 16 hours after operation (32) and is probably caused by diaphragmatic dysfunction initiated by neural reflexes from the surgical area (33). The decreased lung volume leads to a decrease in functional residual capacity, bringing normal breathing below closing volume of the lungs (Fig. 4). When the closing volume exceeds functional residual capacity, regions with low ventilation/perfusion ratios develop, leading to impaired gas exchange with gas trapping, atelectasis, and arterial hypoxemia (of the constant type) (32).

The ventilatory pattern behind postoperative episodic hypoxemia needs to be evaluated in order to rationalize therapy and prevention. The study by Catley et al. showed that episodes of hypoxemia during the first 16 hours after operation (and occurring primarily during the first 8 hours after operation) were mostly due to obstructive apneas, central apneas, and paradoxic breathing (34). From the late postoperative period in the surgical ward, however, few data are available. Preliminary observations found episodic hypoxemia on the second and third nights after major abdominal surgery, primarily due to hypopneas and central and obstructive apneas (35). However, the study comprised only eight patients of whom two probably had sleep apnea syndrome preoperatively (35). Further studies on the precise postoperative nocturnal ventilatory pattern and the effect of different analgesic regimens are needed to allow definite conclusions.

Postoperative Sleep Disturbances

Sleep is divided into two forms: REM sleep and non-REM sleep. REM sleep is the phase of sleep most closely associated with dreaming. It is like full awareness in the variability and rapidity of changes in physiologic state. Thus, there are marked swings in blood pressure and heart rate, alterations in the rate and depth of breathing, and rapid changes in metabolic rate. REM sleep usually disappears on the first and sometimes the second and third postoperative nights (16,36–40). During the following two to four nights, when other sleep abnormalities recover, REM sleep reappears with increased duration (rebound) in most patients (16,38,39).

The postoperative rebound of REM sleep in the middle of the first postoperative week may contribute to the development of sleep disordered breathing and nocturnal hypoxemia (Fig. 5) (16,41). Thus, episodic hypoxemia is more frequent in periods of REM rebound than during other sleep stages in the postoperative period (16).

REM sleep is associated with a profound sympathetic activation and hemodynamic instability on nights with postoperative rebound of REM sleep periods (42), and these hemodynamic changes may be related to the above described hypoxemic episodes (16,41). Therefore, after uncomplicated abdominal surgery, episodic hypoxemia (decreased myocardial oxygen supply) and simultaneous hemodynamic instability (increased myocardial oxygen demand), can be associated with myocardial ischemia (2,31). Because the amount of REM sleep increases in the postoperative period with simultaneous episodic hypoxemia and hemodynamic instability, the postoperative REM sleep rebound may be particularly dangerous and lead to postoperative myocardial ischemia, infarction, and

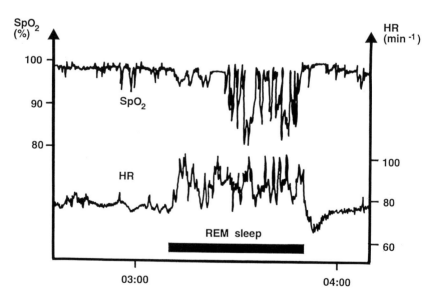

FIG. 5. Episodic hypoxemia (SpO$_2$), heart rate (HR) variations, and associated rebound of rapid eye movement (REM) sleep on the second night after laparotomy in a 36-year-old woman. Reproduced with permission (16).

eventually to unexpected postoperative death (43). This hypothesis warrants further study but is supported by the finding that the majority of unexpected postoperative deaths occurred during the night (44).

Effect of Postoperative Analgesic Technique

High doses of opioids given for pain relief may in selected patients play a role in the production of apneas and episodic hypoxemia (34), but opioid administration is unlikely to be a key pathogenic factor in all patients (45). Thus, in a study of 60 patients undergoing laparotomy and receiving intramuscular opioids for postoperative pain relief, we found a weak (and therefore clinically irrelevant) correlation between opioid dose on day 2 and the number of hypoxemic events on the second postoperative night (Fig. 6A), and the correlation between opioid dose on day 2 and the mean SpO_2 on the second postoperative night did not even reach statistical significance (Fig. 6B) (45).

On the other hand, several studies have shown an increased incidence and severity of both episodic and constant hypoxemia with opioid analgesia compared with regional anesthesia with local anesthetics (34,46). Also, equivalent analgesia with less need for opioids and less constant hypoxemia has been achieved by adding clonidine to opioid regimens (47,48). The opioid-sparing effect of treatment with nonsteroidal anti-inflammatory drugs may improve respiratory function and constant hypoxemia, although this was only demonstrated in two of 15 controlled studies (49). Aside from avoiding the direct effect of opioids on ventilation, another mechanism may be the avoidance of opioid-induced REM sleep suppression with subsequent rebound and episodic hypoxemia (43). Thus, efforts to prevent or reduce postoperative hypoxemia should include an opioid-sparing or opioid-free postoperative pain treatment whenever possible (49).

Studies with continuous-pulse oximetry (and thereby the ability to uncover episodic hypoxemia) and comparing different analgesic techniques in the late postoperative period are limited. We have in Table 1 summarized the three available studies with continuous pulse oximetry monitoring on the second and/or third postoperative night comparing different analgesic techniques.

The study by Entwistle et al. (14) found comparable patterns of oxygenation with paravertebral bupivacaine infusion compared with placebo (additional papaveretum was given as required in both groups) on nights 1–4 after thoracotomy. Owen et al. (10), when comparing three different ways of administering fentanyl epidurally (with or without background infusion and patient controlled analgesia; see Table 1), found no difference in oxygenation between groups on day 2 after operation, and overall there was no correlation between total fentanyl dose and oxygen saturation values (10). The study by van Lersberghe et al. (50) found more constant hypoxemia with epidural fentanyl compared with intravenous or transdermal fentanyl. The occurrence of hypoxemia was related to increased plasma concentration of fentanyl in the epidural infusion group, thus

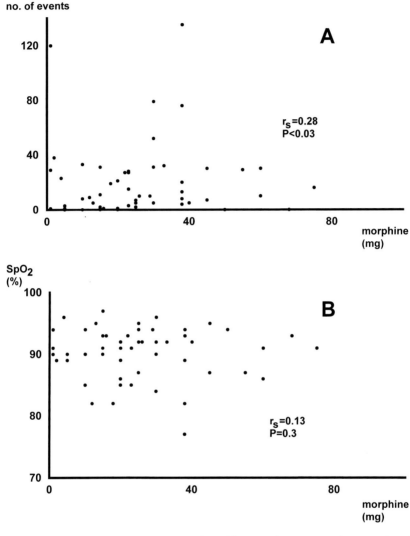

FIG. 6. A: Opioid dose on day 2 versus number of hypoxemic events on the second postoperative night in patients undergoing laparotomy (n = 60). **B:** Opioid dose on day 2 versus mean oxygen saturation (SpO₂) on the second postoperative night in patients undergoing laparotomy (n = 60). Data from Rosenberg et al. (45).

reflecting special pharmacokinetics for fentanyl by this mode of administration (50). Future studies are needed to compare the effect of different analgesic techniques in the late postoperative period on ventilatory disturbances and nocturnal episodic hypoxemia, and such studies are crucial to further the understanding of the effects of postoperative hypoxemia on organ dysfunction.

TABLE 1. *Studies with continuous pulse oximetry monitoring on the second and/or third postoperative night comparing different analgesic regimens*

Study	Patients	Duration of study	Treatment groups	Arterial oxygenation	Comment
Entwistle et al. (14)	20 patients after thoracotomy	First 4 nights after operation	Paravertebral bupivacaine infusion vs. placebo(all received papaveretum as required)	No difference between groups	No data on episodic hypoxemia
Owen et al. (10)	43 patients after abdominal surgery	First 48 hours after operation	Epidural fentanyl: infusion + bolus on demand vs. PCA without background infusion vs. PCA with background infusion	Day 1: more constant hypoxemia in the infusion-bolus group. Day 2: no differences between groups	No data on episodic hypoxemia
Lersberghe et al. (50)	54 patients after lower major abdominal, gynecologic, or urologic surgery	First 72 hours after operation	Epidural fentanyl infusion vs. i.v. fentanyl infusion vs. transdermal fentanyl patch	More constant hypoxemia in the epidural group compared with i.v. or transdermal	No data on episodic hypoxemia

Effect of Anesthetic Technique

Some of the previous studies on the effect of regional versus general anesthesia on the occurrence of late postoperative hypoxemia cannot be interpreted because the regional anesthetic technique has been used for pain relief in the postoperative period in only one of the treatment groups (24,34). However, the available data point in the direction of a difference in postoperative oxygenation in favor of intra- and postoperative regional anesthesia compared with general anesthesia and postoperative opioid analgesia (24,34). Pooling of data from controlled studies shows that postoperative pulmonary function (lung volumes) is improved with regional compared with general anesthetic techniques (1), and an improvement in levels of postoperative hypoxemia would therefore be expected. The optimal design would be intraoperative regional anesthesia compared with general anesthesia, and using the same regimen for postoperative analgesia with continuous monitoring of hypoxemia in the late postoperative period.

Two studies have compared different techniques of general anesthesia and with similar postoperative analgesic regimens (17,51). One study compared propofol with isoflurane in 50 patients undergoing open cholecystectomy, and postoperative analgesia consisted of intramuscular morphine on demand in both groups (17). Patients were monitored with a pulse oximeter on the preoperative night and the first three nights after operation and studied without oxygen therapy, and episodic hypoxemia was defined as a reversible reduction in saturation of 5% or more from baseline occurring within 2 minutes, with a decrease to less than 90%

and lasting at least 32 seconds (17). The main finding of the study was higher mean and minimum SpO$_2$ in the first 8 hours after operation and a higher minimum SpO$_2$ on the first postoperative night in patients receiving propofol compared with the isoflurane group, but oxygenation values on nights 2 and 3 did not differ between the two groups (17). Thus, although the general anesthetic technique per se may be important for the development of hypoxemia in the recovery period, it may not be an important pathogenic factor in the development of hypoxemia in the late postoperative period in the surgical ward. Another study compared the effect of intraoperative air in oxygen (F$_i$O$_2$ = 0.33) versus nitrous oxide in oxygen (F$_i$O$_2$ = 0.33) on the degree of postoperative hypoxemia in 30 patients undergoing laparoscopic cholecystectomy (51). Postoperative analgesia consisted of indomethacin in both groups, and doses did not differ between groups. Postoperative hypoxemia, evaluated by arterial blood gases (giving information on levels of constant hypoxemia) at 24 and 48 hours after surgery, showed improved oxygenation in patients ventilated with air in oxygen during the operation (51).

Effect of Surgical Technique

Minimal invasive surgery leads to major improvement in postoperative pulmonary function and postoperative oxygenation compared with open procedures (Table 2). Effect parameters in these studies have been lung volumes and spot checks of postoperative oxygenation (thus evaluating constant hypoxemia). No

TABLE 2. *The effect of laparoscopic versus open cholecystectomy on postoperative pulmonary function and hypoxemia*

Study	Duration of study	Pulmonary function	Arterial oxygenation	Comment
Frazee et al.(52)	24 h	VC, FEV$_1$		No data on episodic hypoxemia
Joris et al. (53)	48 h	VC, FEV$_1$	lap. > open	No data on episodic hypoxemia
Mealy et al. (54)	24 h	VC, FEV$_1$	lap. = open	No data on episodic hypoxemia
Putensen-Himmer et al. (55)	72 h	VC, FEV$_1$, FRC	lap. > open	No data on episodic hypoxemia
Rademaker et al. (56)	24 h	VC, peak flow, FEV$_1$		No data on episodic hypoxemia
Schauer et al. (57)	12 days	VC, peak flow, FEV$_1$	lap. > open	No data on episodic hypoxemia
McMahon et al. (58)	48 h	VC, peak flow, FEV$_1$	lap. > open	No data on episodic hypoxemia
Redmond et al. (59)	24 h		lap. > open	No data on episodic hypoxemia

VC, vital capacity; FEV$_1$, forced expired volume in first second; FRC, functional residual capacity. All lung volume parameters given in the table were higher after laparoscopic compared with open procedure.

data are available in the literature on the effect of minimal invasive surgery on the development of episodic hypoxemia in the late postoperative period.

Episodic Hypoxemia Induced by Constant Hypoxemia

Hypobaric hypoxia (i.e., constant hypoxemia at high altitude) may trigger the development of apneas, periodic breathing, and subsequent episodic hypoxemia (60,61). Therefore, it is hypothesized that constant hypoxemia per se (as a result of atelectasis after operation) may trigger the development of ventilatory disturbances and episodic hypoxemia after major surgery. We have approached this question in a study comparing supplementary oxygen therapy with placebo (air) on the second night after hip surgery and found that oxygen therapy increased levels of constant hypoxemia but had no effect on the number of hypoxemic episodes on the second postoperative night (62). Thus, the hypothesis that constant hypoxemia may trigger episodic hypoxemia does not seem to apply for the average surgical patient, although it was observed in one of 35 patients (Fig. 7).

However, prediction of patients who may respond with less episodic desaturation after oxygen therapy is not possible at present and should be an issue for future studies. The clinical implications are important because it would mean that episodic hypoxemia in selected patients could be treated by the simple administration of oxygen (by relieving constant hypoxemia).

EFFECTS OF HYPOXEMIA ON POSTOPERATIVE OUTCOME

Cardiac Morbidity

Several studies have demonstrated a temporal relationship between postoperative hypoxemia and atrioventricular block (9,63), ventricular ectopic beats

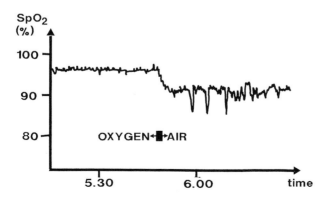

FIG. 7. Changes in oxygen saturation (SpO$_2$) with and without 37% oxygen by face mask on the second night after hip surgery in an 81-year-old female.

(5,64), and episodic tachycardia (5,9). Furthermore, in patients with no symptoms of coronary heart disease, a temporal relationship between episodic hypoxemia and myocardial ischemia in the late postoperative period has been demonstrated in studies with small patient samples (9,65,66). Also, experimental data (67) and early observations in humans (68) have shown that arterial hypoxemia may directly reduce myocardial oxygen supply and thereby cause ischemia. Experimental studies have suggested that in the already ischemic myocardium, superimposed episodic hypoxemia may worsen ischemia (69), and repeated ischemic challenges may progressively impair ventricular function and lead to infarction (70). These findings have been confirmed in a recent clinical study where most postoperative myocardial infarctions were non–Q-wave infarctions caused by subendocardial ischemia of long duration rather than coronary thrombosis (71). Hypoxemia may therefore represent an important risk factor after noncardiac surgery at a time where demand is increased because of the surgical trauma with sympathetic stimulation (72).

Recently, we have studied the effect of oxygen therapy on tachycardia in 12 patients with hypoxemia and randomly allocated to blinded air or oxygen by face mask on the second or third day after major surgery (73). All patients responded similarly to oxygen therapy with an increase in arterial oxygen saturation and a decrease in heart rate (73). Thus, hypoxemia per se may induce increased oxygen demands on the myocardium (tachycardia), and postoperative supplementary oxygen has a positive effect on the overall cardiac oxygen supply and demand balance.

Postoperative myocardial ischemia has been shown to be a strong predictor of postoperative cardiac complications after noncardiac operations (71,74). A number of factors may be involved in the development of myocardial ischemia, such as constant postoperative tachycardia induced by pain and surgical stress (1,9), disruption of fluid and electrolyte homeostasis (75), and arterial hypoxemia (9,66,72,76). Episodes of arterial hypoxemia may be particularly harmful for the heart (9,66,72), because they are often accompanied by sudden increases in heart rate (5,9,66) and blood pressure (77,78), leading to a marked increase in the rate–pressure product. However, the relative importance of all these pathogenic factors to postoperative myocardial infarction and death (and thereby the role of postoperative hypoxemia) needs further study.

Postoperative severe episodic changes in arterial oxygen saturation are especially seen in the sleep apnea syndrome (Fig. 8), which may prove to be an important surgical risk factor (77,79,80). The prevalence of the sleep apnea syndrome in the surgical population is unknown but may be as much as 10%, especially in old age (81). Lying supine, as in the postoperative period because of pain, aggravates the ventilatory disturbance with pronounced apnea and worsened episodic oxygen desaturation (82). Snoring is associated with increased morbidity and mortality in nonsurgical patients (80,83–85), and patients with obstructive sleep apnea are more likely to die during their sleep (86). In a recent study, heavy snorers were identified preoperatively by a simple questionnaire, and these patients had more episodic and constant hypoxemia during the first

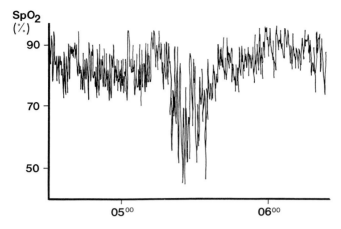

FIG. 8. Pulse oximetry oxygen saturation (SpO₂) on the second night after hip surgery in a patient with sleep apnea syndrome. Reproduced with permission (79).

postoperative night compared with light snorers or nonsnorers (87). The history of snoring should be taken into consideration in future studies on late postoperative hypoxemia.

Wound Complications

Postoperative wound infection is mainly caused by bacterial contamination, impaired host defense, and local factors in the wound, such as type of suture material, hemostasis, etc. Some of these factors can be eliminated by careful surgical technique and the use of antibiotic prophylaxis, but the rate of wound infection and dehiscence still remains a clinical problem (88). Thus, despite antibiotic prophylaxis, wound infection rates are still about 5–10% in colorectal operations, 2–10% in open cholecystectomy, and 4% in vascular surgery (89).

Reduced supply of oxygen to the surgical wound impairs healing (production of collagen) and lowers resistance against bacterial wound infection in experimental and clinical studies (90–92). Observations made during the second and third postoperative nights have suggested that after elective uncomplicated laparotomy arterial oxygen saturation may be a critical determinant of subcutaneous oxygen tension in the area of the wound (25,93). An epidural blockade providing an assumed sympathetic block did not increase subcutaneous oxygen tension nor the effectiveness of treatment with oxygen in stable postoperative patients without complications or cardiovascular disturbances (93), suggesting that perfusion was not a clinical problem in these patients. Postoperative treatment with oxygen usually produces a significant increase in arterial as well as in subcutaneous oxygen tension (25,90,93,94). The dose relationship between arterial and subcutaneous oxygenation (25,93) after elective surgery in patients who

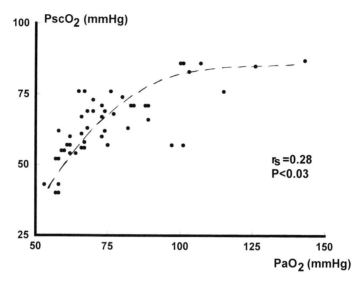

FIG. 9. Arterial oxygen tension (PaO_2) versus subcutaneous oxygen tension ($PscO_2$) during various interventions (epidural blockade, fluid administration, oxygen therapy) in eight patients on the first day after colorectal operation. Adapted with permission (93).

have no circulatory disturbances and are adequately hydrated suggests that wound oxygenation is more dependent on pulmonary oxygenation than wound perfusion, with a breakpoint close to a PaO_2 of 100 mmHg under which tissue oxygen tension is more dependent on arterial oxygen tension (93) (Fig. 9). Thus, based on these data it would seem that a goal of maintaining arterial oxygen tension at a level of 100 mmHg or above after major surgery is appropriate. No data are available addressing the effect of late postoperative episodic hypoxemia on wound oxygenation and metabolism.

Postoperative dehydration may reduce subcutaneous oxygen tension and impair wound healing (90,94,95), and beneficial effects on wound healing can be obtained by optimizing fluid maintenance postoperatively on the basis of measurements of subcutaneous oxygen tension (94). In an experimental model of central hypovolemia using head-up tilt in volunteers, subcutaneous oxygen tension was a more sensitive marker of impaired tissue oxygenation than was arterial oxygen tension (96). Thus, routine measurements of subcutaneous oxygen tension after major operations may guide fluid and transfusion therapy and thereby potentially decrease wound infection and dehiscence.

Cerebral Dysfunction

Impaired cognitive function and surgical delirium is common after major non-cardiac surgery with incidences around 5–10% dependent on the population studied (97,98). The risk factors generally identified include age, dementia, severe illness, metabolic and electrolyte imbalance, use of alcohol and psychoactive drugs, and infections (98–100), whereas type of anesthesia (1,101) and postoperative analgesia (102) may be of less importance. None of these large-scale studies have focused on arterial oxygenation as a risk factor for postoperative delirium, and only a few studies have systematically investigated the effect of postoperative hypoxemia on cognitive function and delirium.

An early study found a correlation between confusion in the recovery room and the degree of arterial hypoxemia 30 minutes after operation and general anesthesia (103). We have previously found that mental function on the third day after laparotomy correlated with mean oxygen saturation on the preceding night (104), and without relationship between mental function and other perioperative variables such as age, duration of surgery, and postoperative doses of opioids (104). A study in a mixed group of 92 surgical patients found that delirium occurred in 42% of patients, was most often diagnosed on the second postoperative day, and correlated significantly with age and degree of hypoxemia on day 1 (100).

The importance of arterial oxygenation in the preservation of cerebral function after operation also has been suggested in two studies with small patient samples in which postoperative delirium was treated successfully with supplementary oxygen after noncardiac thoracotomy (97) and hip surgery (105). A study using an intervention program that included oxygen therapy, early surgery, prevention and treatment of perioperative hypotension, and treatment of postoperative complications reduced the incidence, severity, and duration of acute confusional states in an elderly population undergoing surgery for femoral neck fractures (106). In conclusion, hypoxemia may therefore represent an important risk factor for the development of cerebral dysfunction in the late postoperative period in the surgical ward, although further systematic studies on this relationship are warranted.

TREATMENT

Pharmacologic Intervention

Treatment or prevention of postoperative hypoxemia may be performed using a variety of pharmacologic agents. These include doxapram (stimulates central ventilation), aminophylline (improves diaphragmatic function), naloxone (reduces morphine-induced respiratory depression), almitrine (increases hypoxic pulmonary vasoconstriction and thereby decreases pulmonary shunt), and azetazolamide (produces a slight acidosis and thereby stimulates respiration). So far, only doxapram has been evaluated in the late postoperative period (107,108). In a study using arterial blood gases, doxapram improved the awake arterial oxygen tension in the first 5 days after upper abdominal surgery (108). Unfortunately, a recent study using continuous overnight pulse oximetry had to be terminated prematurely because of adverse events (107). These included agitation, dizziness, palpitation, sweating, muscular fasciculations, tachycardia, and mental confusion, and one patient developed a cerebrovascular incident (107). Therefore, the study comprised only 2 × 9 patients (but aimed at 2 × 20 patients) receiving doxapram or placebo as a continuous infusion for three nights after laparotomy (the dose of doxapram was 2.5 mg/kg/hour during the first hour of infusion and 1 mg/kg/hour for the subsequent hours). However, in this limited patient sample we found an insignificant trend toward higher mean oxygen saturation in the doxapram group on all study nights and a statistically significant higher minimum oxygen saturation and reduced number of hypoxemic events on the first postoperative night (107). Although these preliminary data on the effect of doxapram on postoperative hypoxemia seem promising, further studies on the effect of continuous nocturnal postoperative doxapram infusion on levels of arterial oxygen saturation should be postponed until more knowledge about the pharmacokinetics of doxapram in this particular clinical situation has been gathered.

Prolonged Postoperative Oxygen Treatment

There is only one controlled study available with continuous pulse oximetry for evaluation of the effect of oxygen therapy after the first postoperative night (62). This study evaluated the effect of supplementary oxygen (37% oxygen versus air by Hudson face mask in a double-blind randomized design) on the occurrence of episodic and constant hypoxemia on the second night after total hip replacement. The results showed that the level of constant hypoxemia improved with oxygen therapy, but the number of hypoxemic events was unchanged (62). Thus, the basic mechanism behind episodic hypoxemia in the late postoperative period was not influenced by oxygen therapy. There is a need for further controlled trials evaluating oxygenation with different dosing regimens for oxygen therapy and in different patient categories, as well as the effect of prolonged postoperative oxygen therapy on outcome (109).

Another unsolved question is how to administer oxygen in the late postoperative period. Nolan et al. have used video surveillance on the first postoperative night to demonstrate that the face mask was frequently removed (for several hours in some patients) for various reasons, including routine nursing tasks, and that a nasal cannula was less likely to be removed (110). Treatment with 2 L/min with the nasal cannula gave a similar increase in SpO$_2$ compared with oxygen 4 L/min by face mask (110). We have evaluated three different devices for oxygen administration in the surgical ward, the Hudson face mask (3 L/min oxygen and 12 L/min air), the single lumen nasal prong (3 L/min oxygen), and the double lumen binasal catheter (3 L/min oxygen) (111). Oxygen saturation was slightly lower with the Hudson face mask compared with the binasal catheter and the nasal prong, but the highest degree of comfort was found with the binasal catheter, primarily because the Hudson face mask made it difficult to eat or drink (111).

In the surgical or anesthesiologic literature there are no data on the effect of prolonged postoperative oxygen therapy on morbidity or mortality. However, there are a few studies on the effect on organ function. In patients with late post-operative hypoxemia we have studied the effect of oxygen therapy on tachycardia (73). Twelve patients were randomly allocated to blinded air or oxygen by face mask on the second or third day after major surgery, and all patients responded similarly to oxygen therapy with an increase in arterial oxygen saturation and a decrease in heart rate (73). Thus, postoperative supplementary oxygen had a positive effect on the cardiac oxygen supply (by increasing arterial oxygen saturation) and demand (by decreasing heart rate) balance. There are no studies available on the effect of supplemental oxygen on other variables of cardiopulmonary function after major surgery, and this should therefore be included in future trials.

A study in mice investigated the effect of hyperoxia on bacterial translocation and mortality during gut-derived sepsis in a clinically relevent model of infection (113). The mice were gavaged with 10^9 *Escherichia coli* and subjected to a 20% burn injury and randomized to hyperoxia for different periods of time. Hyperoxia treatment preserved gut morphology and improved gut barrier function and decreased the amount of bacterial translocation. Furthermore, short-term (8 hours) treatment with 100% oxygen after the insult, followed by 5 days of treatment with 40% oxygen improved survival compared with control (70% versus 30% survival, $p < 0.05$) (113).

It has previously been shown that supplementary oxygen therapy may be a successful treatment of delirium or confusion after thoracotomy (97) or hip surgery (105,106), thereby reducing the use of psychoactive drugs in this clinical situation. Oxygen doses used have been oxygen 5 L/min and air 10 L/min by Hudson face mask or nasal catheter (97), oxygen 2 L/min by nasal catheter (105), or oxygen 1 L/min by nasal catheter (106). Controlled studies evaluating the effect of different dosing regimens for oxygen therapy on incidences and duration of postoperative delirium and involving different patient categories are needed.

In conclusion, experimental data are available to suggest a beneficial effect of prolonged postoperative oxygen therapy on morbidity and mortality after major surgery, but the final proof from controlled studies in humans is still awaited.

Nasal Continuous Positive Airway Pressure

The first report of treatment of obstructive sleep apnea syndrome (OSAS) with nasal continuous positive airway pressure (CPAP) was published in 1981 (114), and this treatment is now widely used and accepted as a standard of care for patients with OSAS (115). If episodic hypoxemia in the late postoperative period primarily is due to obstructive apneas, nasal CPAP would be a treatment option and should be evaluated scientifically in this clinical situation. No studies are available in patients undergoing major noncardiac surgery on the effect of nasal CPAP on oxygenation in the late postoperative period. Studies from patients with OSAS have shown patient compliance rates as low as 65%–83%

(116), and these patients are motivated for the treatment because of daytime symptoms. Thus, in postoperative patients it would probably be wise to choose a system with fewer side effects and thereby a higher patient compliance rate compared with that of regular nasal CPAP. Such a system could be a form of intelligent CPAP, called BiPAP, which senses apnea, snoring, and flow limitation, and adjusts CPAP accordingly, with increased patient compliance (115). Furthermore, because the most often reported side effects of conventional CPAP are dry throat and nose and sore eyes (116), future studies with nasal CPAP in the postoperative setting should use humidification of the air.

In volunteers and in patients with OSAS, nasal CPAP had no effect on heart rate, pulmonary artery pressure, ventricular size, or cardiac index, evaluated by echocardiography (117). However, in patients on artificial ventilation, positive end-expiratory pressure may cause a decrease in cardiac output because of decreased venous return or impaired left ventricular function (117). In the postoperative period, during which patients may have tachycardia and hyperdynamic circulation, the effect of nasal CPAP or BiPAP on hemodynamic variables is unknown and should be evaluated before general implementation of the method. In patients with known OSAS undergoing major surgery, another option may be to perform a prophylactic minitracheotomy during general anesthesia. This technique is safe and effective against episodic hypoxemia in patients with OSAS (118).

FUTURE RESEARCH STRATEGIES

The available data suggest that hypoxemia in the late postoperative period may be an important pathogenic factor in the development of cardiac (arrhythmias, myocardial ischemia, infarction, and eventually sudden death), wound (impaired healing and resistance against bacterial wound infections), and cerebral (confusion and delirium) dysfunction and/or complications. However, large-scale clinical studies are needed to verify the relative role of hypoxemia versus other risk factors in these postoperative morbidity parameters. Episodic hypoxemia in the surgical ward may be related to rebound of REM sleep, but otherwise we have no clear understanding of the pathogenesis of postoperative sleep disturbances. An important area for future research would be ways of preventing the abnormal sleep pattern and REM rebound and episodic hypoxemia in the late postoperative period (43). Furthermore, studies to establish preoperative risk indices for the development of late postoperative hypoxemia are warranted. Therapeutic measures against episodic hypoxemia such as nasal CPAP, pharmacologic interventions, and alternative modes of treating postoperative pain with less opioid should be evaluated. Oxygen therapy does not alter the basic mechanism leading to episodic hypoxemia but increases mean arterial oxygen saturation in the late postoperative period (62) and may therefore have an impact on postoperative organ dysfunction and morbidity. However, well-designed controlled studies on different modes of oxygen administration as well as different oxygen dose regimens are necessary before general implementation in the care of the routine surgical patient (109). Recent findings of preservation of lung volume after operation by means of administering a single high dose of steroid before surgery (119,120) should be further explored with regard to the effect on postoperative hypoxemia and morbidity. Use of pain-relieving techniques without opioids, i.e., techniques with continuous epidural infusions of local anesthetics and nonsteroidal anti-inflammatory drugs, may reduce the incidence and severity of postoperative desaturation because opioid-induced respiratory depression and postoperative sleep disturbances (121,122) may be reduced, with a potential beneficial effect on postoperative hypoxemia (16). Furthermore, the improved pain relief may be used to ambulate the patient, which in itself may increase postoperative oxygenation (123). Finally, techniques that imply a reduction of the surgical stress response may have a positive effect on postoperative hypoxemia because of less reduction of postoperative pulmonary function and less trauma-induced postoperative sleep disturbance (43).

IMPACT ON CLINICAL PRACTICE

Despite the lack of final documentation of the relationship between hypoxemia and postoperative outcome, the existing data may have consequences on routine postoperative oxygen therapy and monitoring. Although the decision to treat hypoxemia with supplementary oxygen is not based on scientific evidence, because no controlled studies have shown that treatment will reduce morbidity and mortality, we recommend that high-risk patients receive "prophylactic" oxygen therapy in the late postoperative period (i.e., for 2–4 days). Other patients should receive supplemental oxygen therapy only when hypoxemia (e.g., SpO_2 below 90%) has been verified by routine pulse oximetry monitoring. In the surgical ward, arterial oxygenation is usually measured by drawing an arterial blood sample, but because postoperative hypoxemia is only rarely accompanied by hypercapnia, and because intermittent pulse oximetry monitoring is cheaper, safer, and noninvasive, most arterial blood tests could be replaced by intermittent pulse oximetry (124). We suggest that intermittent monitoring of arterial oxygen saturation with a pulse oximeter should be performed in all patients after major operations, whereas continuous and overnight monitoring may be indicated only in high-risk patients.

In summary, arterial hypoxemia is common after otherwise uncomplicated surgery and may be either constant or episodic in nature. The incidence of episodic hypoxemia has a peak on the second and third nights after operation, and the mean oxygen saturation (i.e., the level of constant hypoxemia) is lowest on the second night after major surgery. The pathogenesis of late postoperative episodic hypoxemia includes pain- or stress-induced sleep disturbances with suppression of rapid eye movement sleep with a subsequent rebound on the second and third nights after operation resulting in ventilatory dysrhythmias and episodic hypoxemia. In selected patients, opioid-induced ventilatory disturbance with intermittent hypoventilation and central or obstructive apneas may produce episodic hypoxemia. Late postoperative constant hypoxemia is primarily due to an increased pulmonary shunt because of the obligatory lung volume reduction after major surgery. The available data strongly suggest that late postoperative hypoxemia is involved in the pathogenesis of cardiac, cerebral, and wound complications/dysfunction after major surgery. Future studies should further evaluate the pathogenesis of postoperative sleep disturbances and episodic hypoxemia, and regimens for prevention and therapy of late postoperative hypoxemia should be developed.

REFERENCES

1. Kehlet H. Modification of responses to surgery by neural blockade: clinical implications. In: Cousins MJ, Bridenbaugh PO, eds. *Neural blockade in clinical anesthesia and management of pain.* 2nd ed. Philadelphia: JB Lippincott; 1988:145–188.
2. Rosenberg J. Hypoxaemia in the general surgical ward—a potential risk factor? *Eur J Surg* 1994; 160:657–661.
3. Møller JT, Wittrup M, Johansen SH. Hypoxemia in the postanesthesia care unit: an observer study. *Anesthesiology* 1990;73:890–895.
4. Rosenberg J, Ullstad T, Rasmussen J, et al. Time course of postoperative hypoxaemia. *Eur J Surg* 1994;160:137–143.
5. Rosenberg J, Dirkes W, Kehlet H. Late postoperative episodic oxygen desaturation and heart rate variations following major abdominal surgery. *Br J Anaesth* 1989;63:651–654.
6. Frater RAS, Moores MA, Parry P, Hanning CD. Analgesia-induced respiratory depression: comparison of meptazinol and morphine in the postoperative period. *Br J Anaesth* 1989;63:260–265.
7. Knill RL, Moote CA, Rose EA, Skinner MI. Marked hypoxemia after gastroplasty due to disorders of breathing in REM sleep. *Anesthesiology* 1987;67:A552.
8. Rosenberg J, Pedersen MH, Ullstad T, et al. Incidence of arterial hypoxemia after laparotomy. *Surg Forum* 1992;43:35–37.
9. Rosenberg J, Rasmussen V, von Jessen F, et al. Late postoperative episodic and constant hypoxaemia and associated ECG-abnormalities. *Br J Anaesth* 1990;65:684–691.
10. Owen H, Kluger MT, Ilsley AH, et al. The effect of fentanyl administered epidurally by patient-controlled analgesia, continuous infusion, or a combined technique of oxyhaemoglobin saturation after abdominal surgery. *Anaesthesia* 1993;48:20–25.
11. Wheatley RG, Somerville ID, Sapsford DJ, Jones JG. Postoperative hypoxaemia: comparison of extradural, i.m. and patient-controlled opioid analgesia. *Br J Anaesth* 1990;64:267–275.
12. Wheatley RG, Shepherd D, Jackson IJB, et al. Hypoxaemia and pain relief after upper abdominal surgery: comparison of i.m. and patient-controlled analgesia. *Br J Anaesth* 1992;69:558–561.
13. Madej TH, Wheatley RG, Jackson IJB, Hunter D. Hypoxaemia and pain relief after lower abdominal surgery: comparison of extradural and patient-controlled analgesia. *Br J Anaesth* 1992;69: 554–557.
14. Entwistle MD, Roe PG, Sapsford DJ, et al. Patterns of oxygenation after thoracotomy. *Br J Anaesth* 1991;67:704–711.
15. Reeder MK, Goldman MD, Loh L, et al. Late postoperative nocturnal dips in oxygen saturation in patients undergoing major abdominal vascular surgery. *Anaesthesia* 1992;47:110–115.
16. Rosenberg J, Wildschiødtz G, Pedersen MH, et al. Late postoperative nocturnal episodic hypoxaemia and associated sleep pattern. *Br J Anaesth* 1994;72:145–150.
17. Georgiou LG, Vourlioti AN, Kremastinou FI, et al. Influence of anesthetic technique on early postoperative hypoxemia. *Acta Anaesthesiol Scand* 1996;40:75–80.
18. Knudsen J. Duration of hypoxaemia after uncomplicated upper abdominal and thoraco-abdominal operations. *Anaesthesia* 1970;25:372–377.

19. Lahnborg G, Lagergren H, Hedenstierna G. Effect of low-dose heparin prophylaxis on arterial oxygen tension after high laparotomy. *Lancet* 1976;i:54–56.
20. Parfrey PS, Harte PJ, Quinlan JP, Brady MP. Postoperative hypoxaemia and oxygen therapy. *Br J Surg* 1977;64:390–393.
21. Hennek K, Sydow F-W. Die thorakale periduralanaesthesie zur intra- und postoperativen analgesia bei lungenresektionen. *Regional-Anaesthesie* 1984;7:115–124.
22. Singh NP, Vargas FS, Cukier A, et al. Arterial blood gases after coronary artery bypass surgery. *Chest* 1992;102:1337–1341.
23. Bishop DGM, McKeown KC. Postoperative hypoxaemia: oesophagectomy with gastric replacement. *Br J Surg* 1979;66:810–812.
24. Modig J. Respiration and circulation after total hip replacement surgery: a comparison between parenteral analgesics and continuous lumbar epidural block. *Acta Anaesthesiol Scand* 1976;20:225–236.
25. Rosenberg J, Ullstad T, Larsen PN, et al. Continuous assessment of oxygen saturation and subcutaneous oxygen tension following abdominal surgery. *Acta Chir Scand* 1990;156:585–590.
26. Reeder MK, Goldman MD, Loh L, et al. Postoperative hypoxaemia after major abdominal vascular surgery. *Br J Anaesth* 1992;68:23–26.
27. Beydon L, Hassapoulos J, Quera M-A, et al. Risk factors for oxygen desaturation during sleep, after abdominal surgery. *Br J Anaesth* 1992;69:137–142.
28. Stevens JD, Braithwaite P, Corke CF, et al. Double-blind comparison of epidural diamorphine and intramuscular morphine after elective caesarean section, with computerised analysis of continuous pulse oximetry. *Anaesthesia* 1991;46:256–259.
29. Brose WG, Cohen SE. Oxyhemoglobin saturation following cesarean section in patients receiving epidural morphine, PCA, or im meperidine analgesia. *Anesthesiology* 1989;70:948–953.
30. Jones JG, Sapsford DJ, Wheatley RG. Postoperative hypoxaemia: mechanisms and time course. *Anaesthesia* 1990;45:566–573.
31. Rosenberg J. Late postoperative hypoxaemia: mechanisms and clinical implications. *Dan Med Bull* 1995;42:40–46.
32. Craig DB. Postoperative recovery of pulmonary function. *Anesth Analg* 1981;60:46–52.
33. Mankikian B, Cantineau JP, Bertrand M, et al. Improvement of diaphragmatic function by a thoracic extradural block after upper abdominal surgery. *Anesthesiology* 1988;68:379–386.
34. Catley DM, Thorton C, Jordan C, et al. Pronounced episodic oxygen desaturation in the postoperative period: its association with ventilatory pattern and analgesic regimen. *Anesthesiology* 1985;63: 20–28.
35. Corsten SA, de Ruijter WJM, Scheffer GJ, et al. Late postoperative nocturnal hypoxaemia and associated ventilatory pattern. *Br J Anaesth* 1995;74(suppl 1):51.
36. Aurell J, Elmqvist D. Sleep in the surgical intensive care unit: continuous polygraphic recording of sleep in nine patients receiving postoperative care. *Br Med J* 1985;290:1029–1032.
37. Ellis BW, Dudley HAF. Some aspects of sleep research in surgical stress. *J Psychosom Res* 1976; 20:303–308.
38. Knill RL, Moote CA, Skinner MI, Rose EA. Anesthesia with abdominal surgery leads to intense REM sleep during the first postoperative week. *Anesthesiology* 1990;73:52–61.
39. Kavey NB, Altshuler KZ. Sleep in herniorrhaphy patients. *Am J Surg* 1979;138:682–687.
40. Lehmkuhl P, Prass D, Pichlmayr I. General anaesthesia and postnarcotic sleep disorders. *Neuropsychobiology* 1987;18:37–42.
41. Knill RL, Moote CA, Rose EA, Skinner MI. Marked hypoxemia after gastroplasty due to disorders of breathing in REM sleep. *Anesthesiology* 1987;67:3A.
42. Knill RL, Skinner MI, Novick T, et al. The night of intense REM sleep after anaesthesia and surgery increases urinary catecholamines. *Can J Anaesth* 1990;37:S12.
43. Rosenberg-Adamsen S, Kehlet H, Dodds C, Rosenberg J. Postoperative sleep disturbances—mechanisms and clinical implications. *Br J Anaesth* 1996;76:552–559.
44. Rosenberg J, Pedersen MH, Ramsing T, Kehlet H. Circadian variation in unexpected postoperative deaths. *Br J Surg* 1992;79:1300–1302.
45. Rosenberg J, Oturai P, Erichsen CJ, et al. Effect of general anesthesia and major versus minor surgery on late postoperative episodic and constant hypoxaemia. *J Clin Anesth* 1994;6:212–216.
46. Modig J. Respiration and circulation after total hip replacement surgery. *Acta Anaesthesiol Scand* 1976;20:225–236.
47. Delaunay L, Leppert C, Dechaubry V, et al. Epidural clonidine decreases postoperative requirements for epidural fentanyl. *Reg Anesth* 1993;18:176–180.

48. Bernard J-M, Lagarde D, Souron R. Balanced postoperative analgesia:effect of intravenous clonidine on blood gases and pharmacokinetics of intravenous fentanyl. *Anesth Analg* 1994;79:1126–1132.
49. Kehlet H, Rung GW, Callesen T. Postoperative opioid analgesia—time for a reconsideration? *J Clin Anesth* 1996;8:441–445.
50. van Lersberghe C, Camu F, de Keersmaecker E, Sacré S. Continuous administration of fentanyl for postoperative pain: a comparison of the epidural, intravenous, and transdermal routes. *J Clin Anesth* 1994;6:308–314.
51. Fujii Y, Tanaka H, Toyooka H. Intraoperative ventilation with air and oxygen during laparoscopic cholecystectomy decreases the degree of postoperative hypoxaemia. *Anaesth Intens Care* 1996;24: 42–44.
52. Frazee RC, Roberts JW, Okeson GC, et al. Open versus laparoscopic cholecystectomy. *Ann Surg* 1991;213:651–654.
53. Joris J, Cigarini I, Legrand M, et al. Metabolic and respiratory changes after cholecystectomy performed via laparotomy or laparoscopy. *Br J Anaesth* 1992;69:341–345.
54. Mealy K, Gallagher H, Barry M, et al. Physiological and metabolic responses to open and laparoscopic cholecystectomy. *Br J Surg* 1992;79:1061–1064.
55. Putensen-Himmer G, Putesen C, Lammer H, et al. Comparison of postoperative respiratory function after laparoscopy or open laparotomy for cholecystectomy. *Anesthesiology* 1992;77:675–680.
56. Rademaker B, Ringers J, Joseph A, et al. Pulmonary function and stress responses after laparoscopic cholecystectomy: comparison with subcostal incision and influence of thoracic epidural analgesia. *Anesth Analg* 1992;75:381–385.
57. Schauer PR, Luna J, Ghiatas AA, et al. Pulmonary function after laparoscopic cholecystectomy. *Surgery* 1993;114:389–399.
58. McMahon AJ, Russell I, Ramsay G, et al. Laparoscopic and minilaparotomy cholecystectomy: a randomized trial comparing postoperative pain and pulmonary function. *Surgery* 1994;115:533–539.
59. Redmond HP, Watson WG, Houghton T, et al. Immune function in patients undergoing open vs. laparoscopic cholecystectomy. *Arch Surg* 1994;129:1240–1246.
60. Berssenbrugge A, Dempsey J, Iber C, et al. Mechanisms of hypoxia-induced periodic breathing during sleep in humans. *J Physiol Lond* 1983;343:507–524.
61. Normand H, Barragan M, Benoit O, et al. Periodic breathing and O_2 saturation in relation to sleep stages at high altitude. *Aviat Space Environ Med* 1990;61:229–235.
62. Rosenberg J, Pedersen MH, Gebuhr P, Kehlet H. Effect of oxygen therapy on late postoperative episodic and constant hypoxaemia. *Br J Anaesth* 1992;68:18–22.
63. Lewis T, Mathison GC. Auriculo-ventricular heart-block as a result of asphyxia. *Heart* 1910;2: 47–53.
64. Ayres SM, Grace WJ. Inappropriate ventilation and hypoxemia as causes of cardiac arrhythmias: the control of arrhythmias without antiarrhythmic drugs. *Am J Med* 1969;46:495–505.
65. Gill NP, Wright B, Reilly CS. Relationship between hypoxaemic and cardiac ischaemic events in the perioperative period. *Br J Anaesth* 1992;68:471–473.
66. Reeder MK, Muir AD, Foëx P, et al. Postoperative myocardial ischaemia: temporal association with nocturnal hypoxaemia. *Br J Anaesth* 1991;67:626–631.
67. Scharf SM, Graver M, Balaban K. Cardiovascular effects of periodic occlusions of the upper airways in dogs. *Am Rev Respir Dis* 1992;146:321–329.
68. Rothschild MA, Kissin M. Induced general anoxemia causing S-T deviation in the electrocardiogram. *Am Heart J* 1933;8:745–754.
69. Coetze A, Foex P, Holland D, et al. Effect of hypoxia on the normal and ischemic myocardium. *Crit Care Med* 1984;12:1027–1031.
70. Geft IL, Fishbein MC, Ninomiya K, et al. Intermittent brief periods of ischemia have a cumulative effect and may cause myocardial necrosis. *Circulation* 1982;66:1150–1153.
71. Landesberg G, Luria MH, Cotev S, et al. Importance of long-duration postoperative ST-segment depression in cardiac morbidity after vascular surgery. *Lancet* 1993;341:715–719.
72. Pateman JA, Hanning CD. Postoperative myocardial infarction and episodic hypoxaemia. *Br J Anaesth* 1989;63:648–650.
73. Stausholm K, Kehlet H, Rosenberg J. Oxygen therapy reduces postoperative tachycardia. *Anaesthesia* 1995;50:737–739.
74. Mangano DT, Browner WS, Hollenberg M, et al. Association of perioperative myocardial ischemia with cardiac morbidity and mortality in men undergoing noncardiac surgery. *N Engl J Med* 1990; 323:1781–1788.

75. Shires GT. Important factors in the management of homeostasis in the surgical patient. *Acta Chir Scand* 1988;(suppl 550):29–35.
76. Tirlapur VG, Mir MA. Nocturnal hypoxemia and associated electrocardiographic changes in patients with chronic obstructive airways disease. *N Engl J Med* 1982;306:125–130.
77. Reeder MK, Goldman MD, Loh L, et al. Postoperative obstructive sleep apnoea: haemodynamic effects of treatment with nasal CPAP. *Anaesthesia* 1991;46;849–853.
78. Reeder MK, Goldman MD, Loh L, et al. Haemodynamic effects of periodic ventilation: abolition with supplementary oxygen. *Br J Anaesth* 1991;67:326–328.
79. Rosenberg J, Kehlet H. Postoperative episodic oxygen desaturation in the sleep apnoea syndrome. *Acta Anaesthesiol Scand* 1991;35:368–369.
80. Hanning CD. Obstructive sleep apnoea. *Br J Anaesth* 1989;63:477–488.
81. Guilleminault C. Obstructive sleep apnea syndrome: a review. *Psychiatr Clin North Am* 1987;10: 607–621.
82. Miki H, Hida W, Kikuchi Y, Takishima T. Effect of sleep position on obstructive sleep apnea. *Tohoku J Exp Med* 1988;156:143–149.
83. Rees J. Snoring. *Br Med J* 1991;302:860–861.
84. Guilleminault C, Connolly SJ, Winkle RA. Cardiac arrhythmia and conduction disturbances during sleep in 400 patients with sleep apnea syndrome. *Am J Cardiol* 1983;52:490–494.
85. D'Alessandro R, Magelli C, Gamberini G, et al. Snoring every night as a risk factor for myocardial infarction:a case-control study. *Br Med J* 1990;300:1557–1558.
86. Ancoli-Israel S, Klauber MR, Kripke DF, et al. Sleep apnea in female patients in a nursing home: increased risk of mortality. *Chest* 1989;96:1054–1058.
87. Gentil B, Lienhart A, Fleury B. Enhancement of postoperative desaturation in heavy snorers. *Anesth Analg* 1995;81:389–392.
88. Riou JPA, Cohen JR, Johnson H Jr. Factors influencing wound dehiscence. *Am J Surg* 1992;163: 324–330.
89. Condon RE, Wittmann DH. Surgical infections. In: Morris PJ, Malt RA, eds. *Oxford textbook of surgery.* New York: Oxford University Press; 1994:27–43.
90. Jönsson K, Jensen JA, Goodson WH III, et al. Tissue oxygenation, anemia, and perfusion in relation to wound healing in surgical patients. *Ann Surg* 1991;214:605–613.
91. Knighton DR, Fiegel VD, Halverson T, et al. Oxygen as an antibiotic: the effect of inspired oxygen on bacterial clearance. *Arch Surg* 1990;125:97–100.
92. Orgill D, Demling RH. Current concepts and approaches to wound healing. *Crit Care Med* 1988;16: 899–908.
93. Rosenberg J, Pedersen U, Erichsen CJ, et al. Effect of epidural blockade on changes in subcutaneous oxygen tension during oxygen therapy following elective uncomplicated major abdominal surgery. *J Surg Res* 1994;56:72–76.
94. Hartmann M, Jönsson K, Zederfeldt B. Effect of tissue perfusion and oxygenation on accumulation of collagen in healing wounds: randomized study in patients after major abdominal operations. *Eur J Surg* 1992;158:521–526.
95. Hartmann M, Jönsson K, Zederfeldt B. Importance of dehydration in anastomotic and subcutaneous wound healing: an experimental study in rats. *Eur J Surg* 1992;158:79–82.
96. Larsen PN, Moesgaard F, Madsen P, et al. Subcutaneous oxygen and carbon dioxide tensions during head-up tilt-induced central hypovolaemia in humans. *Scand J Clin Lab Invest* 1996;56:17–24.
97. Aakerlund L, Rosenberg J. Postoperative delirium: treatment with supplementary oxygen. *Br J Anaesth* 1994;72:286–290.
98. Marcantonio ER, Goldman L, Mangione CM, et al. A clinical prediction rule for delirium after elective noncardiac surgery. *JAMA* 1994;271:134–139.
99. Schor JD, Levkoff SE, Lipsitz LA, et al. Risk factors for delirium in hospitalized elderly. *JAMA* 1992;267:827–831.
100. Dieckelmann A, Haupts M, Kaliwoda A, et al. Akute postoperative psychosyndrome: eine prospektive studie und multivariate analyse von risikofaktoren. *Chirurg* 1989;60:470–474.
101. Ghoneim MM, Hinrichs JV, O'Hara MWO, et al. Comparison of psychologic and cognitive functions after general or regional anesthesia. *Anesthesiology* 1988;69:507–515.
102. Williams-Russo P, Urquhart BL, Sharrock NE, Charlson ME. Post-operative delirium: predictors and prognosis in elderly orthopedic patients. *J Am Geriatr Soc* 1992;40:759–767.
103. Berggren D, Gustafson Y, Eriksson B, et al. Postoperative confusion after anesthesia in elderly patients with femoral neck fractures. *Anesth Analg* 1987;66:497–504.

104. Rosenberg J, Kehlet H. Postoperative mental confusion—association with postoperative hypoxemia. *Surgery* 1993;114:76–81.
105. Krasheninnikoff M, Ellitsgaard N, Rude C, Moller JT. Hypoxaemia after osteosynthesis of hip fractures. *Int Orthop* 1993;17:27–29.
106. Gustafson Y, Brännström B, Berggren D, et al. A geriatric-anesthesiologic program to reduce acute confusional states in elderly patients treated for femoral neck fractures. *J Am Geriatr Soc* 1991;39: 655–62.
107. Rosenberg J, Kristensen PA, Pedersen MH, Overgaard H. Adverse events with continuous doxapram infusion against late postoperative hypoxaemia. *Eur J Clin Pharmacol* 1996;50:191–194.
108. Jansen JE, Sørensen AI, Naesh O, et al. Effect of doxapram on postoperative pulmonary complications after upper abdominal surgery in high risk patients. *Lancet* 1990;335:936–938.
109. Hanning CD. Prolonged postoperative oxygen therapy. *Br J Anaesth* 1992;69:115–116.
110. Nolan KM, Winyard JA, Goldhill DR. Comparison of nasal cannulae with face mask for oxygen administration to postoperative patients. *Br J Anaesth* 1993;70:440–442.
111. Stausholm K, Rosenberg-Adamsen S, Skriver M, et al. Comparison of three devices for oxygen administration in the late postoperative period. *Br J Anaesth* 1995;74:607–609.
112. Hunt TK, Conolly WB, Aronson SB, Goldstein P. Anaerobic metabolism and wound healing: an hypothesis for the initiation and cessation of collagen synthesis in wounds. *Am J Surg* 1978;135: 328–332.
113. Gennari R, Alexander JW. Effects of hyperoxia on bacterial translocation and mortality during gut-derived sepsis. *Arch Surg* 1996;131:57–62.
114. Sullivan CE, Issa FG, Berthon-Jones M, Eves L. Reversal of obstructive sleep apnoea by continuous positive pressure applied through the nares. *Lancet* 1981;i:862–865.
115. Polo O, Berthon-Jones M, Douglas NJ, Sullivan CE. Management of obstructive sleep apnoea/hypopnoea syndrome. *Lancet* 1994;344:656–660.
116. Nino-Murcia G, McCann CC, Bliwise DL, et al. Compliance and side effects in sleep apnea patients treated with nasal continuous positive airway pressure. *West J Med* 1989;150:165–169.
117. Leech JA, Ascah KJ. Hemodynamic effects of nasal CPAP examined by Doppler echocardiography. *Chest* 1991;99:323–326.
118. Hasan A, McGuigan J, Morgan MDL, Matthews HR. Minitracheotomy: a simple alternative to tracheostomy in obstructive sleep apnoea. *Thorax* 1989;44:224–225.
119. Schulze S, Sommer P, Bigler D, et al. Effect of combined prednisolone, epidural analgesia, and indomethacin on the systemic response after colonic surgery. *Arch Surg* 1992;127:325–331.
120. Möiniche S, Dahl JB, Rosenberg J, Kehlet H. Colonic resection with early discharge after combined subarachnoid-epidural analgesia, preoperative glucocorticoids, and early postoperative mobilization and feeding in a pulmonary high-risk patient. *Reg Anesth* 1994;19:352–356.
121. Moote CA, Knill RL, Skinner MI, Rose EA. Morphine disrupts nocturnal sleep in a dose-dependent fashion. *Anesth Analg* 1989;68:S200.
122. Knill RL, Moote CA, Skinner MI, Rose EA. Anesthesia with abdominal surgery leads to intense REM sleep during the first postoperative week. *Anesthesiology* 1990;73:52–61.
123. Mynster T, Jensen LM, Jensen FG, et al. The effect of posture on late postoperative oxygenation. *Anaesthesia* 1996;51:225–227.
124. Rosenberg J, Koch J, Kirchhoff-Jensen R. Pulse oximetry in the general surgical ward—is it worthwhile? *Surg Forum* 1994;45:637–638.

Physiology, Stress, and Malnutrition: Functional
Correlates, Nutritional Intervention,
edited by J.M. Kinney and H.N. Tucker.
Lippincott–Raven Publishers © 1997.

Significance of Intraoperative Thermal Metabolism

Francesco Carli

*Department of Anesthesia, McGill University, Royal Victoria Hospital, Montreal,
Quebec H3A 1A1, Canada*

Hypothermia is the most common disorder of temperature homeostasis during injury, particularly during surgery. It can be of two types: the first is intentional and is routinely used to protect the vital organs during operative procedures when ischemia is anticipated. The second type of hypothermia can occur inadvertently in approximately 50–80% of surgical procedures.

This chapter provides an insight to some understanding of thermal homeostasis during anesthesia and surgery. What is the mechanism of hypothermia during anesthesia? Is hypothermia deleterious to body functions during the perioperative period? Should hypothermia be prevented or treated?

BODY HEAT DISTRIBUTION

Core temperature does not reliably reflect the body's heat content, particularly during incipient hypothermia. Body heat is unequally distributed between an inner, warm, heat-producing core and an outer, colder, insulating shell. When normothermic, the core:shell ratio of body mass is 0.66:0.34. But this ratio is dynamic. During warming, it changes to 0.9:0.1 as the core proportion of body mass increases, and during cooling to 0.5:0.5 as the shell proportion increases. The clinical implication of this is that humans can lose a lot of heat from the shell without a decrease in core temperature.

It is theoretically possible to derive an equation to calculate body heat content (HC). This requires an estimate of the mean body temperature (Tmb), which is the core temperature (Tc) and the shell temperature (taken as equal to mean skin temperature, Tsk) weighted according to their respective body mass proportions. Thus, Tmb = 0.66 Tc + 0.34 Tsk. Body heat content, then, is Tmb × body thermal capacity (3.47 kJ/kg). Originally, Tsk was the average of 26 separate skin temperature measurements. Now only four sites are used, so the accuracy of measurements of Tsk have a major influence on the estimate of Tmb. An additional source of error is that the equation is invariably used without any allowance for changes in the core:shell ratio or body mass proportions. So, although very important in emphasizing the concept of body heat content, and particularly stressing the importance of mean skin temperature, the formula's accuracy has not been verified in surgical patients. In all probability this equation underestimates the changes in body heat content simply because is does not account for changes in the core:shell ratio.

THERMAL BALANCE DURING ANESTHESIA AND SURGERY

Net thermal balance (NTB) is the balance between the metabolic heat production and environmental heat exchange. During surgery, the NTB is negative: metabolic heat production is reduced by anesthetic agents, whereas heat loss is increased when patients are exposed without adequate insulation in a cold environment.

Heat Production

Heat production can be calculated from oxygen consumption ($\dot{V}O_2$), whose energy equivalent is 21 kJ/L. Heat production is expressed in terms of body surface area, 1.8 m^2 for a 70-kg adult. The normal basal metabolic $\dot{V}O_2$ is 250 ml/min, giving a basal metabolic heat production of 48 WaHs/m^2. During anesthesia, metabolism is reduced to at least 80% of basal, approximately 40 W/m^2. In the postoperative period $\dot{V}O_2$ increases dramatically in order to generate more heat and replace that which has been lost. It is the respiratory and cardiac consequences of supporting this increase in $\dot{V}O_2$ that pose a grave risk to the patient. Increases in $\dot{V}O_2$ on the order of two to four times are reported. These estimates are based on the study of young, healthy subjects, not a population that represents the average surgical patient (1).

Heat Loss

Environmental heat loss occurs in four ways: convection, radiation, evaporation, and conduction. There are two other sources of heat loss to consider in surgical patients: respiratory losses and the heat debt incurred by infusing fluids at room temperature.

In an exposed patient the heat loss for radiation and convection is 10 W/m^2 °C, and if Tsk-Ta is more than 4°C, more heat will be lost than produced, NTB will be negative, and the patient will steadily cool.

Breathing dry gas, the respiratory system must evaporate 44 mg/L for full humidification, and the latent heat of evaporation is 2.45 kJ/g. Assuming a minute volume of 8 L/min, the evaporating respiratory heat loss is 8 W/m^2. Realistically, in partial rebreathing circuits the gases are 50% humidified and the respiratory heat loss is 4 W/m^2.

There is also heat debt associated with administration of fluids intravenously. For example, 1 L of crystalloid solution costs 71 kJ to warm from 20°C to 37°C and 1 L of blood 95 kJ. If crystalloids are infused unwarmed, in 1 hour the heat loss rate is approximately 11 W/m^2.

The magnitude of evaporative loss from the surgical incision is also relevant. Although it takes only 4.18 J/g to heat water through 1°C, evaporation requires 2.45 kJ/g. Evaporative losses account for over 70% of heat loss from the abdominal cavity.

Pattern of Thermoregulation

General anesthesia decreases the activation thresholds for responses to hypothermia by 2–3°C and increases those responses defending against hyperthermia. The widening of the interthreshold range produces a broad temperature range over which active thermoregulatory responses are absent. Within this range, body temperature changes are determined passively by redistribution of heat within the body and the difference between heat production and heat loss to the environment. Most induction agents and volatile general anesthetics produce a similar pattern and magnitude of thermoregulatory impairment (2,3). The extent to which core temperature decreases seems to be dose dependent (4). Opioids inhibit thermoregulatory control in a similar fashion. Regional anesthesia per se significantly impairs thermoregulatory control to some extent (5); although central thermoregulation remains intact and therefore provides some protection against hypothermia, local anesthetics are responsible for impaired regional thermal sensation, increased heat loss to environment, and regional inhibition of vasoconstriction and shivering.

The typical pattern of intraoperative hypothermia includes an initial phase of precipitous decrease in core temperature (1 hour) followed by a slow decrease (2–3 hours) and plateau. The initial core hypothermia results from a 15–20% decrease in metabolic heat production and an increased loss of radiant body heat. Nonetheless, these two factors cannot explain entirely the initial core hypothermia that follows induction of general anesthesia. The slow decrease in core temperature likely results from heat loss exceeding metabolic heat production. When patients become hypothermic, this plateau is often accompanied by active thermoregulatory vasoconstriction, thereby decreasing cutaneous heat loss and constraining metabolic heat to the relatively small core compartment.

The contribution of surgical stress and painful stimuli to these aspects of impaired thermoregulation are not well defined; in healthy volunteers anesthetized with enflurane (0.8 minimal alveolar concentration [MAC]) the thermoregulatory threshold for vasoconstriction was found to be 35.1°C without electrical stimulation and 35.5°C during painful electrical stimulation, demonstrating a slight and insignificant effect of nociceptive stimuli in offsetting anesthetic-induced thermoregulatory inhibition (6). Whether the thermoregulatory threshold for vasoconstriction is modulated by the hormonal and cytokine responses to surgical incision remains unknown.

The impaired ability of the infant to withstand cold results from an abnormal pattern of behavior, limited motor development, and poor thermal insulation. The central temperature at which thermoregulatory threshold triggers peripheral vasoconstriction is agent and dose dependent.

Thermoregulation is progressively impaired with old age. Both metabolic and vasomotor responses are reduced in the elderly, resulting in more dependence on behavioral thermoregulation. Heat production is limited as a result of decreased muscle mass and muscle tone; this might explain why shivering is rarely visible in the elderly. A decline in sensitivity appears to result from changes in the nervous system, thereby influencing thermal perception.

Hypothermia is common in traumatized patients (7). The impairment of thermoregulation during the immediate phase after injury is such that, if ambient temperature is below the thermoneutral zone, core temperature starts to decrease. These patients do not shiver despite a body temperature below the threshold for shivering.

Underfeeding for a prolonged period of time has marked effects on thermoregulation (8) and the thermic response to glucose and insulin infusion (9). The defect in cold-induced thermogenesis after weight loss is due to a change in central control mechanisms of thermoregulation and not tissue responsiveness.

We should not forget that medical disorders such as hypothyroidism, hypopituitarism, and diabetes cause some impairment in the control of body temperature. Similarly, drugs such as psychotropics, sedatives, and β-blockers act directly on the thermoregulatory center, induce cutaneous vasodilatation, reduce thermogenic shivering, and lower metabolic rate.

The thermal imbalance continues well into the immediate postoperative period. In the study by Vaughan et al., 60% of patients undergoing a range of elective surgeries had a core temperature below 36.0°C on arrival in the recovery room, and 17% had a core temperature below 35.0 °C. Eighteen percent of patients had a core temperature below 36°C after an average stay in the recovery room of 82 minutes (10). The most important factors that affect the body temperature in the recovery room are the age of the patient and the type of anesthesia.

CONSEQUENCES OF ALTERED THERMAL HOMEOSTASIS

Because this review is confined to perioperative thermal stress, emphasis will be placed on describing the consequences of mild and moderate hypothermia (core temperature below 37.0°C and above 32.0°C) on body functions in the surgical setting. It is not the intention of this review to discuss other thermal disturbances such as accidental and induced hypothermia or malignant hyperpyrexia.

Intraoperative

Mild hypothermia provides substantial protection against central nervous system ischemia and hypoxia (11). The benefits of mild hypothermia have been shown in animal models of cerebral ischemia, focal lesions, hemorrhagic shock, combined hypoxia, and ischemia (12). The cerebral protective mechanism of such technique is more effective than that provided by drugs such as barbiturates and might be explained on the basis of an inhibitory role of hypothermia on the release of excitatory amino acids from the injured brain. Similar conclusions cannot be drawn from human studies; although not proved, mild hypothermia might confer some protection in particular cases such as neurosurgery when tissue ischemia is anticipated.

A moderate decrease in body temperature impairs platelet function (13), and this appears to be related to local temperature and not core temperature. Also, there appears to be an impairment of the extrinsic and intrinsic clotting (14). For a small decrease in body temperature (0.5–1.0°C), there is an increase in the hematocrit by 7% and in platelet count and blood viscosity by 25% (15).

Basal metabolism decreases by approximately 5–10% per 1°C decrease in body temperature. Carbohydrate metabolism is decreased when core temperature decreases below 34.0°C. Glycogen stores in the liver become depleted with lowering of body temperature. Hyperglycemia occurs as a result of either decreased insulin activity or enhanced stimulation of catecholamines, and consequently increased hepatic glycogenolysis and gluconeogenesis.

Cold exposure of rats has been shown to produce some changes in protein metabolism, such as weight loss and increased urinary nitrogen excretion (16). It was speculated that the stimulus for these changes could well be the increased sympathetic activity, which depresses insulin activity to levels that may acutely alter the oxidative and synthetic components of protein metabolism. However, this sustained influence of catecholamines on body protein kinetics has not been confirmed.

The effect of hypothermic bypass (28.0°C) on protein metabolism had been studied in dogs by Johnson et al. (17), who were able to show a significantly decreased protein breakdown as a result of hypothermia, opioid anesthesia, and neuromuscular blockade. More recently, Taggard et al. (18) used two levels of intraoperative hypothermia (20.0 and 28.0°C) to modify the catabolic response associated with coronary artery surgery. A more profound hypothermia did not contribute to a significant attenuation of postoperative muscle breakdown. Normothermic bypass is being advocated lately in view of the findings that such approach is associated with less metabolic and hemodynamic disturbances (19). There is an urgent need to clarify the separate role of temperature on intermediary metabolism during cardiopulmonary bypass.

Moderate perioperative hypothermia and its effect on postoperative protein metabolism have been studied in the abdominal and orthopedic surgical models (20,21). The findings indicate that active maintenance of perioperative normothermia results in a significant attenuation of amino acid oxidation and protein breakdown. Similar results were reported when nursing hypothermic surgical patients at an elevated ambient temperature environment (22).

The effects of mild hypothermia on drug pharmacokinetics and pharmacodynamics were investigated recently, but the study was limited only to volatile anesthetics and muscle relaxants. Although solubility of volatile anesthetics increases in hypothermic tissues, the delayed washout is not clinically relevant (23). Mild hypothermia also decreases twitch height in response to supramaximal stimulation of the ulnar nerve at the wrist (24), but it is unlikely that this represents a serious clinical problem during the recovery if adequate monitoring is available.

Hypothermia has a mild effect on somatosensory evoked potentials, but the changes are unlikely to alter clinical management. Neither hypothermia nor hyperthermia significantly alter electroencephalographic values (25).

In summary, it is not possible at the present stage to identify grossly deleterious effects of moderate hypothermia on body functions during anesthesia and surgery. The reason could be that anesthetized patients receive adequate oxygenation, fluid replenishment, cardiovascular support, and brain protection.

Rewarming Phase

The most severe consequences of intraoperative cooling occur during the postoperative period, especially when rewarming is incomplete.

During the initial postoperative period, anesthetic concentrations in the brain decrease rapidly, allowing reemergence of those thermoregulatory responses such as vasoconstriction and shivering, which were inhibited during general anesthesia. These physiologic responses aim to decrease cutaneous heat dissipation and increase metabolic heat production. They result in a rapid increase in core temperature while the patient regains consciousness. However, normothermia cannot be reestablished if a large heat debt has been accumulated during surgery. The presence of residual anesthetic agents and muscle relaxants, administration of opioids for control of wound pain, and prolonged intraoperative hypothermia could alter the effectiveness of thermoregulatory responses as demonstrated by the slow return of core temperature in hypothermic patients.

The normal response to hypothermia includes activation of the sympathetic nervous system. Studies in healthy volunteers have demonstrated that even small changes in core temperature (0.2–0.4°C) are associated with thermoregulatory vasoconstriction. With exposure to cold ambient temperatures, circulating concentrations of adrenaline and noradrenaline are significantly increased. Two studies in patients undergoing major surgery have reported significantly increased circulating levels of plasma adrenaline and noradrenaline in hypothermic patients compared with those who were maintained normothermic throughout surgery (26,27).

One of the most powerful thermoregulatory responses in the hypothermic awakening subject is peripheral vasoconstriction, mediated primarily in the extremities. It derives that systolic arterial blood pressure is increased after hypothermic anesthesia without changes in heart rate (23). The increase in systemic blood pressure has not been universally reported, and this might be due to the type of patients studied and the sedation and analgesia used in the immediate postoperative period, which could effectively inhibit thermoregulatory vasoconstriction (28). The awareness of the detrimental effects caused by exaggerated sympathetic stimulation on the cardiovascular system and the availability of drugs aiming at modulating this response have influenced our clinical practice, particularly in the immediate perioperative period. Nonetheless, hypothermia appears to increase the incidence of postoperative myocardial ischemia (29). The published data suggest an increased incidence of early postoperative cardiac ischemia in vascular surgery patients with core temperatures below 35.0°C, although the mechanism remains to be determined. The reported high mortality in hypothermic patients (30) could be well explained by the excess perioperative myocardial ischemia. At present, it is premature to conclude that such association exists. In fact, the available data are retrospective and do not compensate for differences within the observed populations.

Shivering is one of the most common mechanisms adopted by the hypothermic patient to increase body temperature. A shiverlike tremor occurs in approximately 40% of the patients recovering from general anesthesia and is preceded by central hypothermia and peripheral vasoconstriction, indicating that it is thermoregulatory in origin. Although there may be some doubt that hypothermia per se is a causative factor, it is true that hypothermic patients shiver for longer periods than do those who are normothermic at the end of surgery.

The tonic pattern of shivering, which represents a simple thermoregulatory response to hypothermia, is alternated by a clonic pattern. It has been speculated that the tremor pattern results from anesthetic-induced disinhibition of normal descending control over spinal reflexes.

A number of studies reported poor correlation between postoperative temperatures and incidence of shivering temperatures; however, no preoperative temperatures had been recorded. In addition the sites where temperatures were recorded were not rigorously selected. This is of great importance because shivering can occur with decreased skin surface temperature even if core temperature is 36.0°C.

From a thermodynamic point of view, shivering is more efficient than voluntary muscle contraction. However, shivering muscles require an increased blood flow that increases convective heat loss, and their activation threshold is below that for vasoconstriction and nonshivering thermogenesis. Shivering is associated with a significant increase in oxygen consumption, and this occurs at a time when pulmonary reserve is diminished, frequently resulting in arterial desaturation and lactic acidemia. Cardiac output is increased to compensate for the increased requirement for oxygen delivery. Dysrhythmias may appear in hypothermic patients in the recovery period, with hypokalemia being a contributing factor (31).

Minute ventilation increases in association with the increase in carbon dioxide production (32), which could contribute to pulmonary hypertension and mixed venous oxygen desaturation in patients with severe underlying pulmonary disease. Tissue hypoxia after severe vasoconstriction causes an increase in anaerobic metabolism.

Thermal discomfort is often mentioned by patients during the immediate postoperative period (23,28). The vigorous muscular activity associated with shivering can exacerbate postoperative pain; in fact, at times it persists even when optimal pain relief is provided (33). Although a direct synergism between shivering and pain perception cannot be confirmed, a similar neuronal traffic could be implicated.

The effect of hypothermia on development of wound infection has received particular attention recently because it could represent a serious postoperative complication. Mild hypothermia has been reported to impair various nonspecific immune functions such as mobility and chemotactic migration of leukocytes and phagocytosis (34). It is not clear to what extent vasoconstriction, by decreasing tissue oxygen tension, could contribute to the development of wound infections (35). Similarly, factors such as nutritional status, pyrexia, and concurrent diseases might influence the wound's immune function. Although perioperative hypothermia may contribute to infections, these are not detected until several days after surgery. The data on altered immune functions currently are too scarce to establish a direct correlation between hypothermia and impaired wound healing.

THERMOGENESIS AFTER SURGERY

The presence of fever after surgery is an accepted phenomenon and regarded as a physiologic response to a pathologic process. Although a decrease in body temperature has been described in animals and humans after accidental injury (ebb phase) (7), there is no evidence of this occurring after surgery. Indeed, the increase in core temperature starts in the immediate postoperative period. In an analysis of 97 patients (age range 25–72 years) undergoing a variety of surgical procedures, receiving either general or regional anesthesia, aural canal temperature reached a mean peak of 37.5°C 14 hours after the end of surgery (range 8–16 hours). A second peak of 37.4°C was reached 32 hours after the end of surgery (36). The increase in body temperature was independent of age, gender, and type of anesthesia. The extent of febrile response could have been related to the intensity of surgical trauma, although a definition of intensity is purely anecdotal. The suggestion that the high fever at times observed in some groups of patients could represent a response to the degree of peripheral vasoconstriction and the duration of intraoperative hypothermia awaits to be proved.

HYPOTHERMIA AND OUTCOME

Although several studies have clearly shown immediate and delayed physiologic perturbations of mild intraoperative hypothermia on organ function such as excessive sympathetic stimulation, interference with drug metabolism, impaired clotting cascade, altered immune system with risk of wound infection, and delayed wound healing, these data do not yet allow us to conclude that hypothermia per se is responsible for any adverse outcome.

I can only trace two studies that have addressed the effect of moderate hypothermia on mortality and morbidity. In an analysis of 100 consecutive patients admitted to a surgical critical care unit after major abdominal, thoracic, or vascular operations, a significantly increased mortality rate during the first 8 hours of postoperative care was observed in a group of patients admitted with a core temperature below 36.0°C. These patients were also hypotensive during this period (systolic blood pressure below 100 mmHg), indicating the inability of these subjects to mount a thermogenic response (30).

The second study was conducted in a group of 100 patients undergoing lower extremity vascular reconstruction, with similar preoperative risk factors for perioperative cardiac morbidity and receiving continuous Holter monitoring throughout the first 24 postoperative hours (29). A greater percentage of patients with electrocardiographic changes consistent with myocardial ischemia was identified in the hypothermic group (36%) compared with those in the normothermic group (p = 0.008). The incidence of low PaO_2 was significantly greater in the hypothermic group, indicating the potential role of hypoxia in the development of cardiac ischemia. From present reports it is likely that excess sympathetic activation in a group of hypothermic patients at risk, such as elderly patients with cardiorespiratory and metabolic disorders, will lead to a greater probability of perioperative myocardial ischemia and incidence of myocardial infarction and postoperative mortality. Unfortunately, the available studies are retrospective and do not compensate for differences within the observed populations. For example, elderly patients, malnourished or with preexisting diseases, undergoing large and long procedures are most likely to become hypothermic. Similarly, patients having severe trauma arrive in the emergency room hypothermic. However, these data per se do not allow the conclusion that hypothermia causes an adverse outcome. Even well designed, prospective, interventional studies of hypothermia and postoperative mortality may not prove a causal effect.

The difficulty in identifying moderate hypothermia as a single perioperative factor modulating outcome lies in the consideration that the current monitoring of vital functions such as the cardiovascular or central nervous system is not designed to differentiate the moderate decrease in body temperature among several other factors associated with surgical stress, e.g., pain and dehydration. From a critical analysis of the pathophysiologic changes resulting from thermal stress, there is a need to address this particular question within the wide concept of the response to surgical stress.

THERAPEUTIC STRATEGIES

Detection of Hypothermia

Hypothermia can be detected only by monitoring body temperature. What we measure as core temperature is actually a representation of deep tissue with supposedly a constant and uniform temperature. This can be achieved by inserting a temperature probe in natural orifices based on accessibility, safety, and comfort. Numerous studies have compared different body sites to identify either correlation or lack of correlation of temperature measurements. It is now apparent that the best sites for determining central or core temperature are the pulmonary artery blood, the tympanic membrane, and the distal esophagus (37). Measurement of skin surface temperature alone is not a reliable indicator because it is affected by vasoconstriction and environmental factors. Accurate estimation of mean skin temperature require measurement at multiple sites, and the recent development of portable infrared thermometers has made this clinically feasible.

The loss of heat from the body is of great importance when therapeutic strategies are to be developed, and this can be calculated from core and mean skin temperatures or measured directly using heat flux transducers. These transducers allow direct measurement of cutaneous heat loss or gain via radiation, convection, conduction, and evaporation. Recent studies have been conducted using 10 or 15 skin surface sites to measure heat loss in watts per square meter of surface area. Transducers are placed on the known sites and flux values converted into watts per site by multiplying the calculated surface area and taking into consideration the gradient temperature and the heat exchange coefficient.

In a pig model (38), the heat loss was measured and the exposed skin surface area together with that of the abdominal cavity exposed through a surgical incision calculated. In this model the abdominal contents were confined within the limits of the surgical incision. The heat loss (radiation, convection, and evaporation) from the abdominal cavity exceeded that from the skin by a factor of five. However, the area of exposed skin was 15 times that of the exposed abdominal cavity. The net result: approximately 75% of the heat loss occurred from the skin. Although it is difficult to reduce heat loss from the abdominal cavity, it is simple to reduce heat loss from the skin and even use the skin surface area as a heat exchange device.

The flux measurements need to be validated in a range of clinical situations and correlated with metabolic rate and the heat calculated using core and mean skin temperature. Based on this innovative technology and according to known parameters (body surface area, patient's body composition, extent of vasoconstriction, type of environment, etc.), one could estimate the loss of heat and gain from the body and plan a rationale of intervention. Measurement of body heat content could then consolidate the present monitoring of core temperature, which has major drawbacks in predicting the distribution of body heat.

Prevention of Hypothermia

Providing thermal neutrality during anesthesia and surgery is beneficial. Although we know that intraoperative thermoregulatory vasoconstriction is remarkably effective in preventing further core hypothermia, patients behave as if they are poikilothermic and therefore largely dependent on the physician's intervention before they reach that thermoregulatory threshold. The sudden decrease in core temperature during the first hour of anesthesia and surgery is accompanied by an increased cutaneous vasodilatation. However, the increased heat loss from the skin and the small decrease in body production do not explain entirely the observed hypothermia. It derives that preventive measures adopted before or during surgery may not necessarily achieve their desired effect.

Most preventive methods advocated aim to reduce the temperature gradient between the patient's core and the immediate environment by reducing losses via all routes. Skin surface warming before induction of anesthesia (39,40) does not alter core temperature much because this remains well regulated, but it does increase body heat content. The increase is mostly in the legs, which are an important component of the peripheral thermoregulatory compartment. When peripheral tissues are warm, subsequent inhibition of normal tonic thermoregulatory vasoconstriction produces little redistribution hypothermia because heat flows only down a temperature gradient. Another method suggested to reduce the core-to-peripheral gradient is to induce vasodilatation pharmacologically (41,42). In this way redistribution hypothermia is minimal.

The preventive measures need to be continued throughout the duration of surgery, and active warming of the core and skin can be achieved with several methods available. Airway heating and humidification, intravenous fluid warmers, and cutaneous warming (43) are some of the interventional strategies currently used. From a clinical point of view the relative efficacy of these treatments needs to be established, together with their relative cost and safety.

Treatment of Established Hypothermia

The large majority of patients intentionally and aggressively maintained normothermic during surgery arrive in the recovery room well vasodilated, with no evidence of shivering and increased metabolic rate. However, intraoperative active warming is not universally advocated and at times it has proved very difficult or impossible to provide thermal neutrality due to several circumstances. If residual hypothermia is present at the end of surgery, the physician has the alternative strategy of treating this residual heat debt. Body rewarming can be achieved by the patient himself using the restored thermoregulatory response, but only healthy patients can face the cardiovascular and metabolic challenge of shivering and severe vasoconstriction. Conversely, active physiologic and pharmacologic measures can be instituted. Cutaneous surface active warming has been shown to be very effective in treating postoperative shivering and increased sympathetic stimulation. Pharmacologic intervention such as high-dose opioids (44), vasodilators (41), and muscle relaxants (45) have been advocated to attenuate the physiologic response associated with shivering and the rewarming phase. These methods have been shown to reduce the work of breathing, the increase in energy expenditure and the production of lactic acid. Reanesthetizing and ventilating hypothermic patients may seem extreme, but in some selected patients with cardiovascular and metabolic abnormalities it can be life saving and less hazardous that shivering.

Alternative Strategies

Increased Body Heat Production

The possible interference of anesthetic agents and surgical stress with normal hypothalamic thermoregulation has focused interest on heat dissipation mechanisms, in part because of the low operating room temperatures used.

This concept is based on the observation that even with heat dissipation maintained at preanesthesia level, the marked decrease in heat production during anesthesia may be expected to cause substantial hypothermia. It has been shown that administration of nutrients, especially proteins and amino acids, stimulates resting energy expenditure and therefore thermogenesis. Either oral or intravenous administration of proteins is accompanied by over a 20% increase in energy expenditure and an increase in blood temperature. Sellden et al. (46,47) have infused a mixture of amino acids intravenously before and during anesthesia and surgery with the intent of stimulating heat generation and whole-body oxidative metabolism, which otherwise would be depressed as a result of anesthesia. In the mind of these investigators, such a stimulation would counteract the perioperative loss of body heat and maintain the patient normothermic. The amount of amino acids infused over 2 hours by theses investigators was equivalent to the ingestion of 28 g of proteins, i.e., approximately half of the daily requirements. Thus, some of the responses observed are likely to be due to an excessive rate of supply of amino acids rather than a normally recruited physiologic mechanism. This is even more likely given that the response observed in the patients studied was much larger that that seen in healthy subjects and septic patients (48). It is not clear whether the preoperative medication and/or anesthesia were responsible for this enhanced response to intravenous amino acids. The increase in metabolic rate was accompanied by an increase in body temperature.

It seems unlikely that this increase in temperature is entirely due to increased thermogenesis; it is highly probable that there was also a reduction in heat loss compared with the control subjects. Any decrease in body heat loss is likely to be achieved by a lower peripheral blood flow, presumably due to increased vascular tone, although this cannot be confirmed because of the lack of appropriate measurements. Almost half of the thermogenesis caused by the amino acid infusion occurs in the splanchnic tissue. This represents the energy costs of protein synthesis, deamination, and decarboxylation of amino acids, gluconeogenesis, and urea synthesis. Although it is not clear which substrate is mainly used for such energy-requiring processes, it is speculated that amino acid oxidation contributes to a large extent. Such an effect, combined with increased vasoconstriction, would represent a considerable cardiovascular challenge to the stressed patient. Such an increase in oxidative metabolism continues in the immediate postoperative period with values up to 50–60% above baseline.

The choice of administering an amino acid mixture as a way of increasing heat production and balancing out the dissipation of body heat caused by anesthesia and surgery over a certain period of time poses some relevant questions; could the protective effect of hypothermia on body functions be disrupted by an increased metabolic demand, raised splanchnic blood flow, and cardiovascular overload? What would be the role of amino acid infusion in providing energy at times of maximal stress? A detailed evaluation of this method on the distribution of body heat in the anesthetized patient and on the thermogenic interactions with different anesthetic techniques is needed.

Sympathetic Deafferentation

The use of regional blockade during the perioperative period is based on the concept that this technique is valuable as it attenuates the sympathetic activation of surgery, maintains cardiovascular stability, induces peripheral vasodilatation, and delays the rewarming phase.

This might be seen as a paradox because it is well recognized that hypothermia is commonly observed when epidural or spinal blocks are administered (49,50). Increased cutaneous heat loss secondary to anesthetic-induced vasodilatation (51) below the level of the block was initially proposed as the etiology of this decrease in core temperature. In fact, skin temperature does increase with the induction of regional anesthesia. However, cutaneous heat loss increases by a small amount, from approximately 100 W to 115 W.

The most likely mechanism whereby regional anesthesia impairs thermoregulation is by blockade of afferent thermal cutaneous input (52). The neural traffic blockade in this situation could be tonic cold signals. This would result in the thermoregulatory system perceiving a lack of tonic cold input as an increase in apparent leg temperature (53). Such phenomena could result in a decrease in cold response threshold, vasoconstriction, and shivering (54). Regional anesthesia would also interfere with efferent response below the level of blockade. Despite the fractional contribution to redistribution during epidural anesthesia, core temperature decreases only by half as much as during general anesthesia because metabolic rate is maintained and the upper limbs are vasoconstricted. The response to surgery and/or hypothermia includes sympathetic activation, and one might propose the hypothesis that an effective epidural blockade would provide sympathetic deafferentation not only to nociceptive stimuli of surgical origin, but also to tonic cold signals. Although this would imply peripheral vasodilatation and loss of heat, it would also mean minimizing the thermogenic response during the immediate postoperative period when the body tries to repay the heat debt. Based on this hypothesis, a sensory blockade (T4–S5) was established with local anesthetics injected in the epidural space before surgery and maintained during the postoperative period (26). General anesthesia was also used. Hypothermia was a feature in all these patients. During the postoperative period (Figs. 1–4) the circulating concentrations of adrenaline and noradrenaline were not significantly changed compared with preoperative levels. Similarly, values of VO$_2$ were low, and the postoperative increase in body temperature was delayed. This was in

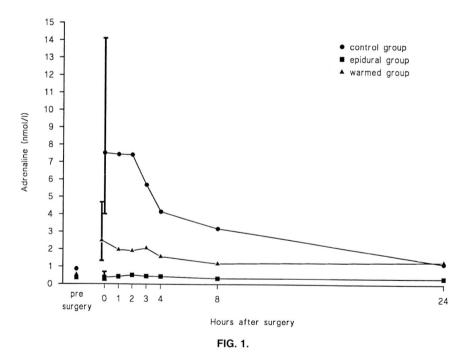

FIG. 1.

FIGS. 1–4. Circulating levels of plasma adrenaline, noradrenaline, and oxygen consumption and dorsum hand temperature during the postoperative period in three groups of patients receiving respectively either routine care, or active warming or epidural anesthesia. All three groups received general anesthesia (26).

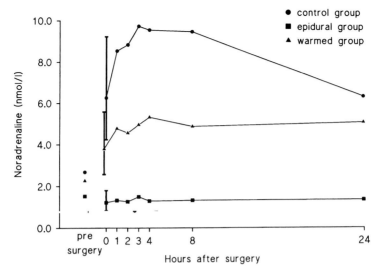

FIG. 2.

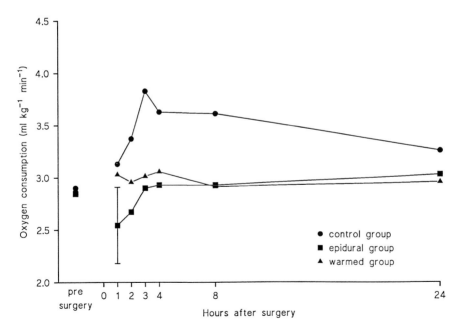

FIG. 3.

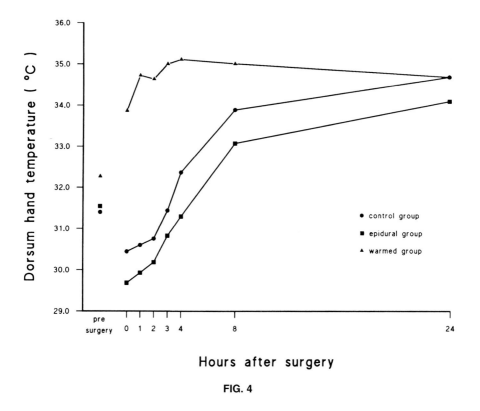

Hours after surgery

FIG. 4

contrast with the increase in catecholamines and metabolic rate observed in a group of hypothermic patients who received only general anesthesia. The question remained as to whether epidural blockade would attenuate or abolish the thermogenic response in a group of hypothermic patients at the end of operation. Therefore, in a subsequent study (55), local anesthetics were administered via the epidural route at the end of surgery, once the hypothermia was achieved (<35.0°C) and the surgical insult established. Extended sensory block (T4–S5) was obtained. The result was a significantly inhibitory effect on the elevated plasma concentrations of catecholamines, together with a delayed rewarming (Figs. 5 and 6) More recently our group has been interested in examining whether metabolic advantages can be identified by combining epidural blockade and active surface warming. It is apparent from preliminary results that there are no additional advantages in providing thermoneutrality when effective sympathetic deafferentation is achieved.

Some questions remain to be addressed in this particular area. What is the role of epidural opioids as adjuvant to local anesthetics in the modulation of afferent cold signals and nociceptive stimuli? Does pain relief as obtained with epidural analgesia attenuate the thermogenic response?

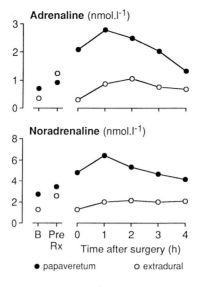

FIG. 5.

FIGS. 5–6. Circulating levels of adrenaline and noradrenaline, and core, mean skin and hand temperature during the first postoperative hours in two groups of patients who at the end of surgery received either opioids or epidural (55).

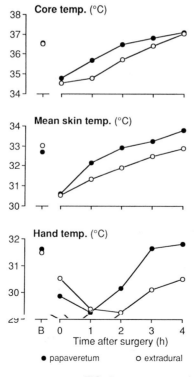

FIG. 6.

CONCLUSIONS

Although mild and moderate hypothermia have been reported to provide organ protection against tissue ischemia, this concept has now been challenged in many settings. Consequences of unintentional hypothermia in either the operating room or emergency department are harmful, and reports linking hypothermia to myocardial ischemia, prolonged duration of drug action, impaired coagulation, and reduced resistance to surgical wound infection (56) are on the increase.

The stress associated with temperature disturbances should be considered part of the overall response to surgical injury; therefore, every effort should be made to provide a global therapy throughout the perioperative period.

REFERENCES

1. English MJM, Farmer C, Scott WAC. Heat loss in exposed volunteers. *J Trauma* 1990;30:422–425.
2. Sessler DI, Olofsson CI, Rubinstein EH, et al. The thermoregulatory threshold in humans during halothane anesthesia. *Anesthesiology* 1988;68:836–842.
3. Sessler DI, Olofsson CI, Rubinstein EH, et al. The thermoregulatory threshold in humans during nitrous oxide-fentanyl anesthesia. *Anesthesiology* 1988;69:357–364.
4. Ramachandra V, Moore C, Kaur N, Carli F. Effect of halothane, enflurane and isoflurane on body temperature during and after surgery. *Br J Anaesth* 1989;62:409–414.
5. Joris J, Ozaki M, Sessler DI, et al. Epidural anesthesia impairs both central and peripheral thermoregulatory control during general anesthesia. *Anesthesiology* 1994;80:268–277.
6. Washington DE, Sessler DI, McGuire J, et al. Painful stimulation minimally increases the thermoregulatory threshold for vasoconstriction during enflurane anesthesia in humans. *Anesthesiology* 1992;77: 286–290.
7. Little JM, Stoner HB. Body temperature after accidental injury. *Br J Surg* 1981;68:221–224.
8. Fellows IW, Macdonald IA, Bennett T, Allison SP. The effects of undernutrition on thermoregulation in the elderly. *Clin Sci* 1985;69:525–532.
9. Galen IW, Macdonald IA. The effects of underfeeding for 7 d on the thermogenic and physiological response to glucose and insulin infusion. *Br J Nutr* 1990;64:427–437.
10. Vaughan MS, Vaughan RW, Cork RC. Postoperative hypothermia in adults: relationship of age, anesthesia and shivering in rewarming. *Anesth Analg* 1981;60:746–751.
11. Busto R, Globus MY, Dietrich WD, et al. Effect of mild hypothermia on ischemia-induced release of neurotransmitters and free fatty acids in rat brain. *Stroke* 1989;20:904–910.
12. Minamisawa H, Smith M, Siesjo BK. The effect of mild hypothermia and hypothermia on brain damage following 5, 10 and 15 minutes of forebrain ischemia. *Ann Neurol* 1990;28:26–33.
13. Valeri CR, Feingold H, Cassidy G, et al. Hypothermia-induced reversible platelet dysfunction. *Ann Surg* 1987;205:175–181.
14. Roher M, Natale A. Effect of hypothermia on the coagulation cascade. *Crit Care Med* 1992;20: 1402–1405.
15. Keatinge WR, Coleshaw SRK, Cotter F. Increase in platelet and red cell counts, blood viscosity and arterial pressure during mild surface cooling. Factors in morbidity from coronary and cerebral thrombosis in winter. *Br Med J* 1984;289:1405–1408.
16. Smith OLK, Huszar G, Davidson SB, Davis E. Effect of cold exposure on muscle aminoacids and proteins in rats. *J Appl Physiol* 1982;52:1250–1256.
17. Johnson DI, Brooks DC, Pressler VM, et al. Hypothermic anesthesia attenuates postoperative proteolysis. *Ann Surg* 1986;204:419–429.
18. Taggart DP, McMillam DC, Preston T, et al. Effect of surgical injury and intraoperative hypothermia on whole body protein metabolism. *Am J Physiol* 1991;260:E118–E125.
19. Tsubo T, Oka Y, Matsuki A, Oyama T. Comparison of hypothermia and normothermia methods of cardiopulmonary bypass: haemodynamic and hormonal responses. *Masui* 1984;33:1180–1186.

20. Carli F, Webster J, Pearson M, et al. Postoperative protein metabolism: effect of nursing elderly patients for 24 h after abdominal surgery in a thermoneutral environment. *Br J Anaesth* 1991;66:292–299.
21. Carli F, Emery PW, Freemantle CA. Effect of peroperative normothermia on postoperative protein metabolism in elderly patients undergoing hip arthroplasty. *Br J Anaesth* 1989;63:276–282.
22. Ryan DW, Clague MB. Nitrogen sparing and the catabolic hormones in patients nursed at an elevated ambient temperature following major surgery. *Intensive Care Med* 1990;16:287–290.
23. Sessler DI, Rubinstein EH, Moayeri A. Physiologic responses to mild perianesthetic hypothermia in humans. *Anesthesiology* 1991;75:594–610.
24. Heier T, Caldwell JE, Sessler DI, Miller RD. Mild intraoperative hypothermia increases duration of action and spontaneous recovery of vecuronium blockade during nitrous oxide-isoflurane anesthesia in humans. *Anesthesiology* 1991;74:815–819.
25. Leslie K, Sessler DI, Bjorksten AR, Moayeri A. Mild hypothermia alters propofol pharmacokinetics and increases the duration of action of atracurium. *Anesth Analg* 1995;81:376–381.
26. Carli F, Webster J, Nandi P, et al. Thermogenesis after surgery:effect of perioperative heat conservation and epidural anesthesia. *Am J Physiol* 1992;263:E441–E447.
27. Frank SM, Higgins M, Breslow MJ, et al. The catecholamines, cortisol and hemodynamic responses to mild hypothermia. A randomized clinical trial. *Anesthesiology* 1995;82:83–93.
28. Kurtz A, Sessler DI, Narzt E, et al. Postoperative hemodynamic and thermoregulatory consequence of intraoperative core hypothermia. *J Clin Anesth* 1995;7:359–366.
29. Frank SM, Beattie C, Christopherson R, et al. Unintentional hypothermia is associated with postoperative myocardial ischemia. *Anesthesiology* 1993;78:468–476.
30. Slotman GJ, Jed EH, Burchard KW. Adverse effects of hypothermia in postoperative patients. *Am J Surg* 1985;149:4095–501.
31. Boelhouwer RU, Bruining HA, Ong GL. Correlations of serum potassium fluctuations with body temperature after major surgery. *Crit Care Med* 1987;15:310–312.
32. Ciofolo MJ, Clergue F, Devillers C, et al. Changes in ventilation, oxygen uptake and carbon dioxide output during recovery from isoflurane anesthesia. *Anesthesiology* 1989;70:737–742.
33. Hines R, Barash PG, Watrous PG, O'Connor T. Complications occurring in the post-anesthesia care unit. A survey. *Anesth Analg* 1992;74:503–509.
34. Van Oss CJ, Absolam DR, Moore LL, et al. Effect of temperature on the chemotaxos, phagocytic engulfment, digestion and O_2 consumption of human polymorphonuclear leukocytes. *J Reticuloendothel Soc* 1980;27:561–565.
35. Sheffield CW, Sessler DI, Hunt TK. Mild hypothermia during isoflurane anesthesia decreases resistance to *E. coli* infection in guinea pigs. *Acta Anaesthesiol Scand* 1994;38:201–205.
36. Carli F, Aber VR. Thermogenesis after major elective surgical procedures. *Br J Surg* 1987;74: 1041–1045.
37. Cork RC, Vaughan RW, Humphrey LS. Precision and accuracy of intraoperaive temperature monitoring. *Anesth Analg* 1983;62:211–214.
38. English MJM, Papenberg R, Scott WAC. Heat loss in an animal experimental model. *J Trauma* 1991; 31:36–38.
39. Just B, Trevien V, Delva E, Lienhart A. Prevention of intraoperative hypothermia by preoperative skin-surface warming. *Anesthesiology* 1993;79:214–218.
40. Hynson JM, Sessler DI, Moayeri A, et al. The effects of pre-induction warming on temperature and blood pressure during propofol/nitrous oxide anesthesia. *Anesthesiology* 1993;79:219–228.
41. Joris J, Banache M, Bonnet F, Sessler DI, Lamy M. Clonidine and ketanserin both are effective treatment for postanesthetic shivering. *Anesthesiology* 1993;79:532–539.
42. Delaunay L, Bonnet F, Liu N, et al. Clonidine comparably decreases the thermoregulatory thresholds for vasoconstriction and shivering in humans. *Anesthesiology* 1993;79:470–474.
43. Hynson JM, Sessler DI. Intraoperative warming therapies: a comparison of three devices. *J Clin Anesth* 1992;4:194–199.
44. Rodriguez Jl, Weissman C, Damask MC, et al. Morphine and postoperative rewarming in critically ill patients. *Circulation* 1983;68:1238–1246.
45. Rodriguez JL, Weissman C, Damask MC, et al. Physiologic requirements during rewarming: suppression of the shivering response. *Crit Care Med* 1983;11:490–497.
46. Sellden E, Brundin T, Wahren J. Augmented thermic effect of amino acids under general anaesthesia: a mechanism useful for prevention of anaesthesia-induced hypothermia. *Clin Sci* 1994;86:611–618.
47. Sellden E, Branstrom R, Brundin T. Preoperative infusion of amino acids prevents postoperative hypothermia. *Br J Anaesth* 1996;76:227–234.

48. Carlson GL, Gray P, Arnold L, et al. Thermogenic, hormonal and metabolic effects of a TPN mixture. Influences of glucose and amino acids. *Am J Physiol* 1994;266:E845–E851.
49. Frank SM, Beattie C, Christopherson R, et al. Epidural versus general anesthesia, ambient operating room temperature and patient age as predictors of inadvertent hypothermia. *Anesthesiology* 1992;77:252–257.
50. Vassilieff N, Rosencher N, Sessler DI, Conseillier C. Shivering threshold during spinal anesthesia is reduced in elderly patients. *Anesthesiology* 1995;82:1162–1166.
51. Matsukawa T, Sessler DI, Christensen R, et al. Heat flow and distribution during epidural anesthesia. *Anesthesiology* 1995;83:961–967.
52. Pierau FK, Wurster RD. Primary afferent input from cutaneous thermoreceptors. *Fed Proc* 1981;40: 2819–2824.
53. Emerick TH, Ozaki M, Sessler DI, et al. Epidural anesthesia increases apparent leg temperature and decreases the shivering threshold. *Anesthesiology* 1994;81:289–298.
54. Giesbrecht GG. Human thermoregulatory inhibition by regional anesthesia. *Anesthesiology* 1994;81: 277–281.
55. Carli F, Kulkarni P, Webster JD, Macdonald IA. Post-surgery epidural blockade with local anaesthetics attenuates the catecholamine and thermogenic response to perioperative hypothermia. *Acta Anaesthesiol Scand* 1995;39:1041–1047.
56. Kurz A, Sessler DJ, Lenhardt R. Perioperative normothermia to reduce the incidence of surgical-wound infection and shorten hospitalization. *N Engl J Med* 1996;334:1209–1215.

Physiology, Stress, and Malnutrition: Functional Correlates, Nutritional Intervention,
edited by J.M. Kinney and H.N. Tucker.
Lippincott–Raven Publishers © 1997.

Dietary Thermogenesis and Cardiovascular Response

Ian A. Macdonald, E.M.M.A. Habas, Mark T. Kearney, and Tracy A. Stubbs

Departments of Physiology and Pharmacology, University of Nottingham Medical School, Nottingham N67 2UH, United Kingdom

The ingestion, digestion, and absorption of food and the distribution of nutrients to the organs and tissues impose substantial metabolic and cardiovascular demands on the body. The primary objective of this review is to consider the factors that affect the cardiovascular responses to nutrient ingestion and whether the cardiovascular and thermogenic response are linked. Some of the apparently inconsistent responses to nutrients that have been described in the literature are likely due to differences in meal composition; in addition, some investigators have used solid food in their studies, whereas others have used drinks. Thus, a secondary objective is to identify the major differences in response to solid and liquid nutrient intake.

CARDIOVASCULAR RESPONSE TO NUTRIENTS

Food ingestion is associated with changes in heart rate, stroke volume, blood pressure, and peripheral blood flow. One of the earliest experimental investigations of this phenomenon was described by Grollman (1) and showed substantial increases in resting cardiac output and heart rate, with minimal disturbance of blood pressure. The main drawback of many of the early studies of the cardiovascular responses to food was the use of invasive techniques and the variable detail concerning the amount and type of food consumed. In the past 10 years, a number of noninvasive techniques for assessing cardiovascular responses have become widely available (2) and have been used to assess the responses to food ingestion. In particular, the use of Doppler ultrasound to measure gastrointestinal blood flow (3,4) in combination with a variety of methods to assess cardiac output and peripheral blood flow has allowed the integrated cardiovascular response to food to be determined.

In healthy young subjects, the cardiovascular response to food is characterized by an increase in gastrointestinal blood flow and cardiac output, with little change in mean arterial blood pressure. The magnitude and time course of these changes are affected by meal size and composition, as discussed below. The peripheral (i.e., limb) blood flow response to meals is more complex, with both decreases and increases in blood flow being observed. This variation in response is partly related to meal composition and the duration of the postprandial measurements, but there also appears to be differences between the effects of solid food and nutrient containing drinks.

Effects of Meal Composition on the Cardiovascular Responses to Nutrients

Qamar et al. (4) measured the superior mesenteric artery (SMA) blood flow response to isoenergetic drinks containing carbohydrate, fat, or protein compared with an equal volume of water. The greatest SMA blood flow response was seen after carbohydrate ingestion, with fat producing a greater response than protein. Waaler and Eriksen (5) studied the effects of isoenergetic and isovolemic drinks containing 4 MJ as either pure protein, carbohydrate or fat on cardiac output and SMA blood flow in healthy young subjects. They also found that the carbohydrate drink produced the greatest cardiac output and SMA blood flow responses and that none of the responses had diminished by the end of the 2-hour measurement period. It was also of interest that the increase in SMA blood flow had commenced within 2–3 minutes of completing the drink and preceded the initial increase in cardiac output by 10–15 minutes. A similar pattern was observed after the fat and protein drinks.

The observations of Waaler and Eriksen (5) are interesting but of limited practical relevance because humans do not usually consume meals of single nutrients. Thus, more useful information can be derived from studies of the effects of mixed nutrient meals with different macronutrient composition. Moreover, the effects of solid food may be of more physiologic relevance than nutrient liquids. Sidery et al. (6) studied the cardiac output, SMA, and calf blood flow response of healthy young subjects to isoenergetic (2.5 MJ) meals that were high in either fat or carbohydrate. On one occasion, 70% of the energy was from fat and on the other occasion 70% was from carbohydrate. In this study, the high-carbohydrate meal increased cardiac output by 32%, which was greater than the 22% increase observed after the high-fat meal. The increase in SMA blood flow was more rapid after the high-carbohydrate meal than after the high-fat meal, but the peak response was larger after the high-fat meal (+122%) than after the high-carbohydrate meal (+87%). With the high-carbohydrate meal, SMA blood flow had almost returned to baseline by 60 minutes postprandium, whereas it remained elevated after the high-fat meal. Conversely, the cardiac output had almost returned to baseline 60 minutes after the high-fat meal but remained elevated after the high-carbohydrate meal.

The different patterns of SMA blood flow response to high-fat and high-carbohydrate meals are not entirely explained by differences in the rate of emptying of

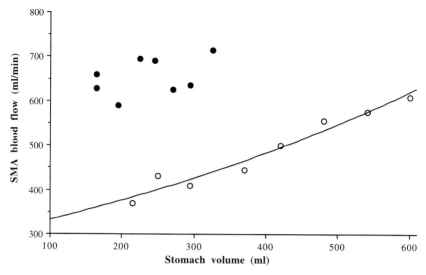

FIG. 1. Relationship between stomach volume and SMA blood flow after a high-carbohydrate (open symbols) or a high-fat meal (filled symbols). Values are means for eight healthy young men; the relationship for the high carbohydrate meal was significant. Reproduced with permission (7).

food from the stomach. Sidery et al. (7) showed a clear, curvilinear relationship between the emptying of the carbohydrate meal from the stomach and the SMA blood flow response, but there was no such relationship for the high-fat meal (Fig. 1). Thus, with a high-carbohydrate meal, the degree of intestinal hyperemia is related to the delivery of nutrients to the intestine and possibly to the extent of gastric distention, but after a high-fat meal other mechanisms must operate.

Effects of Meal Size on Cardiovascular Responses

Many early studies described studying the cardiovascular effects of large or small meals, but the absence of any detail concerning the actual energy content makes them of little value. More recently, Waaler et al. (8) compared the effects of 2- and 5-MJ solid food meals on cardiac output and blood pressure for 2 hours in four healthy young subjects. This rather preliminary study showed that the peak cardiac output response to the large meal was greater and more sustained than to the small meal. They also found that in some subjects there was a decrease in mean arterial blood pressure, especially after the large meal.

A more extensive study of the cardiovascular responses to high-carbohydrate meals of different sizes (1, 2, and 3 MJ) was undertaken by Sidery et al. (9) in a group of eight healthy young women. Postprandial measurements were continued for 3 hours, but after the 3-MJ meal most variables had still not returned to baseline by the end of the period of observation. There was a linear relationship between the peak SMA blood flow response and meal size, as well as between the overall cardiac output (total increase over the 3-hour postprandial period) and meal size (Fig. 2). The mean increase in cardiac output after the 3-MJ meal represented a 50% increase above the fasting value and presents a substantial challenge to cardiovascular homeostasis. The changes in calf blood flow after the different size meals showed an early vasoconstriction followed by a return to, or above, baseline values 2 hours postprandium.

Peripheral (Limb) Blood Flow Responses to Nutrient Ingestion

The greatest inconsistency in the literature on cardiovascular responses to food is in the changes in limb (either calf or forearm) blood flow that occur. Many studies have administered either pure nutrient (usually glucose) or mixed nutrient drinks and shown that limb blood flow increases during the postprandial period (10,11). By contrast, studies using solid food usually report a decrease in limb blood flow during the early postprandial period. For example, 15 minutes after a high-carbohydrate, solid meal there is a decrease in calf blood flow before a recovery to, or above, fasting values, whereas after a high-fat meal, calf blood flow is reduced below baseline for 30–60 minutes (Fig. 3) (6).

An early decrease in limb blood flow after food ingestion would contribute to a redistribution of cardiac output toward the splanchnic bed, and thus would enable the splanchnic hyperemic response to be achieved with a smaller overall increase in cardiac output. As the postprandial period proceeds and the products of digestion are absorbed, an increase in limb blood flow would be of value in ensuring the efficient distribution of nutrients to the peripheral tissues. Thus, the sustained cardiac output seen after ingestion of large meals is likely to supply the extra blood needed by the splanchnic tissues in the early postprandial period and that needed by the peripheral tissues in the later stages. It is possible that with nutrient-containing drinks, the more rapid gastric emptying and nutrient absorption leads to a transient or absent limb vasoconstrictor response, and that only the second phase of increased limb blood flow is observed. This is illustrated by a recent unpublished study in which we gave isoenergetic (2.1 MJ), high-carbohydrate drinks or solid food to healthy subjects and observed a decrease in forearm blood flow after the solid food and an increase after the liquid.

Mechanisms of Postprandial Cardiovascular Responses

The mechanisms responsible for the cardiovascular responses to nutrient ingestion have not been fully elucidated, but the problems that arise in patients with severe autonomic dysfunction suggest an important role for the autonomic nervous system. In addition, some of the gastrointestinal and pancreatic

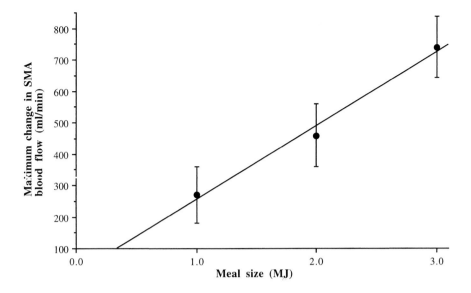

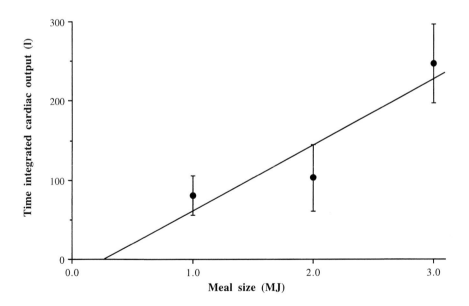

FIG. 2. Influence of meal size on SMA blood flow and cardiac output in healthy young women. All meals had a high carbohydrate content, values plotted are means ± SEM for eight subjects. Reproduced with permission (9).

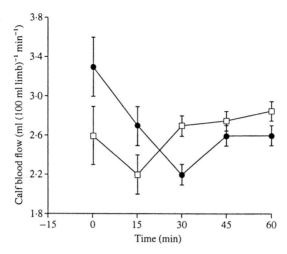

FIG. 3. Effect of high-carbohydrate (open symbols) or high-fat (filled symbols) meals on calf blood flow in healthy young subjects. Values are means ± SEM. Reproduced with permission (6).

hormones released after nutrient ingestion may have important roles in mediating the cardiovascular responses.

Cardiac Responses

Kelbaek et al. (12) showed that acute autonomic blockade, achieved with intravenous metoprolol and atropine given immediately after a meal, prevented the postprandial increase in stroke volume but did not affect the increase in heart rate. However, the study design was rather weak, with no appropriate measurements of the effects of autonomic blockade in the fasting state. Nevertheless, the results would be consistent with a humoral effect on heart rate in the postprandial period.

Other studies have identified the importance of cardiac sympathetic activation and parasympathetic withdrawal in association with the heart rate and cardiac output response to nutrients. Spectral analysis of heart rate variability has been used to provide an indirect assessment of cardiac autonomic nerve activity and has shown reduced parasympathetic and increased sympathetic activity after meals in healthy young subjects (13). However, Ryan et al. (14) only observed an increase in sympathetic activity in their study. A recent study by Cox et al. (15) using invasive venous catheterization techniques cast doubt on these spectral analysis results. They found no increase in noradrenaline spillover from the heart in the postprandial period, which is contrary to what would be expected if cardiac sympathetic activity increased. A further complication is introduced by a recent study of ours (16), which showed that cardiac transplant recipients had normal heart rate and cardiac output responses to a high-carbohydrate meal. It was interesting that they also had a normal heart rate, but not cardiac output, response to a high-fat meal (Fig. 4). Because the plasma insulin responses to the two meals were substantially different, it is possible that the differential cardiac responses resulted from low plasma insulin concentrations being chronotropic, whereas high concentrations may be inotropic (17).

Gastrointestinal Blood Flow

The increase in splanchnic blood flow during the postprandial period is likely to be partly a consequence of parasympathetic nervous stimulation of gastrointestinal motor function, together with effects of the gastrointestinal hormones and nutrient absorption. In primates, the postprandial intestinal hyperemia is prevented by atropine (18), but because atropine also delays gastric emptying, it affects any hyperemia due to nutrient digestion and absorption. There is little doubt that an atropine-sensitive mechanism is involved in the postprandial intestinal hyperemic response because similar effects have been observed in humans (19), but it is unclear whether this is due to the extrinsic parasympathetic nerves or to the intrinsic intestinal neural network. It is also clear that an increase in plasma adrenaline can increase SMA blood flow (20), but this is unlikely to contribute to postprandial intestinal hyperemia, because plasma adrenaline usually decreases after food ingestion.

It is likely that increased intestinal metabolism during nutrient digestion and absorption releases mediators that produce a local vasodilator response. Fara et al. (21) showed, in animals, a linear relationship between jejunal oxygen consumption and blood flow when nutrients were delivered to the intestinal lumen. In addition, several of the gastrointestinal peptides—cholecystokinin (21), gastric inhibitory peptide (22), and vasoactive intestinal peptide (VIP)—produced marked intestinal or generalized vasodilatation in animals. Although VIP would be a strong candidate for mediating postprandial intestinal hyperemia, it cannot do so by acting as a hormone because plasma VIP concentration does not increase after a meal (23) but may act as a neurotransmitter.

In healthy subjects in the fasting state, insulin does not appear to affect SMA blood flow, although this conclusion is only based on a preliminary study of ours (24). However, observations in patients with autonomic failure would indicate that in the absence of normal sympathetic function, insulin can cause SMA vasodilatation and reduce blood pressure (25). We have recently observed that insulin may induce SMA vasodilatation in the postprandial period. Healthy elderly subjects were given a high-fat meal with or without a concomitant insulin infusion, which reproduced the plasma insulin profile seen after a high-carbohydrate meal. The high-fat meal alone decreased SMA vascular resistance by 50 U, whereas concomitant hyperinsulinemia reduced SMA vascular resistance by 70 U.

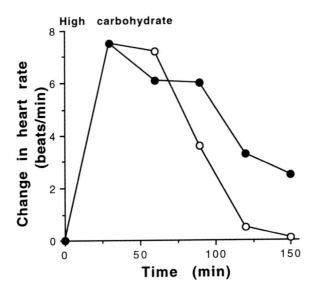

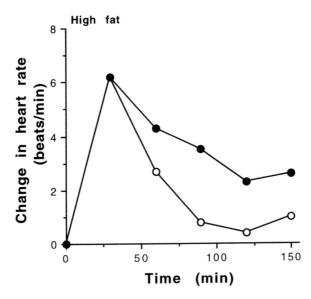

FIG. 4. Heart rate and cardiac output responses to high fat and high carbohydrate meals in healthy subjects (open symbols) and cardiac transplant recipients (filled symbols). Values are means for nine subjects in each group. Reproduced with permission (16).

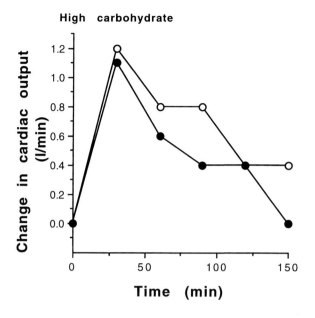

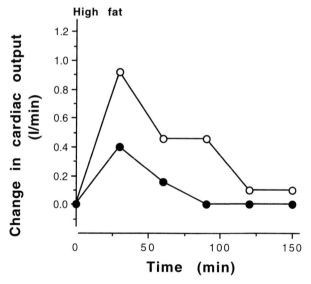

FIG. 4. *Continued.*

Limb Blood Flow

Food ingestion, particularly high-carbohydrate, is associated with an increase in sympathetic nervous system activity. This is manifested by increases in plasma noradrenaline and the noradrenaline spillover rate (15) and by an increase in the muscle sympathetic nerve firing rate (26). This latter response represents an increase in muscle vasoconstrictor nerve activity and may explain the limb vasoconstrictor response seen in the early stages after food ingestion. However, it is also clear that the insulin response to a high-carbohydrate meal may affect limb blood flow. Insulin infusion increases limb blood flow (27), and we have recently observed that the normal sustained limb vasoconstriction seen after a high-fat solid meal can be prevented by the infusion of insulin (Fig. 5) (28). Thus, the early limb vasoconstrictor response seen after food is likely to be mediated by the sympathetic nervous system and contribute to a redistribution of cardiac output, whereas the later limb vasodilatation is probably a result of the vascular effects of insulin and occurs despite a continued increase in muscle sympathetic nerve activity. Further evidence of increased sympathetic nerve activity associated with eating comes from studies on cats by Matsukawa and Ninomiya (29). They observed that both heart rate and renal sympathetic nerve activity increased within 2 seconds of the onset of eating. Although this response is likely to be at least partly related to the physical act of eating, it is consistent with the increased sympathetic activity observed in humans by Cox et al. (15).

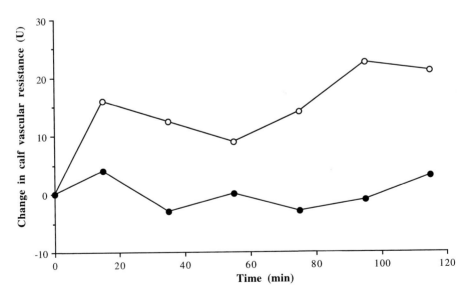

FIG. 5. Calf vasoconstrictor responses to a high-fat meal (open symbols) or to a high-fat meal with a concomitant insulin infusion (filled symbols) in healthy subjects. Adapted from Ref. 28.

Overall Regulation

It seems highly likely that the various postprandial cardiovascular responses described above are part of an overall regulatory process designed to maintain arterial blood pressure. Thus, postprandial intestinal hyperemia is sustained by a combination of an increase in cardiac output and a redistribution of it. As the postprandial period proceeds, this redistribution of cardiac output is modified, enabling delivery of the absorbed nutrients to the peripheral tissues. It is not clear what primary signals are responsible for initiating the normal physiologic response to food ingestion, although venous return to the heart, splanchnic blood volume, and arterial blood pressure are likely to be of major importance. However, it is clear that patients with defective autonomic function, with cardiac insufficiency and the elderly with an age-related decline in autonomic function have significantly disturbed cardiovascular responses to food ingestion.

Defective Cardiovascular Responses to Nutrient Ingestion

Autonomic Failure

A number of degenerative, neurologic diseases lead to a progressive loss of autonomic nervous function. It has been known for many years that such patients are unable to maintain blood pressure when upright. However, it is only relatively recently that these patients were found to experience a decrease in blood pressure postprandially, especially after a meal high in carbohydrates (30). The autonomic dysfunction in these patients means that the postprandial intestinal hyperemia is accompanied by a failure to vasoconstrict the limbs and other vascular beds and a poor, or absent, cardiac response such that blood pressure decreases substantially.

Cardiac Disease

Patients with chronic congestive heart failure have the capacity to increase cardiac output after food ingestion (31,32), which usually maintains blood pressure while total peripheral resistance decreases. Similarly, individuals with angina pectoris also are able to increase resting cardiac output after food ingestion (33). However, in both types of patient the ingestion of food has a detrimental effect on exercise capacity, with both heart failure (34) and angina (33) patients having a significant reduction in symptom-limited exercise tolerance after food ingestion. We have recently extended these observations in patients with angina and found that the effect of food to reduce exercise tolerance is a consequence of its carbohydrate content; a high-fat meal has no such effect (35).

Aging and Autonomic Function

A decline in autonomic nervous system function is a characteristic feature of the aging process, but it is only in the past 15 years that it has become apparent that this may affect the maintenance of arterial blood pressure after meals. Lipsitz et al. (36) demonstrated postprandial declines in blood pressure in the elderly, and it soon became apparent that those most at risk were older, frail, institutionalized individuals. Potter et al. (37) showed that the reduction in blood pressure was more marked after a high-carbohydrate meal than after a high-fat meal, and Sidery et al. (38) found that the decrease in blood pressure was mainly due to an impaired ability to increase cardiac output as compared with the same ability in younger subjects (Fig. 6).

These observations of postprandial hypotension in the elderly have been extended by recent studies by Tamburini et al. (39). They found postprandial reductions of 10–15 mm Hg in systolic blood pressure of elderly subjects who had normal blood pressure responses to standing, but those who had impaired responses to standing (but did not have symptoms of postural dizziness) had decreases in systolic blood pressure of 25 mm Hg after food. Similarly, Goldstein et al. (40) showed that although systolic blood pressure increased after a meal in young subjects, it decreased in the elderly. Furthermore, although food had no effect on the mean arterial blood pressure response to standing in the young, it reduced mean arterial pressure in the elderly.

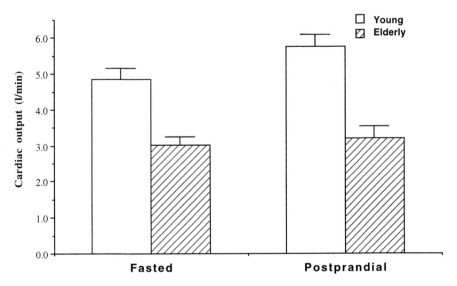

FIG. 6. Cardiac output before and after a high-carbohydrate meal in healthy young and elderly subjects. Values are means ± SEM. Adapted from Refs. 6,38.

Thus, the ingestion of nutrients leads to substantial cardiovascular responses that are affected by meal size and composition and can lead to problems in patients with disturbed cardiac or autonomic nervous function.

DIETARY THERMOGENESIS

There is an extensive body of literature on the factors affecting dietary thermogenesis, a review of which is beyond the scope of this chapter. Instead, the effects of meal size and composition on whole body thermogenesis and differences in the regional responses are considered here in more detail.

Meal Size

One of the main problems in drawing conclusions about possible differences in thermogenic responses to different sized meals is the long duration of response to large meals. Thus, Belko and Barbieri (41) gave subjects their total daily energy requirements (12 MJ) over a 10-hour period either as two large or four smaller (but still substantial) meals. They found similar integrated responses over 10 hours with both feed regimens, but in both cases metabolic rate was not returning toward baseline values after 10 hours. Moreover, the peak increase in metabolic rate was similar after the large and smaller meals (approximately 25–30%), suggesting that a maximum stimulation of thermogenesis had been reached with the 3.1-MJ meal and that larger meals simply prolong the response.

Tai et al. (42) measured the thermogenic response over a 5-hour period after consumption of a single 3.1-MJ meal, or after the consumption of six meals, each of 0.52 MJ, at 30-minute intervals. They found a smaller thermogenic response over the 5-hour period with the smaller meals than after the large one. However, this may in part be a consequence of the intermittent nature of the measurements and the difficulty in measuring smaller peak responses as accurately as larger ones. A similar (although nonsignificant) effect was observed by Vaz et al. (43), who found a smaller thermogenic response over 2 hours when three 1.05-MJ meals were consumed in the first 60 minutes, compared with one 3.15-MJ meal at the beginning of the 2-hour period. However, the responses to both meal patterns had not reached a maximum by 2 hours, and the measurements of metabolic rate were made for 10–12 minutes in every 30. Thus, some caution is needed before firmly concluding that small meals are associated with smaller overall thermogenic responses.

Meal Type and Composition

There is some evidence that solid food meals produce a higher thermogenic effect than do homogenized liquids with the same nutrient content (44,45). This has been attributed to the solid food being more palatable and producing a hedonistic response that increases the activation of the sympathetic nervous system.

The individual nutrients produce different thermogenic responses, with protein having a much greater effect than carbohydrate or fat. Many studies have addressed this topic, but a large proportion of them had a rather unsatisfactory design, which weakens the conclusions. For example, Swaminathan et al. (46) compared single nutrient drinks (protein, carbohydrate, or fat) with an isoenergetic (1.7 MJ) mixed nutrient solid meal and only measured the thermogenic response for 2 hours. The response to protein was greater than the response to fat or carbohydrate, but slightly less than the response to the solid mixed meal.

Kinabo and Durnin (47) found that varying the fat and carbohydrate contents of a 2.5- and 5-MJ meal had no effect on the thermogenic response measured over 5 hours. The changes in composition were substantial (70% carbohydrate to 65% fat) and would have produced different postprandial cardiovascular responses (see above).

Although the overall fat content of a mixed nutrient meal may not affect the thermogenic response, there is some evidence that the type of fat is of importance. Scalfi et al. (48) showed that replacing most of the long-chain triglycerides in a mixed nutrient solid food meal (30% total energy as fat) with medium-chain triglycerides increased the thermogenic response. The two meals were substantial (over 5 MJ) and produced sustained increases in metabolic rate for at least 6 hours; thus, the total response was not determined for either meal. Nevertheless, the long-chain triglyceride meal increased metabolic rate by 15% over the 6 hours, whereas the response to the medium-chain triglyceride meal was 22%. This increased thermogenic response was accompanied by a substantially lower plasma glucose response, indicating some stimulation of carbohydrate metabolism.

Regional Thermogenic Responses to Nutrient Ingestion

There have been very few studies in humans of individual organ and tissue thermogenic responses to nutrient ingestion. The major reason for this is the invasive nature of such studies and the concern that this may disturb the subjects and produce some artefacts in the results. Aksnes et al. (49) infused intravenously 0.6 MJ of amino acids over 2.5 hours and found that whole-body thermogenesis increased by 19% and that the splanchnic tissues accounted for approximately one half of this response. Although cardiac output increased by approximately 15%, there was no increase in splanchnic blood flow. By contrast, the oral ingestion of fructose or glucose (in drinks) stimulates whole-body thermogenesis without increasing splanchnic thermogenesis (50). This indicates that the thermogenic response occurs in extra-splanchnic tissues, and it is likely that skeletal muscle is a major contributor to such a response because forearm oxygen consumption increases during a hyperinsulinemic, euglycemic clamp (51).

It is interesting that whereas the glucose drink produced a substantial (20–25%) increase in cardiac output and a small increase in splanchnic blood flow, the fructose drink did not, despite producing a slightly larger thermogenic response.

Cox et al. (15) studied the whole-body and regional cardiovascular and thermogenic responses to a mixed nutrient, 2.9-MJ liquid meal. Whole-body thermogenesis increased by 16–22% over the 90-minute period of measurements, with significant increases in renal and splanchnic, but no change in cardiac, oxygen consumption (Fig. 7). The increases in renal and splanchnic oxygen consumption only accounted for 22% of the whole-body response, implying a substantial contribution from other (including muscle) tissues. It is of great interest that the 26% increase in renal oxygen consumption occurred despite an 11% decrease in renal blood flow, whereas there were increases in both blood flow and oxygen consumption in the splanchnic bed.

Vaz et al. (43) attempted to measure the forearm oxygen consumption response to a large (3.15 MJ) mixed meal, which increased whole-body thermogenesis by 22%. They failed to observe any significant increase in forearm oxygen consumption, although the numerical increase amounted to a 30% increase during the 2-hour postprandial period of measurement. Vaz et al. (43) obtained the forearm venous blood sample from a superficial vein, and because most of the forearm oxygen consumption occurs in the deep, muscle tissues, if the venous drainage is incompletely mixed, or the muscle tissue does not drain into the superficial vein, serious errors could arise in estimating forearm oxygen consumption.

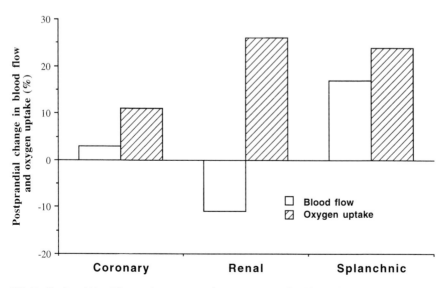

FIG. 7. Regional blood flow and oxygen uptake responses to food ingestion in healthy subjects. Adapted from Ref. 15.

On the basis of the study by Cox et al. (15), the same group as Vaz et al. (43), approximately 80% of the whole-body thermogenic response to food occurs in tissues other than the splanchnic and renal areas. If the whole-body thermogenic response is equivalent to 60 ml oxygen/min, this means that approximately 48 ml/min is in tissues such as skeletal muscle, skin, and adipose tissue. In an 80-kg person, the skeletal muscle would constitute approximately 30 kg and would have a resting oxygen consumption of approximately 2 ml/kg/min. Thus, a 30% increase in muscle oxygen consumption after a meal would account for one third of the nonsplanchnic, nonrenal response.

Role of the Autonomic System in the Regulation of Dietary Thermogenesis

It was clear that the autonomic (especially the sympathetic) nervous system plays an important role in regulating the cardiovascular response to nutrient ingestion, and a similar role can be identified in relation to the thermogenic response. Nacht et al. (52) infused the muscarinic antagonist atropine into healthy subjects and showed a significant blunting of the thermogenic response to a mixed nutrient drink. Although they showed that little of the original drink remained in the stomach 6 hours later, it is highly likely that atropine disturbed vagally mediated gastric emptying and gastrointestinal secretions and motility and retarded nutrient absorption.

This interpretation is supported by subsequent work from the same group, who showed that parasympathetic blockade with atropine had no effect on the thermogenic response to the hyperinsulinemic, euglycemic clamp, where the glucose is administered intravenously (53). Thus, any parasympathetic nervous system effects on dietary thermogenesis are likely to be mediated through alterations in nutrient delivery due to changes in gastrointestinal motility and secretions.

There is a widely held belief that the sympathetic nervous system contributes to the thermogenic response to nutrient ingestion. This is exemplified by the observations of Schwartz et al. (54), who found a correlation between the thermogenic response to a meal and the increase in plasma noradrenaline appearance rate (an index of sympathetic activation) in healthy young subjects. They also observed that the blunted thermogenic response in elderly subjects was accompanied by a lower degree of sympathetic activation and that there was no correlation between thermogenesis and sympathetic activation in the elderly. Vaz et al. (43) found no correlation between the thermogenic response to a meal and the whole-body plasma noradrenaline appearance rate for the 10 young subjects studied. However, the time courses of the mean values for thermogenic and sympathetic responses were similar and were also similar to the heart rate response, so a link between thermogenic, cardiac, and sympathetic nervous responses cannot be ruled out. Cox et al. (15) found no correlation between the oxygen consumption and noradrenaline spillover responses to food in the splanchnic or renal areas for nine subjects, but again there were similar increases in the mean values over the postprandial period.

Some doubt must be cast on any proposal that sympathetic activation is responsible for a major component of the thermogenic response to nutrient ingestion because Nacht et al. (52) found no diminution of the thermogenic response during the infusion of the β-adrenoceptor antagonist propranolol, and a similar observation was made by Morgan et al. (55). Furthermore, patients with complete spinal cord transection at the cervical level have normal thermogenic responses to a mixed nutrient test drink (56). The latter observation appears to provide clear evidence of the unimportance of efferent sympathetic outflow from the central nervous system in mediating thermogenic responses to food. However, it is somewhat surprising that these patients did not have a postprandial decrease in blood pressure. Such tetraplegic patients can retain spinal sympathetic reflexes, so one cannot rule out an involvement of the sympathetic nervous system in their thermogenic response to food.

Thus, there is some doubt concerning the direct role of the autonomic nervous system in the thermogenic response to nutrient ingestion. On the basis of the evidence reviewed above, it seems most likely that the autonomic nervous system is more important for controlling the gastrointestinal and cardiovascular responses to food and that any effect on thermogenesis is likely to be indirect.

INTEGRATION OF CARDIOVASCULAR AND THERMOGENIC RESPONSES TO NUTRIENTS

The overall response to nutrient ingestion involves an increase in splanchnic blood flow, to facilitate digestion and absorption; an eventual increase in limb and organ blood flow, to enable nutrient distribution; and an increase in whole-body thermogenesis. The thermogenic response reflects the metabolic cost of digestion, absorption, and use of nutrients, and it is of interest to determine whether this thermogenesis is linked in any way to the cardiovascular response.

Cardiac Output

It is well established that during aerobic exercise there is a direct relationship between the increases in whole-body oxygen consumption and cardiac output. This relationship is understandable given the need to deliver more oxygen to, and remove waste products from, the metabolically active tissues. Although one might intuitively feel that such a relationship would also be a part of the physiologic response to nutrient ingestion, it would appear from the literature that this is not so.

Brundin and Wahren (53) showed that oral intake of glucose increases whole-body oxygen uptake by 8.8% and cardiac output by 28%, whereas an isoenergetic amount of fructose had a similar effect on oxygen uptake but did not

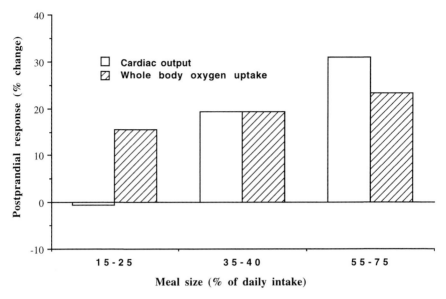

FIG. 8. Cardiac output and whole-body oxygen uptake responses to different size meals in healthy subjects. Adapted from Ref. 57.

increase cardiac output. Previously, Bagatell and Heymsfield (57) had studied the cardiac output and whole-body oxygen consumption responses to mixed nutrient solid food meals of different energy contents, ranging from 15% to 75% of daily energy requirements in a single meal. They found that although meals providing 15–25% of daily energy requirements had a substantial effect on oxygen uptake, there was no change in heart rate or cardiac output. By contrast, the medium-size and large meals had small, additional effects on oxygen uptake but much larger cardiac effects (Fig. 8). The results of Bagatell and Heymsfield (57) are somewhat surprising because others have found that meals containing 25% of daily energy requirements have significant effects on cardiac output, which may reflect the insensitivity of the earlier echocardiographic technique that they used. Thus, it would appear that in some circumstances there is no direct link between the cardiac and whole-body thermogenic responses to nutrient ingestion.

Splanchnic Blood Flow

There is no doubt that splanchnic blood flow increases after food ingestion, although Brundin and Wahren (53) observed no splanchnic hyperemia after oral fructose intake. It is also clear that most of this hyperemic response to food is likely to be related more to the requirements for digestive secretions and nutrient absorption rather than being directly linked to splanchnic thermogenesis. Cox et al. (15) observed that a mixed nutrient drink increased splanchnic blood flow and oxygen uptake by similar amounts, whereas Brundin and Wahren (58) found that a mixed meal increased splanchnic blood flow by 50% and oxygen uptake by 30%. Interestingly, a high-protein meal produced a similar increase in splanchnic oxygen uptake without any increase in blood flow (59).

The intestinal hyperemic response to nutrients appears to be directly related to the rate of nutrient administration, whereas the whole-body thermogenic response is only apparent after a minimum rate of nutrient delivery has been exceeded. This is the conclusion of a study we performed of the responses of healthy volunteers to feeding via a nasogastric tube. Administration of a standard enteral feeding mixture (4.2 kJ/ml) at rates from 100 to 300 ml/h produced a linear increase in SMA blood flow, but there was a significant thermogenic response only to the highest rate of feeding (9) (Fig. 9). We have recently extended this study and examined the cardiac output, SMA blood flow, and whole-body thermogenic response to either oral ingestion of 1.67 MJ of enteral feed or to nasogastric infusion of this amount over 2 hours (60). Oral feeding increased cardiac output by 25% and produced significant increases in SMA blood flow and whole-body thermogenesis. By contrast, the nasogastric feed had much smaller effects on cardiac output and SMA blood flow and did not stimulate thermogenesis (Fig. 10).

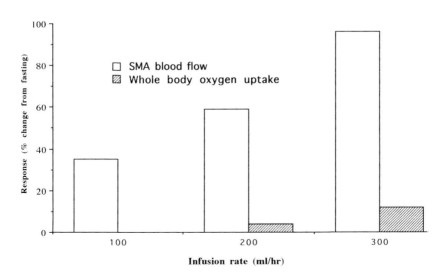

FIG. 9. SMA blood flow and whole-body oxygen uptake responses to nasogastric infusion of an enteral feed in healthy young subjects. Adapted from Ref. 9.

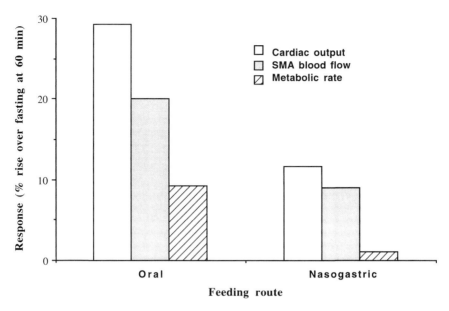

FIG. 10. Comparison of cardiac output, SMA blood flow, and metabolic rate responses to oral feeding or nasogastric infusion in healthy young subjects. Adapted from Ref. 60.

Other Regions

Cox et al. (15) showed that the small increase in renal oxygen consumption occurring after nutrient ingestion occurred despite a 10% decrease in blood flow. However, because renal blood flow is normally very high, fulfilling roles in cardiovascular and electrolyte homeostasis rather than simply meeting the metabolic demands of the kidneys, it is not surprising that a small increase in oxygen consumption can be achieved by simply increasing the oxygen extraction (i.e., the arteriovenous oxygen difference). On this basis, one would expect that tissues that normally have a high oxygen extraction in the fasting state (e.g., the heart and resting skeletal muscle) would require an increase in blood flow if their oxygen uptake increased after nutrient ingestion.

There have been no studies of muscle blood flow and oxygen consumption after solid food meals, but it would be particularly interesting to know whether the early and late postprandial phases showed different relationships between blood flow and oxygen uptake. With liquid meals there appears to be a qualitative relationship between increases in skeletal muscle blood flow and oxygen uptake, but further studies are needed with more reliable techniques. Similarly, there is little information concerning coronary blood flow and oxygen uptake responses to meals, but given the invasive nature of such studies, this is hardly surprising. Cox et al. (15) reported no increase in coronary blood flow or oxygen uptake after a mixed nutrient drink, which is not surprising because they also found no heart rate response to the meal.

CONCLUSION

An important aspect of the physiologic response to nutrient ingestion is whether the cardiovascular and metabolic (including thermogenic) components are integrated as part of an overall regulatory system. From the evidence presented above, it is apparent that although nutrient intake can produce substantial cardiovascular and thermogenic responses, there appears to be little direct relationship between the two. It seems probable that the cardiovascular response to nutrients is primarily organized to facilitate digestion, absorption, and distribution to the tissues while maintaining blood pressure and cerebral blood flow. The thermogenic response is principally a consequence of the use of nutrients by tissues for energy metabolism, synthesis, and storage. In many tissues, this thermogenic function can probably be achieved without substantial increases in blood flow, as well as oxygen delivery, simply by increasing oxygen extraction. The cardiovascular response to food can be substantial and in some clinical situations may disturb cardiovascular homeostasis, lowering blood pressure and organ/tissue blood flow. It is not known what effect such cardiovascular disturbances might have on the metabolic and thermogenic response to nutrients, but care should be taken when providing nutritional support to patients with abnormal cardiac or autonomic nervous system function. Little is known of the cardiovascular consequences of parenteral feeding, although in a preliminary study we showed substantial increases in SMA blood flow during infusion of a total parenteral nutrient mixture (9). Thus, further studies are needed to establish the extent to which the responses to enteral feeding described above also occur during parenteral feeding.

ACKNOWLEDGMENTS

Studies described from the authors' laboratory were supported by Project Grants from the Wellcome Trust. We thank Kirsty Hitt for her expert assistance in the preparation of this manuscript.

REFERENCES

1. Grollman A. Physiological variations in cardiac output in man III. Effect of the ingestion of food on the cardiac output, pulse rate, blood pressure and oxygen consumption of man. *Am J Physiol* 1929; 39:366–370.
2. Kearney MT, Cowley AJ, Macdonald IA. The cardiovascular responses to feeding in man. *Exp Physiol* 1995;80:683–700.
3. Qamar MI, Read AE, Skidmore R, Evans JM, Williamson JCN. Transcutaneous Doppler ultrasound measurement of coeliac axis blood flow in man. *Br J Surg* 1985;72:391–393.

4. Qamar MI, Read AC. Effects of ingestion of carbohydrate, fat, protein and water on the mesenteric blood flow in man. *Scand J Gastroenterol* 1988;23:26–30.
5. Waaler BA, Eriksen M. Post-prandial cardiovascular responses in man after ingestion of carbohydrate, protein or fat. *Acta Physiol Scand* 1992;146:321–327.
6. Sidery MB, Macdonald IA, Cowley AJ, Fullwood LF. Cardiovascular responses to high fat and high carbohydrate meals in young subjects. *Br J Nutr* 1991;261:H1430–1436.
7. Sidery MB, Macdonald IA, Blackshaw PE. Superior mesenteric artery blood flow and gastric emptying in humans and the differential effects of high fat and high carbohydrate meals. *Gut* 1994;35:186–190.
8. Waaler BA, Eriksen M, Toska K. The effect of meal size on postprandial increase in cardiac output. *Acta Physiol Scand* 1991;142:33–39.
9. Sidery MB, Allison SP, Macdonald IA. The acute cardiovascular and metabolic responses to enteral and parenteral nutrition. *Clin Nutr* 1994;13:51–52.
10. Mansell PI, Macdonald IA. The effect of underfeeding on the physiological responses to food ingestion in normal weight women. *Br J Nutr* 1988;60:39–48.
11. Sidery MB, Gallen IW, Macdonald IA. The initial physiological responses to glucose ingestion in normal subjects are modified by a 3d high-fat diet. *Br J Nutr* 1990;64:705–713.
12. Kelbaek H, Munck O, Christensen NJ, Godtfredsen J. Autonomic nervous control of postprandial haemodynamic changes at rest and upright exercise. *J Appl Physiol* 1987;63:1862–1865.
13. Hayano J, Sakakibara Y, Yamada M, et al. Diurnal variations in vagal and sympathetic cardiac control. *Am J Physiol* 1990;258:H642–H646.
14. Ryan SM, Goldberger AL, Ruthazer R, Mietus J, Lipsitz LA. Spectral analysis of heart rate dynamics in elderly persons with postprandial hypotension. *Am J Cardiol* 1992;69:201–205.
15. Cox HS, Kaye DM, Thompson JM, et al. Regional sympathetic nervous activation after a large meal in humans. *Clin Sci* 1995;89:145–154.
16. Kearney MT, Cowley AJ, Stubbs TA, Perry AJ, Macdonald IA. Central and peripheral haemodynamic responses to high carbohydrate and high fat meals in human cardiac transplant recipients. *Clin Sci* 1996;90:473–483.
17. Baron AD, Brechtel G. Insulin differentially regulates systemic and skeletal muscle vascular resistance. *Am J Physiol* 1993;265:E61–67.
18. Vatner SF, Patrick TA, Higgins CB, Franklin D. Regional circulatory adjustments to eating and digestion in conscious unrestrained primates. *J Appl Physiol* 1974;36:524–529.
19. Sieber C, Beglinger C, Jaeger K, Hildebrand P, Stalder GA. Regulation of postprandial mesenteric blood flow in humans: evidence for a cholinergic nervous reflex. *Gut* 1991;32:361–366.
20. Braatvedt GD, Flynn MD, Stanners A, Halliwell M, Corrall RJM. Splanchnic blood flow in man: evidence for mediation via a β-adrenergic mechanism. *Clin Sci* 1993;84:201–207.
21. Fara JW, Rubinstein EH, Sonnenschein RR. Intestinal hormones in mesenteric vasodilation after intraduodenal agents. *Am J Physiol* 1972;223:1058–1067.
22. Fara JW, Salazar AM. Gastric inhibitory polypeptide increases mesenteric blood flow. *Proc Soc Exp Biol Med* 1978;158:446–448.
23. Mitchell SJ, Bloom SR. Measurement of fasting and postprandial plasma VIP in man. *Gut* 1978;19: 1043–1048.
24. Gallen IW, Sidery MB, Turrett G, Macdonald IA. The effect of β-adrenoceptor blockade on the cardiovascular response to hyperinsulinaemia. *Diabetic Med* 1990;7(suppl 2):2A.
25. Kooner JS, Da Costa DF, Bannister R, Mathias CJ, Macdonald IA. Insulin induced hypotension in autonomic failure during euglycaemia. *J Physiol* 1987;382:36P.
26. Fagius J, Berne C. Increase in muscle nerve sympathetic activity in humans after food intake. *Clin Sci* 1994;86:159–167.
27. Anderson EA, Hoffman RP, Balon TW, Sinkey CA, Mark AL. Hyperinsulinaemia produces both sympathetic neural activation and vasodilation in normal humans. *J Clin Invest* 1991;87:2246–2252.
28. Kearney MT, Stubbs TA, Cowley AJ, Macdonald IA. Does insulin mediate the haemodynamic response to food ingestion? *J Physiol* 1995;489:42P.
29. Matsukawa K, Ninomiya I. Changes in renal sympathetic nerve activity, heart rate and arterial blood pressure associated with eating in cats. *J Physiol* 1987;390:229–242.
30. Mathias CJ, Bannister R. Post-cibal hypotension in autonomic disorders. In: Bannister R, Mathias CJ, eds. *Autonomic failure: a textbook of clinical disorders of the autonomic nervous system.* 3rd ed. Oxford, England: Oxford University Press; 1992:489–509.

31. Cowley AJ, Stainer K, Murphy DT, Murphy J, Hampton JR. A non-invasive method for measuring cardiac output:the effect of Christmas lunch. *Lancet* 1986;2:1422–1424.
32. Jarvis RC, Green JA, Nara AR, Pospisil R, Kasmer RJ. Effects of food ingestion on haemodynamics in chronic congestive heart failure. *Crit Care Med* 1988;16:491–494.
33. Cowley AJ, Fullwood LJ, Stainer K, Harrison E, Muller AF, Hampton JR. Post-prandial worsening of angina: all due to changes in cardiac output? *Br Heart J* 1991:66:147–150.
34. Muller AF, Hawkins M, Batin P, Evans S, Cowley AJ. Food in chronic heart failure: improvement in central haemodynamics but deleterious effects on exercise tolerance. *Eur Heart J* 1992;13: 1460–1467.
35. Kearney MT, Charlesworth A, Cowley AJ, Macdonald IA. William Hebesden revisited: Postprandial angina-intervals between food and exercise and meal composition are important determinants of time to onset of ischemia and maximal exercise tolerance. *J Am Coll Cardiol* 1997 (in press).
36. Lipsitz LA, Nyquist RP, Wei JY, Rowe JW. Postprandial reduction in blood pressure in the elderly. *N Engl J Med* 1983;309:81–83.
37. Potter JF, Heseltine D, Hartley G, Matthews J, Macdonald IA, James OFW. Effect of meal composition on the post-prandial blood pressure, catecholamine and insulin changes in elderly subjects. *Clin Sci* 1989;77:265–272.
38. Sidery MB, Cowley AF, Macdonald IA. Cardiovascular responses to a high-fat and a high-carbohydrate meal in healthy elderly subjects. *Clin Sci* 1993;84:263–270.
39. Tamburimi C, Poggesi L, Modesti PA. Postprandial cardiovascular response in non-institutionalised, normotensive elderly. *Cardiol Elderly* 1995;3:285–288.
40. Goldstein IB, Shapiro D, Hui KK. Cardiovascular effects of food in young and elderly adults. *J Psychophysiol* 1995;9:221–230.
41. Belko AZ, Barbieri TF. Effect of meal size and frequency on the thermic effect of food. *Nutr Res* 1987;7:237–242.
42. Tai MM, Cartillo P, Pi-Sunyer FX. Meal size and frequency: effect on the thermic effect of food. *Am J Clin Nutr* 1991;54:783–787.
43. Vaz M, Turner A, Kingwell B, et al. Postprandial sympatho-adrenal activity: its relation to metabolic and cardiovascular events and to changes in meal frequency. *Clin Sci* 1995;89:349–357.
44. Brondel I, LeBlanc J. Role of palatability on meal-induced thermogenesis in human subjects. *Am J Physiol* 1985;248:E333–336.
45. Robinson SM, York DA. Cigarette smoking and the thermic responses to isocaloric meals of varying composition and palatability. *Eur J Clin Nutr* 1988;42:551–559.
46. Swaminathan R, King RFGJ, Holmfield J, Siwek RA, Baker M, Wales JK. Thermic effect of feeding carbohydrate, fat, protein and mixed meal in lean and obese subjects. *Am J Clin Nutr* 1985;42: 177–181.
47. Kinabo JL, Durnin JVGA. Thermic effect of food in man: effect of meal composition and energy content. *Br J Nutr* 1990;64:37–44.
48. Scalfi L, Coltorti A, Contaldo F. Post-prandial thermogenesis in lean and obese subjects after meals supplemented with medium-chain and long-chain triglycerides. *Am J Clin Nutr* 1991;53:1130–1133.
49. Aksnes AK, Brundin T, Hjeltnes N, Wahren J. Metabolic, thermal and circulatory effects of intravenous infusion of amino acids in tetraplegic patients. *Clin Physiol* 1995;15:377–396.
50. Brundin T, Wahren J. Whole body and splanchnic oxygen consumption and blood flow after oral ingestion of fructose or glucose. *Am J Physiol* 1993;264:E504–513.
51. Mansell PI, Macdonald IA. Effect of starvation on insulin induced glucose disposal and thermogenesis in man. *Metabolism* 1990;39:502–510.
52. Nacht CA, Christin L, Temler E, Chiolero R, Jequier E, Acheson K. Thermic effect of food: possible implication of parasympathetic nervous system. *Am J Physiol* 1987;253:E481–488.
53. Deriaz O, Nacht CA, Chiolero R, Jequier E, Acheson KJ. The parasympathetic nervous system and the thermic effect of glucose/insulin infusions in humans. *Metabolism* 1989;38:1082–1088.
54. Schwartz RS, Jaeger LF, Veith RC. The thermic effect of feeding in older men: the importance of the sympathetic nervous system. *Metabolism* 1990;39:733–737.
55. Morgan JB, York DA, Wilkin TJ. Influence of propranolol on the acute thermic effect of feeding in man. *Ann Nutr Metab* 1986;30:386–392.
56. Aksnes AK, Brundin T, Hjeltnes N, Maehlum S, Wahren J. Meal-induced rise in resting energy expenditure in patients with complete cervical spinal cord lesions. *Paraplegia* 1993;31:462–472.
57. Bagatell CJ, Heymsfield SB. Effect of meal size on myocardial oxygen requirements: implications for post-myocardial infarction diet. *Am J Clin Nutr* 1984;39:421–426.

58. Brundin T, Wahren J. Influence of a mixed meal on splanchnic and interscapular energy expenditure in man. *Am J Physiol* 1991;260:E232–237.
59. Brundin T, Wahren J. Influence of protein ingestion on human splanchnic and whole-body oxygen consumption, blood flow and blood temperature. *Metabolism* 1994;43:626–632.
60. Stubbs TA, Macdonald IA. Cardiovascular and metabolic responses to nasogastric and oral feeding in healthy, young volunteers. *Proc Nutr Soc* 1997 (in press).

*Physiology, Stress, and Malnutrition: Functional
Correlates, Nutritional Intervention,*
edited by J.M. Kinney and H.N. Tucker.
Lippincott–Raven Publishers © 1997.

Glucose versus Amino Acids: Splanchnic and Total $\dot{V}O_2$ and Blood Flow

Tomas Brundin

*Department of Clinical Physiology, Karolinska Hospital,
S-171 76 Stockholm, Sweden*

BACKGROUND

The increase in resting oxidative metabolism that accompanies the administration of protein or carbohydrates (1), i.e. nutrient-induced thermogenesis (2), starts readily after a meal, reaches a maximum after 1–2 hours, and then declines over 2–5 hours. The so-called thermic effect of nutrients, defined as the increase in whole-body energy expenditure in percentage of the metabolizable energy content of the nutrient given, is 30–40% for protein or balanced amino acid mixtures, 6–9% for carbohydrates, and 0–2% for fat (3). Because of these proportions, the protein-induced thermogenesis dominates quantitatively the total thermogenic response to most mixed diets. Thus, in healthy, normal-weight adults, the thermogenic action exerted by a specific nutrient relates closely to its energy content, irrespective of the size of the individual receiving it.

Because the total nutrient-induced thermogenesis exceeds the calculated so called *obligatory* metabolic costs for absorption, processing, and storage of the nutrients, the term *facultative* thermogenesis (or "Luxuskonsumption") was originated by Neuman in 1902 (4).

The mechanisms whereby nutrient administration stimulates energy expenditure seem to vary between species. In several mammals, e.g. rodents, *facultative* thermogenesis was found to occur in interscapular brown adipose tissue in response to a nutrient-induced central activation of the sympathetic nervous system (for ref. see 5). When thermophotography studies showed a postprandial heat radiation from the interscapular region in adult humans (6,7), it was suggested that the observed heat radiation could emanate from an increased oxidative metabolism in underlying interscapular brown adipose tissue. However, histological studies failed to reveal brown fat in tissue specimen from such "hot" interscapular areas (8,9). Moreover, the venous blood drainage from the back thoracic wall, studied by catheterization of the azygos vein (10,11), showed no signs of increased regional oxygen uptake or heat production after a mixed meal or during intravenous (i.v.) infusion of noradrenaline (12). The mixed meal induced an increased azygos venous blood flow and a reduced venous heat drainage, indicating an increased postprandial heat dissipation from the back thoracic wall, which might well explain the increased heat radiation observed by thermophotography. The findings did not confirm the view that interscapular brown adipose tissue should be the site for the so-called facultative nutrient-induced thermogenesis in adult humans.

Role of the Sympathetic Nervous System

Our understanding of the mechanisms behind human nutrient-induced thermo-genesis seemed to progress when it was found that the ingestion of nutrients, at least carbohydrates, elicits a significant central activation of the sympatho-adrenal system, reflected by increased blood concentrations of catecholamines (13–16) and increased efferent impulse frequencies in peripheral sympathetic nerves (17,18). The well-known stimulatory action of increased sympatho-adrenal activity on muscle oxidative metabolism seemed an attractive and con-ceivable mechanism behind *facultative* nutrient-induced thermogenesis (19–20).

Blood catecholamine concentrations were found to increase significantly also in response to an i.v. bolus dose of glucose (21). However, a continuous i.v. glu-cose infusion did not measurably stimulate efferent sympathetic nervous activity (17). Other conflicting findings appeared. Protein meals, although markedly stim-ulating resting energy expenditure, failed to increase measurably the blood con-centration of catecholamines (15). In a later study, however, the efferent impulse frequency in peripheral sympathetic nerves showed a small but significant increase in response to meat meals (22). The quantitative importance of this small increase for the protein-induced thermogenesis may be questioned (cf. 15).

In attempts to assess quantitatively the sympatho-adrenal contribution to nutri-ent-induced thermogenesis in humans, β-adrenergic receptor inhibition has been used in numerous studies. The results are contradictory. Some demonstrate that propranolol reduces significantly the thermogenic response to oral or i.v. admin-istration of glucose-containing nutrient mixtures (20,23). Others fail to confirm any contribution (24–27). Consistent results were obtained concerning pure glucose meals, the thermic effect of which was not reduced by propranolol (28,29). On the other hand, propranolol reduces significantly the pulmonary oxy-gen uptake during hyperinsulinemic clamp (30–32). Several studies have shown that a hyperinsulinemic clamp increases considerably both the blood concentra-tions of catecholamines (33,34) and the efferent impulse frequency in peripheral sympathetic nerves (34,35). It was even proposed that the blood concentration of insulin should constitute the adequate stimulus whereby nutrients activate the sympatho-adrenal system (17,33). However, because propranolol failed to reduce the thermic effect recorded during endogenous release of considerable amounts of insulin in response to glucose meals of 100–250 g (28,29), the physiological significance of the findings from the hyperinsulinemic clamp studies may be disputed. It is generally agreed that the hyperinsulinemic clamp technique, although an elegant and useful pharmacological model, represents a completely unphysiological situation.

Taken together, literature hitherto gives no conclusive support for the hypothesis that sympatho-adrenal activation plays a quantitatively important role for the nutrient-induced thermogenesis in humans under physiologic conditions. Moreover, a principal question may be raised against the hypothesis. If a substantial part of the nutrient-induced thermogenesis were mediated via sympatho-adrenal stimulation of muscular oxidative metabolism (19–20), then the thermic effect would be expected to vary in proportion to the individual muscle mass. We found no reports supporting this assertion. In contrast, a number of studies of normal weight individuals demonstrate a remarkably consistent magnitude of the thermic effect, irrespective of the individual size of the subjects studied. However, sympatho-adrenal activity may contribute to the splanchnic circulatory response to oral glucose ingestion.

WHOLE-BODY AND REGIONAL SPLANCHNIC STUDIES

Methodology

Obviously, findings from whole-body studies or from separate regional studies have not clarified successfully the mechanisms behind human nutrient-induced thermogenesis. In a different approach, we have measured simultaneously both whole-body and regional splanchnic metabolic, circulatory, and thermal effects of nutrient administration in healthy subjects and patients. The methods required, indirect calorimetry and catheterization techniques, have been in continuous use in our laboratory for 30 years. A computerized device for blood thermometry was developed in 1985 (10,36).

Procedures

Studies of thermogenesis require a well-defined basal state. Our healthy volunteers report to the laboratory in the morning after an overnight fast (12–14 hours). The patients were hospitalized before the day of study. Invasive techniques are necessary for reliable determinations of cardiac output and splanchnic blood flow. Therefore, a right-sided hepatic vein, the pulmonary and a systemic artery have to be catheterized. After the catheterization procedure, the duration of which seldom exceeds 10 minutes, blood is drawn for zero point analysis of indocyanine dye (Cardio-Green, Hynson, Westcott & Dunning Products, Becton Dickinson & Co, Cockeysville, MD), which is then infused at a constant rate into the right atrium via the side hole of the pulmonary artery catheter. The infusion continues for 45–60 minutes in order to achieve steady-state plasma concentrations before the baseline blood samples are drawn. The period of indocyanine infusion serves as a recovery period after catheterization.

The baseline measurements (pulmonary gas exchange for periods of 7–9 minutes and simultaneous blood sampling from the catheters) are performed twice, with a 10-min interval. After that, the nutrient to be studied is administered and the measurements are repeated at timed intervals. If the baseline energy expenditure exceeds the individually predicted basal value (37) by more than 7% or heart rate is >80/min, the study is discarded.

Analytical Methods

After several years with Douglas bags and computerized open-circuit calorimetry and ventilated hood technique, we now measure respiratory gas exchange by means of a continuous breath-by-breath analysis (MEDGRAPH-ICS, System CPX/D, Medical Graphics Corp., St Paul, MN) using a nose-clip and mouth-piece technique with which the subject has previously been made familiar. The coefficient of variation for a single determination of the pulmonary oxygen uptake is <2%. For determination of arterio-pulmonary arterial and arterio-hepatic venous oxygen differences, the blood oxygen content is analyzed oximetrically (OSM 3 HEMOXIMETER, Radiometer, Copenhagen, Denmark). Blood glucose concentrations are analyzed using a glucose dehydrogenase technique (38).

The splanchnic blood flow is estimated from duplicate blood sampling using the classical continuous indocyanine infusion method (39,40). Using a high-performance liquid chromatography technique for the analysis of plasma concentrations of indocyanine (41), the coefficient of variation for a single determination of the splanchnic plasma flow is 0.8–1.2%. The blood temperatures are recorded continuously from thermistor-equipped catheters at a sampling frequency of 1 Hz, as described elsewhere (10,36). The blood thermometer allows the detection of small temperature variations, the absolute measuring accuracy being $\pm 0.001°C$ and the sensitivity $0.0003°C$.

Calculations

Cardiac output, regional splanchnic oxygen uptake, and extra-splanchnic arterio-venous oxygen difference are calculated according to the Fick principle (42). The average values obtained at -10 and 0 minutes are used as basal when calculating changes from the basal state. The values for oxygen uptake and blood flow in extra-splanchnic tissues are calculated from the individual differences between whole-body and splanchnic oxygen uptake and blood flow, respectively. The whole-body accumulation of heat is calculated from individual body weights and increments in mixed venous blood temperature, using the traditional normal value for whole-body specific heat, 3.474 kJ/°C/kg (43).

Ethics

All subjects are informed of the nature, purpose, and possible risks of the study before giving their voluntary consent to participate. The study protocol has to be reviewed and approved by the institutional ethics committee. Most of our invasive studies are limited to 4 hours after the catheterization procedure. During the period allowed we cover the onset, increase, and maximum of nutrient-induced thermogenesis. The later phase of decline cannot be included in our invasive studies.

RESULTS AND COMMENTS

General

It was found that the various nutrients stimulate differently the oxygen uptake, blood flow, and heat accumulation in healthy male subjects (Figs. 1–3). After protein meals or during i.v. infusion of amino acid mixtures, the increase in oxygen consumption was distributed almost equally between the splanchnic and extrasplanchnic parts of the body (44,45). In contrast, orally ingested carbohydrates

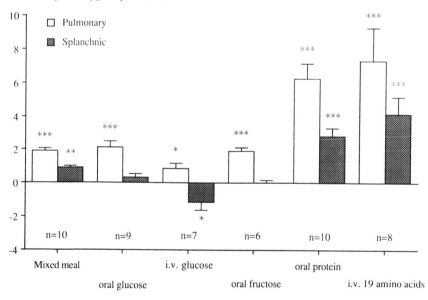

FIG 1. Two-hour changes in pulmonary and splanchnic oxygen uptake in healthy male subjects in response to a mixed meal (3,000 kJ), oral glucose (1,200 kJ), i.v. glucose (1,200 kJ), oral fructose (1,200 kJ), a fish protein meal (900 kJ), and i.v. infusion of a mixture of 19 amino acids (480 kJ). Values are means ±SEM. Asterisks indicate significant difference from the basal state: *p < 0.05, **p < 0.01, ***p < 0.001.

2 h change in cardiac output and splanchnic blood flow, ml/kJ of nutrient administered

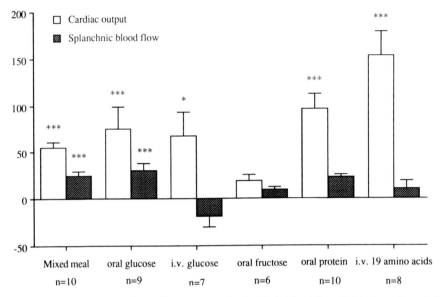

FIG. 2. Two-hour changes in cardiac output and splanchnic blood flow. Nutrients and symbols as in Fig. 1.

2 h change in whole body heat content, J/kJ of nutrient administered

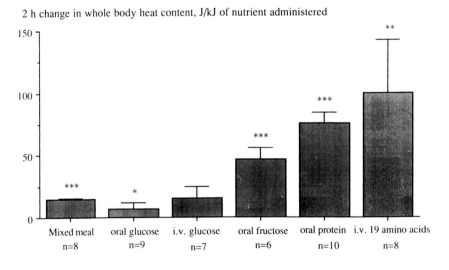

FIG. 3. Two-hour changes in whole-body heat content. Nutrients and symbols as in Fig. 1.

(glucose or fructose) exerted their oxidative stimulation primarily in the extra-splanchnic tissues (46,47). During i.v. glucose infusion, the pulmonary oxygen uptake showed a small but significant increase, whereas the splanchnic oxygen uptake decreased. After a mixed meal (55% glucose + 17% protein + 28% fat) the splanchnic tissues accounted for 40–45% of the whole-body thermogenic response (11,48). Thus, only protein-containing meals were able to stimulate significantly the 2-hour postprandial splanchnic oxygen uptake (Fig. 1). In tetraplegic patients (49–52), the 2-hour thermic effects of a mixed meal, a glucose meal, or an i.v. infused amino acid mixture did not differ significantly from those in healthy controls (Fig. 4.). The splanchnic proportions of the whole-body increase in oxygen consumption were in the tetraplegic patients similar to those in healthy controls. In patients with tetraplegia due to complete cervical spinal cord lesions, the peripheral sympathetic nervous system shows low activity (53,54) and is not accessible for stimulatory impulses from the brain. The findings render little support to the hypothesis that central stimulation of efferent sympatho-adrenal activity is necessary for thermogenic responses of normal magnitude in humans.

Cardiac output is known to increase after meals (55–58). We found it significantly stimulated in healthy subjects (Fig. 2) by mixed meals, oral or i.v. glucose, oral protein, or i.v. amino acid mixtures, but not by oral fructose (11,44,48,59). As described earlier (56), the increase in cardiac output was more prompt and marked after carbohydrates than after protein.

Splanchnic blood flow was not significantly stimulated by oral fructose, oral protein, or i.v. infused glucose or amino acid mixtures in healthy subjects

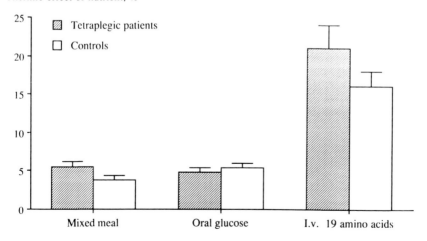

Thermic effect of nutrient, %

FIG. 4. Two-hour thermic effects of a mixed meal (40% of basal 24-h energy requirement, glucose 52% + protein 11% + fat 37%, n = 6/6), 75 g of oral glucose (n = 9/6), and of a 2-h i.v. infusion of a mixture of 19 amino acids (480 kJ, n = 8/8) in tetraplegic male patients and in healthy men. Values are means ±SEM.

(44–47,60). The substantial increase in splanchnic blood flow that accompanies a glucose-containing meal may be of physiological importance because it possibly facilitates the intestinal absorption of nutrients in general. To our knowledge this effect of glucose has not yet been subjected to systematic studies. In tetraplegic patients, oral glucose caused no significant increase in splanchnic blood flow (49,51).

In healthy subjects the blood flow in extra-splanchnic tissues increased significantly in response to glucose, mixed meals, oral protein, and i.v. amino acid mixtures, but not to oral fructose (11,44–48). The postprandial increase in mixed blood temperature, representing the accumulation of heat in the body, differed greatly between the various nutrients studied. Protein or amino acids induced the most marked heat accumulation, whereas i.v. glucose did not increase the blood temperature significantly (Fig. 3).

The marked nutrient-specific differences in metabolic and circulatory stimulation may suggest that the mechanisms behind their stimulatory actions are also nutrient specific.

Glucose

Pulmonary Oxygen Uptake

After oral ingestion of glucose (or fructose), the pulmonary oxygen uptake increases immediately, reaching a maximum after 1–2 hours, and then declines

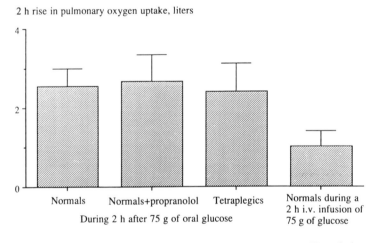

FIG. 5. Two-hour increase in pulmonary oxygen uptake in response to 75 g of glucose: orally ingested in nine normal men, in nine normal men under propranolol (0.2 mg/kg body weight), in six male tetraplegic patients, and during i.v. infusion of 75 g of glucose in seven normal men. Values are means ± SEM.

(46,61). In a recent study (62), we failed to reduce the 2-hour thermic effect of 75 g of oral glucose by propranolol (Fig. 5), thus confirming the findings from earlier studies of pure glucose meals (28,29). When infused i.v., glucose was recently found to exert very low whole-body thermogenesis (Fig. 5). Thus, during a 2-hour i.v. infusion of 75 g of glucose, the increase in pulmonary oxygen uptake was <40% of that measured during 2 hours after 75 g of oral glucose (60). The classical interpretation of this finding would be that the difference represents the so-called *obligatory* metabolic costs for the splanchnic absorption and processing of glucose. As explained below, it is more complicated. In tetraplegic patients, oral glucose stimulated normally the pulmonary oxygen uptake (Fig. 5), although their low arterial plasma concentrations of catecholamines were unaffected (49,51).

Splanchnic Oxygen Consumption

The splanchnic oxygen uptake increases modestly (or tends to increase) during the first 30 minutes after oral ingestion of 75 g of glucose (46,47,60,62). However, the initial increase is transient, and the average 2-hour postprandial splanchnic oxygen uptake is not significantly higher than that in the basal state (Fig. 6).

The absence of a significant net 2-hour increase in splanchnic oxygen uptake after oral glucose may seem controversial. It is well known that glucose

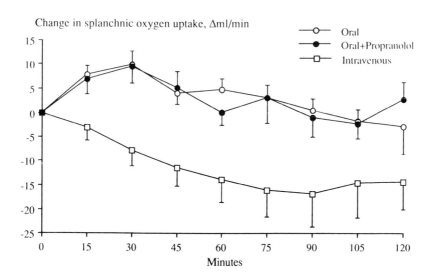

FIG. 6. Changes in splanchnic oxygen uptake in healthy male subjects in response to 75 g of glucose, orally ingested (n = 9), i.v. infused (n = 7), and orally ingested under propranolol, 0.2 mg/kg (n = 9). Values are means ± SEM.

ingestion automatically generates considerable metabolic costs for intestinal absorption [1 mole of adenosine triphosphate (ATP)/mole of glucose absorbed] and for hepatic glycogen formation (2 moles ATP/mole glucose) (63). The findings indicate that the absorption costs were counterbalanced by a simultaneous reduction of other energy-consuming splanchnic processes. The findings from the i.v. glucose study may illustrate this phenomenon. The i.v. administration of glucose was found to reduce significantly the splanchnic oxygen consumption to a level approximately 25% below that in the basal state (Figs. 1 and 6). The reduction in splanchnic oxygen uptake could fully explain why the 2-hour increase in pulmonary oxygen uptake was significantly lower during i.v. than after oral glucose. Our data give no direct information on which of the basal, energy-consuming splanchnic processes was inhibited by glucose administration. However, hepatic gluconeogenesis, recently found to account for approximately half of the total hepatic release of glucose in the basal state (64,65), is known to be a markedly energy-consuming process (for ref. see 63). If the basal gluconeogenesis were completely inhibited, which may be questioned, such an inhibition could largely explain the reduction in splanchnic oxygen consumption observed during the 2-hour i.v. glucose infusion. Irrespective of the mechanism behind the observed reduction in splanchnic oxygen uptake during i.v. glucose infusion, the present findings clearly indicate that the low whole-body thermogenesis reflects the bidirectional metabolic response to glucose infusion. It represents the net result of a reduction in splanchnic uptake and a simultaneous increase in extra-splanchnic oxygen consumption.

After oral glucose ingestion, the metabolic costs for intestinal glucose absorption are most likely offset by a simultaneous reduction of other energy-consuming splanchnic processes, probably in the liver. The early-onset, small increase in splanchnic oxygen uptake, differing from the prompt decrease in splanchnic oxygen uptake observed during i.v. infusion, may reflect the early, not yet counterbalanced metabolic costs for intestinal absorption (Fig. 6). As suggested in the case of i.v. glucose infusion, a reduction (or inhibition) of hepatic gluconeogenesis might well occur after the oral glucose load, thus in part offsetting the metabolic costs for intestinal glucose absorption.

Because the proportion of orally ingested glucose that was absorbed during the postprandial observation period is unknown, the obligatory costs for absorption cannot be calculated accurately. It is therefore unknown if oral glucose reduces the basal oxidative splanchnic (hepatic) metabolism to the same extent as i.v. glucose did. Irrespective of the exact values, the findings show that 75 g of glucose, ingested in the fasting state, cause no significant net 2-hour increase of the splanchnic oxidative metabolism. The results confirm our earlier finding that the net 2-hour thermogenesis in healthy subjects after 75 g of oral glucose (or fructose) occurs in the extra-splanchnic tissues only (46). Likewise, in the tetraplegic patients the splanchnic oxygen uptake was unchanged after 75 g of oral glucose (51).

Extra-Splanchnic Oxygen Consumption

Whether ingested orally or infused i.v., glucose stimulated to a similar extent the extra-splanchnic oxygen uptake in healthy subjects, although the extra-splanchnic disposal of glucose was greater in the i.v. than in the oral group (60). Thus, during the 2-hour i.v. infusion of 75 g of glucose, approximately 58 g were disposed in the extra-splanchnic tissues. For 2 hours after the administration of 75 g of oral glucose, approximately 40 g of the glucose released postprandially via the hepatic veins were disposed in the extra-splanchnic tissues. Although the 2-hour extra-splanchnic glucose uptake was 45% greater during i.v. infusion than after oral ingestion, the simultaneous increase in extra-splanchnic oxygen consumption was only 21% higher (not significant) in the i.v. group than in the oral group (Fig. 7).

In both the oral and i.v. group, the increase in extra-splanchnic oxygen consumption exceeded considerably that necessary to cover the calculated metabolic costs for extra-splanchnic glucose disposal. Thus, the increase in extra-splanchnic oxygen consumption probably included the so-called *facultative* thermogenesis. If this should be secondary to an increased sympatho-adrenal stimulation, one would expect it to be reduced in patients with tetraplegia. However, in such patients the 2-hour stimulation of the extra-splanchnic oxygen uptake after 75 g of oral glucose did not differ from that

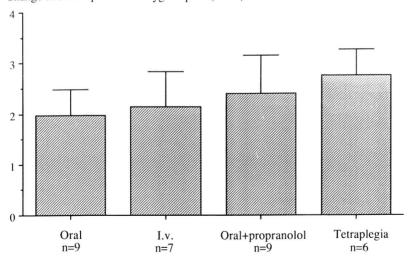

FIG. 7. Two-hour increase in extra-splanchnic oxygen uptake in response to 75 g of glucose: orally ingested, i.v. infused, orally ingested under propranolol in healthy male subjects, and orally ingested in tetraplegic male patients. Values are means ± SEM.

occurring in the control group of healthy individuals (49,51). Propranolol did not reduce the increase in extra-splanchnic oxygen uptake after 75 g of oral glucose in normal individuals (62).

The findings do not support the view that sympatho-adrenal activity contributes importantly to the so-called *facultative* part of the glucose-induced thermogenesis in humans.

Cardiac Output

Cardiac output was stimulated by oral or i.v. glucose, not by oral fructose (46–48,62) (Fig. 2). Propranolol reduced significantly the basal level of cardiac output but did not reduce its increase for 2 hours after the administration of 75 g of oral glucose (62). In tetraplegic patients cardiac output showed a nonsignificant tendency to increase after oral glucose (49,51).

Splanchnic Blood Flow

In healthy subjects, splanchnic blood flow increased promptly in response to oral ingestion of glucose or glucose-containing meals (11,46–48,62) (Fig. 8). As

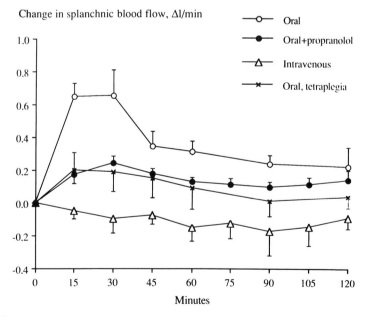

FIG. 8. Changes in splanchnic blood flow in healthy male subjects in response to 75 g of glucose: orally ingested (n = 9), orally ingested under propranolol (0.2 mg/kg body weight, n = 9), i.v. infused (n = 7), and orally ingested in six tetraplegic patients. Values are means ± SEM.

shown earlier (66), i.v. glucose failed to stimulate splanchnic blood flow (60). In patients with tetraplegia, 75 g of oral glucose failed to stimulate splanchnic blood flow (49,51). In addition, we recently found that propranolol reduces largely both the basal splanchnic blood flow and its increase after oral glucose in healthy volunteers (62). The findings indicate that efferent sympathetic activity is necessary for the normal mechanism whereby oral glucose stimulates splanchnic blood flow. However, oral fructose or i.v. glucose infusions, both known to stimulate significantly the sympatho-adrenal system (67,68) did not stimulate splanchnic blood flow in normal individuals (46). Thus, besides an increased sympathetic nervous activity, a permissive action, possibly exerted by intestinal hormones, seems to be needed for the glucose-induced stimulation of splanchnic blood flow.

Extra-Splanchnic Blood Flow

The blood flow in extra-splanchnic tissues increased significantly in response to oral or i.v. infused glucose (46,47,60) (Fig. 9). The increase after oral glucose was not reduced by propranolol (62) and was not subnormal in tetraplegic patients (49,51). Thus, sympatho-adrenal activity seems not to be involved in the mechanisms behind the glucose-induced increase in

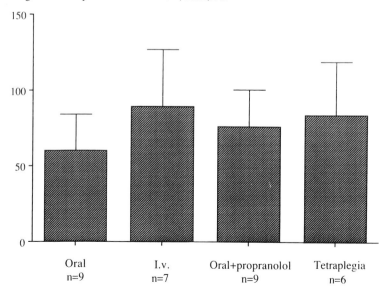

FIG. 9. Two-hour increase in extra-splanchnic blood flow in response to 75 g of glucose. Nutrients, patients, and symbols as in Fig. 8.

extra-splanchnic blood flow. Probably the extra-splanchnic vasodilation response to glucose is mediated by insulin-induced release of endothelial nitric oxide (69,70). In addition, we found that i.v. infusion of large amounts of glucose (0.6 g/min) causes significant hemodilution. The ensuing plasma volume expansion significantly increases heart stroke volume and cardiac output, probably by improving right ventricular filling (60). Spraul et al. (71) recently demonstrated a lack of temporal relationship between insulin-induced skeletal muscle vasodilation and efferent activity in peripheral sympathetic muscle nerves.

Thermal Effects

Oral or i.v. glucose administration exerts no significant thermal effects in normal individuals (50,52) (Fig. 3). The almost unaffected mixed venous blood temperature indicates that increased heat dissipation compensates for the extra postprandial heat production. In tetraplegic patients, however, oral glucose induced a considerable increase in the mixed blood temperature (Fig. 10) (49,51). The abnormal hyperthermic reaction illustrates the defective thermoregulatory control in the state of tetraplegia. In such patients the remaining internal temperature sense is confined to the spinal thermosensors only

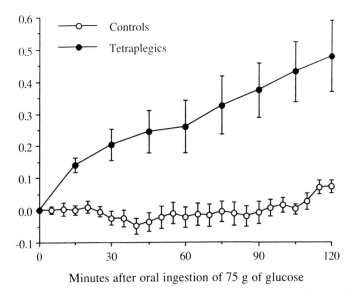

FIG. 10. Changes in mixed blood temperature in six healthy men and in six tetraplegic male patients after oral ingestion of 75 g of glucose. Values are means ± SEM.

because the efferent signals from the hypothalamic thermosensors are blocked by the spinal cord injury (72).

Protein and Amino Acids

Pulmonary Oxygen Uptake

It has been shown (1–3,15,44,45,56,59,61,73) that, compared with carbohydrates, protein or amino acid mixtures cause a more marked and long-lasting stimulation of whole-body oxygen consumption (Fig. 1). We found a thermic effect of $13 \pm 3\%$ during 2 hours after a fish meal (900 kJ of protein), and $16 \pm 1\%$ during 2.5 hours of i.v. infusion of a mixture of 19 amino acids (600 kJ); (VAMIN, 18 g N/l, Pharmacia Hospital Care, Stockholm, Sweden). Thus, unlike glucose, protein or amino acids exerted similar thermic effects whether ingested orally or infused i.v. In tetraplegic patients, the thermic effect of the i.v. amino acid mixture tended to be higher, $21 \pm 3\%$ (Fig. 4), but the difference from the healthy controls was not statistically significant (49,52). The increase in pulmonary oxygen uptake proceeds gradually, showing no tendency to level off during 3 hours of i.v. infusion of 4 kJ/min of a balanced amino acid mixture (59). When the infusion ceases, the oxygen uptake declines slowly, still being considerably elevated above the basal level 2 hours after the infusion (74).

Splanchnic Oxygen Consumption

During 2 hours after a protein (fish) meal, the splanchnic organs accounted for $43 \pm 8\%$ of the increase in whole-body oxygen consumption (Fig. 1) (44), the splanchnic proportion of the whole-body thermogenesis being similar to that observed after a mixed meal (cf.11,48,75). During 2.5 hours of i.v. infusion of the amino acid mixture, the corresponding value was $51 \pm 8\%$, statistically not significantly different from that after the fish meal (45). In the tetraplegic patients, the splanchnic proportion of whole-body thermogenesis during i.v. infusion of the amino acid mixture was similar to that in normal individuals (52).

A protein meal, the only nutrient able to significantly stimulate splanchnic oxidative metabolism, seems not to cause measurable costs for intestinal absorption. Neither its whole-body thermic effect nor its stimulation of splanchnic oxygen uptake differed significantly from those observed during i.v. infusion of amino acid mixtures. Thus, the considerable increase in splanchnic oxidative metabolism that accompanies a protein meal probably represents the metabolic costs for hepatic processing of amino acids (compare with Fig. 1). The protein- or amino acid–induced increase in splanchnic oxygen uptake tended to level off after 60–120 minutes (Fig. 11). This finding may possibly reflect a maximum capacity for hepatic processing of amino acids.

Change in oxygen uptake, Δml/min

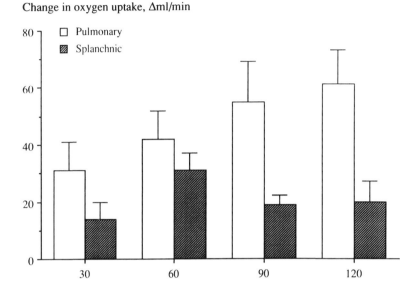

Minutes after a fish meal, 900 kJ

FIG. 11. Changes in pulmonary and splanchnic oxygen uptake in 10 healthy subjects after oral ingestion of a fish meal. Values are means ± SEM.

Extra-Splanchnic Oxygen Uptake

After the fish meal or during i.v. infusion of the amino acid mixture, the extra-splanchnic oxygen uptake increased gradually, showing no tendency to level off during the study period (44,45). It is not known in which organs or tissues the extra-splanchnic half of protein- or amino acid-induced thermogenesis takes place. It seems conceivable that these tissues should be capable of substantial variations in oxygen consumption. Such tissues are the skeletal muscles, kidneys, heart, or brain. In dogs, the oxygen uptake in isolated hindlimb muscles was shown to increase in response to glycine infusions (76). However, in humans no significant increase in leg oxygen uptake was found during 3 hours after a protein meal (77). The kidneys were found not to contribute measurably to whole-body thermogenesis during i.v. infusion of an amino acid mixture (59). The modest increase in cardiac output that accompanies protein meals or amino acid infusions (44,45) may indicate that the heart could, to a limited extent, contribute to the increased oxidative metabolism. Because the respiratory exchange ratio does not increase in healthy individuals after protein meals (44) or during amino acid infusions (45,59), the brain, mainly oxidizing carbohydrates, would hardly be suspected of an important contribution.

It is not known by which processes, or signals, protein or amino acid mixtures stimulate the extra-splanchnic oxidative metabolism. The finding of an amino acid-induced thermic effect, augmented rather than reduced in tetraplegic patients, does not favour the view that central activation of the peripheral nervous system should constitute a necessary step in the mechanisms behind amino acid-induced thermogenesis. Possibly the stimulation occurs directly in the peripheral cells in response to elevated extracellular amino acid concentrations or via a second messenger system. If so, inhibiting thermoregulatory signals, keeping the peripheral cellular oxidation within acceptable limits, would be needed for prevention of hyperthermia. Such efferent signals from the central thermosensors, as shown in animals, are able to suppress the metabolic rate when the arterial blood temperature exceeds the ambient set point (78,79). Indirectly, a similar mechanism was demonstrated in humans, in whom the meal-induced thermogenesis decreased when the normal heat dissipation across the abdominal wall was prevented by thermal insulation (48). If thermoregulatory processes can affect the magnitude of the amino acid-induced thermogenesis in humans by inhibitory signals, then supranormal thermic effects would be expected if the central thermosensors are partly or totally silenced.

Cardiac Output

Cardiac output is known to increase after meals (55–58). We found it moderately stimulated by 0.8–1.2 L/min after a fish meal (44) and during i.v. infusion of the amino acid mixture (45,59). The whole-body arterio-venous oxygen difference did not change from its basal level, i.e.. the systemic circulation remained normokinetic. In tetraplegic patients, cardiac output increased normally during i.v. amino acid infusion (49,52).

Splanchnic Blood Flow

As demonstrated earlier, splanchnic blood flow is unaffected by a meat meal (77). The entire increase in splanchnic oxygen uptake that occurs is fully explained by an increased oxygen extraction from the splanchnic blood (77). We found the same in response to a fish meal and to i.v. infusion of an amino acid mixture (44,45). Thus, the splanchnic circulation became markedly hypokinetic after a protein meal or during i.v. amino acid infusion.

Extra-Splanchnic Blood Flow

In the extra-splanchnic tissues the blood flow increased moderately after a fish meal and during i.v. infusion of an amino acid mixture (44,45). We have no information on whether the increase in blood flow is equally distributed over the extra-splanchnic tissues.

Thermal Effects

Unlike glucose, protein or amino acid mixtures increase the body temperature when administered (compare with Fig. 3). Thus, the pulmonary arterial blood

Change in arterial temperature, Δ°C

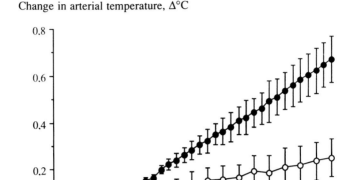

Minutes of i.v. infusion of amino acids, 240 kJ/h

FIG. 12. Changes in blood temperature in five male tetraplegic patients ● and in eight healthy men ○ during i.v. infusion of a mixture of 19 amino acids, 240 kJ/min. Values are means ± SEM.

temperature increased by 0.25–0.3°C during 2 hours after a fish meal or during an amino acid infusion (44,45,59). Also after a mixed, protein-containing meal, the mixed blood temperature increased by approximately 0.2°C (11,48). The increased accumulation of heat, not counter-regulated by the central thermosensors, indicates that protein or amino acids can adjust upward the central nervous temperature set point (80). In tetraplegic patients (52), amino acid infusion caused a supranormal increase in blood temperature, almost three times that seen in healthy individuals (Fig. 12). The 2.5-hour thermic effect of i.v. amino acids was 21 ± 3% in the tetraplegic patients and 16 ± 2% in normals (compare with Fig. 4). The difference did not attain statistical significance.

General Anesthesia

In patients subjected to premedication (lorazepam) and anesthesia (isoflurane) for abdominal surgery, infusions of an amino acid mixture exerted a remarkably augmented thermic effect (81). Thus, the thermic effect of such infusions, 4 kJ/min, was fivefold greater than that observed in unanesthetized individuals (45,59). The effect was most marked at emergence from anesthesia when the pulmonary oxygen uptake increased to 71 ± 21% above the preanesthesia levels (Fig. 13). Moreover, it was found that the amino acid mixture, when infused after premedication but before the onset of isoflurane anesthesia, exerted a similarly

Change in pulmonary oxygen uptake, Δml/min

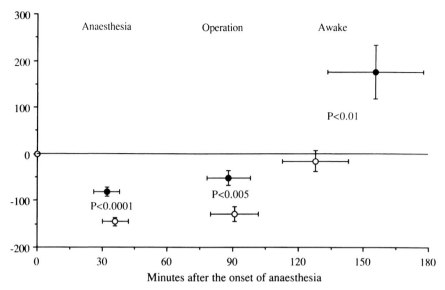

FIG. 13. Changes in pulmonary oxygen uptake during anesthesia, operation, and awakening in 11 control patients (○) and in 10 patients (●) receiving an i.v. infusion of an amino acid mixture (4 kJ/min), started at the onset of anesthesia. Vertical bars indicate SEM of mean changes. Horizontal bars indicate SEM of time after the onset of anesthesia.

Blood temperature changes, Δ°C

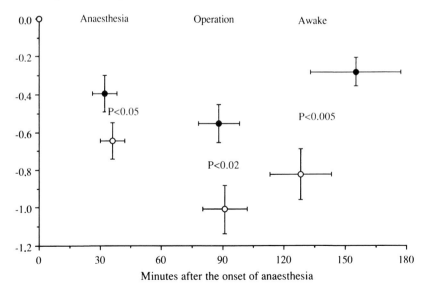

FIG. 14. Changes in blood temperature during anesthesia, operation, and awakening. Patients and symbols as in Fig. 13.

augmented thermic effect that reached a delayed maximum at emergence from anesthesia (74). The augmented thermic effect of amino acids was found to occur almost exclusively in the extra-splanchnic tissues (82). The heat accumulation induced by preoperative or intraoperative amino acid infusions was found to effectively prevent postoperative hypothermia (Fig. 14). The mechanism whereby the amino acid–induced thermogenesis is enhanced under general anesthesia is hitherto unknown.

HYPOTHESIS

The nature of so-called *facultative* thermogenesis, induced by carbohydrate administration, has been debated. Even the existence of a "Luxuskonsumption" has been questioned (for ref. see 83). The present findings fail to confirm the view that efferent central nervous stimulation should be involved in the mechanisms behind carbohydrate-induced thermogenesis. It seems remarkable that the increased central activation of the sympatho-adrenal system, which undoubtedly follows upon carbohydrate administration, fails to exert consistently measurable effects on whole-body oxygen uptake. According to the view proposed by Newsholme and others, the entire thermogenesis might be explained by the metabolic costs associated with the absorption, processing, and storage of the nutrients administered. When including the costs for the mechanisms necessary for the control of nutrient processing (83), there may be no room for *facultative* thermogenesis.

Considering a possible involvement of central thermoregulation, suggested above, the following findings may be listed:

1. The thermic effect of amino acids was augmented rather than reduced in tetraplegic patients in whom central thermoregulation is incomplete (72).
2. Hyperthermia accompanied both a glucose meal and i.v. infusions of amino acids in tetraplegic patients.
3. The extra-splanchnic thermic effect of amino acids was considerably supranormal in anesthetized patients in whom central thermoregulation is completely silenced (84).
4. The amino acid-induced heat accumulation exceeded considerably that observed in the unanesthetized state.

These findings suggest that the central thermosensors, partly blocked in tetraplegia and totally silenced under anesthesia, normally exert an inhibitory action on the amino acid-induced peripheral heat generation. In addition, it seems likely that the extra-splanchnic energy expenditure for processing of amino acids starts directly in the peripheral tissues, possibly in response to increased extracellular concentrations of amino acids. If so, the peripheral heat generation would, if uncontrolled, accelerate and cause hyperthermia. Postprandial hyperthermia occurred in the tetraplegic patients. During anesthesia, no net hyperthermia was apparent because the heat generation was offset by the pharmacological suppression exerted by the anesthetic agent on the whole-body metabolic rate.

The findings and considerations led to the hypothesis that the central nervous system does not contribute to nutrient-induced thermogenesis by a stimulatory action. In contrast, its main role seems to be inhibitory in character.

SUMMARY AND CONCLUSIONS

The present findings do not support the classical hypothesis on the mechanisms behind nutrient-induced thermogenesis. It seems difficult to believe that the increase in oxidative metabolism that accompanies nutrient administration results from efferent stimulation from the central nervous system. In particular, the findings in tetraplegic patients, and those in normal individuals under ß-adrenergic receptor inhibition, contradict that the sympathetic nervous system, necessary for oxidative heat generation in response to cooling, plays a quantitatively important role for nutrient-induced thermogenesis. However, sympathoadrenal activation seems to participate in the mechanisms whereby orally ingested glucose stimulates the splanchnic blood flow.

The extra-splanchnic half of the increased heat production in response to the administration of protein or amino acids occurs in hitherto unidentified tissues. There are no reasons to believe that this extra heat production results from central nervous stimulation. In contrast, the findings from individuals under anesthesia suggest that the amino acid–induced heat generation accelerates when the normal central nervous inhibitory control is silenced by anesthesia. Consequently, the major role of the central nervous system for the nutrient-induced thermogenesis seems to be inhibitory in character, not stimulatory.

ACKNOWLEDGMENTS

These studies were supported by grants from the Swedish Medical Research Council, project 3108; Magnus Bergvalls Stiftelse; Fredrik och Ingrid Thurings Stiftelse; Pharmacia Hospital Care, Stockholm, Sweden; Finnsugar Xyrofin Ltd., UK; Karolinska Institute; and Sunnaas Hospital, Oslo, Norway.

REFERENCES

1. Rubner, M. *Die Gesetze des Energieverbrauchs bei der Ernährung*. Leipzig & Vienna: Franz Deuticker; 1902.
2. James WPT. From SDA to DIT to TEF. In: Kinney JM, Tucker HN, eds. *Energy metabolism: tissue determinants and cellular corollaries*. New York: Raven; 1992:163–186.
3. Jéquier E. The influence of nutrient administration on energy expenditure in man. *Clin Nutr* 1986;5: 181–186.

4. Neumann RA. Experimentelle Beiträge zur Lehre von dem täglichen Nahrungsbedarf des Menschen unter besonderer Berüksichtigung der notwendigen Eiweissmenge. *Arch Hyg Bakt* 1902;45:1–87.
5. Himms-Hagen J. Thermogenesis in brown adipose tissue as an energy buffer. Implications for obesity. *N Engl J Med* 1984;311:1549–1558.
6. Rothwell N, Stock M. A role for brown adipose tissue in diet-induced thermogenesis. *Nature (Lond)* 1979;281:31–35.
7. Lev-Bari E, Horwitz VC, Shilo R. Diet-induced thermogenesis visualized by thermography. *Isr J Med Sci* 1982;18:889–890.
8. Astrup A, Bülow J, Christensen NJ. Ephedrine-induced thermogenesis in man: no role for interscapular brown adipose tissue. *Clin Sci* 1984;66:179–186.
9. Astrup A. Thermogenesis in human brown adipose tissue and skeletal muscle induced by sympathomimetic stimulation. *Acta Endocrinol* 1986;278(suppl):1–32.
10. Brundin T, Hagenfeldt L, Söderberg R, Wahren J. Blood flow substrate utilization and heat generation in tissues drained by the azygos vein in man. *Clin Physiol (Oxf)* 1987;7:481–491.
11. Brundin T, Wahren J. Influence of a mixed meal on splanchnic and interscapular energy expenditure in man. *Am J Physiol* 1991;260:E232–E237.
12. Brundin T, Söderberg R, Wahren J. Heat production in tissues drained by the azygos vein. In: Christiansen C, Juel Riis B, eds. *Highlights on endocrinology. Proc Eur Congr Endocrinol 1st* Copenhagen 1987;379–384.
13. Young JB, Landsberg L. Stimulation of the sympathetic nervous system during sucrose feeding. *Nature (Lond)* 1977;269:615–617.
14. Welle S, Lilavivat U, Campbell RG. Increased plasma norepinephrine concentrations and metabolic rates following glucose ingestion in man. *Metabolism* 1980;29:806–809.
15. Welle S, Lilavivat U, Campbell RG. Increased plasma norepinephrine levels following glucose but not protein or fat consumption. *Metabolism* 1981;30:953–958.
16. Kleinbaum J, Schamoon H. Selective counterregulatory hormone response after oral glucose in man. *J Clin Endocrinol Metab* 1982;55:787–790.
17. Berne C, Fagius J, Niklasson F. Sympathetic response to oral carbohydrate administration. Evidence from microelectrode nerve recordings. *J Clin Invest* 1989;84:1403–1409.
18. Spraul M, Anderson EA, Bogardus C, Ravussin E. Muscle sympathetic nerve activity in response to glucose ingestion. *Diabetes* 1994;43:191–196.
19. Astrup A, Bülow J, Christensen NJ, et al. Facultative thermogenesis induced by carbohydrate: a skeletal muscle component mediated by epinephrine. *Am J Physiol* 1986;250:E226–E229.
20. Astrup A, Simonsen L, Bülow J, et al. Epinephrine mediates facultative carbohydrate-induced thermogenesis in human skeletal muscle. *Am J Physiol* 1989;257:E340–E345.
21. Robertson RP, Porte D Jr. Plasma catecholamine responses to intravenous glucose in normal man. *J Clin Endocrin Metab* 1974;38:403–405.
22. Fagius J, Berne C. Increase in muscle nerve sympathetic activity in humans after food intake. *Clin Sci* 1994;86:159–167.
23. Welle S, Campbell RG. Stimulation of thermogenesis by carbohydrate overfeeding. Evidence against sympathetic nervous system mediation. *J Clin Invest* 1983;71:916–925.
24. Zed C, James WPT. Dietary thermogenesis in obesity. Response to carbohydrate and protein meals: the effect of ß-adrenergic blockade and semistarvation. *Int J Obesity* 1986;10:391–405.
25. Vernet O, Nacht C-A, Christin L, et al. ß-adrenergic blockade and intravenous nutrient-induced thermogenesis in lean and obese women. *Am J Physiol* 1987;253:E65–E71.
26. Welle SL, Nair KS, Campbell RG. Failure of chronic ß-adrenergic blockade to inhibit overfeeding-induced thermogenesis in humans. *Am J Physiol* 1989;256:R653–R658.
27. Thörne A, Wahren J. Beta-adrenergic blockade does not influence the thermogenic response to a mixed meal in man. *Clin Physiol (Oxf)* 1989;9:321–332.
28. Zwillich C, Martin B, Hofeldt F, et al. Lack of effects of beta sympathetic blockade on the metabolic and respiratory responses to carbohydrate feeding. *Metabolism* 1981;30:451–456.
29. Seaton T, Welle S, Alex S, et al. The effect of adrenergic blockade on glucose-induced thermogenesis. *Metabolism* 1984;33:415–419.
30. Acheson K, Jéquier E, Wahren J. Influence of ß-adrenergic blockade on glucose-induced thermogenesis in man. *J Clin Invest* 1983;72:981–986.
31. DeFronzo RA, Thorin D, Felber JP, et al. Effect of beta and alpha adrenergic blockade on glucose-induced thermogenesis in man. *J Clin Invest* 1984;73:634–639.
32. Ravussin E, Acheson K, Vernet O, et al. Evidence that insulin resistance is responsible for the decreased thermic effect of glucose in human obesity. *J Clin Invest* 1985;76:1268–1273.

33. Rowe JW, Young JB, Minaker KL, et al. Effect of insulin and glucose infusions on sympathetic nervous system activity in normal man. *Diabetes* 1981;30:219–225.
34. Berne C, Fagius J, Pollare T, Hjemdahl P. The sympathetic response to euglycaemic hyperinsulinaemia. Evidence from microelectrode nerve recordings in healthy subjects. *Diabetologia* 1992;35: 873–879.
35. Anderson EA, Hoffman RP, Balon TW, et al. Hyperinsulinemia produces both sympathetic neural activation and vasodilation in normal humans. *J Clin Invest* 1991;87:2246–2252.
36. Brundin T, Söderberg R, Wahren J. A versatile technique for multi-channel, digital blood temperature recording in man. *Clin Physiol (Oxf)* 1987;7:537–539.
37. Harris JA, Benedict FG. *A biometric study of basal metabolism in man.* Publication no. 279. Washington, DC: Carnegie Institution of Washington; 1919:1–266.
38. Banauch D, Brümmer W, Ebeling W, et al. Eine Glucose-Dehydrogenase für die Glucose-Bestimmung in Körperflüssigkeiten. *Z Klin Chem Klin Biochem* 1975;13:101–107.
39. Bradley SE, Ingelfinger FJ, Bradley GP, Curry JJ. The estimation of hepatic blood flow in man. *J Clin Invest* 1945;24:890–897.
40. Rowell LB, Blackmon JR, Bruce RA. Indocyanine green clearance and estimated hepatic blood flow during mild to maximal exercise in upright man. *J Clin Invest* 1964;43:1677–1690.
41. Burns E, Ball CE, Christie JP, et al. Direct and indirect measurement of the hepatic extraction ratio of indocyanine green in the rat. *Clin Sci* 1989;76:503–508.
42. Fick A. Über die Messung des Blutquantums in den Herzventrikeln. In: *Sitzungsberichte der physmed Ges zu Würzburg.* XIV. Sitzung am 9. Juli 1870:16.
43. Minard D. Body heat content. In: Hardy JD, Gagge AP, Stolwijk JAJ, eds. *Physiological and behavioral temperature regulation.* Springfield, IL: Charles C Thomas; 1970:345–357.
44. Brundin T, Wahren J. Influence of protein ingestion on human splanchnic and whole body oxygen consumption, blood flow and blood temperature. *Metabolism* 1994;43:626–632.
45. Brundin T, Wahren J. Effects of i.v. amino acids on human splanchnic and whole body oxygen consumption, blood flow and blood temperatures. *Am J Physiol* 1994;266:E396–E402.
46. Brundin T, Wahren J. Whole-body and splanchnic oxygen consumption and blood flow after oral ingestion of fructose or glucose. *Am J Physiol* 1993;264:E504–E513.
47. Brundin T. Mechanisms of nutrient-induced thermogenesis—total and splanchnic oxygen consumption and blood flow. *Int J Obesity* 1993;17(suppl 3):S52–S55.
48. Brundin T, Thörne A, Wahren J. Heat leakage across the abdominal wall and meal-induced thermogenesis in normal weight and obese subjects. *Metabolism* 1992;41:49–55.
49. Aksnes A-K. Metabolic, circulatory and thermal effects of nutrients in patients with complete cervical spinal cord lesions [Thesis]. Stockholm, Sweden: Karolinska Institute; 1995:1–40.
50. Aksnes A-K, Brundin T, Hjeltnes N, et al. Meal-induced rise in resting energy expenditure in patients with complete cervical spinal cord lesions. *Paraplegia* 1993;31:462–472.
51. Aksnes A-K, Brundin T, Hjeltnes N, Wahren J. Glucose-induced thermogenesis in tetraplegic patients with low sympatho-adrenal activity. *Am J Physiol* 1994;266:E161–E170.
52. Aksnes A-K, Brundin T, Hjeltnes N, Wahren J. Metabolic, thermal and circulatory effects of intravenous infusion of amino acids in tetraplegic patients. *Clin Physiol (Oxf)* 1995;15:377–396.
53. Claus-Walker J, Halsted LS. Metabolic and endocrine changes in spinal cord injury: I. The nervous system before and after transection of the spinal cord. *Arch Phys Med Rehabil* 1981;62:595–601.
54. Wallin G, Stjernberg L. Sympathetic activity in man after spinal cord injury. *Brain* 1984;107: 183–198.
55. Collett ME, Liljestrand G. Variations in the resting minute volume of the heart in man. *Scand Arch Physiol* 1924;45:17–28.
56. Aperia A, Carlens E. Vergleich zwischen der Wirkung von Fett, Kohlenhydrat und Eiweiss auf den Kreislauf des Menschen. *Scand Arch Physiol* 1931;63:151–163.
57. Grollman A. Physiological variations in the cardiac output of man. III. The effect of the ingestion of food on the cardiac output, pulse rate, blood pressure, and oxygen consumption of man. *Am J Physiol* 1929;89:366–370.
58. Gladstone SA. Cardiac output and related functions under basal and postprandial conditions. *Arch Intern Med* 1935;55:533–546.
59. Brundin T, Wahren J. Renal oxygen consumption, thermogenesis and amino acid utilization during i.v. infusion of amino acids in man. *Am J Physiol* 1994;267:E648–E655.
60. Brundin T, Bränström R, Wahren J. Effects of intravenous versus oral glucose administration on oxygen consumption and blood flow in splanchnic and extra-splanchnic tissues. *Am J Physiol* 1996; 271:E496–E504.

61. Pittet P, Gygax PH, Jéquier E. Thermic effect of glucose and amino acids in man studied by direct and indirect calorimetry. *Br J Nutr* 1974;31:343–349.
62. Brundin T, Aksnes A-K, Wahren J. Whole body and splanchnic metabolic and circulatory effects of glucose during β-adrenergic receptor inhibition. *Am J Physiol* 1997;272.
63. Flatt JP. Energy costs of ATP synthesis. In: Kinney JM, Tucker HN, eds. *Energy metabolism: tissue determinants and cellular corollaries.* New York: Raven; 1992:319–342.
64. Landau BR, Wahren J, Chandramouli V, et al. Use of ^2H_2O for estimating rates of gluconeogenesis. Application to the fasted state. *J Clin Invest* 1995;95:172–178.
65. Landau BR, Wahren J, Chandramouli V, et al. Contributions of gluconeogenesis to glucose production in the fasted state. *J Clin Invest* 1996;98:378–385.
66. Felig P, Wahren J. Influence of endogenous insulin secretion on splanchnic glucose and amino acid metabolism in man. *J Clin Invest* 1971;50:1702–1711.
67. Tappy L, Randin JP, Felber JP, et al. Comparison of thermogenic effect of fructose and glucose in normal humans. *Am J Physiol* 1986;250:E718–E724.
68. Schwartz J-M, Acheson K, Tappy L, et al. Thermogenesis and fructose metabolism in humans. *Am J Physiol* 1992;262:E591–E598.
69. Steinberg HO, Brechtel G, Johnson A, et al. Insulin-mediated skeletal muscle vasodilation is nitric oxide dependent. A novel action of insulin to increase nitric oxide release. *J Clin Invest* 1994;94:1172–1179.
70. Scherrer U, Randin D, Vollenweider P, et al. Nitric oxide release accounts for insulin's vascular effects in humans. *J Clin Invest* 1994;94:2511–2515.
71. Spraul M, Ravussin E, Baron AD. Lack of relationship between muscle sympathetic nerve activity and skeletal muscle vasodilation in response to insulin infusion. *Diabetologia* 1996;39:91–96.
72. Thauer R. Thermosensitivity of the spinal cord In: Hardy JD, Gagge AP, Stolwijk JAJ, eds. *Physiological and behavioral temperature regulation.* Springfield, IL: Charles C Thomas; 1970:472–492.
73. Lusk G. The specific dynamic action. *J Nutr* 1930;3:519–530.
74. Selldén E, Bränström R, Brundin T. Pre-operative infusion of amino acids prevents post-operative hypothermia. *Br J Anaesth* 1996;96:227–234.
75. Jensen MD, Johnson CM, Cryer PE, Murray MJ. Thermogenesis after a mixed meal: role of leg and splanchnic tissues in men and women. *Am J Physiol* 1995;268:E433–E438.
76. Rapport D, Katz LN. The effect of glycine upon the metabolism of isolated perfused muscle. *Am J Physiol* 1927;80:185–199.
77. Wahren J, Felig P, Hagenfeldt L. Effect of protein ingestion on splanchnic and leg metabolism in normal man and in patients with diabetes mellitus. *J Clin Invest* 1976;57:987–999.
78. Downey JA, Mottram RF, Pickering GW. The location by regional cooling of central temperature receptors in the conscious rabbit. *J Physiol (Lond)* 1964;170:415–441.
79. Eisenman JS, Depression of preoptic thermosensitivity by bacterial pyrogen in rabbits. *J Appl Physiol* 1974;227:1067–1073.
80. Benzinger TH, Kitzinger C, Pratt AW. The human thermostat. In: Herzfeld CM, ed. *Temperature. Its measurement and control. Science and industry, part 3.* New York: Reinhold; 1963:637–665.
81. Selldén E, Brundin T, Wahren J. Augmented thermic effect of amino acids under general anaesthesia. A mechanism useful for prevention of anaesthesia-induced hypothermia. *Clin Sci* 1994;86:611–618.
82. Selldén E, Bränström R, Brundin T. Augmented thermic effect of amino acids under general anaesthesia occurs predominantly in extra-splanchnic tissues. *Clin Sci* 1996;91:431–439.
83. Newsholme EA, Crabtree B, Parry-Billings M. The energetic cost of regulation: an analysis based on the principles of metabolic-control-logic. In: Kinney JM, Tucker HN, eds. *Energy metabolism: tissue determinants and cellular corollaries.* New York: Raven; 1992:467–493.
84. Sessler DI. Central thermoregulatory inhibition by general anesthesia. *Anesthesiology* 1991;75:557–559.

Physiology, Stress, and Malnutrition: Functional Correlates, Nutritional Intervention,
edited by J.M. Kinney and H.N. Tucker.
Lippincott–Raven Publishers © 1997.

Overview of Nutrients, Thermogenesis, and Stress

John Wahren

Section of Clinical Physiology, Department of Surgical Sciences, Karolinska Hospital, S-171 77 Stockholm, Sweden

The section on nutrients, thermogenesis and stress has facilitated discussion of an assembly of different issues related to substrate supply, pulmonary function, thermoregulation and energy expenditure in perioperative patients. It is the purpose of this chapter to provide a brief review of the major points raised by each of the authors and to offer a personal perspective on the possible relevance of some of the recent developments in this field. Four different themes have been discussed in the preceding chapters: anorexia, hypoxemia, hypothermia, and thermogenesis. They are addressed separately in the following sections.

ANOREXIA

The relatively high incidence of malnutrition in the elderly and in surgical patients (1) is a cause of concern and may be seen as a neglected clinical problem, especially in view of the apparent association with poor clinical outcome (2,3). Part of the reason that the problem of malnutrition has received relatively little scientific attention may be the lack of generally agreed upon, consistent measures of nutritional status. Such measures would facilitate both comparisons between study groups and the evaluation of different treatment modalities. At this time it appears that formulation of appropriate nutritional and anthropometric measurements should be given a high priority.

As outlined in the presentation by Susan Jebb, the causes of weight loss in most anorectic patients may be sought both in changes in energy expenditure and a diminished food intake. The underlying disorder may increase the patient's resting energy expenditure—although possibly not as much as previously believed—but the accompanying relative physical inactivity most often results in an unchanged or even diminished total energy expenditure. A number of variables, all of which may be influenced by disease, regulate food intake. A markedly diminished food intake due to anorexia of disease as well as to physical limitations results in a gradual breakdown of energy homeostasis with catabolism of body fuel stores. Unavoidably, not only adipose tissue but also protein stores are broken down, with resultant loss of vital body functions. Thus, in the management of anorexia, improvement of food intake by means of dietary advice, sip feeds, artificial nutrition, or specific substrates are important features.

The ability of humans to tolerate long periods of partial or total food deprivation is predicated upon several important metabolic adjustments. Thus, long-term fasting is characterized by diminished glucose turnover and reduced hepatic gluconeogenesis from amino acids, as evidenced by decreased urinary excretion of nitrogenous products, primarily urea (4). The keto acids, 3-hydroxybutyrate and acetoacetate, become increasingly available during progressive fasting and, because they are water soluble and able to cross the blood–brain barrier (5), they serve as major fuels for the brain in the prolonged fasted state, thereby reducing the body's glucose requirements (6).

Although the metabolic adaptation to prolonged fasting is relatively well understood, less attention has been directed to the metabolic changes that occur during the first 2–3 days of fasting. The initial metabolic changes are of particular interest in the context of patients with anorexia or malnutrition because these patients may eat intermittently and/or ingest insufficient amounts of nutrients, thereby placing themselves in a situation similar to that for short-term starvation. After 60–72 hours of fasting, hepatic glucose production is decreased (7), most likely because of diminished hepatic glycogen depots (8). At this time glucose homeostasis is maintained solely by gluconeogenesis, and an augmented hepatic uptake of amino acids and other gluconeogenic precursors takes place (7). The amino acids, in turn, are being mobilized primarily from muscle tissue at a substantially greater rate than after an overnight fast; net release of amino acids from skeletal muscle is increased by 70% (9), and urinary excretion of 3-methyl histidine reflecting muscle proteolysis is markedly augmented during the first 2–3 days of fasting (10,11). Amino acid extraction by the liver is augmented (7), and hepatic gluconeogenesis is accelerated, as evidenced by increased rates of hepatic urea formation and urinary excretion during the first days of fasting (10,11). Even though some of the amino acids initially derive from the intracellular free amino acid pool in muscle (11), repletion of this tightly regulated pool during fasting will have to derive from breakdown of muscle protein. The accelerated rate of protein catabolism persists until fasting progresses beyond the initial phase to the fully adapted state; during continued fasting the ketoacid concentrations increase and the rates of amino acid mobilization and muscle proteolysis again decrease to and below the levels observed after an overnight fast, allowing the subjects to preserve body protein stores (6). This line of reasoning may help explain the often very marked rate of protein loss in malnourished or anorectic patients whose metabolic situation will in part be similar to that for early starvation.

The physiologic mechanism by which the body is able to spare body protein effectively during prolonged fasting as distinct from short-term starvation has not been determined. However, it may be hypothesized that the elevated levels of keto acids that normally occur during fasting serve to decrease net muscle protein breakdown (12). Investigations of the possible role of keto acids in this context have been hampered by difficulties related to the administration of keto acids. Being fairly strong acids, the keto acids cannot be conveniently administered in acid form. Likewise, infusion of the keto acid sodium salts results in sodium overload (12). However, an alternative substrate, 1,3-butanediol mono- or diesters of keto acids, may offer new possibilities (13). The 1,3-butanediol diester of acetoacetate is a water-soluble, sodium-free, diffusible precursor of the physiologic keto acids. Its metabolism is indicated below:

1,3-butanediol diacetoacetate → 1,3-butanediol + 2 acetoacetate →
$$3 \text{ 3-hydroxybutyrate}$$

Hydrolysis to butanediol and acetoacetate occurs by nonspecific esterases in plasma and tissues. Butanediol is subsequently oxidized in the liver to 3-hydroxybutyrate with generation of 2 NADH. The reducing equivalents are then trapped as acetoacetate is converted to 3-hydroxybutyrate in the liver, leaving hepatic redox state unchanged (14). Administration of butanediol diesters to animals and humans is accompanied by mild to modest hyperketonemia (13,15). Further work will be required to establish whether this substrate can be used in experimental work aimed at defining the possible role of keto acids in the metabolic adaptation to prolonged fasting and, possibly, in parenteral and/or enteral nutrition.

HYPOXEMIA

In the presentation by Jacob Rosenberg, it was emphasized that episodic or constant arterial hypoxemia occurs frequently after otherwise uncomplicated surgery. The incidence of episodic hypoxemia shows a peak during the second or third night after the surgical procedure. Pain and stress-induced sleep disturbances with suppression of rapid eye movement sleep may be factors of importance for subsequent episodic hypoxemia; there may be a rebound of rapid eye movement sleep on the second or third night after surgery, giving rise to ventilatory dysrhythmias and episodes of hypoxemia. Likewise, opioid-containing analgesics may precipitate intermittent hypoventilation, and episodes of central apnea also may elicit periods of hypoxemia. Constant hypoxemia during the early postoperative course is most often due to uneven ventilation/perfusion distribution due to the lung volume reduction, diaphragm dysfunction, and mechanical limitations imposed after abdominal surgery in particular. There is now a wealth of data to indicate that hypoxemia in the postoperative period is a major factor in the pathogenesis of cardiac and cerebral dysfunction as well as in the development of wound complications. Clearly, there is a need to explore how postoperative sleep disturbances may be avoided and to develop improved regimens for postoperative pulmonary care.

The hypoxic ventilatory reflex mechanism is considered to be of importance for the protection against hypoxemia in the early postoperative period. Recently, the seemingly established concept that volatile anesthetic agents such as halothane, enflurane, and isoflurane depress or abolish the hypoxic reflex mechanism (16) has received renewed attention. Thus, 0.2% isoflurane (end-tidal) is reported not to influence the ventilatory response to mild isocapnic hypoxia nor to mild hyper-capnic challenge (17). Likewise, the poikilocapnic (CO_2 not controlled) ventila-tory response to hypoxia is uninfluenced by 0.85 minimum alveolar concentration (MAC) isoflurane (18). The earlier investigations on hypoxic ventilatory reflexes and anesthetic agents were mostly conducted using halothane (16). Thus, the new findings suggest that there may be differences between the different anesthetic agents. Nevertheless, the present evidence indicates that the specific depressant effect of isoflurane on the hypoxic ventilatory response may be substantially less than previously believed and constitutes a possible clinical advantage.

The effect of muscle relaxants on the hypoxic ventilatory response has been examined recently. A diminished hypoxic response has been reported for human subjects partially paralyzed with vecuronium. Thus, both with a poikilocapnic and an isocapnic test procedure, the hypoxic response was found to be reduced after vecuronium administration (19,20). Hypoxic stimulation can be expected to act either on the glomus cells of the carotid bodies or directly on the carotid body nerve terminals eliciting release of acetylcholine, catecholamines, or neu-ropeptides, but the exact mechanisms by which the carotid body converts a hypoxic stimulus into an afferent signal to the central nervous system is not fully understood. Alternatively, the observed effect of vecuronium could be explained by an influence of the muscle relaxant on stretch receptors or muscle spindles in striated respiratory muscles or, possibly, as a direct effect on the central nervous system. However, the latter possibilities are unlikely to be of major importance because direct recordings of phrenic nerve activity demonstrate that vecuronium markedly reduces the hypoxia-induced increase in phrenic nerve activity in the rabbit (21). Further studies will be required to delineate the possible role of this mechanism in early postoperative hypoxemia.

In the treatment of postoperative hypoxemia, measures such as artificial ven-tilation, oxygen therapy, positive end-expiratory pressure, etc. are well estab-lished. Twenty years ago a change of body position from the supine position to the prone was shown to exert a beneficial effect on oxygenation in patients with acute respiratory failure (22). Since then, few clinical reports have addressed the possible advantages of the prone position for pulmonary exchange. However, a recent study from the Karolinska Hospital, Stockholm, has reexamined pul-monary gas exchange in the prone and supine positions in a group of patients with severe lung disorders (S. Lindahl, personal communication). Eleven patients with acute pulmonary insufficiency caused by trauma, septicemia, aspi-ration, or burn injury were studied during mechanical ventilation in both the supine and prone positions. Ten of the 11 patients responded positively with improved arterial oxygenation in the prone position. At unchanged ventilatory parameters, the average arterial oxygen partial pressure increased by 40% in the prone position (Fig. 1), despite a decrease in the fraction of inspired oxygen. The oxygen index (P_aO_2/FiO_2) increased by 150% in the prone position, whereas the arterial partial pressure for carbon dioxide remained unchanged. The survival rate for the above patients treated in the prone position was 64% as compared with only 35% in a group of previously studied and clinically similar patients that received extracorporal membrane oxygenator treatment (23).

The reason for the patients' improvement in pulmonary function in the prone position is not apparent. The conventional wisdom is that pulmonary perfusion is largely dependent on gravity. Accordingly, the distribution of ventilation/perfusion ratios can be expected to be similar for the supine and prone positions, thereby minimizing the incentive to explore possible pulmonary function benefits in the prone body position. However, in recent years it has been suggested that gravity may be only a minor determinant of pulmonary blood distribution (24); vascular conductance is greater in the dorsal parts of the lung as compared with the ventral region, independent of body position (25). Irrespective of the mechanism behind the observed improvement in oxygenation in the prone position, it appears that shifting patients to the prone position may be a form of treatment that can be attempted before extracorporeal membrane oxygenator or NO therapy is commenced.

HYPOTHERMIA

The most common disorder of temperature homeostasis after trauma or surgery is hypothermia. It usually occurs inadvertently and in as many as 50–80% of all surgical procedures. In the presentation by Franco Carli, thermal balance during anesthesia was discussed and the consequences of perioperative hypothermia were presented. Heat production is decreased during anesthesia secondary to reduced tissue metabolism. At the same time, heat loss may be augmented because of cutaneous vasodilatation, and thermoregulation is often impaired due to influences on the central nervous system from the anesthetic agents. All of the above factors contribute to the development of perioperative hypothermia, often amounting to 1.5–2.0°C or more. Although mild to modest intraoperative hypothermia may provide protection against central nervous system ischemia, the negative consequences of hypothermia in the immediate postoperative period, including impaired blood coagulation, negative nitrogen balance, and reduced resistance to wound infection, have been emphasized recently (26). As the effects of the anesthesia wear off and the thermoregulatory center again becomes functional, sympathoadrenal activation occurs with increases in heart rate and blood pressure, and there may be intense shivering. The cardiovascular changes increase the risk of hypoxemia and myocardial ischemia (27). In addition, shivering is very uncomfortable to most patients. Even mild hypothermia has been shown to increase blood loss and transfusion requirements during total hip arthroplasty, possibly because of

PaO$_2$, kPa

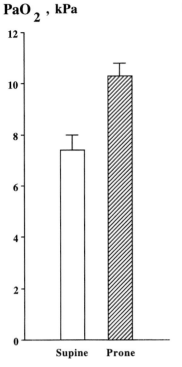

Oxygen Index

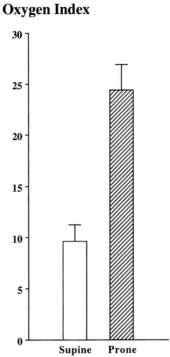

PaCO$_2$, kPa

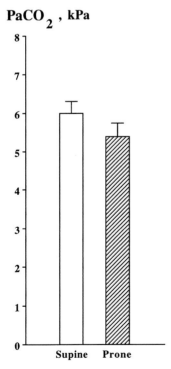

FIG. 1. Arterial partial pressure for oxygen (PaO$_2$) and carbon dioxide (PaCO$_2$) and oxygen index (PO$_2$/FiO$_2$) in 11 patients with severe lung disorders requiring intensive care. Measurements were made in the supine and prone positions. Values for oxygen index and PaO$_2$ in the prone position are significantly greater than the corresponding values in the supine position ($p < 0.005$). Values are means ±SE.

hypothermia-related coagulation disorders (28). The clinical significance of perioperative hypothermia has been further emphasized in a recent U.S. multicenter study (29). The findings indicate that hypothermia during anesthesia and colorectal surgery may significantly delay wound healing and predispose patients to wound infections and prolonged hospitalization as compared with patients that were at normothermia during surgery (29).

Perioperative hypothermia remains common even though several methods of warming are available. Thermal neutrality in the operating room, skin surface warming, airway heating and humidification, and forced air heating (30) have all been tried with varying degrees of success. More recently, an alternative procedure based on the thermogenic effect of amino acids has been presented (31,32). The thermic effect of amino acids is high in comparison with that of other nutrients and may account for 30–40% of the energy content. Therefore i.v. infusion of a mixture of amino acids during surgery stimulates whole-body oxidative metabolism, and it can be shown to effectively reduce or prevent perioperative hypothermia (31,32). Once awake, the patients given amino acids, unlike controls, did not shiver and had pulmonary oxygen uptakes and cardiac outputs above the preoperative basal levels. In addition, the patients' baseline temperatures were restored more quickly than were those of the controls (31). Starting the amino acid infusion 1–2 hours before surgery prevented any significant decrease in rectal temperature in patients undergoing hysterectomy (32). Remarkably, the thermic effect of amino acids in anesthetized patients (volatile anesthetic agents and benzodiazepine premedication) was found to be substantially augmented as compared with that observed in awake controls, a finding for which there is no immediate explanation at this time. Further observations in connection with amino acid infusions may help in elucidating the mechanism of heat loss in the perioperative period and assist in establishing appropriate procedures to minimize hypothermia during anesthesia and surgery.

Several different thermometry techniques are in use for the evaluation of patients' thermal balance. Thus, so-called body core thermometry with measurements in the esophagus, rectum, or colon or on the tympanic membrane is often combined with skin thermometry to describe the whole-body temperature. However, the heat content of the body is probably best reflected by the temperature of the mixed blood (arterial or pulmonary arterial), which can be measured accurately by use of commercially available thermistor-equipped catheters. It has the advantage of representing the temperature of the entire body, not only the body core. In addition, it follows with a short time-constant change in thermal balance, for example, during physical exercise (33) (Fig. 2).

THERMOGENESIS

Ingestion of food and the subsequent distribution of nutrients from the gastrointestinal tract to the various tissues and organs influence markedly both

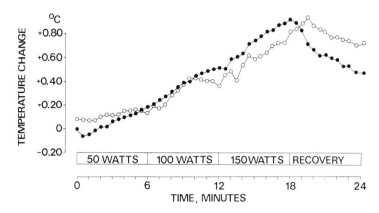

FIG. 2. Temperature of mixed venous blood (pulmonary artery) (●) and in the esophagus (○) at rest, during exercise, and during recovery. Mean values for seven individuals are indicated. Data from Brundin (33).

circulation and metabolism of the body. These aspects are covered in the chapters by Ian Macdonald and Tomas Brundin and are discussed together.

Interesting observations were presented concerning the thermic response to a meal administered slowly via a nasogastric tube. The response was greatly reduced as compared with that observed after oral ingestion of an identical meal. Thus, a meal of 1.67 MJ, infused over 2 hours via a nasogastric tube, caused no significant thermic effect (34). Although tube feeding is very unlike normal ingestion of food, the finding seems remarkable. The authors point out the probable importance of palatability for the physiologic responses to food ingestion, as demonstrated earlier by LeBlanc and Brondel. In this context, it should be mentioned that central activation of the parasympathetic nervous system might affect at least the upper part of the gastrointestinal tract, reached by vagal innervation. An increased release of acetylcholine might possibly induce a local intestinal release of nitric oxide, which in turn, may reduce the intestinal vascular resistance. However, significant increments of the entire splanchnic blood flow after pure fructose meals or protein meals (fish or meat) have been observed (35,36).

New information was provided on the limb blood flow responses to solid versus liquid meals. Thus, an initial reduction of limb blood flow has been found to follow the ingestion of solid, mixed meals (37), whereas a similar flow reduction is not always obvious after liquid meals (38). The authors suggest that the early blood flow reduction reflects an increased vascular resistance in skeletal muscle, induced by central activation of the muscular sympathetic nerves that accompanies the meal ingestion. After a liquid meal, possibly absorbed more rapidly, vasodilatory mechanisms may start earlier and thus conceal an initial limb vasoconstriction. The explanation proposed by the authors may be in line with the recent findings that postprandial muscular vasodilatation is probably mediated by an insulin-induced release of nitric oxide (39).

The cardiovascular response to ingestion of a mixed meal is characterized by an increase in cardiac output and little if any change in arterial blood pressure. Splanchnic blood flow increases markedly after ingestion of glucose-containing meals but not after oral administration of fructose (35). Intravenous infusion of glucose or amino acids do not stimulate splanchnic flow (40,41). Propranolol partly abolishes the glucose-induced increase in splanchnic blood flow (42). Likewise, in patients with complete cervical spinal cord lesions—and no efferent central sympathetic activity—glucose ingestion results in a diminished hepatic blood flow response compared with healthy controls (43). Taken together, the findings suggest that increased sympathetic nervous activity contributes to the mechanisms whereby glucose-containing meals stimulate splanchnic blood flow.

Although there is good agreement in the literature regarding the gastrointestinal blood flow response to glucose administration, divergent results are reported for protein ingestion or amino acid administration. Thus, superior mesenteric artery blood flow, as evaluated by transcutaneous Doppler ultrasound technique, is reported to increase by up to 60% after ingestion of a liquid protein meal (44,45). In contrast, neither protein ingestion nor intravenous amino acid infusion have been found to increase total splanchnic blood flow measured by the indocyanine green constant rate infusion technique (36,41,46). The different results may be related to the well-known difficulties in obtaining quantitative blood flow data using the ultrasound Doppler technique; these are related to the problems in reproducibly assessing the vessel transectional area and the angle of the Doppler probe to the direction of the blood flow. There are few studies on the circulatory response to fat ingestion, probably because of the minimal thermogenic response that accompanies intake of fat. However, reports are available suggesting an increase in both cardiac output and superior mesenteric artery blood flow using the ultrasound Doppler technique after a fat-containing meal (37,44,45). These results should be interpreted with caution because of the inherent difficulties with the ultrasound methodology as regards quantitative flow measurements.

The studies concerning whole-body and splanchnic thermogenic responses to oral and intravenous glucose, respectively, have shown that the whole body thermic effect of glucose may represent the net result of regional bidirectional changes. Thus, after intravenous glucose infusion in healthy subjects, splanchnic oxygen uptake decreased by approximately 20%, probably reflecting a reduction of hepatic gluconeogenesis, whereas simultaneous extra-splanchnic oxygen uptake increased by 10%; the resultant whole-body thermic effect of intravenous glucose amounted to less than 3% (40). Similarly, after oral glucose ingestion, splanchnic oxygen uptake remained essentially unchanged (small initial increase followed by a decline), extra-splanchnic oxygen uptake increased by 9%, and the whole body response was an 8% increase (35). It is noteworthy that the extra-splanchnic increase in oxygen uptake was similar for intravenous and oral glucose administration. In contrast, splanchnic energy expenditure differed markedly, perhaps as a result of greater energy costs for absorption and transport of oral as compared with intravenous glucose. These findings thus suggest that measurements of regional quantitative changes induced by nutrient intake may facilitate an improved understanding of the complex mechanisms involved in the regulation of nutrient-induced thermogenesis.

Currently available data regarding the influence of individual nutrients on whole-body and regional energy expenditure are compatible with the notion that the absorption and metabolic processing of the nutrients may be the dominating component in the increase in energy expenditure. Although the "obligatory" costs thus may become better defined with regional measurements for individual substrates, the facultative component remains ill understood. Sympathetic nervous activation of brown adipose tissue was long thought to be important in this context, but it has not proven possible to demonstrate the presence of metabolically active brown adipose tissue in adult humans (47,48). The role of the sympathetic nervous system in regulating nutrient-induced thermogenesis is also being questioned. In several studies, nutrient-induced thermogenesis of normal magnitude was demonstrated in subjects given beta receptor blocking agents, as well as in patients with complete cervical spinal cord lesions in whom the pathways for central activation of the peripheral sympathetic nerves were severed. Together, these findings indicate that increased sympathetic activity is of little or no importance for the nutrient-induced increase in energy expenditure (42,43,49–51). However, the central nervous system appears to be involved in the regulation of nutrient-induced thermogenesis. When the abdominal area was thermally insulated in normal-weight subjects, the nutrient-induced increase in whole-body oxygen uptake was diminished in comparison with that for noninsulated subjects and became similar to

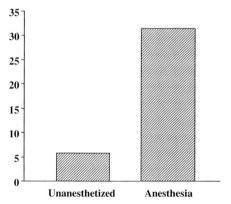

Thermic Effect of Amino Acids

FIG. 3. Mean thermic effect of amino acids during 30-min intravenous infusion in 10 patients under general anesthesia (isoflurane) and in eight unanesthetized subjects. Data from Selldén et al. (31).

that observed in obese individuals (52,53). In accordance with these observations, when obese patients lose weight and reduce their abdominal insulation, they also normalize their previously reduced thermogenic response to a meal (54). Whether this phenomenon occurs via blood temperature changes recorded by the central thermosensors or otherwise has not been determined. However, irrespective of the mechanism involved, the findings imply that the central nervous system is able to suppress the whole-body thermogenic response to nutrients. This formulation receives further support from studies in patients whose central thermosensors have been rendered nonfunctional by general anesthesia (31,32). Thus, during isoflurane anesthesia, i.v. infused amino acids elicited a fivefold increase in energy expenditure compared with in the nonanesthetized state (Fig. 3). The combined findings thus suggested that the role of the central nervous system for the nutrient-induced thermogenesis is restraining rather than stimulatory in nature.

REFERENCES

1. McWhirter JP, Pennington CR. Incidence and recognition of malnutrition in hospital. *Br Med J* 1994;308:945–948.
2. Larsson J, Unosson M, Ek A-C, et al. Effect of dietary supplement on nutritional status and clinical outcome in 501 geriatric patients—a randomized study. *Clin Nutr* 1990;9:170–184.
3. Lumbers M, Driver LT, Howland RJ, Older MWJ, Williams CM. Nutritional status and clinical outcome in elderly female surgical orthopaedic patients. *Clin Nutr* 1996;15:101–107.
4. Owen OE, Felig P, Morgan AP, et al. Liver and kidney metabolism during prolonged starvation. *J Clin Invest* 1969;48:574–583.
5. Hasselbalch SG, Knudsen GM, Jakobsen J, et al. Blood-brain barrier permeability of glucose and ketone bodies during short-term starvation on humans. *Am J Physiol* 1995;268:E1161–1166.
6. Owen OE, Morgan AP, Kemp HG, et al. Brain metabolism during fasting. *J Clin Invest* 1967;46:1589–1595.
7. Wahren J, Efendic S, Luft R, et al. Influence of somatostatin on splanchnic glucose metabolism in postoperative and 60-hour fasted humans. *J Clin Invest* 1977;59:299–307.
8. Nilsson L, Hudson, Hultman E. Liver glycogen in man—the effect of total starvation or a carbohydrate-poor diet followed by carbohydrate refeeding. *Scand J Clin Lab Invest* 1973;32:325–330.
9. Pozefsky T, Tancredi RG, Moxley RT, et al. Effects of brief starvation on muscle amino acid metabolism in nonobese man. *J Clin Invest* 1976;57:444–449.
10. Garty R, Vaisman H, Trostler N. Excretion of 3-methylhistidine in nonobese fasting subject. *Isr J Med Sci* 1985;21:817–821.
11. Giesecke K, Magnusson I, Ahlberg M, et al. Protein and amino acid metabolism during early starvation as reflected by excretion of urea and methylhistidines. *Metabolism* 1989;38:1196–1200.
12. Sherwin RS, Hendler RG, Felig P. Effect of diabetes mellitus and insulin on the turnover and metabolic response to ketones in man. *Diabetes* 1976;25:776–784.
13. Desrochers S, Dubreuil P, Brunet J, et al. Metabolism of (R,S)-1,3-butanediol acetoacetate esters, potential parenteral and enteral nutrients in conscious pigs. *Am J Physiol* 1995;268:E660–E667.
14. Desrochers S, David F, Garneau M, et al. Metabolism of R- and S-1,3-butanediol in perfused livers from meal-fed and starved rats. *Biochem J* 1992;285:647–653.
15. Tobin RB, Mehlman MA, Kies C, Fox HM, Soeldner JS. Nutritional and metabolic studies in humans with 1,3-butanediol. *Fed Proc* 1975;34:2171–2176.
16. Knill RI, Gelb AW. Ventilatory responses to hypoxia and hypercapnia during halothane sedation and anesthesia in man. *Anesthesiology* 1978;49:244–251.
17. Sollevi A, Lindahl SGE. Hypoxic and hypercapnic ventilatory responses during isoflurane sedation and anaesthesia in women. *Acta Anaesthesiol Scand* 1995;39:931–938.

18. Sjögren D, Sollevi A, Ebberyd A, Lindahl S. Poikilocapnic hypoxic ventilatory response in humans during 0.85 MAC isoflurane anesthesia. *Acta Anaesthesiol Scand* 1994;38:149–155.
19. Eriksson LI, Lennmarken C, Wyon N, Johnson A. Attenuated ventilatory response to hypoxaemia at vecuronium-induced partial neuromuscular block. *Acta Anaesthesiol Scand* 1992;36:710–715.
20. Eriksson LI, Sato M, Severinghaus JW. Effect of a vecuronium-induced partial neuromuscular block on hypxic ventilatory response. *Anesthesiology* 1993;78:693–699.
21. Wyon N, Eriksson LI, Yamanoto Y, Lindahl S. Vecuronium-induced depression of phrenic nerve activity during hypoxia in the rabbit. *Anesth Analg* 1996;82:1252–1256.
22. Piehl MA, Brown RS. Use of extreme position changes in acute respiratory failure. *Crit Care Med* 1976;4:13–14.
23. Brunet F. Extracorporeal and intravascular lung support in the treatment of ARDS. *Acta Anaesthesiol Scand* 1993;37:159–164.
24. Glenny RW, Lamm WJE, Albert RK, Robertson HT. Gravity is a minor determinant of pulmonary blood flow distribution. *J Appl Physiol* 1991;71:620–629.
25. Beck KC, Rehder K. Differences in regional vascular conductances in isolated dog lungs. *J Appl Physiol* 1986;64:350–538.
26. Mortensen D, Garrard CS, Phil D. Colorectal surgery comes in from the cold. *N Engl J Med* 1996;334:1263.
27. Frank SM, Beattie C, Christopherson R, Noris EJ, Perler BA. Unnintentional hypothermia is associated with postoperative myocardial ischemia. The perioperative ischemia randomized anesthesia trial study group. *Anesthesiology* 1993;78:468–476.
28. Schmied H, Kurz A, Sessler DI, Kozek S, Reiter A. Mild hypothermia increases blood loss and transfusion requirements during total hip arthroplasty. *Lancet* 1996;347:289–292.
29. Kurz A, Sessler DI, Lenhardt R. Perioperative normothermia to reduce the incidence of surgical-wound infection and shorten hospitalization. Study of wound infection and temperature group. *N Engl J Med* 1996;334:1209–1215.
30. Kurz A, Kurz M, Poeschl G, et al. Forced-air warming maintains intraoperative normothermia better than circulating-water mattresses. *Anesth Analg* 1993;77:89–95.
31. Selldén E, Brundin T, Wahren J. Augmented thermic effect of amino acids under general anaesthesia. A mechanism useful for prevention of anaesthesia-induced hypothermia. *Clin Sci* 1994;86:611–618.
32. Selldén E, Bränström R, Brundin T. Preoperative infusion of amino acids prevents postoperative hypothermia. *Br J Anaesth* 1996;96:227–234.
33. Brundin T. Temperature of mixed venous blood during exercise. *Scand J Clin Lab Invest* 1975;35:599–543.
34. Stubbs TA, MacDonald IA. Cardiovascular and metabolic responses to nasogastric and oral feeding in healthy, young volunteers. *Proceedings of the Nutrition Society.* 1997 (in press).
35. Brundin T, Wahren J. Whole-body and splanchnic oxygen consumption and blood flow after oral ingestion of fructose or glucose. *Am J Physiol* 1993;264:E504–E513.
36. Wahren J, Felig P, Hagenfeldt L. Effect of protein ingestion on splanchnic and leg metabolism in normal man and in patients with diabetes mellitus. *J Clin Invest* 1976;57:987–999.
37. Sidery MB, MacDonald AJ, Cowley AJ, Fullwood LJ. Cardiovascular responses to high-fat and high-carbohydrate meals in young subjects. *Am J Physiol* 1991;261:H1430–H1436.
38. Mansell PI, MacDonald IA. The effect of underfeeding on the physiological responses to food ingestion in normal weight women. *Br J Nutr* 1988;60:39–48.
39. Spraul M, Ravussin E, Baron AD. Lack of relationship between muscle sympathetic nerve activity and skeletal muscle vasodilation in response to insulin infusion. *Diabetologia* 1996;39:91–96.
40. Brundin T, Bränström R, Wahren J. Effects of intravenous versus oral glucose administration on oxygen consumption and blood flow in splanchnic and extra-splanchnic tissues. *Am J Physiol* 1996;271:E496–E504.
41. Brundin T, Wahren J. Effects of i.v. amino acids on human splanchnic and whole body oxygen consumption, blood flow and blood temperatures. *Am J Physiol* 1994;266:E396–E402.
42. Brundin T, Aksnes A-K, Wahren J. Influence of a non-selective b-adrenergic receptor blockade on whole body and splanchnic circulatory and metabolic response to glucose ingestion in man. *Am J Physiol* 1997 (in press).
43. Aksnes A-K, Brundin T, Hjeltnes N, Wahren J. Glucose-induced thermogenesis in tetraplegic patients with low sympatho-adrenal activity. *Am J Physiol* 1994;266:E161–E170.
44. Qamar MI, Read AE. Effects of ingestion of carbohydrate fat, protein, and water on the mesenteric blood flow in man. *Scand J Gastrenterol* 1988;23:26–30.

45. Waaler BA, Eriksen M. Post-prandial cardiovascular responses in man after ingestion of carbohydrate, protein or fat. *Acta Physiol Scand* 1992;146:321–327.
46. Brundin T, Wahren J. Influence of protein ingestion on human splanchnic and whole body oxygen consumption, blood flow and blood temperature. *Metabolism* 1994;43:626–632.
47. Brundin T, Hagenfeldt L, Söderberg R, Wahren J. Blood flow, substrate utilization and heat generation in tissues drained by the azygos vein in man. *Clin Physiol* 1987;7:481–491.
48. Brundin T, Wahren J. Influence of a mixed meal on splanchnic and interscapular energy expenditure in humans. *Am J Physiol* 1991;260:E232–237.
49. Thörne A, Wahren J. Beta-adrenergic blockade does not influence the thermogenic response to a mixed meal in man. *Clin Physiol* 1989;9:321–332.
50. Aksnes A-K, Brundin T, Hjeltnes N, Wahren J. Metabolic, thermal and circulatory effects of intravenous infusion of amino acids in tetraplegic patients. *Clin Physiol* 1995;15:377–396.
51. Aksnes A-K, Brundin T, Hjeltnes N, Maehlum S, Wahren J. Meal-induced rise in resting energy expenditure in patients with complete cervical spinal cord lesions. *Paraplegia* 1993;31:462–472.
52. Brundin T, Thörne A, Wahren J. Heat leakage across the abdominal wall and meal-induced thermogenesis in normal-weight and obese subjects. *Metab Clin Exp* 1992;41:49–55.
53. Thörne A, Hallberg D, Wahren J. Meal-induced thermogenesis in obese patients before and after weight reduction. *Clin Physiol* 1989;9:481–498.
54. Thörne A, Näslund I, Wahren J. Meal-induced thermogenesis in previously obese patients. *Clin Physiol* 1990;10:99–109.

Physiology, Stress, and Malnutrition: Functional Correlates, Nutritional Intervention,
edited by J.M. Kinney and H.N. Tucker.
Lippincott–Raven Publishers © 1997.

Pancreatic Islet B-Cell Responsiveness During Starvation

Willy J. Malaisse

Laboratory of Experimental Medicine, Brussels Free University, Brussels B-1070, Belgium

The secretion of insulin by the pancreas plays a key role in fuel homeostasis, and the metabolism of nutrients in islet B cells plays a key role in the regulation of their secretory activity. The endocrine pancreas can thus be viewed both as a sensor and a regulator of extracellular fuel availability.

Such a dual role is operative not solely in the rapid adjustment of extracellular nutrient concentration, for instance after food intake or during muscular exercise, but also participates in the long-term control of fuel homeostasis in situations such as growth, pregnancy, or starvation.

The major aim of the present report is to review current knowledge on the mechanisms by which the insulin-producing cells adapt their responsiveness to selected secretagogues in starvation.

STARVATION-INDUCED CHANGES IN B-CELL SECRETORY RESPONSIVENESS

In rats, the amount of insulin stored in the pancreas remains fairly stable for at least 2 days after the onset of starvation, and only decreases thereafter (1). In animals injected with guinea pig anti-insulin serum, the secretion of insulin, as judged from the progressive neutralization of the antibodies, is already decreased after 24 hours of starvation, even when the fed and fasted rats are examined at comparable plasma sugar concentrations (1).

Likewise, in pieces of pancreatic tissue removed from rats deprived of food for 1 or 2 days and incubated at a fixed concentration of D-glucose (11.1 or 27.8 mmol/L), the secretion of insulin occurs at a much lower rate than in pancreatic fragments prepared from fed animals, whereas the basal insulin output, as measured in the presence of 5.6 mmol/L D-glucose, is little affected (1). In vitro, the secretory response to other nutrient or non-nutrient secretagogues, such as D-glyceraldehyde, L-leucine, β-hydroxybutyrate, hypoglycemic sulfonylurea, or theophylline, is also little or not affected by starvation (2) (Fig. 1). Fasting not only decreases the maximal secretory response evoked by high concentrations of

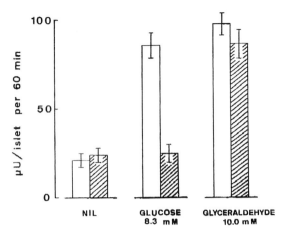

FIG. 1. Insulin output by islets removed from fed rats (open columns) and animals starved for 48 hours (hatched columns) and incubated in the absence of any exogenous nutrient or presence of either 8.3 mM D-glucose or 10.0 mM D-glyceraldehyde (2).

D-glucose (e.g., 27.8 mmol/L), but the concentration of the hexose required to cause half-maximal stimulation of insulin release is also higher in islets from fasted, as compared with fed, rats (3) (Fig. 2). Moreover, in glucose-stimulated islets, starvation increases the time required to reach a sustained secretory level (1).

These findings indicate that fasting can be considered a model for altered recognition of D-glucose by the pancreatic islet B-cell.

MECHANISM OF THE STARVATION EFFECT

Several mechanisms could conceivably account for the starvation-induced change in the B-cell secretory responsiveness to D-glucose. For instance, because the hypothalamus exerts a long-term control on pancreatic islet function and because the ingestion of noncaloric sweet-tasting drinks provides a feeling of well-being in human subjects undergoing total starvation, it was investigated whether the decrease in the insulin secretory response to D-glucose normally seen in fasted rats may be prevented by allowing the animals access to drinking water containing saccharin (3). In rats fasted for 24 or 48 hours, however, ingestion of the sweet drinking water failed to affect the fasting-induced changes in body weight, plasma insulin concentration, and insulin output from isolated islets incubated at increasing concentrations of D-glucose.

The effect of starvation upon the secretory behavior of the endocrine pancreas may be explained in part by an increase in the plasma concentration of free fatty acids, leading to the operation of a glucose fatty acid cycle in the islet B cells. However, methyl pyruvate, an inhibitor of the carnitine-dependent oxidation of

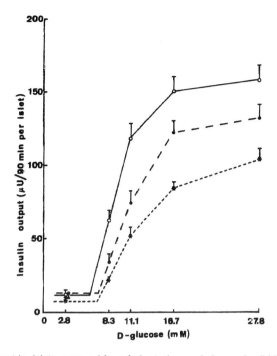

FIG. 2. Insulin output by islets removed from fed rats (open circles and solid line) and animals fasted for either 24 hours (closed circles and dashed lines) or 48 hours (asterisks and dotted line) (3).

long-chain fatty acids, fails to augment, and actually inhibits, insulin release evoked by D-glucose (16.7 mmol/L) in islets removed from 48-hour fasted rats. This occurred despite the fact that the concentration of methyl pyruvate (0.1 mmol/L) used in these experiments was sufficient to suppress the oxidation of exogenous [U-^{14}C]palmitate and to inhibit $^{14}CO_2$ output from islets prelabeled with [U-^{14}C]palmitate (4).

A better understanding of the mechanism by which starvation affects the secretory behavior of the B cell emerged from metabolic studies conducted in islets from either fed or starved rats, as indicated in the next section of this review.

METABOLIC STUDIES

The finding previously mentioned that starvation decreases the B-cell secretory response to D-glucose but fails to affect the insulinotropic action of D-glyceraldehyde represented a first indication that fasting may be associated with a block of D-glucose metabolism in the early steps of glycolysis, before the triose phosphate step (2). This view was further supported by the observation that starvation fails to affect either the oxidation of D-glyceraldehyde or the production of lactate by islets exposed to this triose, while decreasing the uptake of D-glucose and its oxidation and conversion to lactate (2).

Further studies indicated that starvation also affects the mitochondrial oxidative response of the islets to D-glucose. For instance, starvation decreases the ratio between D-[U-^{14}C]glucose oxidation and either D-[5-^{3}H]glucose use or the generation of ^{14}C-labeled acidic metabolites from the former tracer, this decrease being observed both at low and high concentrations of hexose (5). By comparing the fate of D-[5-^{3}H]glucose, D-[3,4-^{14}C]glucose, D-[6-^{14}C]glucose, and D-[2-^{14}C]glucose in islets from fed and starved rats, it was shown that starvation indeed decreases oxidative glycolysis more severely than nonoxidative glycolysis, impairs the preferential stimulation of D-[3,4-^{14}C]glucose oxidation relative to D-[5-^{3}H]glucose use as normally observed in response to an increase in hexose concentration, and lowers the ratio between D-[6-^{14}C]glucose oxidation and hexose use (6).

It should be stressed that these anomalies in the oxidative response of the islets to D-glucose do not necessarily imply a primary alteration of mitochondrial behavior. Indeed, in islets from fed rats, the preferential stimulation of mitochondrial oxidative events caused by an increase in D-glucose concentration involves the activation by either cytosolic or mitochondrial Ca^{2+} of key mitochondrial dehydrogenases, including FAD-linked glycerophosphate dehydrogenase (7), NAD-isocitrate dehydrogenase (8), and the 2-ketoglutarate dehydrogenase complex (9). Because starvation decreases the effect of D-glucose to stimulate [45]Ca net uptake by isolated pancreatic islets (2), this cationic defect, which is itself attributable to the impaired metabolism of D-glucose in islets from starved rats may partially account for the perturbation of the B-cell mitochondrial oxidative response in these same islets.

ENZYMATIC DATA

The experimental data reviewed so far suggest that a major primary determinant of the starvation-induced changes in B-cell function consists of an impairment of D-glucose metabolism in the early steps of glycolysis, this defect leading in turn to secretory changes in the mitochondrial steps of hexose catabolism.

It could be argued that even the alteration of D-glucose uptake and phosphorylation in islets from starved rats is secondary to a decreased functional response of the islets and, hence, a lesser consumption of adenosine triphosphate (ATP) by the energy-requiring processes of proinsulin biosynthesis and insulin release (2). Therefore, we considered that it would be more credible that the impairment of glycolysis represents a primary event if fasting were to be associated with a reduced activity of key glycolytic enzymes in islet homogenates. A decreased activity of glucokinase was indeed observed in homogenates of islets from fasted, as compared with fed, rats (10) (Fig. 3). The activity of the low-Km hexokinase and that of phosphoglucoisomerase were little or not affected. A

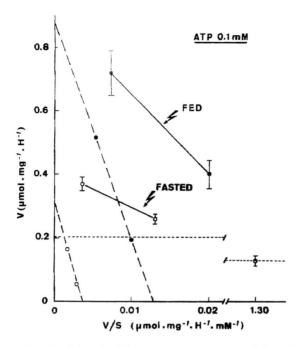

FIG. 3. Glucose phosphorylation by islet homogenates prepared from fed rats (closed circles) or animals starved for 48 hours (open circles). After correction for the contribution of the high affinity hexokinase (dotted lines), the residual values were plotted (dashed lines) to document the fasting-induced decrease in Vmax without change in Km of low affinity glucokinase (10).

modest decrease of phosphofructokinase activity also was observed in islets from starved rats.

The starvation-induced decrease in glucokinase activity was confirmed in subsequent reports (5,11). In addition to the incorporation of D-glucose 6-phosphate in the assay medium to inhibit the low-Km hexokinase preferentially, D-fructose 1-phosphate was used to relieve glucokinase from the potential inhibitory action of D-fructose 6-phosphate generated from exogenous D-glucose 6-phosphate.

In our most recent work, the decrease of glucokinase activity in islet homogenates prepared from rats starved for 48 hours was found to coincide with a lower glucokinase content, as documented in Western blots in which glucokinase was detected with a polyclonal sheep antiserum against an *Escherichia coli*–derived B1 isoform of rat glucokinase (11) (Fig. 4).

At variance with the finding of a decrease in glucokinase content and activity, starvation fails to affect the activity of key mitochondrial dehydrogenases in islet homogenates, including FAD-linked glycerophosphate dehydrogenase, 2-ketoglutarate dehydrogenase, and glutamate dehydrogenase. The specific activity of

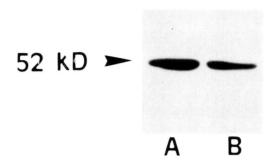

FIG. 4. Western blot for glucokinase in islets from fed rats (A) and animals starved for 48 hours (B) (11).

lactate dehydrogenase also fails to be significantly different in islets from fed and starved rats (12).

In starvation, a specific, or at least preferential, repression of glucokinase in the islet cells may obviously account for a decrease in D-glucose phosphorylation. However, this enzymatic adaptation may have a number of other metabolic consequences in intact islets. For instance, in pancreatic islets from rats fasted for 48 hours, the decrease in glucose-stimulated insulin release coincides with a suppression of the glucose-induced increment in both D-glucose 1,6-bisphosphate content and pyruvate and lactate output, despite unaltered activity of phosphoglucomutase (13). These findings suggest that, in islets from fasted rats, a reduced availability of D-fructose-1,6-bisphosphate and/or 1,3-diphospho-D-glycerate, secondary to both the repression of glucokinase and phosphofructokinase and the poor activation of the latter enzyme, may hamper the synthesis of D-glucose-1,6-bisphosphate. Such an interpretation is supported by the fact that in mouse islets exposed to 16.7 mmol/L D-glucose, fasting decreases the tissue content in D-fructose 1,6-bisphosphate and triose phosphates even when the D-glucose 6-phosphate content appears unaffected (14,15). The fasting-induced alteration of islet D-glucose metabolism would thus be due to impairment of the dual role of the hexose as a precursor of both glycolytic intermediates and suitable activator(s) of phosphofructokinase.

In this respect, it is interesting to note that starvation tends to minimize the anomeric preference of the B cell for α-D-glucose. There is indeed a trend toward a lesser secretory potential of α-D-glucose, relative to β-D-glucose, in the perfused pancreas of fasted, as distinct from fed, rats (16). This is compatible with an impaired activation of phosphofructokinase by D-glucose 1,6-bisphosphate in the islets of starved rats, because the process of D-glucose 1,6-bisphosphate synthesis, as catalyzed by the α-stereospecific phosphoglucomutase, participates in the anomeric specificity of the metabolic and, hence, secretory response to D-glucose (17).

A further example of a cause-to-effect link between the decrease in D-glucose phosphorylation by glucokinase and the alteration of more distal metabolic events in islets from starved rats relates to the impairment of the B-cell oxidative response to D-glucose, as described in the preceding section of this review. In this case again, the insufficient activation by Ca^{2+} of key mitochondrial dehydrogenases probably represents the mere consequence of the primary decrease in D-glucose phosphorylation.

To summarize the metabolic and enzymatic information so far provided in this review, it could be stated that, in the islets of starved rats, the repression of glucokinase and resulting decrease in D-glucose phosphorylation impedes subsequent regulatory mechanisms, such as the activation of phosphofructokinase or the preferential stimulation of mitochondrial oxidative events, that are otherwise operative in glucose-stimulated B cells and normally account for the high efficiency of their glucose-sensing device.

DETERMINANTS OF GLUCOKINASE REPRESSION

The apparent repression of B-cell glucokinase in starvation is most probably attributable to a lowering of plasma glucose concentration. The B-cell glucokinase, as distinct from liver glucokinase, is indeed currently considered as a glucose-inducible, rather than insulin-inducible, enzyme.

More precisely, the suppression of B-cell glucokinase in starvation may be due to the absence of the hyperglycemic waves that are normally associated with food intake. In support of such a view, it was reported, more than 25 years ago, that the intravenous administration of D-glucose loads and resulting burst of hyperglycemia prevent the starvation-induced decrease in B-cell secretory activity, even when the amount of D-glucose given could be considered as negligible in terms of caloric supply (18).

As reviewed in detail elsewhere, the long-term regulation of pancreatic B-cell responsiveness to D-glucose by food availability, feeding schedule and diet composition also supports the above-mentioned proposal (19). Thus, the results of experiments conducted in starved rats, in animals exposed to an altered feeding schedule, and in rats given free access to a high-carbohydrate, high-protein, or high-lipid, as distinct from balanced, diet all suggest that a sufficient prandial hyperglycemia is essential for maintenance of an optimal metabolic and secretory behavior of the islet B cell in response to an increase in D-glucose concentration (19).

In order to further explore this issue, attempts were made to simulate in vitro the situation encountered in starvation, as indicated in the next section of this review.

IN VITRO MODELS OF GLUCOSE DEPRIVATION

Two models were developed to study in vitro the consequences of glucose deprivation. In the first model, pancreatic islets are preincubated for 180 minutes at increasing concentrations of D-glucose before assessing their secretory responsiveness to the hexose. Under these conditions, a concentration-related priming action of D-glucose is observed (20). Like in starvation, the response to D-glucose (16.7 mmol/L) is indeed much lower after preincubation at low (2.8 mmol/L), as distinct from high (16.7 mmol/L), hexose concentration. This contrasts with the fact that, during the final incubation, both the basal insulin output and the release of insulin provoked by 2-ketoisocaproate, taken as representative of a nonglucidic nutrient, are nearly identical in islets first preincubated at either low or high D-glucose concentration (20,21).

The concentration of D-glucose used during the preincubation period also affects the metabolic behavior of the islets. Indeed, the oxidation of D-[U-^{14}C]glucose, relative to either the use of D-[5-^{3}H]glucose or the generation of ^{14}C-labeled acidic metabolites, is lower in islets preincubated at 2.8 mmol/L D-glucose than in the islets preincubated at 16.7 mmol/L D-glucose (5).

In the second model, islets are cultured for 20–72 hours at increasing concentrations of D-glucose and then examined for their metabolic and secretory behavior (5,21). The release of insulin measured over 60–90 minutes incubation in the presence of D-glucose (16.7 mmol/L) is again increased as a function of the hexose concentration (2.8 to 11.1 mmol/L) in the culture medium (21,22). Likewise, the use of D-[5-^{3}H]glucose and oxidation of D-[6-^{14}C]glucose during the final incubation of 90 minutes increases as a function of the hexose concentration present in the culture medium during the initial 72-hour period (5). This coincides with a preferential increase of glucokinase, relative to hexokinase, activity in the islets first cultured at a high concentration of D-glucose (5). Once again, the secretory response of the islets to the nonglucidic nutrient 2-ketoisocaproate, as distinct from that evoked by D-glucose, is not increased after culturing the islets at high, rather than low, hexose concentration (21).

These data indicate that it is indeed feasible to simulate in vitro, by exposing the islets to low or high concentrations of D-glucose for a sufficient length of time, the changes in secretory, metabolic, and enzymatic activities otherwise caused by starvation.

PREVENTION OF THE EFFECTS CAUSED BY HEXOSE DEPRIVATION OR STARVATION

In several animal models of non–insulin-dependent diabetes mellitus, the B cell often displays a preferential alteration of its secretory response to D-glucose, as distinct from other nutrient or non-nutrient secretagogues (23,24). This situation is comparable with that found in starvation. The models of starvation or hexose deprivation could thus be used to explore the long-term effects on B-cell function of selected agents that are contemplated as possible tools to restore the secretory potential of the endocrine pancreas in type 2 diabetes.

Along this line of thinking, we have recently investigated whether nonglucidic nutrients, especially the esters of succinic acid, are able to protect the B-cell against the unfavorable effects of starvation and glucose deprivation.

The selection of the esters of succinic acid for such a purpose is motivated by two major considerations. First, at variance with succinic acid itself, its esters penetrate efficiently into islet cells, in which they undergo hydrolysis, so that succinic acid then becomes readily available for mitochondrial metabolism (25,26). Second, succinic acid, considered as a mitochondrial fuel, is well suited to bypass those site-specific defects in hexose transport, phosphorylation, and further metabolism currently held responsible for the preferential alteration of the B-cell response to D-glucose in non–insulin-dependent diabetes (24).

The monomethyl ester of succinic acid (SAM) was indeed found to protect the B cell against the impairment of glucose-stimulated insulin release caused by either glucose deprivation or starvation (21). This was documented in three distinct experimental models (Fig. 5). In the first model, preincubation of the islets for 180 minutes at low glucose concentration in the presence of SAM prevented

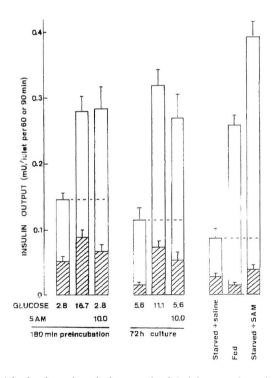

FIG. 5. Basal (hatched columns) and glucose-stimulated (open columns) insulin release in islets preincubated for 180 minutes (left panel) at low (2.8 mM) or high (16.7 mM) hexose concentration in the absence or presence of the monomethyl ester of succinic acid (SAM; 10 mM), in islets first cultured for 72 hours (middle panel) at low (5.6 mM) or high (11.1 mM) hexose concentration in the absence or presence of SAM (10 mM), and in islets removed from fed rats and starved animals infused for 3 days with either saline or an isotonic solution of SAM sodium salt (60µmol/g body wt per day) (21).

the decrease in the secretory response to D-glucose otherwise observed during a subsequent incubation. In the second model, an impaired secretory response to D-glucose was observed after a 3-day culture at low (2.8 or 5.6 mmol/L) as distinct from high (11.1 mmol/L) hexose concentration and the presence of SAM in the culture medium again protected against this anomaly. In the third model, the infusion of SAM for 3 days to starved rats restored the secretory potential of isolated islets to a level comparable with that found in fed rats.

In a further study, the metabolic determinants of this protective effect of SAM were explored (5) (Fig. 6). Within limits, SAM was found to improve the metabolic behavior of the islets in the three experimental models mentioned above. To cite only one example, the infusion of SAM to starved rats prevented the decrease in islet glucokinase activity that was otherwise observed when comparing fed rats to starved animals (5).

The infusion of the dimethyl ester of succinic acid (SAD) to starved rats also prevents the starvation-induced B-cell desensitization to D-glucose (27). The finding that SAD, like SAM, exerts a long-term positive effect on the secretory potential of insulin-producing cells was considered of interest because SAD offers the far-from-negligible advantage over SAM of remaining efficient as an insulinotropic agent when administered enterally (28,29). However, the conduct of experiments including the oral intake of SAD over several days was hampered by the apparent unpalatability of the ester (30). This was eventually overcome by

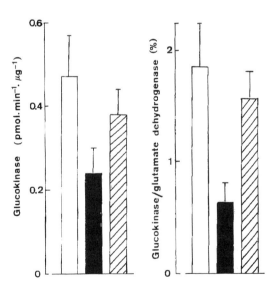

FIG. 6. Glucokinase activity in islet homogenates from fed rats (open columns) and starved animals infused with either saline (solid columns) or the monomethyl ester of succinic acid (hatched columns). The results are expressed in absolute terms (left) or relative to the paired measurement of glutamate dehydrogenase activity (right) (5).

conditioning normal rats to the oral administration of SAD (31). Even so, the oral intake of SAD by the conditioned rats failed to prevent the starvation-induced impairment of glucose-stimulated insulin release in these animals (32). This appears attributable to the fact that, under these experimental conditions, the absorption of SAD from the gastrointestinal tract is too low to duplicate a rate of SAD delivery into the bloodstream comparable with that achieved in SAD-infused rats.

Despite the latter limitation, the use of SAM, SAD, and other esters of succinic acid (33–35) as possible tools in the treatment of type 2 diabetes remains, at least from the conceptual standpoint, an interesting perspective.

Moreover, the knowledge that these esters are efficiently metabolized in islet cells raises the question whether they could also be used in other cell types endangered by an imbalance between ATP synthesis and breakdown.

METABOLIC, HORMONAL, AND ENZYMATIC EFFECTS OF SAD IN STARVED RATS

In order to answer the latter question, we have first documented that SAD supports ATP generation in isolated hepatocytes (36) and colonocytes (37) while being less efficiently metabolized in muscle (38) or neural (39) cells. The overall nutritional value of SAD in the whole organism was eventually assessed by infusing the ester at a rate of 80 μmol/g body weight for either 2 or 4 days in starved rats (40). The ester failed to prevent the starvation-induced decrease in body weight, paraovarian fat mass, and liver or muscle protein content. However, the infusion of SAD minimized the decrease in plasma glucose and insulin concentrations, liver glycogen content, hepatic glucokinase activity, and, as expected, islet secretory responsiveness to D-glucose, otherwise caused by starvation. Likewise, the infusion of SAD delayed the increase in free fatty acid and β-hydroxybutyrate plasma concentration occurring during starvation.

CONCLUDING REMARKS

The starvation-induced change in the responsiveness of the pancreatic islet B cell may appear at the first glance to be a rather narrow topic. Yet, the present review illustrates that a number of lessons can be drawn from the study of this phenomenon. It is relevant to the regulation of fuel homeostasis both in the whole organism and at the B-cell level. It provides essential information concerning the organization of the B-cell glucose-sensing device, with emphasis on the role of both glucokinase and more distal regulatory steps in the control of D-glucose metabolism. It simulates the preferential impairment of the B-cell secretory response to D-glucose in non–insulin-dependent diabetes. As such, it provides a model to study the immediate and long-term effects on the endocrine pancreas of other nutrients, such as the esters of succinic acid, that could be used to bypass site-specific defects of hexose metabolism in the diabetic B cell. The usefulness of such alternative nutrients may not be restricted to islet cells, whether in starvation or other situations in which fuel availability represents a critical issue. In fact, it was recently proposed that the esters of succinic acid may be helpful in the treatment of endotoxemia and multiple organ failure (41), a long way, indeed, from the impairment of insulin release in starved rats.

ACKNOWLEDGMENTS

Recent experimental work mentioned in this review was supported by grants from the Belgian Foundation for Scientific Medical Research and a Concerted Research Action of the French Community of Belgium. I thank C. Demesmaeker for secretarial help.

REFERENCES

1. Malaisse WJ, Malaisse-Lagae F, Wright PH. Effect of fasting upon insulin secretion in the rat. *Am J Physiol* 1967;213:843–848.
2. Levy J, Herchuelz A, Sener A, Malaisse WJ. The stimulus-secretion coupling of glucose-induced insulin release. XX. Fasting: a model for altered glucose recognition by the B-cell. *Metabolism* 1976; 25:583–591.
3. Segura MC, Malaisse WJ. Failure of noncaloric sweet drinking to prevent the fasting-induced inhibition of insulin release. *Ann Nutr Metab* 1987;31:272–275.
4. Malaisse WJ, Malaisse-Lagae F, Sener A, Hellerström C. Participation of endogenous fatty acids in the secretory activity of the pancreatic B-cell. *Biochem J* 1985;227:995–1002.
5. Eizirik DL, Welsh N, Sener A, Malaisse WJ. Protective action of succinic acid monomethyl ester against the impairment of glucose-stimulated insulin release caused by glucopenia or starvation :metabolic determinants. *Biochem Med Metab Biol* 1994;53:34–45.
6. Malaisse WJ, Malaisse-Lagae F. Hexose metabolism in pancreatic islets. Oxidative response to D-glucose in fed and starved rats. *Acta Diabetol* 1992;29:94–98.
7. Rasschaert J, Malaisse WJ. Hexose metabolism in pancreatic islets. Glucose-induced and Ca^{2+}-dependent activation of FAD-glycerophosphate dehydrogenase. *Biochem J* 1991;278:335–340.
8. Rasschaert J, Malaisse WJ. Hexose metabolism in pancreatic islets. Regulation of NAD-isocitrate dehydrogenase activity. *Biochem Med Metab Biol* 1992;48:32–40.
9. Sener A, Rasschaert J, Malaisse WJ. Hexose metabolism in pancreatic islets. Participation of Ca^{2+}-sensitive 2-ketoglutarate dehydrogenase in the regulation of mitochondrial function. *Biochim Biophys Acta* 1990;1019:42–50.
10. Malaisse WJ, Sener A, Levy J. The stimulus-secretion coupling of glucose-induced insulin release. XXI. Fasting-induced adaptation of key glycolytic enzymes in isolated islets. *J Biol Chem* 1996;251:1731–1737.
11. Gasa R, Sener A, Malaisse WJ, Gomis R. Apparent starvation-induced repression of pancreatic islet glucokinase. *Biochem Mol Med* 1995;56:99–103.
12. Rasschaert J, Malaisse WJ. Activity of key mitochondrial dehydrogenases in pancreatic islets of starved rats. *Med Sci Res* 1994;22:339–340.
13. Giroix M-H, Dufrane SP, Malaisse-Lagae F, et al. Fasting-induced impairment of glucose-1,6-bisphosphate synthesis in pancreatic islets. *Biochem Biophys Res Commun* 1984;119:543–548.
14. Idahl L-A. Dynamics of pancreatic β-cell responses to glucose. *Diabetologia* 1973;9:403–412.
15. Hedeskov CJ, Capito K. The effect of starvation in insulin secretion and glucose metabolism in mouse pancreatic islets. *Biochem J* 1974;140:423–433.
16. Leclercq-Meyer V, Marchand J, Malaisse WJ. Effect of starvation upon the anomeric specificity of glucose-induced insulin release. *Diab Nutr Metab* 1993;6:129–134.

17. Malaisse-Lagae F, Sener A, Malaisse WJ. Phospho-glucomutase: its role in the response of pancreatic islets to glucose epimers and anomers. *Biochimie* 1982;64:1059–1063.
18. Grey NJ, Goldring S, Kipnis DH. The effects of fasting, diet and actinomycin D on insulin secretion in the rat. *J Clin Invest* 1970;49:881–889.
19. Carpinelli AR, Curi R, Malaisse WJ. Long-term regulation of pancreatic B-cell responsiveness to D-glucose by food availability, feeding schedule, and diet composition. *Physiol Behav* 1992;52: 1193–1196.
20. Malaisse WJ, Sener A. Interaction between D-glucose and Ca^{2+} in the priming of the pancreatic B-cell. *Diab Res* 1987;4:5–8.
21. Conget I, Zhang T-M, Eizirik DL, Malaisse WJ. SAM prevents impairment of glucose-stimulated insulin secretion caused by hexose deprivation or starvation. *Am J Physiol* 1995;268:E580–E587.
22. Malaisse-Lagae F, Sener A, Malaisse WJ. Can desensitization of the B-cell to D-glucose be simulated in cultured pancreatic islets? *Acta Diabetol Lat* 1987;24:17–25.
23. Malaisse WJ. Alteration of pancreatic B-cell D-glucose metabolism in type 2 diabetes: the G quintet. *Endocrinologia* 1993;40:309–313.
24. Malaisse WJ. The beta cell in non-insulin-dependent diabetes: giving light to the blind. *Diabetologia* 1994;37(suppl 2):S36–S42.
25. Malaisse WJ, Rasschaert J, Villanueva-Peñacarrillo ML, Valverde I. Respiratory, ionic and functional effects of succinate esters in pancreatic islets. *Am J Physiol* 1993;264:E428–E433.
26. Malaisse WJ, Sener A. Metabolic effects and fate of succinate esters in pancreatic islets. *Am J Physiol* 1993;264:E434–E440.
27. Malaisse WJ. Prevention of starvation-induced B-cell desensitisation to D-glucose by infusion of succinic acid dimethyl ester. *Med Sci Res* 1995;23:375–376.
28. Malaisse-Lagae F, Zhang T-M, Bakkali Nadi A, Malaisse WJ. Insulinotropic efficiency of enterally administered succinic acid dimethyl ester. *Med Sci Res* 1994;22:365–367.
29. Malaisse-Lagae F, Bakkali Nadi A, Malaisse WJ. Insulinotropic response to enterally administered succinic and glutamic acid methyl esters. *Arch Int Pharmacodyn* 1994;328:235–242.
30. Malaisse-Lagae F, Malaisse WJ. Apparent unpalatability of succinic acid dimethyl ester. *Med Sci Res* 1995;23:131–132.
31. Malaisse-Lagae F, Bakkali Nadi A, Zhang T-M, Malaisse WJ. Conditioning of normal rats to the oral administration of succinic acid dimethyl ester. *Med Sci Res* 1995;23:435–438.
32. Malaisse-Lagae F, Zhang T-M, Bakkali Nadi A, Malaisse WJ. Failure of succinic acid dimethyl ester oral intake to prevent the starvation-induced impairment of glucose-stimulated insulin release. *Diab Res* 1995;28:111–119.
33. Malaisse WJ, Zhang T-M, Leclercq-Meyer V, Sener A, Björkling F. Insulinotropic action of the D-glucosyl and 3-O-methyl-D-glucosyl monomethyl esters of succinic acid. *Diab Res* 1994;25:93–105.
34. Malaisse WJ, Blaehr L, Björkling F. Insulinotropic action of new succinic acid esters. *Med Sci Res* 1995;23:9–10.
35. Björkling F, Malaisse-Lagae F, Malaisse WJ. Insulinotropic action of novel succinic acid esters. *Pharmacol Res* 1996;33:273–275.
36. Zhang T-M, Sener A, Malaisse WJ. Metabolic effects and fate of succinic acid methyl esters in rat hepatocytes. *Arch Biochem Biophys* 1994;314:186–192.
37. Zhang T-M, Jijakli H, Malaisse WJ. Nutritional efficiency of succinic acid and glutamic acid dimethyl esters in colon carcinoma cells. *Am J Physiol* 1996;270:G852–G859.
38. Zhang T-M, Rasschaert J, Malaisse WJ. Metabolism of succinic acid methyl esters in myocytes. *Clin Nutr* 1995;14:166–170.
39. Zhang T-M, Rasschaert J, Malaisse WJ. Metabolism of succinic acid methyl ester in neural cells. *Biochem Mol Med* 1995;54:112–116.
40. Ladrière L, Zhang T-M, Malaisse WJ. Effects of succinic acid dimethyl ester infusion upon metabolic, hormonal and enzymatic variables in starved rats. *J Parent Enter Nutr* 1996;20:251–256.
41. Malaisse WJ, Bakkali Nadi A, Ladrière L, Zhang T-M. Protective effects of succinic acid dimethyl ester infusion in experimental endotoxemia. *Nutrition* 1997 (in press).

Physiology, Stress, and Malnutrition: Functional Correlates, Nutritional Intervention, edited by J.M. Kinney and H.N. Tucker. Lippincott–Raven Publishers © 1997.

Extracellular Metabolic Regulation in Adipose Tissue

Keith N. Frayn, Barbara A. Fielding, Jaswinder S. Samra, and Lucinda K. M. Summers

Oxford Lipid Metabolism Group, Radcliffe Infirmary, Oxford OX2 6HE, United Kingdom

White adipose tissue is important in the regulation of whole-body energy metabolism, particularly of whole-body lipid metabolism. Just as the insulin responsiveness of glucose metabolism in skeletal muscle determines the whole-body sensitivity of glucose metabolism to insulin, so it may be argued that the sensitivity to insulin of metabolic processes in white adipose tissue determines many aspects of whole-body lipid metabolism (1).

Unlike skeletal muscle, adipose tissue is predominantly involved in exchange with the blood of hydrophobic and insoluble metabolites, nonesterified fatty acids (NEFA) and triacylglycerol (TAG), in both the fasting and fed states. It is now appreciated that regulation of the perfusion of skeletal muscle may play an important role in modulation of glucose metabolism (2,3). In the case of a tissue whose major exchanges are of hydrophobic substances, unable to diffuse through any distance without specialized carrier systems, it seems a priori even more probable that there will be intimate relationships between blood flow and metabolic regulation. The essential relationships between the vascular system and the metabolism of adipose tissue are highlighted by considering the enzyme lipoprotein lipase (LPL), a key enzyme in the delivery of fatty acids to the tissue for storage. Although this enzyme is synthesized within adipocytes, it must act on TAG in lipoprotein particles, which are too large to cross the endothelial barrier. LPL is therefore exported from the adipocytes to the capillaries, where it is attached to the luminal side of the endothelial cells so as to act upon passing lipoprotein particles. Thus, a key enzyme in adipose tissue metabolic regulation and a key target for insulin action is situated in an extracellular environment.

Two seminal papers that drew attention to the possibility of extracellular metabolic regulation in adipose tissue were published from the laboratory of Jules Hirsch about 6 years ago (4,5). It is well known that fatty acids released from stored, intracellular TAG may be re-esterified within the tissue. It has usually been assumed that this happens within the adipocyte cytosol. In those papers, however, fatty acids were shown to follow an extracellular pathway before re-esterification. Thus, their fate might be determined by blood flow through the tissue as well as by purely metabolic (intracellular) events. Superficially this seems an unnecessarily complicated metabolic pathway. In this review we shall add additional evidence for this extracellular pathway and try to build it into a picture of metabolism and metabolic regulation in adipose tissue in which the close relationship between metabolism and blood flow plays a central role.

MICROANATOMY OF ADIPOSE TISSUE METABOLISM

Vascularity

Adipose tissue is relatively well vascularized, at least in relation to its volume of cytoplasm (6). At least one capillary appears to make contact with each cell (7). Resting blood flow in subcutaneous white adipose tissue is typically 3–4 ml/100 g tissue/min, to be compared with around 1.5 ml/100 ml tissue/min for resting skeletal muscle (8). This blood flow might seem excessive if viewed in relation to the oxygen consumption of the tissue (Table 1), but this emphasizes the fact that adipose tissue is involved primarily in the exchange with blood of hydrophobic substrates, and O_2 consumption is not a major feature of adipose tissue metabolism (9).

Fat Deposition

The major route for fat deposition in adipocytes, at least in humans on a typical Western diet in which fat supplies a large proportion of energy, is the uptake of preformed fatty acids from the plasma TAG-rich lipoproteins. These comprise chylomicrons, the largest of the lipoprotein particles, which carry dietary fat absorbed in the small intestine, and very low density lipoproteins (VLDLs), which carry endogenous TAG secreted from the liver. Within the capillaries of adipose tissue these particles interact with LPL molecules (actually homo-dimers) attached to heparan sulphate glycosaminoglycan chains forming the

TABLE 1. *Blood flow in relation to oxygen consumption in various tissues*

	Skeletal muscle (resting)	Skeletal muscle (maximal work)	Brain	Liver	Adipose tissue
Blood flow (ml/min/kg wet weight)	15	1,100	540	1,000	30
O_2 consumption (ml/min/kg wet weight)	3	125	34	44	0.3
Blood flow per unit O_2 delivered to tissue (ml blood/ml O_2)	5	9	16	23	100

Data from various sources (8,10–12).

endothelial glycocalyx (Fig. 1). It is known from the kinetic properties of purified LPL that around 40 molecules of LPL must act on a particle at one time to achieve maximal rates of TAG hydrolysis (14,15). It is also known that, at least in vitro, LPL is specific for the *sn*-1 and *sn*-3 positions on a TAG molecule, and the resultant *sn*-2 monoacylglcyerol (MAG) can be hydrolyzed by LPL only after isomerization to the *sn*-1(3)-MAG (15,16). The use of TAG molecules labeled in both the fatty acid and glycerol moieties has shown that hydrolysis by LPL is a prerequisite for uptake by adipose tissue (17,18), also confirming that the monoacylglycerol esterification pathway is of minor significance in adipocytes (19,20). The latter point is not surprising in view of the high activities of monoacylglycerol lipase present both extracellularly (21) and intracellularly (22). In our own studies of LPL action in human subcutaneous adipose tissue in vivo, discussed further below, we have found no liberation of MAG into the adipose-venous plasma even during the highest rates of LPL action (prolonged insulin infusion after a high-fat meal), showing that if MAG is not taken up into adipocytes (for which there is no direct evidence), it is hydrolyzed very efficiently somewhere in the extracellular space (23,24).

The fatty acids released by the action of LPL may therefore be taken up by adipocytes for activation [formation of the coenzyme A (CoA)-ester], esterification by the phosphatidic acid pathway, and storage as TAG. The route by which LPL-released fatty acids reach the adipocytes is of great interest, but far from clear. They are unlikely to diffuse freely from the site of LPL action, through the endothelium to the adipocytes. This problem was investigated by Scow et al. in the 1960s and 1970s (25). By studies of the physiology of fat deposition (e.g., using perfused adipose tissue preparations) and by electron microscopy, they developed a model in which fatty acids were sequentially removed from a TAG

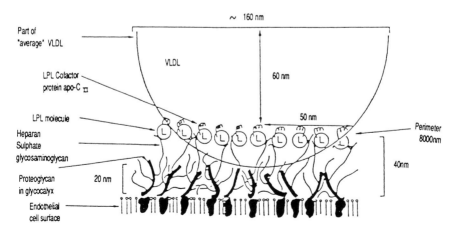

FIG. 1. Relationship of lipoprotein lipase (circles marked L) to endothelial cell surface and to a lipoprotein particle (a VLDL particle is shown). Reproduced with permission (13).

molecule (14). This model suggested that the *sn*-1 and *sn*-3 fatty acids were removed in the capillary lumen and during passage through endothelial cell fenestrations, leaving a MAG molecule that was hydrolyzed in the subendothelial space (although the enzyme responsible for hydrolysis of this last fatty acid was uncertain) (14,18). The fatty acids released from TAG hydrolysis were thought to flow by diffusion in membranous structures, which formed extensions of the adipocyte cell membrane (14). An alternative suggestion to the membranous arrangement suggested by Scow et al. is the presence of a relatively structured environment in which albumin is sequestered, through which fatty acids can move by virtue of their binding affinity for albumin (26). There has been considerable interest in links between albumin binding sites on adipocytes or endothelial cells and the transport of fatty acids in adipose tissue (27–30), although the position is still not clear.

Whatever the precise structural basis for the movement of fatty acids from the site of LPL action to the adipocyte, some major points are clear. The process appears to be one of facilitated diffusion: there is no evidence for active transport of fatty acids, which seem to follow concentration gradients between capillaries and cells (31). Not all the fatty acids released by LPL enter the adipocytes: a proportion are always released into the venous plasma. This has long been clear from animal studies (20,32) and has been confirmed in a number of ways in humans, most clearly by the use of isotopic tracers to follow TAG-fatty acids. Such studies show the rapid entry of TAG-fatty acids into the plasma NEFA pool, at an enrichment that is far too great for them to have entered the TAG storage pool en route (33–35). On the other hand, LPL-derived fatty acids do not appear to be in equilibrium initially with plasma NEFA. There is no evidence for net uptake of plasma NEFA into adipose tissue. Labeled fatty acids injected directly into the extracellular compartment of adipose tissue equilibrate rapidly with a cellular fatty acid pool and may be taken up by adipocytes and esterified, but they do not exchange rapidly with the intravascular pool (36). Studies with cell preparations (mammary cells) show that the LPL-derived fatty acids that are taken up into the cells for esterification do not equilibrate with NEFA in the medium (37). Our own studies, in which we have looked at regulation of the partitioning of LPL-derived fatty acids between tissue uptake and release into plasma, are discussed further below.

Because this loss of fatty acids into the venous plasma occurs at a time when one would expect, a priori, that the metabolic drive in adipocytes would be toward fat storage, it might appear a wasteful process. However, it appears to be tissue specific. Skeletal muscle and myocardium both express LPL at high activities, but there is no evidence that either of these tissues releases NEFA into the circulation during the hydrolysis of circulating TAG. [Some net release of NEFA across typical muscle preparations such as the human forearm is explained by the contribution of small numbers of adipocytes to the venous drainage (38,39).] This suggests that the loss of LPL-derived fatty acids has a functional role in adipose tissue. It has been argued that it constitutes a metabolic branch-point, conferring additional precision on the regulation of net fatty acid storage (40).

Fat Mobilization

The process of liberation of fatty acids from the TAG droplet within adipocytes is initiated by the enzyme hormone-sensitive lipase (HSL). HSL is an intracellular enzyme, unrelated structurally to LPL, and regulated on a minute-to-minute basis by reversible phosphorylation at a single serine residue (41). Phosphorylation of the enzyme is mediated by the cyclic adenosine monophosphate (cAMP)-dependent protein kinase, protein kinase A, in response to an elevation in the cAMP concentration. This in turn is brought about by the binding to receptors of hormones that activate adenylate cyclase. In human adipose tissue, the major regulators are probably epinephrine and norepinephrine (42). In many physiologic situations it appears that HSL is regulated more by inhibitory influences, including insulin, α_2-agonists, and adenosine, all of which act by lowering the cellular cAMP concentration (43–45).

The phosphorylation of HSL may affect its intracellular location. There is evidence that phosphorylation leads to translocation of the enzyme to the surface of the TAG droplet (46). Other proteins such as the perilipins may be involved in this process (47–49). HSL acts on the stored TAG, liberating fatty acids. Again there is evidence that in vitro HSL action results in generation of a MAG, which would be hydrolyzed by the very active intracellular MAG-lipase of adipose tissue (22). During high rates of catecholamine-stimulated lipolysis, intracellular MAG and DAG may accumulate (50), but this must be only temporary because there is no net release of either MAG or DAG from adipose tissue (23). Thus, three fatty acids and one molecule of glycerol are liberated from each molecule of TAG hydrolyzed.

The fate of these fatty acids is determined by the nutritional and hormonal state. A proportion may be re-esterified within the tissue in an apparently futile cycle, although again it can be argued that the existence of such a cycle would give very precise control to the process of fat mobilization. It is this step, of re-esterification, that Edens et al. suggested to occur via an extracellular pathway (5), raising again the possibility of extracellular metabolic regulation in adipose tissue. There is additional evidence for this suggestion from studies of differentiated adipocytes in culture (51). Labeled fatty acids present in the medium are taken up and esterified to TAG, but there is almost no mixing with intracellular fatty acids released in lipolysis: it was estimated that > 99% of endogenous intracellular fatty acids were excluded from the esterification pathway. Again, these results would be neatly explained if entry to the esterification pathway was via a separate pool requiring export from the cell and re-entry across the cell membrane.

Relationships Between Fat Storage and Fat Mobilization: Pools of Fatty Acids Within Adipose Tissue

Fatty acids must therefore flow both into and out of adipocytes, and indeed into and out of adipose tissue as a whole. In general, fat mobilization tends to be active in situations such as starvation and exercise, when fat deposition is likely to be low, and vice versa, but it is not plausible to suggest that only one process or the other can occur at any one time. In the situation of transition from fasting to fed state after a meal, for instance, there is likely to be a smooth transition from a state of mainly fat mobilization to one in which fat deposition predominates. Our own estimates of the rates of action in vivo of the enzymes HSL and LPL (Fig. 2) bear out the idea that both may be active simultaneously. This raises the question of how the movement of fatty acids is controlled. In principle there might be separate channeling of HSL-derived fatty acids, moving from cells into capillaries, and of LPL-derived fatty acids moving in the opposite direction. No structural basis for such channeling has ever been produced. Instead, all the evidence suggests a common pool of HSL- and LPL-derived fatty acids.

Our studies of human adipose tissue metabolism in vivo have provided some information on this subject. The principle of these studies, based on selective catheterization of a vein draining the subcutaneous adipose tissue of the anterior

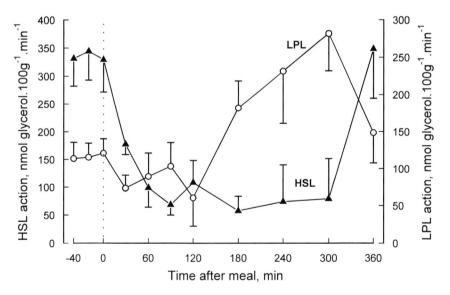

FIG. 2. Rates of action of hormone-sensitive lipase (HSL) and lipoprotein lipase (LPL) in subcutaneous adipose tissue in vivo in 13 normal subjects, before and after eating a mixed meal. The rate of action of LPL is calculated from the extraction of plasma TAG across the tissue. The rate of action of HSL is assumed to represent the difference between LPL-derived glycerol and total glycerol efflux from the tissue, assuming that each lipase releases glycerol mole for mole with TAG hydrolysis (31). Reproduced with permission (9).

abdominal wall, was outlined in an earlier volume in this series (12). Considerable evidence shows that the blood obtained in this way represents relatively pure drainage from adipose tissue (52). As already discussed, our studies show that LPL and HSL are usually simultaneously active (Fig. 2), although as expected HSL predominates in the postabsorptive state (after overnight fast) and LPL in the postprandial state. It is clear from measurement of the fatty acids released into the venous plasma that in the postprandial state, especially, the rate of action of HSL is not sufficient to account for all NEFA release. A proportion of LPL-derived fatty acids must therefore "escape" by this route (31,53). It is possible to estimate the proportion of fatty acids liberated from TAG that are re-esterified in the tissue, based on the assumption that glycerol released in the process of TAG hydrolysis is not reused in the tissue (54,55); if there were no re-esterification, the ratio of NEFA to glycerol release from the tissue would be 3:1, and departures from this ratio indicate the extent of re-esterification. The proportion of fatty acids re-esterified within the tissue is dependent on the nutritional state and changes with time after a meal (Fig. 3). This figure for proportional re-esterification applies to the sum of LPL- and HSL-derived fatty acids. We have tried to estimate separately the proportion of LPL-derived fatty acids that are re-esterified by making extreme assumptions about the fate of HSL-derived fatty acids (e.g., all escape re-esterification, or 100% re-esterification). Only one assumption

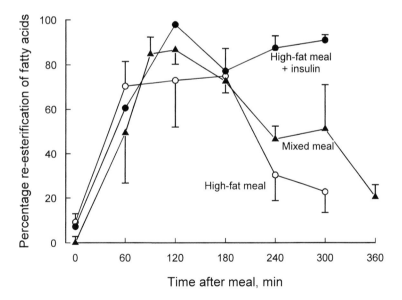

FIG. 3. Percentage re-esterification of fatty acids in subcutaneous adipose tissue in vivo in normal subjects after overnight fast (time zero) and after eating a mixed meal (3.1 MJ, 33 g fat) (▲) or a high-fat meal (4.7 MJ, 80 g fat) (○). In some experiments additional insulin was infused from 30 min after the high-fat meal (●). Percentage re-esterification is calculated from the ratio of non-esterified fatty acid to glycerol release (31). Reproduced with permission (40).

produces consistently plausible results in all physiologic situations in which we have applied it: that there is equal proportional re-esterification of HSL- and LPL-derived fatty acids (31). This does not, of course, prove, but it is entirely consistent with, a model in which HSL- and LPL-derived fatty acids enter a common pool from which esterification takes place.

The studies summarized above lead to some conclusions about the distribution of fatty acids within adipose tissue. Fatty acids released in intracellular lipolysis by HSL must apparently leave the adipocyte before re-esterification, and clearly before release into the plasma as NEFA. LPL-derived fatty acids may be released as NEFA into the plasma but appear initially to enter a pool that is not in equilibrium with plasma NEFA. Our own data fit with the idea that there is a common pool of fatty acids released from both HSL and LPL action, from which fatty acids may be drawn for esterification or for release as plasma NEFA. We have no direct information on the location of any such pool. Esterification is, of course, a cytosolic process, whereas LPL-derived fatty acids are, at least initially, in the extracellular space. From the various lines of evidence presented earlier, it is possible that this pool exists somewhere in the extracellular environment, perhaps in equilibrium with an intracellular pool by means of an adipocyte fatty acid transporter (56,57). The situation is summarized schematically in Fig. 4.

If this common pool of fatty acids is indeed, as proposed by Edens et al. (5), in the extracellular space, then the possibility exists that it will be affected by tissue perfusion. This possibility is discussed further below.

RELATIONSHIPS BETWEEN BLOOD FLOW AND METABOLISM IN WHITE ADIPOSE TISSUE

Adipose tissue blood flow is regulated by a large number of effectors (Table 2). It also varies considerably in different physiologic states (Table 3). Adipose tissue blood flow is increased in states of both fat mobilization (starvation, exercise) and fat deposition (glucose ingestion, feeding). This is entirely consistent with the idea developed earlier that in both these conditions there is a need for coordination of blood flow and metabolism, either to carry away NEFA, the product of fat mobilization, or to deliver lipoprotein-TAG, the substrate for fat deposition.

Fat Mobilization

The intimate relationship between increased blood flow and increased lipolysis has become increasingly apparent with the development of new techniques for studying these processes. In particular, the technique of microdialysis (see Hellmér and Arner, this volume) allows both lipolysis and nutritive blood flow to be followed simultaneously, the former by measurement of interstitial glycerol

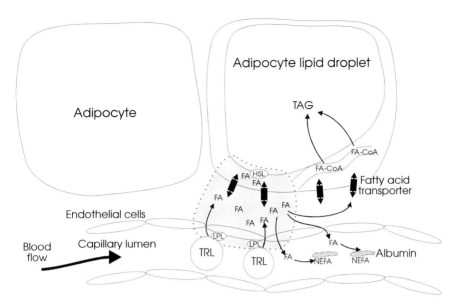

FIG. 4. Schematic representation of possible compartmentalization of fatty acids in adipose tissue. Fatty acids (FAs) released by the action of hormone-sensitive lipase (HSL) on intracellular triacylglycerol (TAG), and fatty acids released by the action of lipoprotein lipase (LPL) on the circulating TAG-rich lipoproteins (TRL particles: chylomicrons and VLDL) enter a common, extracellular pool (gray area enclosed in dotted line). From this pool, FAs may either enter the pathway of esterification or enter the plasma as nonesterified fatty acids (NEFAs), bound to plasma albumin (hatched shapes). There is no evidence that the latter route is reversible in a net sense (i.e., there is always a net efflux of NEFA from adipose tissue in vivo), implying that the effective FA concentration in the shaded pool is always greater than that in plasma. This scheme offers the possibility that the fate of fatty acids within the shaded pool is affected by the rate of blood flow, as suggested by other investigators (5,58). Black boxes with arrows represent the putative fatty acid transporter (59), although it is also possible that fatty acids cross the cell membrane by passive diffusion (30). Scheme based in part on Edens et al. (5).

concentrations and the latter by measurement of the escape of a nonmetabolized marker such as ethanol from the dialysate (45,61,62). Agents affecting lipolysis may be added directly to the perfusate, and by diffusion into the tissue around the probe they cause local rather than systemic changes. In a series of studies there has been almost universal correspondence between lipolysis and local blood flow: when lipolysis is stimulated, for instance by ß-adrenergic agents, blood flow is increased; when lipolysis is inhibited, by α_2-adrenergic agents, blood flow is decreased (45,63,64). In the physiologic states of starvation and exercise, the same correspondence holds true (Table 3).

There are two possible explanations for these observations. Either lipolytic agents may independently act as vasodilators, or some product of lipolysis has a vasodilatory action. Although the former is undoubtedly to some extent true, at least in the case of catecholamines, it is difficult to suppose that all lipolytic and

TABLE 2. *Endogenous regulators of adipose tissue blood flow*

Regulator	Effect	Notes	Local to adipose tissue?
Sympathetic stimulation	Vasodilatation	β-Adrenergic effect; may become α-mediated vasoconstriction at high intensity/frequency	No
Epinephrine	Vasodilatation	β-Adrenergic effect; may become α-mediated vasoconstriction at high concentrations	No
Insulin	Vasoconstriction?	Direct effect uncertain; may be mediated via effects on prostaglandin or adenosine release Physiologic relevance uncertain because blood flow increases after a meal	No
Thyroid hormones	Vasodilatation	Chronic effect	No
Vasopressin	Vasoconstriction	May only apply at very high concentrations	No
Adenosine	Vasodilatation		Yes
Prostaglandins	Vasodilatation		Yes
Angiotensin-II	?	Effects on blood flow not shown	Possibly (angiotensinogen produced by adipocytes)
Nonesterified fatty acids	Vasoconstriction at high concentrations (relative to albumin)		Yes

Based in part on Frayn and Macdonald (60).

antilipolytic agents act directly on the vasculature in this way. It seems more plausible that the latter mechanism is present, even if mainly as "fine-tuning." Candidates for a vasoactive lipolytic product are fatty acids themselves, or other compounds whose production increases with stimulation of lipolysis such as prostacyclin (PGI_2) (65), PGE_2 (66), or adenosine. There is supporting evidence for each of these candidates. Insulin exerts an antilipolytic action in adipose tissue, and reduces catecholamine-induced PGI_2 and PGE_2 production (67). Both adenosine and PGE_2 act directly as potent antilipolytic agents and could be seen as exerting feedback restraint on lipolysis (Fig. 5) and effectively "closing the loop" (66–68).

The need for such coordination between lipolysis and blood flow has been highlighted in studies in which catecholamines have been infused into normal volunteers. For instance, Kurpad et al. infused norepinephrine at 0.42 nmol/kg/min and assessed lipolysis by catheterization of the subcutaneous adipose tissue venous

TABLE 3. *Changes in adipose tissue blood flow in various acute physiologic states, in relation to requirements for lipolysis or substrate delivery*

State	Adipose tissue blood flow	Lipolysis	Substrate delivery
Starvation	↑	↑	↔
Exercise	↑	↑	↔
Hypoglycemia	↑	↑	↔
Feeding	↑	↓	↑
Standing	↓	↔	↔
Mental stress	↑	↑	↔

Based in part on Frayn and Macdonald (60).

drainage (69). Although the net release of NEFA from the tissue increased fivefold after 30 minutes, the adipose tissue venous NEFA concentration increased by only 2.7-fold because of an associated twofold increase in blood flow. Elia has pointed out that, had blood flow not increased in a coordinated manner, the venous plasma NEFA concentration would have considerably exceeded the binding capacity of albumin with potential adverse consequences (70). In a similar study, we infused epinephrine at a rate of 0.14 nmol/kg/min (71). NEFA efflux from adipose tissue increased fivefold and remained relatively constant throughout the 60-min infusion period. Again, however, a coordinated increase in blood flow kept the adipose venous NEFA concentration below 3 mmol/L (Fig. 6), the level above which the proportion of fatty acids bound to albumin increases sharply.

There are also situations in which restricted perfusion of adipose tissue may limit the release of NEFA into the systemic circulation. This is clearly seen during endurance exercise. Although adipose tissue blood flow increases during endurance exercise, concomitant with increased delivery of NEFA to the circulation (72), it does not increase in proportion to the systemic NEFA concentration. Thus, it could be argued that the increase in blood flow is not appropriate to the degree of stimulation of lipolysis. The rate of delivery of

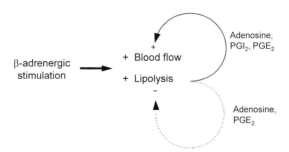

FIG. 5. Scheme for coordinated regulation of adipose tissue blood flow and lipolysis. Stimulation of lipolysis (e.g., by β-adrenergic stimulation) leads to production of vasodilator substances. In turn, adenosine and PGE$_2$ have antipolytic effects.

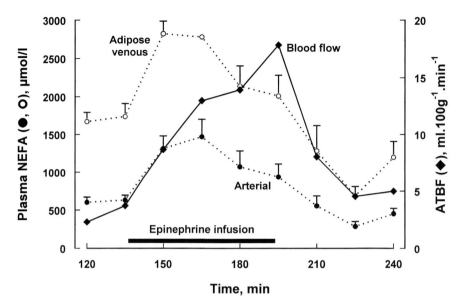

FIG. 6. Effects of epinephrine infusion (25 ng/kg/min) on adipose tissue blood flow (ATBF), and on arterial(ized) and adipose tissue venous nonesterified fatty acid (NEFA) concentrations, in six normal subjects. As the NEFA concentration in the venous plasma approached 3 mmol/L, so increased blood flow prevented a further increase despite continued NEFA efflux at a high rate. Based on data in Samra et al. (71).

fatty acids does not increase consistently with increasing intensity of exercise. Rather, fatty acid delivery is surprisingly low during high-intensity exercise (e.g., rate of systemic fatty acid delivery at 25% VO₂max 26 μmol/kg/min; at 85% VO₂max 17 μmol/kg/min) (73). It seems that adipose tissue blood flow does not increase sufficiently to remove all the fatty acids liberated by lipolysis during strenuous exercise. This is shown particularly clearly by the sudden release of fatty acids, not accompanied by glycerol, from adipose tissue when exercise ceases (74): these appear to be fatty acids that have accumulated in the tissue because of inadequate perfusion during exercise. Bülow et al. (75,76) have suggested that a relative vasoconstriction results from the exceptionally high NEFA:albumin ratios that exist in adipose tissue vasculature during exercise (74).

A similar phenomenon has been observed in hypovolemic shock in the dog. Arterial NEFA concentrations fail to increase as might be expected for the degree of lipolytic drive: removal of adipose tissue vasoconstriction with the α-adrenergic blocker phenoxybenzamine allows greater fat mobilization (77). Although the dog may be particularly susceptible to catecholamine-induced vasoconstriction in adipose tissue, such mechanisms also may occur in humans. Systemic plasma NEFA concentrations are not as high after severe physical injuries as might be expected from the degree of neurohumoral response; in fact, they reach their highest levels after injuries of moderate severity (78).

Fat Deposition

Adipose tissue blood flow increases with glucose or carbohydrate ingestion (79,80). However, much larger effects appear to be produced by ingestion of mixed meals containing carbohydrate, fat, and protein (53,81,82) (Fig. 7), although there has as yet been no attempt to dissect out the individual contributions of the macronutrients. Again, such coordination makes sense if it is seen as increasing the delivery of substrate (chylomicron-TAG) to adipose tissue LPL for storage. The mediators of this increase in blood flow are not known, but the sympatho-adrenal response to feeding is almost certainly involved because the timing of the increased blood flow (peak at 30–60 minutes after eating) (Fig. 7) coincides with maximal norepinephrine concentrations and spillover into the circulation (83,84). In addition, the increase is blunted or abolished by propranolol (80). Other signals such as gastrointestinal hormones or metabolites may be involved but have not been investigated.

The link between substrate delivery to LPL and its rate of action has been illustrated in two ways. Firstly, administration of an intravenous bolus of heparin displaces LPL from its endothelial binding sites in all tissues so that LPL is present in the systemic circulation. This is accompanied by rapid

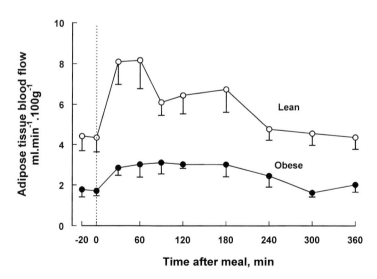

FIG. 7. Subcutaneous abdominal adipose tissue blood flow after overnight fast and after a mixed meal (1.6 MJ, 60 g fat), in 10 lean subjects (body mass index <25 kg/m²) and six obese subjects (body mass index >30 kg/m²). Reproduced with permission (82).

hydrolysis of plasma TAG with production of NEFA. Typically the plasma TAG concentration decreases by 50% within 15 minutes of administration of 50 U/kg of heparin, and the plasma NEFA concentration increases three- to four-fold (85). There is no suggestion in this situation that the total amount of LPL has increased; it has simply been distributed in the circulation so that more substrate can gain access.

Secondly, we have investigated the rate of action of adipose tissue LPL in vivo during epinephrine infusion. This is of interest because of considerable evidence from cellular and molecular studies that epinephrine suppresses the expression of LPL in adipose tissue (86). However, we found that in vivo epi-nephrine infusion markedly increased the rate of action of adipose tissue LPL (Fig. 8), assessed as the rate of TAG extraction across the tissue. The increased rate of LPL action paralleled almost exactly the increase in adipose tissue blood flow (Fig. 8). It seems clear that increased blood flow results in greater sub-strate delivery to LPL and that this effect, at least in such an acute situation, out-weighs any suppressive effect of the catecholamine on LPL expression.

However, it is of interest to ask what happens to the fatty acids released by LPL under these conditions. The ratio of NEFA to glycerol release during epi-nephrine or norepinephrine infusion increases to significantly greater than 3:1 (69,71), probably reflecting the temporary intracellular accumulation of MAG and DAG under these conditions of rapid lipolysis. Therefore, it is unlikely that there is any concomitant esterification of fatty acids, and we must assume that

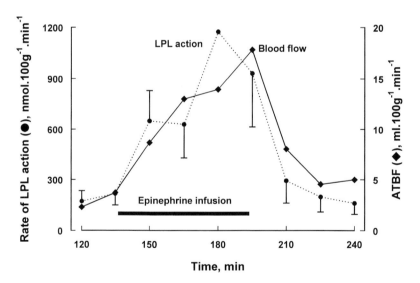

FIG. 8. Effects of epinephrine infusion (25 ng/kg/min) on the rate of action of lipoprotein lipase (LPL) in subcutaneous adipose tissue, and on adipose tissue blood flow (ATBF), in six normal subjects. LPL action is taken as equal to TAG extraction across the tissue. Based on Samra et al. (71).

the LPL-derived fatty acids follow the mass flow of fatty acids out of the tissue, i.e. that they are quantitatively released into the venous plasma. The increased adipose tissue blood flow also could be seen as removing fatty acids from the tissue, reducing their retention by esterification. Thus, although catecholamine infusion may markedly increase LPL action, it does not in itself result in increased fat deposition. Whether increased fat deposition could be brought about in this situation by addition of other hormones, particularly insulin, is not known.

There is another potential benefit of the association between increased adipose tissue blood flow and LPL action. Fatty acids released by the action of LPL can cause product inhibition of the enzyme (87) and may lead to its release from the endothelial binding sites into the circulation (88,89). An increased blood flow may assist in removing these fatty acids, so allowing maximal LPL activity. The corollary, however, may be that a proportion of the fatty acids released by LPL will inevitably be lost to the systemic circulation, as observed.

METABOLIC AND VASCULAR INTEGRATION IN PHYSIOLOGIC SITUATIONS

The discussion above leads to a picture of highly coordinated metabolism and blood flow in adipose tissue. After an overnight fast it may be that adipose tissue blood flow is at its lowest level during normal situations. If fasting continues, adipose tissue blood flow is likely to increase gradually as fat mobilization increases, a process that becomes increasingly important over the period from about 12–24 hours of starvation (90,91). The increased blood flow thus allows the transport out of adipose tissue of fatty acids released in lipolysis. Alternatively, if a meal is taken, then blood flow also increases in response to the meal, allowing the delivery of more substrate to LPL.

However, in the postprandial state this simplistic picture does not hold true. The increase in adipose tissue blood flow after a mixed meal peaks at 30–60 minutes after the meal and, as discussed earlier, coincides with both the peak in plasma insulin concentrations and the sympathetic response. The activation of adipose tissue LPL by insulin is a relatively slow process (92,93), taking a matter of 5–6 hours even during constant infusion of insulin. In vivo, the peak of LPL action occurs 4–5 hours after a typical mixed meal, at a time when the plasma TAG concentration is maximal (Fig. 2) (31,94). It might be thought that it would be more sensible physiologically if the increase in blood flow occurred at this time, bringing more substrate for LPL to act upon, and removing its products. We believe that these apparently discrepant time courses may reflect a metabolic compromise. The net movement of fatty acids into adipose tissue after a mixed meal occurs remarkably steadily over a period of several hours (40), despite the underlying divergent time courses of the activation of esterification (Fig. 3) and LPL (Fig. 2). If the suggestion made earlier, and by

Edens et al. (5), that blood flow may affect the partitioning of LPL-derived fatty acids is true, then it also may be true that it would be deleterious to fat storage if adipose tissue blood flow were excessive at the time of maximal LPL action. As in the case of epinephrine infusion, LPL-derived fatty acids might be effectively washed away rather than taken up by the tissue for storage. We have remarked previously that the smooth pattern of overall fatty acid or substrate-carbon flows in and out of adipose tissue before and after a meal is made up from a number of different processes, each with its own characteristic time course (53,95). Perhaps the temporal pattern of blood flow in the tissue is yet another component of that coordinated system.

In support of the view that a metabolic compromise underlies the pattern of blood flow after a meal are some recent observations of postprandial metabolism after sequential fatty meals (96). In these studies we fed subjects a breakfast containing 54 g fat and a lunch 5 hours later. The pattern of lipemia after the lunch was unlike the usual pattern observed after an overnight fast, with an early sharp peak (at 60 minutes) of both plasma and chylomicron-TAG concentrations. Although we did not measure blood flow, it seems likely that this coincided with peak adipose tissue blood flow. Of great interest was the behavior of the plasma NEFA fraction. Unlike the usual situation after a meal in which NEFA concentrations decrease, in some subjects they increased markedly, following closely the pattern of chylomicron-TAG concentrations. Analysis of specific fatty acids in the NEFA fraction showed that these NEFAs arose largely from LPL action on the chylomicron-TAG. Thus, in that situation there was considerable spillover of LPL-derived fatty acids, and it seems possible that this reflected the coincidence of peak blood flow and peak chylomicron-TAG concentrations. This seems to emphasize the normal close coordination of metabolic and circulatory events, and perhaps the disadvantages of sequential fatty meals that have become a feature of the Western diet.

POSSIBILITIES OF PATHOLOGIC REGULATION OF BLOOD FLOW AND METABOLISM

It has been suggested that resistance to the vasodilatory effect of insulin in skeletal muscle may underlie, at least in part, resistance to insulin-mediated glucose uptake in obesity and non–insulin-dependent diabetes mellitus (97–99). Could the same be true in adipose tissue? There is some controversy about the absolute magnitude of adipose tissue blood flow in obesity, confounded by the difficulty of knowing whether to express it per cell or per unit weight of tissue (60). In humans, subcutaneous adipose tissue blood flow per unit weight of tissue appears to be decreased in obesity (82,94). However, there is a complication in that the partition coefficient between adipose tissue and blood for xenon, the most widely used indicator for adipose tissue blood flow, varies with the degree of adiposity and is not accurately known in obese subjects. It has been suggested that the commonly used value of 10 ml/g is not widely inaccurate in both normal and obese subjects (100), but even if the greater differences between lean and obese suggested by Jelnes et al. (101) were to apply, it is still probable that subcutaneous adipose tissue blood flow is decreased in obesity. More important than the absolute difference between lean and obese might be their different pattern of response to a meal (82,94). The obese fail to show the sharp increase seen in lean subjects (Fig. 7). Although this may represent resistance to β-adrenergic stimulation (102) rather than resistance to insulin, there is a clear parallel with the impairment of skeletal muscle blood flow regulation in obesity (97).

What effects might this have on metabolic regulation in adipose tissue? A superficial response is to reiterate the idea that increased adipose tissue blood flow after a meal might serve to wash away fatty acids otherwise destined for re-esterification: thus, reduced adipose tissue blood flow in the obese in the post-prandial period might account for their tendency to accumulate fat. However, it seems most likely that the resistance of adipose tissue blood flow is a secondary consequence of obesity. However, it may well affect the normally precise temporal coordination of postprandial metabolism, and this may have adverse effects in terms of generation of an atherogenic lipoprotein profile (1).

CONCLUSION

We conclude that in adipose tissue, perhaps more than in any other tissue, there are intimate connections between blood flow and metabolism. Some important metabolic pathways in adipose tissue are located in an extracellular environment (e.g., the action of LPL on lipoprotein-TAG), and there are real and obvious possibilities for metabolic regulation to occur in the extracellular compartment.

ACKNOWLEDGMENTS

We thank Drs. Max Lafontan and Pierre Barbe of INSERM Unité 82 317, Toulouse, France, and Drs. Steffan Enoksson and Peter Arner of Huddinge University Hospital, Huddinge, Sweden, for sharing their data on blood flow and lipolysis with us. The Oxford Lipid Metabolism Group, INSERM Unité 82 317 and the Department of Medicine at Huddinge are part of the European Commission BIOMED 1 Concerted Action on the Impairment of Adipose Tissue Metabolic Regulation as a Generator of Risk Factors for Cardiovascular Disease (EUROLIP). Our own studies presented in this chapter were supported by the Wellcome Trust and the Ministry of Agriculture, Fisheries and Food. The Oxford Lipid Metabolism Group (OXLIP) is supported by the Oxford Diabetes Trust. We thank Dr. Simon Coppack, Sandy Humphreys, and other members of OXLIP whose work is referred to in this chapter.

REFERENCES

1. Frayn KN. Insulin resistance and lipid metabolism. *Curr Opin Lipidol* 1993;4:197–204.
2. Baron AD. Hemodynamic actions of insulin. *Am J Physiol* 1994;267:E187–E202.
3. Clark MG, Colquhoun EQ, Rattigan S, et al. Vascular and endocrine control of muscle metabolism. *Am J Physiol* 1995;268:E797–E812.
4. Leibel RL, Forse RA, Hirsch J. Effects of rapid glucose infusion on in vivo and in vitro free fatty acid re-esterification by adipose tissue of fasted obese subjects. *Int J Obesity* 1989;13:661–671.
5. Edens NK, Leibel RL, Hirsch J. Mechanism of free fatty acid re-esterification in human adipocytes in vitro. *J Lipid Res* 1990;31:1423–1431.
6. Gersh I, Still MA. Blood vessels in fat tissue. Relation to problems of gas exchange. *J Exp Med* 1945;81:219–232.
7. Ryan TJ, Curri SB. Blood vessels and lymphatics. *Clin Dermatol* 1989;7:25–36.
8. Elia M, Kurpad A. What is the blood flow to resting human muscle? *Clin Sci* 1993;84:559–563.
9. Frayn KN, Humphreys SM, Coppack SW. Fuel selection in white adipose tissue. *Proc Nutr Soc* 1995;54:177–189.
10. Rowe GG, Maxwell GM, Castillo CA, Freeman DJ, Crumpton CW. A study in man of cerebral blood flow and cerebral glucose, lactate and pyruvate metabolism before and after eating. *J Clin Invest* 1959;38:2154–2158.
11. Savard G, Kiens B, Saltin B. Central cardiovascular factors as limits to endurance; with a note on the distinction between maximal oxygen uptake and endurance fitness. In: Macleod D, Maughan R, Nimmo M, Reilly T, Williams C, eds. *Exercise: benefits, limits and adaptations*. London: Spon; 1987:162–177.
12. Frayn KN. Studies of human adipose tissue in vivo. In: Kinney JM, Tucker HN, eds. *Energy metabolism: tissue determinants and cellular corollaries*. New York: Raven; 1992:267–295.
13. Cryer A. Tissue lipoprotein lipase activity and its action in lipoprotein metabolism. *Int J Biochem* 1981;13:525–541.
14. Scow RO, Blanchette-Mackie EJ, Smith LC. Role of capillary endothelium in the clearance of chylomicrons. A model for lipid transport from blood by lateral diffusion in cell membranes. *Circ Res* 1976;39:149–162.
15. Scow RO, Olivecrona T. Effect of albumin on products formed from chylomicron triacylglycerol by lipoprotein lipase in vitro. *Biochim Biophys Acta* 1977;487:472–486.
16. Nilsson-Ehle P, Egelrud T, Belfrage P, Olivecrona T, Borgström B. Positional specificity of purified milk lipoprotein lipase. *J Biol Chem* 1973;248:6734–6737.
17. Jones NL, Havel RJ. Metabolism of free fatty acids and chylomicron triglycerides during exercise in rats. *Am J Physiol* 1967;213:824–828.
18. Scow RO, Hamosh M, Blanchette-Mackie EJ, Evans AJ. Uptake of blood triglyceride by various tissues. *Lipids* 1972;7:497–505.
19. Scow RO, Chernick SS, Fleck TR. Lipoprotein lipase and uptake of triacylglycerol, cholesterol and phosphatidylcholine from chylomicrons by mammary and adipose tissue of lactating rats in vivo. *Biochim Biophys Acta* 1977;487:297–306.
20. Scow RO. Metabolism of chylomicrons in perfused adipose and mammary tissue of the rat. *Federation Proc* 1977;36:182–185.
21. Verine A, Boyer J. Lipases operative at the fat cell surface: attempt at an integrated approach. *Cell Biochem Function* 1987;5:175–181.
22. Fredrikson G, Tornqvist H, Belfrage P. Hormone-sensitive lipase and monoacylglycerol lipase are both required for complete degradation of adipocyte triacylglycerol. *Biochim Biophys Acta* 1986;876:288–293.
23. Fielding BA, Humphreys SM, Shadid S, Frayn KN. Arterio-venous differences across human adipose tissue for mono-, di- and tri-acylglycerols before and after a high-fat meal. *Endocrinol Metab* 1995;2:13–17.
24. Fielding BA, Humphreys SM, Shadid S, Frayn KN. Plasma mono-, di- and triacylglycerol measurements in a study of fat uptake by human adipose tissue in vivo. *Biochem Soc Trans* 1995;23(suppl):487.
25. Scow RO, Blanchette-Mackie EJ. Why fatty acids flow in cell membranes. *Prog Lipid Res* 1985;24:197–241.
26. Saggerson ED. Hormonal regulation of biosynthetic activities in white adipose tissue. In: Cryer A, Van RLR, eds. *New perspectives in adipose tissue*. London: Butterworths; 1985:87–120.

27. Brandes R, Ockner RK, Weisiger RA, Lysenko N. Specific and saturable binding of albumin to rat adipocytes: modulation by epinephrine and possible role in free fatty acid transfer. *Biochem Biophys Res Commun* 1982;105:821–827.
28. Potter BJ, Sorrentino D, Berk PD. Mechanisms of cellular uptake of free fatty acids. *Annu Rev Nutr* 1989;9:253–270.
29. Trigatti BL, Gerber GE. A direct role for serum albumin in the cellular uptake of long-chain fatty acids. *Biochem J* 1995;308:155–159.
30. Trigatti BL, Gerber GE. The effect of intracellular pH on long-chain fatty acid uptake in 3T3-L1 adipocytes: evidence that uptake involves the passive diffusion of protonated long-chain fatty acids across the plasma membrane. *Biochem J* 1996;313:487–494.
31. Frayn KN, Shadid S, Hamlani R, et al. Regulation of fatty acid movement in human adipose tissue in the postabsorptive-to-postprandial transition. *Am J Physiol* 1994;266:E308–E317.
32. Bergman EN, Havel RJ, Wolfe BM, Bohmer T. Quantitative studies of the metabolism of chylomicron triglycerides and cholesterol by liver and extrahepatic tissues of sheep and dogs. *J Clin Invest* 1971;50:1831–1839.
33. Miller HI, Bortz WM, Durham BC. The rate of appearance of FFA in plasma triglyceride of normal and obese subjects. *Metabolism* 1968;17:515–521.
34. Binnert C, Laville M, Pachiaudi C, Rigalleau V, Beylot M. Use of gas chromatography/isotope ratio-mass spectrometry to study triglyceride metabolism in humans. *Lipids* 1995;30:869–873.
35. Fielding BA, Frayn KN, Halliday D, Bannister PA, Callow J, Venkatesan S. Rapid entry of dietary fatty acids into the plasma non-esterified fatty acid pool. *Proc Nutr Soc* 1996;56:162A.
36. Ookhtens M, Montisano D, Lyon I, Baker N. Transport and metabolism of extracellular free fatty acids in adipose tissue of fed and fasted mice. *J Lipid Res* 1987;28:528–539.
37. Clegg RA. Triacylglycerol hydrolysis by cells isolated from lactating rat mammary gland. *Biochim Biophys Acta* 1981;663:598–612.
38. Baltzan MA, Andres R, Cader G, Zierler KL. Heterogeneity of forearm metabolism with special reference to free fatty acids. *J Clin Invest* 1962;41:116–125.
39. Rabinowitz D, Zierler KL. Role of free fatty acids in forearm metabolism in man, quantitated by use of insulin. *J Clin Invest* 1962;41:2191–2197.
40. Frayn KN, Coppack SW, Fielding BA, Humphreys SM. Coordinated regulation of hormone-sensitive lipase and lipoprotein lipase in human adipose tissue in vivo: implications for the control of fat storage and fat mobilization. *Adv Enzyme Regul* 1995;35:163–178.
41. Langin D, Holm C, Lafontan M. Adipocyte hormone-sensitive lipase: a major regulator of lipid metabolism. *Proc Nutr Soc* 1996;55:93–109.
42. Coppack SW, Jensen MD, Miles JM. In vivo regulation of lipolysis in humans. *J Lipid Res* 1994;35:177–193.
43. Kather H, Bieger W, Aktories K, Jakobs KH. Human fat cell lipolysis is primarily regulated by inhibitory modulators acting through distinct mechanisms. *J Clin Invest* 1985;76:1559–1565.
44. Arner P, Kriegholm E, Engfeldt P, Bolinder J. Adrenergic regulation of lipolysis in situ at rest and during exercise. *J Clin Invest* 1990;85:893–898.
45. Galitzky J, Lafontan M, Nordenström J, Arner P. Role of vascular alpha-2 adrenoceptors in regulating lipid mobilization from human adipose tissue. *J Clin Invest* 1993;91:1997–2003.
46. Egan JJ, Greenberg AS, Chang M-K, Wek SA, Moos MC, Londos C. Mechanism of hormone-stimulated lipolysis in adipocytes: translocation of hormone-sensitive lipase to the lipid storage droplet. *Proc Natl Acad Sci U S A* 1992;89:8537–8541.
47. Greenberg AS, Egan JJ, Wek SA, Garty NB, Blanchette Mackie EJ, Londos C. Perilipin, a major hormonally regulated adipocyte-specific phosphoprotein associated with the periphery of lipid storage droplets. *J Biol Chem* 1991;266:11341–11346.
48. Blanchette Mackie EJ, Dwyer NK, Barber T, et al. Perilipin is located on the surface layer of intracellular lipid droplets in adipocytes. *J Lipid Res* 1995;36:1211–1226.
49. Londos C, Gruia-Gray J, Brasaemle DL, et al. Perilipin: possible roles in sturcture and metabolism of intracellular neutral lipids in adipocytes and steroidogenic cells. *Int J Obesity* 1996; 20(suppl 3):97–101.
50. Arner P, Östman J. Mono- and diacylglycerols in human adipose tissue. *Biochim Biophys Acta* 1974;369:209–221.
51. Abumrad NA, Forest C, Regen DM, Barnella US, Melki SA. Metabolism of oleic acid in differentiating BFC-1 preadipose cells. *Am J Physiol* 1991;261:E76–E86.
52. Frayn KN, Coppack SW, Humphreys SM. Subcutaneous adipose tissue metabolism studied by local catheterization. *Int J Obesity* 1993;17(suppl 3):18–21.

53. Coppack SW, Fisher RM, Gibbons GF, et al. Postprandial substrate deposition in human forearm and adipose tissues in vivo. *Clin Sci* 1990;79:339–348.
54. Vaughan M. The metabolism of adipose tissue in vitro. *J Lipid Res* 1961;2:293–316.
55. Lin ECC. Glycerol utilisation and its regulation in mammals. *Ann Rev Biochem* 1977;46:765–795.
56. Abumrad NA, Park JH, Park CR. Permeation of long-chain fatty acid into adipocytes. Kinetics, specificity, and evidence for involvement of a membrane protein. *J Biol Chem* 1984;259: 8945–8953.
57. Harmon CM, Luce P, Abumrad NA. Labelling of an 88 kDa adipocyte membrane protein by sulpho-N-succinimidyl long-chain fatty acids: inhibition of fatty acid transport. *Biochem Soc Trans* 1992;20:811–813.
58. Leibel RL, Edens NK, Fried SK. Physiologic basis for the control of body fat distribution in humans. *Annu Rev Nutr* 1989;9:417–443.
59. Abumrad NA, el Maghrabi MR, Amri EZ, Lopez E, Grimaldi PA. Cloning of a rat adipocyte membrane protein implicated in binding or transport of long-chain fatty acids that is induced during preadipocyte differentiation. Homology with human CD36. *J Biol Chem* 1993;268:17665–17668.
60. Frayn KN, Macdonald IA. Adipose tissue circulation. In: Bennett T, Gardiner SM, eds. *Nervous control of blood vessels.* Amsterdam: Harwood Academic 1996, pp. 505–539.
61. Fuchi T, Rosdahl H, Hickner RC, Ungerstedt U, Henriksson J. Microdialysis of rat skeletal muscle and adipose tissue: dynamics of the interstitial glucose pool. *Acta Physiol Scand* 1994;151: 249–260.
62. Felländer G, Linde B, Bolinder J. Evaluation of the microdialysis ethanol technique for monitoring of subcutaneous adipose tissue blood flow in humans. *Int J Obesity* 1996;20:220–226.
63. Enoksson S, Nordenström J, Bolinder J, Arner P. Influence of local blood flow on glycerol levels in human adipose tissue. *Int J Obesity* 1995;19:350–354.
64. Barbe P, Millet L, Galitzky J, Lafontan M, Berlan M. In situ assessment of the role of the β1-, β2- and β3-adrenoceptors in the control of lipolysis and nutritive blood flow in human subcutaneous adipose tissue. *Br J Pharmacol* 1996;117:907–913.
65. Axelrod L, Levine L. Prostacyclin production by isolated adipocytes. *Diabetes* 1981;30:163–167.
66. Richelsen B. Release and effects of prostaglandins in adipose tissue. *Prostaglandins Leukot Essent Fatty Acids* 1992;47:171–182.
67. Axelrod L. Insulin, prostaglandins, and the pathogenesis of hypertension. *Diabetes* 1991;40: 1223–1227.
68. Vernon RG, Clegg RA. The metabolism of white adipose tissue in vivo and in vitro. In: Cryer A, Van RLR, eds. *New perspectives in adipose tissue.* London: Butterworths; 1985:65–86.
69. Kurpad A, Khan K, Calder AG, et al. Effect of noradrenaline on glycerol turnover and lipolysis in the whole body and subcutaneous adipose tissue in humans in vivo. *Clin Sci* 1994;86:177–184.
70. Elia M. General integration and regulation of metabolism at the organ level. *Proc Nutr Soc* 1995; 54:213–232.
71. Samra JS, Simpson EJ, Clark ML, et al. Effects of epinephrine infusion on adipose tissue: interactions between blood flow and lipid metabolism. *Am J Physiol* 1996;271:E834–E839.
72. Bülow J, Madsen J. Adipose tissue blood flow during prolonged, heavy exercise. *Pflügers Arch* 1976;363:231–234.
73. Romijn JA, Coyle EF, Sidossis LS, et al. Regulation of endogenous fat and carbohydrate metabolism in relation to exercise intensity and duration. *Am J Physiol* 1993;265:E380–E391.
74. Hodgetts V, Coppack SW, Frayn KN, Hockaday TDR. Factors controlling fat mobilization from human subcutaneous adipose tissue during exercise. *J Appl Physiol* 1991;71:445–451.
75. Bülow J, Madsen J, Astrup A, Christensen NJ. Vasoconstrictor effect of high FFA/albumin ratios in adipose tissue in vivo. *Acta Physiol Scand* 1985;125:661–667.
76. Madsen J, Bülow J, Nielsen NE. Inhibition of fatty acid mobilization by arterial free fatty acid concentration. *Acta Physiol Scand* 1986;127:161–166.
77. Kovách AGB, Rosell S, Sándor P, Koltay E, Kovách E, Tomka N. Blood flow, oxygen consumption, and free fatty acid release in subcutaneous adipose tissue during hemorrhagic shock in control and phenoxybenzamine-treated dogs. *Circ Res* 1970;26:733–741.
78. Stoner HB, Frayn KN, Braton RN, Threlfall CJ, Little RA. The relationships between plasma substrates and hormones and the severity of injury in 277 recently injured patients. *Clin Sci* 1979; 56:563–573.
79. Bülow J, Astrup A, Christensen NJ, Kastrup J. Blood flow in skin, subcutaneous adipose tissue and skeletal muscle in the forearm of normal man during an oral glucose load. *Acta Physiol Scand* 1987;130:657–661.

80. Simonsen L, Bülow J, Astrup A, Madsen J, Christensen NJ. Diet-induced changes in subcutaneous adipose tissue blood flow in man: effect of β-adrenoceptor inhibition. *Acta Physiol Scand* 1990;139:341–346.
81. Samra JS, Frayn KN, Giddings JA, Clark ML, Macdonald IA. Modification and validation of a commercially available portable detector for measurement of adipose tissue blood flow. *Clin Physiol* 1995;15:241–248.
82. Summers LKM, Samra JS, Humphreys SM, Morris RJ, Frayn KN. Subcutaneous abdominal adipose tissue blood flow: variation within and between subjects and relationship to obesity. *Clin Sci* 1996;91:679–683.
83. Welle S, Lilavivathana U, Campbell RG. Increased plasma norepinephrine concentrations and metabolic rates following glucose ingestion in man. *Metabolism* 1980;29:806–809.
84. Cox HS, Kaye DM, Thompson JM, et al. Regional sympathetic nervous activition after a large meal in humans. *Clin Sci* 1995;89:145–154.
85. Fielding BA, Humphreys SM, Allman RFC, Frayn KN. Mono-, di- and triacylglycerol concentrations in human plasma: effects of heparin injection and of a high-fat meal. *Clin Chim Acta* 1993; 216:167–173.
86. Yukht A, Davis RC, Ong JM, Ranganathan G, Kern PA. Regulation of lipoprotein lipase translation by epinephrine in 3T3-L1 cells. Importance of the 3′ untranslated region. *J Clin Invest* 1995; 96:2438–2444.
87. Bengtsson G, Olivecrona T. Lipoprotein lipase. Mechanism of product inhibition. *Eur J Biochem* 1980;106:557–562.
88. Peterson J, Bihain BE, Bengtsson-Olivecrona G, Deckelbaum RJ, Carpentier Y, Olivecrona T. Fatty acid control of lipoprotein lipase: a link between energy metabolism and lipid transport. *Proc Natl Acad Sci U S A* 1990;87:909–913.
89. Karpe F, Olivecrona T, Walldius G, Hamsten A. Lipoprotein lipase in plasma after an oral fat load: relation to free fatty acids. *J Lipid Res* 1992;33:975–984.
90. Klein S, Sakurai Y, Romijn JA, Carroll RM. Progressive alterations in lipid and glucose metabolism during short-term fasting in young adult men. *Am J Physiol* 1993;265:E801–E806.
91. Samra JS, Clark ML, Humphreys SM, Macdonald IA, Frayn KN. Regulation of lipid metabolism in adipose tissue during early starvation. *Am J Physiol* 1996;271:E541–E546.
92. Sadur CN, Eckel RH. Insulin stimulation of adipose tissue lipoprotein lipase. Use of the euglycemic clamp technique. *J Clin Invest* 1982;69:1119–1125.
93. Yki-Järvinen H, Taskinen M-R, Koivisto VA, Nikkilä EA. Response of adipose tissue lipoprotein lipase activity and serum lipoproteins to acute hyperinsulinaemia in man. *Diabetologia* 1984; 27:364–369.
94. Coppack SW, Evans RD, Fisher RM, et al. Adipose tissue metabolism in obesity: lipase action in vivo before and after a mixed meal. *Metabolism* 1992;41:264–272.
95. Frayn KN, Humphreys SM, Coppack SW. Net carbon flux across subcutaneous adipose tissue after a standard meal in normal-weight and insulin-resistant obese subjects. *Int J Obesity* 1996;20:795–800.
96. Fielding BA, Callow J, Owen RM, Samra JS, Matthews DR, Frayn KN. Postprandial lipemia: the origin of an early peak studied by specific dietary fatty acid intake during sequential meals. *Am J Clin Nutr* 1996;63:36–41.
97. Laakso M, Edelman SV, Brechtel G, Baron AD. Decreased effect of insulin to stimulate skeletal muscle blood flow in obese man. A novel mechanism for insulin resistance. *J Clin Invest* 1990;85: 1844–1852.
98. Baron AD, Laakso M, Brechtel G, Edelman SV. Mechanism of insulin resistance in insulin-dependent diabetes mellitus: a major role for reduced skeletal muscle blood flow. *J Clin Endocr Metab* 1991;73:637–643.
99. Baron AD, Steinberg H, Brechtel G, Johnson A. Skeletal muscle blood flow independently modulates insulin-mediated glucose uptake. *Am J Physiol* 1994;266:E248–E253.
100. Jansson P-A, Lönnroth P. Comparison of two methods to assess the tissue/blood partition coefficient for xenon in subcutaneous adipose tissue in man. *Clin Physiol* 1995;15:47–55.
101. Jelnes R, Rasmussen LB, Eickhoff JH. Direct determination of the tissue-to-blood partition coefficient for Xenon in human subcutaneous adipose tissue. *Scand J Clin Lab Invest* 1984;44: 643–647.
102. Blaak EE, van Baak MA, Kemerink GJ, Pakbiers MTW, Heidendal GAK, Saris WHM. β-adrenergic stimulation and abdominal subcutaneous fat blood flow in lean, obese, and reduced-obese subjects. *Metabolism* 1995;44:183–187.

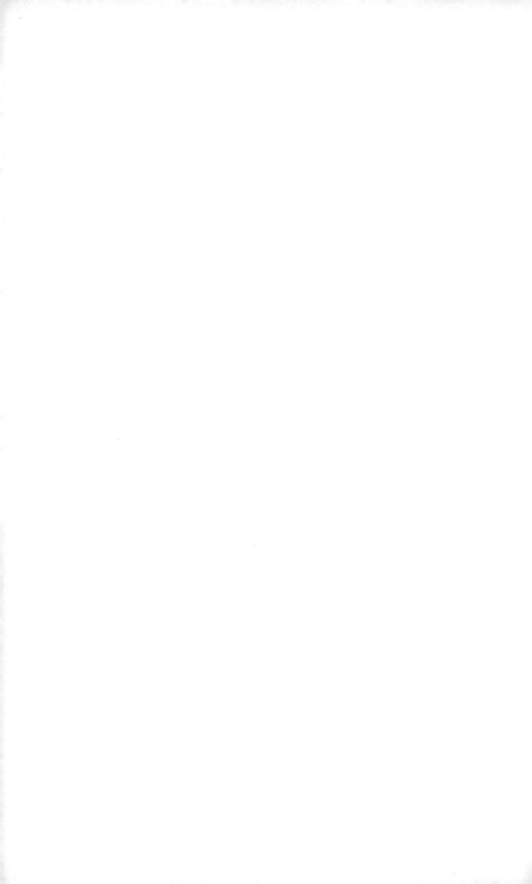

Physiology, Stress, and Malnutrition: Functional Correlates, Nutritional Intervention,
edited by J.M. Kinney and H.N. Tucker.
Lippincott–Raven Publishers © 1997.

Vascular and Metabolic Regulation of Muscle

Michael G. Clark, Stephen Rattigan, Kim A. Dora,
John M. B. Newman, John T. Steen, Kelly A. Miller,
and Michelle A. Vincent

Department of Biochemistry, University of Tasmania, Hobart, TAS 7001 Tasmania, Australia

Our interest for some years has been the role of the vasculature in the control of muscle metabolism by either influencing hormone and nutrient access or by releasing paracrine substances where they may then act to regulate muscle metabolism. This chapter addresses the history of these concepts as well as data we have recently obtained that lends support to the concept of controlled access and implying a paracrine role for the vasculature in influencing surrounding skeletal muscle.

HISTORY AND EVIDENCE FOR THE VASCULAR CONTROL OF MUSCLE METABOLISM THROUGH NUTRIENT AND HORMONE ACCESS

The concept of nutritive and non-nutritive flow in muscle appears to date from the work of Pappenheimer (1). His experiments in 1941 (1) showed that changes, up or down, in oxygen consumption of constant-pressure perfused dog gastrocnemius muscle at rest resulted from infusion of epinephrine or stimulation of vasoconstrictor nerves, respectively. Epinephrine under these conditions was viewed as increasing nutritive flow, whereas stimulation of vasoconstrictor nerves was viewed as increasing non-nutritive flow (1). These concepts were tested in some detail over the following years. A study by Sonnenschein and Hirvonen (2) examining blood flow and maximum force produced by isometric contractions of cat gastrocnemius-soleus muscles showed that reductions in flow by intra-arterial infusion of epinephrine or norepinephrine, clamping of the arterial inflow, or stimulation of the sympathetic chain yielded equivalent reductions in muscle force. Intra-arterial infusion of acetylcholine or of histamine at rates insufficient to produce systemic effects resulted in either of two patterns of response: increase in flow with no change in muscle force, or no change in flow with diminution in muscle force. On the assumption that the maximal muscle force was an index of nutritional flow, it was concluded that norepinephrine and epinephrine produced parallel decreases in nutritional and non-nutritional flow similar to sympathetic stimulation or clamping of the arterial inflow. Acetylcholine or histamine were concluded to have increased non-nutritional flow and/or decreased nutritional flow, provided they had no direct effects on the muscle or on neuromuscular transmission.

Over the period 1940 to the early 1960s, further attempts were made to resolve the relationship between blood flow and clearance of intramuscularly injected markers or contractile performance of working muscle. For example, Hyman et al. (3) noted that in resting muscle stimulation of the sympathetic vasodilator system increased total blood flow but decreased local clearance of intramuscularly injected radioiodide. In contracting muscle, stimulation of the sympathetic vasodilator system seemed to have little effect. Thus, Hirvonen and Sonnenschein (4) noted that neither blood flow nor muscle force were affected and concluded that a fundamental difference appeared to exist in the responses of the vasculature of resting and active muscle where this difference related to the interplay of specialized effects of vasomotor innervations and the action of vasodilator metabolites. Renkin and Rosell (5) studied arteriovenous extraction of rubidium-86 in dog and cat muscle perfused at constant flow. Metabolic vasodilatation due to muscular contractions induced a pronounced decrease in resistance and an increase in transport of Rb^{86} from blood to tissue. Vasodilatation resulting from inhibition of vasoconstrictor tonus produced effects similar those produced by metabolic vasodilatation, but stimulation of vasodilator nerve activity did not increase transport of Rb^{86} from blood to tissue. Thus, by the early 1960s it was clear that control of blood flow within muscle (i.e., the balance between nutritive and non-nutritive flow) determined performance and transcapillary exchange.

The key issue of the non-nutritive vessels as arteriovenous channels or "functional shunts" capable of carrying high flow, with little or no nutrient exchange, presented a challenging concept that still remains unresolved. Arteriovenous communications of small diameter and short length, and hence low resistance, were reported in amphibian skeletal muscle by Zweifach (6). In addition, Saunders (7) claimed the presence of large-caliber shunts in the vascular bed of human skeletal muscle. Dog muscle also seemed to show significant passage (17.5%) of intra-arterially injected 20-μm microspheres (8). However, flow through these shunts in dog muscle appeared to be dependent on a critical arterial pressure, below which the shunts would not permit the passage of beads of 40 μm in size (9). Despite these claims, other workers failed to find large arteriovenous shunts in skeletal muscle. Thus, Piiper and Rosell (10) using 20-, 30-, and 40-μm wax spheres found only negligible venous recovery after intra-arterial injection into cat muscle. In addition, they could find no evidence that vasodilator nerve activity preferentially opened large arteriovenous shunts.

An interesting study by Barlow et al. (11) showed a vascular pathway in muscle not noted by others. The work followed from an earlier careful study by the same investigators (12) that failed to show any anatomic evidence of arteriovenous anastomoses, even though other investigators, including Walder

(13), had noted that intravenous infusions of epinephrine increased muscle blood flow without an increase in the clearance rate of intramuscularly injected radioactive sodium. In their 1961 study, Barlow et al. (12) used a semi-isolated cat biceps preparation, which also displayed flow increase by epinephrine without an increase in [24]Na clearance. Because extramuscular shunting was eliminated by using the semi-isolated biceps and large vessel anastomoses could not be found, it seemed likely that a non-nutritive capillary system was present within the preparation. Epinephrine-mediated changes in capillary permeability or in fixation of [24]Na by muscle cells also was ruled out. Key observations were the [24]Na washout curves, which showed two different rates and were thus suggestive of two compartments. These were identified as two circulations in muscle: one relates to the nutrition of the muscle fibers and the other to the nutrition of the intramuscular septa and tendons. [24]Na clearance was shown to be faster in the former, and the effect of epinephrine on each circulation was different, reflecting a vascular network in the septa, insulated by connective tissue, that had poor nutrient exchange capabilities. These findings were consistent with the earlier proposal of Renkin (14) for two circulatory systems in skeletal muscle. The findings of Barlow et al. (12) and the observation of preferential capillary pathways by Zweifach and Metz (15) at the end of the spinotrapezius muscle of the rat presented an apparent solution to the problem of non-nutritive flow and provided the impetus for the later studies by Lindbom and Arfors (16) to further explore the nature of the nonhomogeneous blood flow distribution in the rabbit tenuissimus muscle. These investigators noted that a majority of the main feeding arterioles (transverse arterioles) continued into adjacent connective tissue after giving off branches (terminal arterioles) within the muscle tissue to supply the muscle capillaries. The transverse arterioles were thus concluded to be supplying two vascular areas, with the major part of the arteriolar flow, under normal resting conditions, being distributed to the muscle capillaries under the control of the terminal arterioles. These investigators also surmised that differential sensitivity of the larger transverse and smaller terminal arterioles to the various stimuli could determine the muscle capillary perfusion (nutritive flow). For the tenuissimus muscle, non-nutritive flow was implied to be that received by the connective tissue at the extremity of the transverse arteriole (16).

Apart from controlling oxygen delivery to support working muscle fibers, the balance of nutritive to non-nutritive blood flow has implications for access of other nutrients and hormones. Factors controlling glucose uptake by skeletal muscle are important to the understanding of diabetes. Muscle represents the major insulin-sensitive organ of the body that can become insulin resistant in many diabetics, and a possible role of the vasculature in the control of glucose uptake by muscle is apparent from several studies. For example, Table 1 shows data from Kern et al. (17) where insulin-mediated 3-O-methylglucose uptake in incubated rat soleus muscle is compared with the same muscle in a perfused rat hindlimb system. Clearly, the muscle receiving nutrient and hormone by the

TABLE 1. *Insulin dose response of 3-O-methylglucose transport rates in soleus muscle as an isolated incubated preparation or a component muscle of the perfused hindlimb.*

| Insulin addition (nmol/L) | Transport rate (nmol/g/min) | |
	Incubated (n = 22)	Perfused (n = 9)
None	124±13	41±10[a]
1	194±13	79±10[a]
10	252±13	571±82[a]
100	313±13	600±51[a]

Modified with permission from ref. (17). Values were given as means with errors often within symbols; interpolated maximum values are thus shown here.
[a]$p < 0.01$ perfused versus incubated.

vascular route has a lower basal rate (perhaps less hypoxia), a higher maximum insulin-mediated rate (optimal access for 3-O-methylglucose and insulin), and an overall greater percentage increase over the full range of insulin concentrations. Similar observations were made when extensor digitorum longus muscles, incubated and perfused, were compared (17).

In a second example, Grubb and Snarr (18) reported that glucose uptake by the perfused rat hindlimb changed in proportion to total flow. Indeed, Fig. 1, which is based on their data, shows that the glucose uptake rate reached a plateau at supraphysiologic flow rates even though carefully conducted controls showed that this was not due to saturation of the uptake process. These investigators concluded that the rate may have declined at high flow because much of the flow was selectively channeled through non-nutritive vessels.

The third example implying vascular regulation of muscle metabolism stems from reports by Laakso et al. (19) of insulin-mediated increases in human leg blood flow in conjunction with increases in glucose uptake (Fig. 2). Although Baron's laboratory (19) was not the first to report that insulin mediated a marked increase in leg blood flow (20), his group was the first to report an impairment of insulin-mediated flow increase along with the loss in glucose uptake in insulin-resistant patients [i.e., those with non–insulin-dependent diabetes mellitus (NIDDM)]. These findings implied that insulin's action to increase flow to skeletal muscle might well form some of the basis by which insulin mediates an increase in glucose uptake by this tissue (Fig. 2). However, not all laboratories agree that insulin's ability to increase muscle blood flow in patients with NIDDM is impaired (21,22). Although there is no evidence as yet that insulin alters the proportion of nutritive to non-nutritive flow within the skeletal muscles, some reports on collected leg muscle lymph suggest that insulin access to muscle is not impeded by vascular defects in NIDDM patients (23).

Taken together, there would appear to be ample evidence to suggest that an important level of control of aerobic performance and metabolism by muscle resides within the vasculature and its determining effect on nutrient access. A

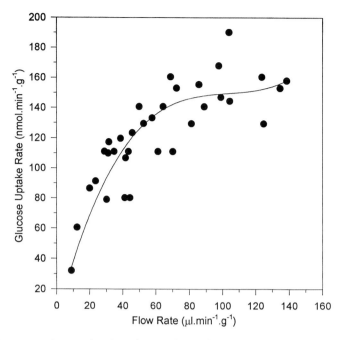

FIG. 1. Glucose uptake as a function of the perfusate flow rate for the constant-flow perfused rat hindlimb. Modified with permission (18).

regulated balance between nutritive and non-nutritive flow would also seem obvious. However, nowadays the notion of a parallel division of the microcirculatory arteriovenous paths into nutritive and non-nutritive vessels is not widely accepted. Indeed, current physiology textbooks regard skeletal muscle as having only a single vascular supply (24), and the phenomenon of a discretely controlled functional vascular shunt is regarded as unlikely (25). Comparisons between arteriovenous equilibration fractions of high and low diffusible substances suggest that limitations of transport from capillary to tissue of slowly diffusing substances is due to the high ratio of Q (flow)/PS (capillary diffusion capacity) that can occur in short arteriovenous paths (25). Implied in this line of thinking is the notion that non-nutritive flow would represent a situation of few open capillaries, a low capillary surface area, and a high capillary flow rate. Until technology exists for determining both flow rate through a particular capillary and the amount of O_2 consumed by parenchymal tissue from that capillary, these matters cannot be resolved. Consequently assumptions have to be made as to what occurs in exchange vessels when complex organs such as the perfused hindlimb are considered. Thus proposed relationships between capillary flow and nutrient exchange become virtually meaningless, more so if exchange in particular capillaries (nutritive) turns out to be regulated by paracrine factors.

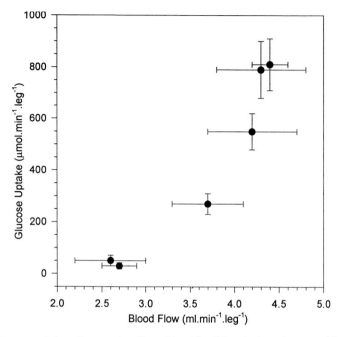

FIG. 2. Glucose uptake rate as a function of leg blood flow in lean humans. Modified with permission (19).

VASCULAR CONTROL OF MUSCLE METABOLISM AND PERFORMANCE: NEW INSIGHTS

The approach we have adopted to explore the relationship between the vasculature and muscle metabolism/performance has focused on the perfused rat hindlimb and the use of agents known to have vascular effects in this organ. The perfusion technique was essentially the same constant-flow system as that developed by Ruderman (26) with red blood cell–containing perfusate at 37°C or as modified by Côté et al. (27), involving erythrocyte-free medium to allow direct recording of venous PO_2. For both, an arterial pressure transducer was fitted in line to monitor changes in vascular resistance. Red blood cells were required to be omitted in some experiments so that interference in vascular space recruitment studies was minimized. Thus, postequilibration efflux of entrapped red blood cells could be measured along with entrapped fluorescently labeled macromolecules, such as dextran. When red blood cells were not used, the perfusate temperature was usually reduced to 25°C; this allowed ample O_2 availability and maintenance of physiologic energy status (e.g., CrP:Cr and adenine nucleotide energy charge).

Two aspects of our initial findings were entirely unexpected. First, because vascular effects of various vasoactive agents had been studied independently of metabolism, we expected that at constant flow, vasoconstrictors such as angiotensin and vasopressin would have strong vasoconstrictor activity with little or no effect on hindlimb metabolism. However, these agents profoundly affected the metabolism of the perfused hindlimb. Second, it was surprising that when various vasoconstrictors were compared, they fell into either of two groups that we have since called type A or type B, depending on whether they stimulated or inhibited $\dot{V}O_2$, respectively. Figure 3 shows typical data for a representative member of each type of vasoconstrictor. In addition to the opposite effects on $\dot{V}O_2$, other indices of metabolism were similarly affected. Thus, type A vasoconstrictors increased lactate, glycerol, urate, uracil, and fatty acid efflux and increased pressure and $\dot{V}O_2$. Type B vasoconstrictors had quite the opposite effect to type A and decreased all these indices of metabolism. It is perhaps important to note that some agents belong in both categories dependent on dose.

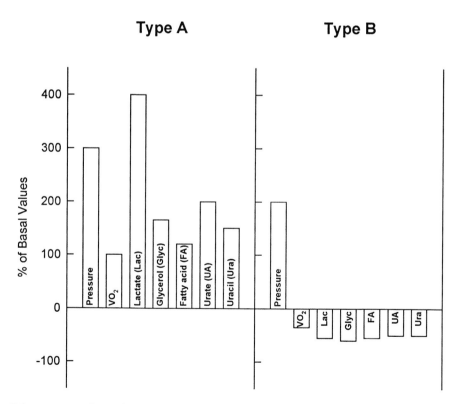

FIG. 3. Typical effects of type A and type B vasoconstrictors on the perfused hindlimb. Data are shown for 100 nmol/L norepinephrine (type A) and for 1 μmol/L 5-HT (type B). Other members of the two groups of vasoconstrictors are listed elsewhere (28). Most values can be found in earlier reports (28,49,63), and discriminating features of the two groups of vasoconstrictors are provided elsewhere (63). The basal value for free-fatty acid release was 0.11 ± 0.04 μmol/g/h.

Thus, for example, norepinephrine at low dose (≤1 µmol/L) is a type A vaso-constrictor and at higher doses is a type B vasoconstrictor (Fig. 4). The various members of each category are listed elsewhere (28) and include those that show dose-dependent dichotomy. Plots of change in $\dot{V}O_2$ as a function of change in perfusion pressure clearly show that there is no straightforward simple relation-ship between the two (Fig. 4).

The notion that the type A and B vasoconstrictor effects result from vascular flow redistribution in muscle becomes particularly persuasive when the issue of aerobic muscle contraction is considered. Aerobic muscle tension development (fatiguing tetanic tension) is well known to be critically dependent on oxygen flow (4). Thus, occlusion of flow to working fibers dramatically reduces tension. Conversely, increasing total flow to a working hindlimb increases tension if prior flow is suboptimal. Figure 5 shows the effect of two type A vasoconstrictors [angiotensin II (AII), low-dose norepinephrine plus propranolol (LNE + Prop)] and one type B vasoconstrictor [serotonin (5-HT)] on tension development and oxygen uptake. Keeping in mind that these data are from constant flow perfused

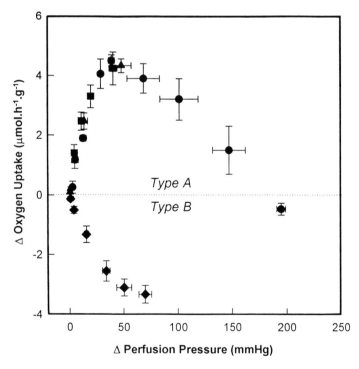

FIG. 4. Changes in oxygen uptake rate plotted against corresponding changes in perfusion pressure for the constant-flow perfused rat hindlimb at 25°C. Data are from earlier reports (64,38,65) and involve dose curves for (■) AII, (▲) vasopressin, (●) norepinephrine, and (◆) 5-HT.

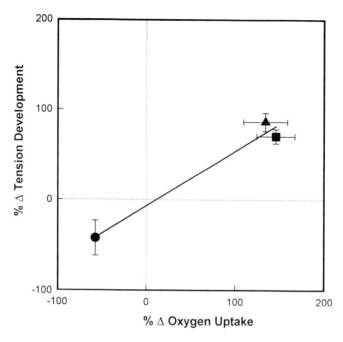

FIG. 5. Changes in aerobic tension development plotted against corresponding oxygen uptake for the constant-flow perfused rat hindlimb at 37°C. Data are from earlier reports (29,30) and unpublished observations. Additions were (●) 0.5 μmol/L 5-HT, (■) low-dose (0.1 μmol/L) norepinephrine + 10 μmol/L (±) propranolol, and (▲) 5 nmol/L AII. All hindlimbs were actively contracting due to stimulation of the sciatic nerve. Experimental details are from Dora et al. (29).

hindlimb and that anaerobic (twitch) tension is not affected by either type A or B vasoconstrictor, it appears likely that perfusate flow within muscle is altered. Thus, type A vasoconstrictors appear to act to increase O_2 supply to the working fibers by diminishing flow elsewhere. Conversely, type B vasoconstrictors, such as 5-HT, decrease O_2 supply to the working fibers and increase flow to functional vascular shunts (non-nutritive vessels). Both of the key studies supporting these findings (29,30) used perfusion medium containing red blood cells (35% hematocrit) at 37°C. Flow rate was high (approximately 1 ml/min/g), and basal perfusion pressure approached a physiologic level (66 ± 3 mmHg). However, once again, when muscles (soleus or extensor digitorum longus) were removed from the rat and incubated, tension development was found to be completely unaffected by the addition of the vasoconstrictor. This implies that the vasoconstrictors have no direct effect on skeletal muscle metabolism to affect contractility; rather, an indirect effect occurs involving the vascular control of oxygen supply that is demonstrable only in perfusion.

In each of the perfusions of Fig. 5 involving type A vasoconstrictors (e.g., low-dose NE + Prop or AII), vasoconstrictor-induced increases in perfusion pressure decreased markedly when motor nerve stimulation commenced to initiate contraction by the calf muscle group. This decrease in pressure would appear to be similar to that occurring in vivo when a muscle group begins to work (exercise) and is often referred to as sympatholysis (31). This is believed to result from a locally released vasodilator from the working fibers that acts against the pre-existing vascular tone to specifically enhance blood flow to the working fibers. Thus, exercising muscle can specifically receive enhanced blood flow (reactive hyperemia) against a global vasoconstrictor tone (32). There appears little doubt that the heterogeneity of red cell distribution and velocities that exist in resting muscle are largely eliminated when muscle contracts. This has been confirmed using in vivo microscopy (33) or direct surface electrode measurement of local hydrogen clearance (34). Moreover, the redistribution of flow observed by Harrison et al. (34) during exercise occurred in the absence of any increase in total flow.

There is some evidence that exercise-mediated release of so-called metabolic vasodilators opens terminal arterioles leading to nutritive capillaries (35). Accordingly, it would seem unlikely that access to nutritive capillaries is directly governed by type B vasoconstrictor sites on terminal arterioles because 5-HT–mediated vasoconstriction is not overcome by skeletal muscle contraction (28). Moreover, there is evidence that 5-HT–mediated vasoconstriction occurs on larger arterioles both from direct observations by others (36) as well as our own findings from vascular casts (37) and lack of dependence on extracellular Ca^{2+} and O_2 (38). Similarly, relaxation of type A sites on terminal arterioles that govern access to non-nutritive capillaries (28) would decrease nutritive flow. Thus, it seems likely that 5-HT (type B) may be acting on larger arterioles (proximal supply arteries) or even feed arteries external to the muscle fibers and not small arterioles (36) to control overall pressure on the nutritive capillary network. Partial or total constriction of these larger vessels would shift the point in the microcirculation that holds the resistance to pressure to larger vessels. Therefore, because the nutritive capillary network is now under lower pressure, those capillaries of higher resistance would cease flow (39). If conditions of constant flow prevail, vasoconstriction at sites on the larger vessels may deflect flow to branch vessels higher up the vascular tree leading to non-nutritive capillaries possibly in nonmuscle tissue (e.g., septa and tendons) (11). In such a model, sites for type A vasoconstrictors that increase nutritive flow could be located on transverse arterioles proximal to low-resistance capillaries supplying connective tissue (16) or on feeding vessels for large capillarylike arteriovenous channels of intermuscular septa and tendon (40). Constriction at either or both of these sites increases pressure in the nutritive capillary network, and more nutritive capillaries of higher resistance begin to carry flow (39). Metabolic vasodilators produced during muscle contraction may dilate terminal arterioles that have neither type A nor type B vasoconstrictor sites.

A recent observation in our laboratory is that 12-μm microspheres (Fig. 6), but neither 24- nor 90-μm microspheres (unpublished observations), partially revert type B metabolic characteristics to type A. This may mean that the 12-μm micros-pheres are able to pass the partly constricted type B sites on the larger arterioles and block the terminal arterioles, increasing the pressure in the nutritive capillary network. This in turn leads to flow being carried by an increased number of nutri-tive capillaries. The response is restricted to a finite number of beads (3×10^6 for a 7-g hindlimb). If this number is exceeded, presumably the beads begin to block vessels leading to capillaries (nutritive and non-nutritive) without discrimination, and thus total flow decreases (Fig. 6). Evidently, larger beads block higher in the vascular tree and lower the pressure on the capillary network.

Glucose uptake by the constant-flow perfused rat hindlimb is responsive to insulin, and type A and B vasoconstrictors have marked effects on glucose uptake by this preparation, particularly when insulin is present (41,42) (Fig. 7). These effects, like those on aerobic tension development, are not apparent when isolated muscles (red or white) are incubated with insulin $\pm$ vasoconstrictors

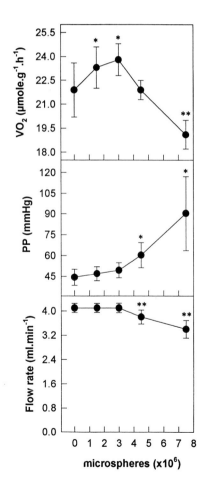

FIG. 6. Effect of microsphere infusion on 5-HT-mediated changes in oxygen uptake, perfusion pressure, and flow rate of the perfused rat hindlimb at 32°C. Pump rate for arterial delivery was constant; actual venous outflow rates are shown. Basal rates, before 5-HT addition, which was maintained throughout were 25.5 ± 1.0 μmol/g/h: $\dot{V}O_2$), 30 ± 0.5 mm Hg (pressure), and 4.2 ± 0.2 ml/min (flow). *p < 0.05, **p < 0.01 when compared with the absence of microspheres using Student's paired *t* test (n = 5) (unpublished data).

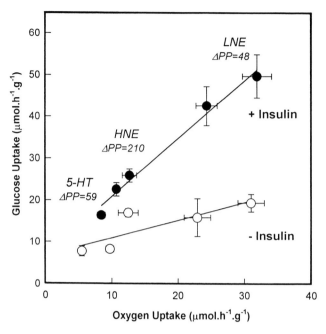

FIG. 7. Glucose uptake rate plotted against oxygen uptake rate for the perfused rat hindlimb at 37°C. Experimental conditions were as described elsewhere (41). Additions were 5-HT (10 μmol/L 5-HT), low-dose norepinephrine (LNE, 1 μmol/L), or high-dose norepinephrine (HNE, 10 μmol/L). Data from earlier reports (41,42).

(41; unpublished observations), so direct effects of the vasoconstrictors on skeletal muscle glucose metabolism are unlikely. Figure 7 shows a positive correlation between the rate of insulin-mediated glucose uptake and the rate of oxygen uptake. It is noteworthy that insulin has almost no effect on oxygen uptake and that because the clearance of glucose is low in the absence of insulin, the type A and B vasoconstrictors have little effect. An explanation to account for the type A and type B vasoconstrictor effects to alter insulin-mediated glucose uptake follows the lines used earlier in this article and focuses on the vasculature. Thus, we would argue that type A vasoconstrictors, by increasing the extent of nutritive flow, increases both insulin and glucose access. Type B vasoconstrictors appear to be the opposite, and by increasing non-nutritive flow, perhaps to septa and tendons (12), reduce access. The possibility that either type A or type B vasoconstrictors have direct effects on muscle to influence glucose uptake or modify insulin action can be assessed by adding vasodilators to the perfused hindlimb that are known to have no direct effects themselves on skeletal muscle. Thus, the inhibition of insulin-mediated glucose uptake by 5-HT was countered by carbachol, which also opposed the effect of 5-HT to increase perfusion pressure and to inhibit oxygen uptake (41).

TABLE 2. *Effects of vasoconstrictors on vascular recruitment in the constant-flow perfused rat hindlimb preparation*

	Type A	Type B	n
Increase in perfusion pressure (mm Hg)	35 ± 5	32 ± 3	3
Volume of blood displaced (µl)	37.9 ± 2.6	0	3
Volume of vascular tree[a] recruited (ml)	0.74 ± 0.14[b]	0	16
Volume of vascular tree[c] derecruited (ml)	0	0.32 ± 0.05[d]	16

Data are from Newman et al. (37).

[a]Volume recruited was determined with FITC dextran (M_r 150,000) by varying the time between successive exposures to 0.1 µmol/L NE, which at this dose is purely a type A vasoconstrictor.

[b]The volume is not static; $t_{0.5}$ = 16 min.

[c]Volume derecruited was determined with FITC dextran by varying the time between successive exposures to 1 µmol/L 5-HT, a type B vasoconstrictor.

[d]The volume is not static; $t_{0.5}$ = 15 min.

EVIDENCE FOR DISTINCT VASCULAR PATHWAYS IN MUSCLE

Evidence that metabolic and contractile effects of the type A and B vasoconstrictors derive from their effects to control different flow routes within muscle has recently been obtained (Table 2) (37). Again, perfusion conditions were constant flow. Cell-free perfusate was deliberately chosen so that efflux by trapped red blood cells could be readily detected. Table 2 shows data for a type A vasoconstrictor (0.1 µmol/L NE) and a type B vasoconstrictor (0.75 µmol/L 5-HT) that gave similar increases in perfusion pressure. Even though the perfusion pressures were similar for NE and 5-HT (e.g., 35 ± 5 (n = 3) and 32 ± 3 (n = 3) mm Hg, respectively), only NE increased the postequilibration red blood cell washout. Estimates indicated the total equivalent volume of blood washed out to be 37.9 ± 2.6 µl. Red blood cells were not washed out even if a higher dose of 5-HT (1 µmol/L) was used that increased pressure by 72 ± 0.7 mm Hg (37).

Additional experiments were then conducted to directly test the notion that NE acts to access additional nutritive vessels within the hindlimb vasculature. To do this, FITC-labeled dextran (M_r 150,000) was infused over a constant period of 35 minutes and NE introduced for 10 minutes in the middle of the labeled-dextran infusion, the rationale being that if NE increased perfusate distribution, these newly recruited vessels would thus be loaded with the marker and trapped when NE was withdrawn. These predictions appeared to be valid, and a significant new space was recruited by NE that was emptied after a second exposure to the catecholamine. By varying the time of exposure between consecutive infusions of NE, it was apparent that the recruited space was slowly cleared. Linear extrapolation to zero time (the time at which the first NE infusion ceased) suggested that the volume recruited could approach as much as 0.74 ± 0.14 ml or 31.4 ± 6.0% of the pre-NE vascular volume. To address the possibility that NE closed off a previously perfused region in conjunction with the recruitment of the new space, a single infusion of NE was made during the period of labeled dextran infusion and continued beyond cessation of the dextran infusion, the rationale being that if NE-mediated vasoconstriction closed off a vascular space, this would be cleared upon cessation of the catecholamine infusion. No evidence could be found for an NE-mediated closure (derecruitment) of a previously perfused vascular space concomitant with the recruitment of the new space (Table 2).

As indicated earlier, 5-HT has been categorized by us (28) as a type B vasoconstrictor of the perfused rat hindlimb and as such produces markedly different effects to NE, a type A vasoconstrictor. Table 2 summarizes data from experiments in which 5-HT replaced NE but which were identical to those described above involving NE. Thus, unlike NE, 5-HT did not recruit a new vascular space that was filled by labeled dextran, but rather, vasoconstriction by this agonist resulted in the closing off of a space. Prior loading of this space with labeled dextran was cleared when 5-HT infusion ceased. By using tactics similar to those used for NE, it was possible to calculate the derecruited space as 0.32 ± 0.05 ml or $13.6 \pm 2.1\%$ of the preserotonin perfused vascular volume. Derecruitment occurred without an accompanying recruitment of new space. Overall, the type B vasoconstrictor 5-HT would appear to be closing down access to nutritive capillaries (the derecruited space) and increasing flow through nonnutritive vessels that were already perfused. The type A vasoconstrictor is apparently recruiting nutritive capillaries, but not at the expense of non-nutritive flow, which decreases but does not stop.

METABOLIC INDICATORS OF NUTRITIVE FLOW

As indicated above, there is now solid evidence that the type A and B vasoconstrictors have opposing effects on metabolism in the constant flow perfused rat hindlimb. Because these opposing effects may result from selective vasoconstriction at different sites to alter nutrient access and possibly nutritive flow, we have attempted to monitor the effect of type A and B vasoconstrictors on the metabolism of an infused substrate known to be metabolized by an endothelial enzyme in this preparation. The rationale for these experiments was that if type A and B vasoconstrictors acted by altering the pattern of perfusate flow within muscle there would be a corresponding change in the exposure of exogenously added substrate to enzyme(s) located in the vasculature. Increased exposure to an endothelial enzyme, for example, might therefore be expected to lead to increased metabolism of the substrate as it passes through the vascular system once.

There were similarities and differences in the approach used by other researchers in the past. Clearance of intramuscular injections of [24]Na or iodide was used by early researchers to measure blood flow. However, when tried in skeletal muscle, it soon became clear that alterations in flow did not coincide under all conditions with the rate of clearance (12 and references therein). It was partly from this divergence that the concepts of nutritive and non-nutritive flow pioneered by Pappenheimer (1) were extended (43). For example, Renkin in 1955 (14) studied the filtration rates of antipyrine, urea, and sucrose in the perfused hindlimb of the cat. These substances were infused intra-arterially and their clearance assessed under a variety of conditions. More recently, evidence for a functional shunt (non-nutritive) of 30–40% in the dog gastrocnemius muscle, both at rest and during stimulation, was obtained via the local xenon clearance method (44) and via inert gas washout (45). Harrison et al. (34) have used both surface and intravenous hydrogen clearance measurements to confirm heterogeneity of flow within dog and rabbit skeletal muscle. During motor nerve stimulation they concluded that oxygenated blood was diverted from high-flow, non-nutritive vessels to normal (nutritive) capillaries to meet the increased local oxygen demand. However, to our knowledge assessment of relative nutritive flow in muscle using metabolism of exogenously applied substrates has not been studied previously.

In choosing the substrate to be infused, it was imperative that three conditions be fulfilled. First, the substrate, at the concentrations used, should be nonvasoactive. Second, the substrate should be converted to only one product by the enzyme in question, and the sum of the substrate and product should be quantitative. Third, the conversion of substrate to product should be catalyzed solely by the enzyme in question.

Our choice of the substrate, 1-methyl xanthine (1-MX), was prompted by the observations by Day et al. (46) that 1-MX, derived from theophylline, could be used as an in vivo biochemical probe of allopurinol efficacy in humans. They reported that 1-MX was converted solely to 1-methyl urate (1-MU), and recoveries of 1-MX + 1-MU were quantitative. In our studies, 1-MX was found to have neither vasoconstrictor nor vasodilator effect in the perfused rat hindlimb over the concentration range at which its metabolism could be readily studied (5–100 µmol/L). This was important because methyl xanthines, as inhibitors of cyclic adenosine monophosphate phosphodiesterases, can alter Ca^{2+} ion transients and as a consequence can have potent relaxing activities on preconstricted smooth muscles (47). They may also increase intracellular Ca^{2+} levels by releasing Ca^{2+} from intracellular and extracellular stores (48). However, the concentration generally required for methyl xanthines to have these effects is 100 µmol/L or greater; thus, the metabolism of 24 µmol/L 1-MX could be studied in the constant flow perfused rat hindlimb without effect on the balance of nutritive to non-nutritive flow.

Fulfillment of the second condition that 1-MX was exclusively metabolized to 1-MU was met and under a variety of perfusion conditions (basal, NE-vasoconstricted, or 5-HT vasoconstricted) the recovery of 1-MX + 1-MU was always 100 ± 5%.

Proof that the 1-MX was metabolized to 1-MU solely by xanthine oxidase was obtained by using allopurinol. At 20 µmol/L this analogue of hypoxanthine completely inhibited the conversion of 1-MX to 1-MU by the perfused hindlimb.

Having met the three stringent conditions that would allow 1-MX metabolism as a qualitative index of nutritive flow, it was of considerable interest to then study the effects of type A and B vasoconstrictors on the rate of metabolism. Table 3 shows the results from such studies as well as the effects of increasing flow rate, which alone had significant effects on the metabolism of 1-MX to 1-MU, increasing from 52 ± 4 to 108 ± 8 nmol/min/g hindlimb muscle as the steady state flow rate was increased from 5 to 12 ml/min. The type B vasoconstrictor 5-HT, infused when the flow rate was 5 ml/min, inhibited the metabolic rate from 52 ± 4 to 36 ± 3 nmol/min/g hindlimb muscle ($p < 0.0001$). The type A vasoconstrictor NE had no significant effect when the flow rate was 5 ml/min. This appeared to be due to competitive inhibition between the infused 1-MX and endogenously produced hypoxanthine and xanthine, which were increased due to the type A vasoconstrictor activity (49). At the higher flow of 12 ml/min this competition was markedly reduced due to the effect of increased flow to decrease the concentration of the endogenously released xanthines. Thus, at 12 ml/min NE significantly increased metabolism of 1-MX from 108 ± 8 to 132 ± 11 nmol/min/g hindlimb muscle ($p < 0.001$). Overall these results support the notion that type A vasoconstrictors increase and type B vasoconstrictors decrease nutritive flow in the constant flow perfused rat hindlimb.

Metabolism of 1-MX in vivo has been successfully used by Birkett et al. (50) as a biochemical probe for studying the efficacy of allopurinol in gout treatment. However, 1-MX is poorly absorbed and has to be administered intravenously. In addition, extensive first-pass metabolism occurs, and the 1-MU/1-MX ratio after intravenous 1-MX is about 2.5. However despite these problems, 1-MX is a successful indicator in vivo, and the 1-MU/1-MX ratio decreases sharply as the concentration of oxypurinol (the product of xanthine oxidase on allopurinol) increases and vice versa (50).

A distinct disadvantage of using 1-MX metabolism as an indicator of skeletal muscle nutritive flow in vivo is the fact that xanthine oxidase, the enzyme

TABLE 3. *Effect of flow rate and vasoconstrictors on metabolism of infused 1-methyl xanthine (1-MX) to 1-methyl urate (1-MU) by the constant-flow perfused rat hindlimb*

Additions	Flow rate (ml/min)	Metabolism of 1-MX to 1-MU (nmol/min/g hindlimb muscle)
None	5 ± 0.1	52 ± 4
None	12 ± 0.2	108 ± 8
NE (0.05 μmol/L)	12 ± 0.2	132 ± 11[a]
5-HT (0.35 μmol/L)	5 ± 0.1	36 ± 3[a]

Hindlimbs were surgically isolated, cannulated, and allowed to equilibrate for 40 min with erythrocyte-free perfusion medium at 25°C. 1-MX was infused at a constant rate to reach approximately 24 μmol/L final concentration. At steady state 1-MX:1-MU ratio, the flow rate was increased or 5-HT was infused. When the flow rate was increased, a new steady state was allowed to occur before infusing NE. Samples were collected from the venous outflow for 1-MX and 1-MU analysis by HPLC. Values are means $\pm$ SEM for $n = 5$.
[a]$p < 0.001$ relative to corresponding "None."

responsible for the metabolism of 1-MX to 1-MU, is low in skeletal muscle relative to other tissues. Thus, although Hellsten-Westing (51) found xanthine oxidase to be localized mainly in the vascular smooth muscle cells and endothelial cells of capillaries and smaller vessels of skeletal muscle, its total activity appeared to be about 1/800 that found in liver.

Despite this drawback, the use of 1-MX in vivo for nutritive flow assessment in skeletal muscle has been instructive. Thus, Fig. 8 shows the effect of insulin infusion in vivo (10 mU/min/kg) on hindlimb metabolism of 1-MX. In these experiments animals were maintained at 37°C under anesthesia with indwelling probes for monitoring femoral artery blood flow, heart rate, and blood pressure. Femoral vein and carotid artery cannulae allowed determination of arteriovenous difference for 1-MX across the hindlimb. The data show that insulin increased 1-MX disappearance. The main contributing factor to the insulin-mediated increase in disappearance was the increase in femoral blood flow from 0.75 to 1.60 ml/min with little change in extraction of 1-MX. These findings suggest that insulin mediated an increase in flow to muscle with a greater exposure to xanthine oxidase (capillary recruitment). By so doing, insulin probably improves access for both itself and glucose to muscle fibers.

Clearly, more experiments are required to validate the in vivo use of indicators of nutritive flow in skeletal muscle. Type A and type B vasoconstrictor effects need to be compared and the findings from the perfused rat hindlimb substantiated.

VASCULAR CONTROL OF SKELETAL MUSCLE BY PARACRINE SIGNALS

We have been intrigued by our own findings (28) and those of others (27,52,53) that type A vasoconstrictors have such marked effects to stimulate

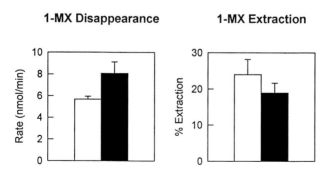

FIG. 8. Effect of insulin infusion in vivo (10 mU/min/kg) on hindlimb metabolism of 1-MX. Animals were anesthetized, and indwelling probes were placed to monitor femoral artery blood flow, heart rate, and blood pressure. Femoral vein and carotid artery cannulae allowed determination of AV difference for 1-MX across the hindlimb. Values are means ± SEM for n = 4 (unpublished data).

basal metabolism by muscle. There is no obvious reason why this should occur, particularly because there is no evidence of pre-existing hypoxia, nor is there evidence that the new steady state of increased metabolism reflects "catch up." Furthermore, increasing the supply of oxygen and nutrients to muscle is not, in itself, a stimulus for increased metabolism [e.g., red blood cell vs. non–red blood cell perfusions (28)]. Thus, we have proposed (28) that site-specific vasoconstriction (e.g., by type A vasoconstrictors) within the hindlimb leads to the release of a signal substance(s). An endocrine relationship between the vasculature and the skeletal muscle fibers is proposed where vasoconstriction and increased flow are the two principal mechanisms for shear stress–dependent endothelial release of paracrine signals.

Evidence already exists that hemodynamic forces, shear stress, and intravascular pressure are regulatory signals of cardiac metabolism and function (54 and references therein). The positive inotropic effect of flow (Gregg effect) (55) is now regarded as being caused by pure hydraulic factors and by an ischemic correction. Thus, only at low perfusion pressures do the metabolic consequences of ischemia superimpose on the inotropism of flow (56). Furthermore, if coronary flow is kept constant, a positive inotropic effect can be induced by increasing the viscosity of the perfusing medium (57). It is also important to note that the hormonelike effect of coronary flow–enhanced contraction appears to result from an elevation of intracellular free calcium (56) and is not the result of an increase in initial muscle length or ventricle cell rigidity (57).

Recent findings by Rubio et al. (54) may further help in the search for paracrine signals of vascular origin controlling skeletal muscle metabolism. These researchers have noted that auricular–ventricular transmission, another calcium-dependent cardiac function, was also stimulated by coronary flow. However, when coronary vascular resistance was altered by dilation (nitroglycerin, bradykinin, nitroprusside, or adenosine) or by constriction (AII), the stimulatory effect of flow remained the same despite wide changes in perfusing pressure (54). These observations imply that flow and not pressure is the key stimulus.

A flow-dependent effect on the isometric twitch tension of blood-perfused canine muscle (58) has been attributed to a mediator that at high flow acts to increase force development (59). According to our observations, we would argue that increasing flow to working muscle may simply increase force development by increasing nutritive flow. However, a flow-induced mediator release also may occur. Interestingly, Murrant and Barclay (59) recently reported that s-nitroso-N-acetyl penicillamine, a source of nitric oxide, increased the developed force of isolated contracting mouse muscles. Nitric oxide also may be involved in exercise-mediated glucose uptake (60) and insulin-mediated vasodilatation (61) of muscle. Such findings support the notion of the vascular control of skeletal muscle by paracrine signals and may help to explain the mechanism by which increased flow (62) or type A vasoconstrictors (28) increase metabolism in perfused rat hindlimb.

SUMMARY

A clear picture is now emerging of the control of skeletal muscle contraction and metabolism by the vasculature. Early observations by other researchers had suggested the presence of two circulation systems (nutritive and non-nutritive) in this tissue where the flow in either had specific but different regulation. Our recent findings indicate that vasoconstriction at specific sites in the vascular tree control the flow to either nutritive or non-nutritive regions. Type A vasoconstrictors improve flow to nutritive regions by constricting transverse arterioles to thus restrict entry to low-resistance capillaries that could be in muscle or connective tissue. Type B vasoconstrictors probably act on larger arterioles to lower pressure on the nutritive capillary network and redirect flow to non-nutritive vessels possibly located in septa and tendons. Evidence is presented for type A vasoconstrictors to improve metabolism, aerobic contraction performance, and hormone access. This appears to be achieved by increasing the perfused space (recruitment of nutritive capillaries) without derecruitment of existing perfused space. Type B vasoconstrictors decrease metabolism, contraction performance, and hormone access by apparently closing off a significant perfusion space; no new space is recruited. Changes in the metabolism of exogenously applied 1-MX to 1-MU, as a putative maker of the capillary network, are consistent with the type A and B vasoconstrictor effects of endogenous metabolism and contraction in the constant-flow perfused hindlimb and the notion of discretely controlled nutritive and non-nutritive flow in skeletal muscle. There is the possibility that these concepts can now be investigated in vivo. Finally there is evidence that paracrine substances of vascular origin influence skeletal muscle contraction. Future studies will show whether they also can mediate metabolism and account for the effects of vasoconstriction.

ACKNOWLEDGMENTS

Research from the authors' laboratory was generously supported by grants from the Australian Research Council, National Health and Medical Research Council, and Australian Mutual Provident Society Medical Research Fund. We thank Andrew Clark and Anita Matthias for helpful discussions during the preparation of this chapter.

REFERENCES

1. Pappenheimer JR. Vasoconstriction nerves and oxygen consumption in the isolated perfused hindlimb muscles of the dog. *J Physiol Lond* 1941;99:182–200.
2. Sonnenschein RR, Hirvonen L. Effects of vasoactive drugs on blood flow and work performance in skeletal muscle. *Biochem Pharmacol* 1961;8:166.
3. Hyman C, Rosell S, Rosén A, et al. Effects of alteration of total muscular blood flow on local tissue clearance of radio-iodide in the cat. *Acta Physiol Scand* 1959;46:358–374.

4. Hirvonen L, Sonnenschein RR. Relation between blood flow and contraction force in active skeletal muscle. *Circ Res* 1961;10:94–104.

5. Renkin EM, Rosell S. Effects of different types of vasodilator mechanisms on vascular tonus and on transcapillary exchange of diffusible material in skeletal muscle. *Acta Physiol Scand* 1962;54:241–251.

6. Zweifach BW. The structure and reactions of the small blood vessels in Amphibia. *Am J Anat* 1937;60: 473–514.

7. Saunders RL de CH, Lawrence J, MacIver DA, et al. Anatomic basis of the peripheral circulation in man. In: Redisch W, Tangco F, eds. *Peripheral circulation in health and disease.* New York: Grune & Stratton; 1957:113–145..

8. Dieter E. Über das Vorkommen arterio-venöser Anastomosen im Skeletmuskel. *Pflügers Arch* 1954;258: 470–474.

9. Kovách AGB, Antal J, Doby T. Haemodynamic regulation of the arteriovenous anastomoses of the limbs in the dog. *Acta Physiol Acad Sci Hung* 1958;14:141–147.

10. Piiper J, Rosell S. Attempt to demonstrate large arteriovenous shunts in skeletal muscle during stimulation of sympathetic vasodilator nerves. *Acta Physiol Scand* 1961;53:214–217.

11. Barlow TE, Haigh AL, Walder DN. Dual circulation in skeletal muscle. *J Physiol Lond* 1959;149: 18–19P.

12. Barlow TE, Haigh AL, Walder DN. A search for arteriovenous anastomoses in skeletal muscle. *J Physiol Lond* 1958;143:80P.

13. Walder DN. The relationship between blood flow, capillary surface area, and sodium clearance in muscle. *Clin Sci* 1955;14:303–315.

14. Renkin EM. Effects of blood flow in diffusion kinetics in isolated perfused hind legs of cats. A double circulation hypothesis. *Am J Physiol* 1955;183:125–136.

15. Zweifach BW, Metz DB. Selective distribution of blood through the terminal vascular bed of mesenteric structure and skeletal muscle. *Angiology* 1955;6:289–290.

16. Lindbom L, Arfors K-E. Non-homogeneous blood flow distribution in the rabbit tenuissimus muscle. *Acta Physiol Scand* 1984;122:225–233.

17. Kern MA, Tapscott EB, Snider RD, Dohm GL. Differences in glucose transport rates between perfused and in vitro incubated muscles. *Horm Metab Res* 1990;22:366–368.

18. Grubb B, Snarr JF. Effect of low flow rate and glucose concentration on glucose uptake rate by the rat limb. *Proc Soc Exp Biol Med* 1977;154:33–36.

19. Laakso M, Edelman SV, Brechtel G, Baron AD. Impaired insulin-mediated skeletal muscle blood flow in patients with NIDDM. *Diabetes* 1992;41:1076–1083.

20. Gelfand RA, Barrett EJ. Effect of physiological hyperinsulinemia on skeletal muscle protein synthesis and breakdown in man. *J Clin Invest* 1987;80:1–6.

21. Della F, Larsen JJ, Mikines KJ, Galbo H. Normal effect of insulin to stimulate leg blood flow in NIDDM. *Diabetes* 1995;44:221–226.

22. Pendergrass M, Fazion E, Collins D, Defronzo RA. Forearm blood flow is not a primary regulator of muscle glucose uptake [Abstract]. *Diabetes* 1995;44(suppl 1):196.

23. Castillo C, Bogardus C, Bergman R, et al. Interstitial insulin concentrations determine glucose uptake rates but not insulin resistance in lean and obese men. *J Clin Invest* 1994;93:10–16.

24. Guyton AC. *Textbook of medical physiology.* 8th ed. Philadelphia: WB Saunders; 1991.

25. Renkin EM. Exchange of substances through capillary walls. In: Wolstenholme GEW, Knight J, eds. *Circulatory and respiratory mass transport.* Boston: Little Brown; 1969:50–66.

26. Ruderman NB, Houghton CRS, Hems R. Evaluation of the isolated perfused rat hindquarter for the study of muscle metabolism. *Biochem J* 1971;124:639–651.

27. Côté C, Thibault MC, Vallières J. Effect of endurance training and chronic isoproterenol treatment on skeletal muscle sensitivity to norepinephrine. *Life Sci* 1985;37:695–701.

28. Clark MG, Colquhoun EQ, Rattigan S, et al. Vascular and endocrine control of muscle metabolism. *Am J Physiol* 1995;268:E797–E812.

29. Dora KA, Rattigan S, Colquhoun EQ, Clark MG. Aerobic muscle contraction impaired by serotonin-mediated vasoconstriction. *J Appl Physiol* 1994;77:277–284.

30. Rattigan S, Dora KA, Tong ACY, Clark MG. Perfused skeletal muscle contraction and metabolism improved by angiotensin II mediated vasoconstriction. *Am J Physiol* 1996;271:E96–E103.

31. Rememsnyder JP, Mitchell JH, Sarnoff SJ. Functional sympatholysis during muscular activity. *Circ Res* 1962;11:370–380.

32. Segal SS. Convection, diffusion and mitochondrial utilization of oxygen during exercise. In: Lamb DR, Gisolfi CV, eds. *Energy metabolism in exercise and sport, perspectives in exercise science and sports medicine.* Vol. 5. Dubuque, IA: Brown & Benchmark; 1992:269–344.

33. Groom AC, Ellis CG, Wrigley SM, Potter RF. Architecture and flow pattern in capillary networks of skeletal muscle in frog and rat. In: Popel AS, Johnson PC, eds. *Microvascular networks: experimental and theoretical studies*. Basel, Switzerland: Karger; 1986:61–76.

34. Harrison DK, Birkenhake S, Knauf SK, Kessler M. Local oxygen supply and blood flow regulation in contracting muscle in dogs and rabbits. *J Physiol Lond* 1990;422:227–243.

35. Lindbom L. Distribution patterns of blood flow in the rabbit tenuissimus muscle in response to brief ischemia and muscular contraction. *Microvasc Res* 1986;31:143–156.

36. Lamping KG, Kanatsuka H, Eastham CL, et al. Nonuniform vasomotor responses of the coronary microcirculation to serotonin and vasopressin. *Circ Res* 1989;65:343–351.

37. Newman JMB, Dora KD, Rattigan S, et al. Norepinephrine and serotonin vasoconstriction in rat hindlimb control different vascular flow routes. *Am J Physiol* 1996;270:E689–E699.

38. Dora KA, Richards SM, Rattigan S, et al. Serotonin and norepinephrine vasoconstriction in rat hindlimb have different oxygen requirements. *Am J Physiol* 1992;262:H698–H703.

39. Lindbom L, Arfors K-E. Mechanisms and site of control for variation in the number of perfused capillaries in skeletal muscle. *Int J Microcirc Clin Exp* 1985;4:19–30.

40. Grant RT, Payling Wright H. Anatomical basis for non-nutritive circulation in skeletal muscle exemplified by blood vessels of rat biceps femoris tendon. *J Anat* 1970;106:125–133.

41. Rattigan S, Dora KA, Colquhoun EQ, Clark MG. Serotonin-mediated acute insulin resistance in the perfused hindlimb but not in incubated muscle: a role for the vascular system. *Life Sci* 1993;53:1545–1557.

42. Rattigan S, Dora KA, Colquhoun EQ, Clark MG. An α-adrenergic vascular effect of norepinephrine to inhibit insulin-mediated glucose uptake in the perfused rat hindlimb. *Am J Physiol* 1995;268: E305–E311.

43. Walder DN. The local clearance of radioactive sodium from muscle in normal subjects and those with peripheral vascular disease. *Clin Sci* 1953;12:153–167.

44. Cerretelli P, Marconi C, Pendergast D, et al. Blood flow in exercising muscle by xenon clearance and by microsphere trapping. *J Appl Physiol* 1984;56:24–30.

45. Piiper J, Meyer M. Diffusion-perfusion relationship in skeletal muscle: models and experimental evidence for inert gas washout. *Adv Exp Med Biol* 1984;69:457–465.

46. Day RO, Miners J, Birkett DJ, et al. Relationship between plasma oxypurinol concentrations and xanthine oxidase activity in volunteers dosed with allopurinol. *Br J Clin Pharmacol* 1988;26:429–434.

47. Leijten PAA, Van Breemen C. The effects of caffeine on the noradrenaline-sensitive calcium store in rabbit aorta. *J Physiol* 1984;357:327–339.

48. Van der Bent V, Bény J-L. Mechanisms controlling caffeine-induced relaxation of coronary artery of the pig. *Br J Pharmacol* 1991;103:1877–1882.

49. Clark MG, Richards SM, Hettiarachchi M, et al. Release of purine and pyrimidine nucleosides and their catabolites from the perfused rat hindlimb in response to noradrenaline, vasopressin, angiotensin II and sciatic-nerve stimulation. *Biochem J* 1990;266:765–770.

50. Birkett DJ, Miners JO, Day RO. 1-methylxanthine derived from theophylline as an in vivo biochemical probe of allopurinol effect. *Br J Clin Pharmacol* 1991;32:238–241.

51. Hellsten-Westing Y. Immunohistochemical localization of xanthine oxidase in human cardiac and skeletal muscle. *Histochemistry* 1993;100:215–222.

52. Grubb B, Folk GE. The role of adrenoceptors in norepinephrine-stimulated V̇O$_2$ in muscle. *Eur J Pharmacol* 1977;43:217–223.

53. Richter EA, Ruderman NB, Gavras H, et al. Muscle glycogenolysis during exercise: dual control by epinephrine and contractions. *Am J Physiol* 1982;242:E25–E32.

54. Rubio R, Ceballos G, Suarez J. Coronary flow stimulates auricular–ventricular transmission in the isolated perfused guinea pig heart. *Am J Physiol* 1995;269:H1177–H1185.

55. Gregg DE, Fisher LC. Blood supply to the heart. In: *Handbook of physiology circulation*. Section 2, Vol. II. Washington, DC: American Physiology Society; 1963:1517–1584.

56. Kitakaze M, Marban E. Cellular mechanisms of the modulation of contractile function by coronary perfusion pressure in ferret hearts. *J Physiol Lond* 1989;414:455–472.

57. Arnold G, Koshe F, Miessner E, et al. The importance of the perfusing pressure in the coronary studies for the contractility and the oxygen consumption of the heart. *Pflugers Arch* 1968;299:339–356.

58. Barclay JK, Stainsby WN. The role of blood flow in limiting maximal metabolic rate in muscle. *Med Sci Sports* 1975;7:116–119.

59. Murrant CL, Barclay JK. Endothelial cell products alter mammalian skeletal muscle function in vitro. *Can J Physiol Pharmacol* 1995;73:736–741.

60. Balon TW, Nadler JL. Nitric oxide release is present from incubated skeletal muscle preparations. *J Appl Physiol* 1994;77:2519–2521.

61. Steinberg HO, Bretchel G, Johnson A, et al. Insulin mediated vasodilation is a determinant of in vivo insulin mediated glucose uptake [Abstract]. *Diabetes* 1995;44(suppl 1):56A.
62. Ye J-M, Colquhoun EQ, Hettiarachchi M, Clark MG. Flow-induced oxygen uptake by the perfused rat hindlimb is inhibited by vasodilators and augmented by norepinephrine: a possible role for the microvasculature in hindlimb thermogenesis. *Can J Physiol Pharmacol* 1990;68:119–125.
63. Clark MG, Colquhoun EQ, Dora KA, et al. Resting muscle: a source of thermogenesis controlled by vasomodulators. In: Milton AS, ed. *Temperature regulation.* Basel, Switzerland: Birkhäuser Verlag; 1994:315–320.
64. Colquhoun EQ, Hettiarachchi M, Ye JM, et al. Vasopressin and angiotensin II stimulate oxygen uptake in the perfused rat hindlimb. *Life Sci* 1988;43:1747–1754.
65. Dora KA, Colquhoun EQ, Hettiarachchi M, et al. The apparent absence of serotonin-mediated vascular thermogenesis in perfused rat hindlimb may result from vascular shunting. *Life Sci* 1991;48: 1555–1564.

Physiology, Stress, and Malnutrition: Functional
Correlates, Nutritional Intervention,
edited by J.M. Kinney and H.N. Tucker.
Lippincott–Raven Publishers © 1997.

Adipose Tissue: Regional Responsiveness

Johan Hellmér and Peter Arner

Division of Endocrinology, Huddinge University Hospital, S-141 86 Huddinge, Sweden

ADIPOSE TISSUE AND ENERGY BALANCE

Body fat in humans consists mainly of white adipose tissue. The total body fat in adult humans normally accounts for about 10% of body weight. Brown fat is present only in small amounts in adults and may play a role in heat production and energy expenditure, but it takes no part in energy storage, which is the main function of white fat (1). Normal amounts of white fat in adults constitute an energy reserve for about 3 months (2). Fat is stored inside the white adipocytes as triglycerides and accounts for 95% of the cell content. Triglycerides consist of a glycerol moiety and three carboxylated fatty acids. The net balance of energy depends mainly on nutritional status and energy expenditure.

The breakdown of triglycerides to glycerol and nonesterified fatty acids (lipolysis) is regulated by circulating hormones, paracrine factors, and norepinephrine from the sympathetic nerve ends. After food intake, triglycerides accumulate in the adipose tissue either through synthesis from carbohydrates (lipogenesis) or through the direct uptake of nonesterified fatty acids from circulating lipoproteins (3). In the fasting state, triglycerides are broken down to nonesterified fatty acids and glycerol by the action of hormone-sensitive lipase and then released into the circulation. Fat cell size seems to vary with nutritional status so that obese patients, for example, have large adipocytes and cell size is also reduced after fasting (4). With increasing obesity, new adipocytes probably develop from fibroblastlike preadipocytes so that in extreme obesity both cell size and cell number are increased (5). Lipolysis regulation is disturbed in many common diseases, such as diabetes, obesity, hyperlipoproteinemia, and thyroid disorders. Marked regional differences in lipolysis regulation in human white adipose tissue have often been noted. Differences are seen between visceral, abdominal subcutaneous, and peripheral subcutaneous fat both at rest and during adaptation to fasting and physical exercise. Furthermore, abdominal (android) but not peripheral (gynoid) obesity is associated with a higher cardiovascular and metabolic morbidity (6–8).

HORMONAL REGULATION OF LIPOLYSIS

Adipocytes in humans show a few marked differences from those in several laboratory animals, including the most common one, the rat. Human adipocytes during in vitro studies have a basal lipolytic activity that is not related to any known hormonal influence. In most animal fat cells no spontaneous lipolysis is detectable (9). Local modulators, such as adenosine and prostaglandins, may play an important role in the regulation of basal lipolysis in human adipose tissue (10,11). In adult human adipose tissue only insulin and catecholamines have an acute and pronounced effect on lipolysis (12). This is in contrast to several other species in which hormones, such as glucagon, ACTH, secretin, luteinizing hormone, follicle-stimulating hormone, and human chorionic gonadotropin, have a lipolytic effect (9,13).

Insulin, the major antilipolytic hormone, reduces the liberation of free fatty acids from the fat cell. The question of how insulin produces its antilipolytic effect is still somewhat controversial. The binding of insulin to its receptor results in the activation of a tyrosine kinase, which then generates intracellular signals (14). Data have been published showing that insulin inhibits adenylate cyclase, stimulates phosphodiesterase, and inhibits hormone-sensitive lipase (15). Catecholamines act through the adenylate cyclase system and exhibit both a lipolytic effect (via beta-receptors) and an antilipolytic effect (via alpha$_2$-receptors) in human fat cells.

CLINICAL ASPECTS ON CENTRAL AND PERIPHERAL OBESITY

Several epidemiologic studies have shown that central obesity, often expressed as an increased waist/hip ratio, is a risk factor for myocardial infarction. A lot of the gender differences in frequency of coronary heart disease are explained if men and women with comparable waist/hip ratios are studied (16,17). Femoral/gluteal subcutaneous fat generally has a slow turnover of triglycerides, except during late pregnancy and lactation, when lipid mobilization is facilitated. Lipoprotein lipase is the key enzyme for lipid uptake from blood, and its activity seems regulated by cortisol and female sex steroid hormones. Because fat cells lack specific sex steroid hormone receptors, it has been suggested that they exert their actions through glucocorticoid receptors (18). This provides one possible explanation for the typical gender difference in adipose tissue localization. Another could be that women show a more pronounced decrease in beta-adrenoceptor activity and an increase in alpha-adrenoceptor activity in femoral/gluteal as compared with abdominal adipose tissue than do men.

Abdominal obesity normally reflects both an increased subcutaneous and visceral adipose mass. The relative amount of each can be determined via computed tomography and via less accurate antropometric measurements. The visceral adipose tissue has the unique property of having direct access to the liver through the portal system. Nonesterified fatty acids could interfere with liver metabolism in many ways. A high influx of nonesterified fatty acids to the liver may (a) cause glucose intolerance through the Randle's cycle as well as increased lipogenesis and (b) cause increased very low density lipoprotein production by the liver because nonesterified free fatty acids are major substrates for triglycerides. Furthermore, nonesterified fatty acids may directly alter hepatic insulin action. They can inhibit insulin clearance by the liver (19) and also cause gluteal insulin resistance due to interactions with insulin receptors in the hepatocytes (20).

Despite some answers, there are still many remaining questions about the metabolic differences of adipose tissue in various locations in the body. Are regional differences due to early determination in stem cells or preadipocytes? Or are they merely a reflection of regional differences in blood flow, innervation, or connective tissue impact?

REGIONAL DIFFERENCES IN VITRO

Adipose tissue metabolism may be of critical importance to the etiology of the metabolic syndrome as discussed previously. A great deal of interest has focused on regional differences, and many modern sophisticated techniques in analytical chemistry, molecular biology, physiology, and radiology have been applied. It is not possible to directly quantify free fatty acid esterification to triglycerides in fat cells. Instead, indirect radioisotope methods must be used. In contrast, the lipolytic cascade, which is initiated by hormone to receptor binding and ends with acceleration or retardation of triglyceride hydrolysis, can be quantified. The end products, glycerol and nonesterified fatty acids, are easily measured, and many of the regulatory enzymes and receptors are purified, sequenced, and cloned. We focus the following discussion on regional differences in lipolysis regulation because this is where in vitro results and microdialysis data can be compared.

It has long been known from in vitro studies that the lipolytic activity varies between adipose depots in humans. This potentially important observation has been the subject of intense research and has been reviewed in detail (21). The highest lipolytic activity is found in visceral adipose tissue followed by subcutaneous abdominal tissue, and the lowest activity is seen in subcutaneous femoral/gluteal depots. The mechanisms behind these variations has been partly explained and involves the actions of insulin and catecholamines, the two major lipolysis-regulating hormones. The antilipolytic action of insulin is higher in visceral as compared with subcutaneous adipose tissue. This difference can be explained by alterations in both insulin receptor affinity and post-receptor mechanisms. As regards the lipolytic action of catecholamines, the pattern seems to be an increasing sensitivity from peripheral to more central fat depots so that visceral fat has the highest and femoral/gluteal fat has the lowest sensitivity. The major molecular mechanism for these differences in sensitivity seems to be a variation in the total amount of cell surface beta-adrenoceptors on the adipocytes. Beta-receptors in visceral fat seem to be 10 times more sensitive than those in subcutaneous abdominal fat and a hundred times more sensitive than those in subcutaneous femoral/gluteal fat. This could in turn be explained by a doubling of the number of cell surface beta-receptors in subcutaneous fat as compared with femoral/gluteal fat and a further doubling in visceral fat (22,23). Similar regional variations in adrenergic control of lipolysis also has been shown in dogs (24). Reciprocal variations in alpha$_2$-receptors also may play a role. The physiologic meaning of this difference is not known. It is possible that in catabolic situations in connection with acute stress (exercise, strain, trauma) when stored energy is needed, it may be advantageous to have easy access to visceral fat with only a moderate increase in catecholamines, thereby saving peripheral fat for more severe and/or prolonged situations with higher catecholamine levels.

MICRODIALYSIS TECHNIQUE

Microdialysis is a technique by which a catheter or a tube partly consisting of a semi-permeable membrane is inserted into an organ or a tissue. If the catheter or tube is then slowly perfused with a physiologic solution, this enables continuous sampling and manipulation of the interstitial fluid. The system could be viewed as a kind of artificial capillary. Any substances able to pass the semi-permeable membrane for reasons of size or chemical properties will equilibrate between the extra-cellular water and the solution inside the membrane. This works both ways so that extracellular metabolites can be assayed in the outgoing solution (called the dialysate) and drugs added to the ingoing solution (called the perfusate) can affect the cells next to the membrane through diffusion in the extra-cellular space (Fig. 1).

The technique has been in use since the 1970s but was used until the late 1980s almost exclusively to investigate neurotransmitters in rat and cat brains (25). Since the first publications (26,27) on its use in human adipose tissue, it has rapidly increased our knowledge on the regulation of adipose tissue metabolism in situ. Microdialysis has since then been applied to human muscle, blood, skin, brain, and kidney, indicating its potential as a useful tool in clinical experimental investigations. As an illustration to its varied use in clinical studies of adipose tissue, it has been used in ambulatory patients with portable pumps to monitor tissue glucose levels for several days (28) as well as in critically ill neonates to continuously monitor metabolic changes (29).

Technically, two different variants have been used in human adipose tissue. One is a commercially available double-lumen catheter in which the perfusate enters through an inner cannula and the dialysate leaves through a sidearm (Fig. 1) (27). The other consists of two separate single-lumen cannulas, connected by dialysis tubing. Both cannulas are inserted into the adipose tissue, and the perfusate enters through one cannula, then passes through the dialysis tubing, and finally

A

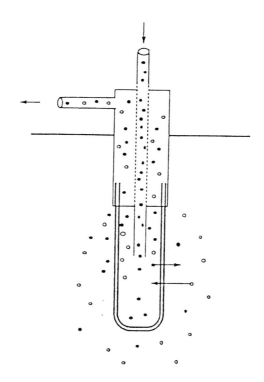

B

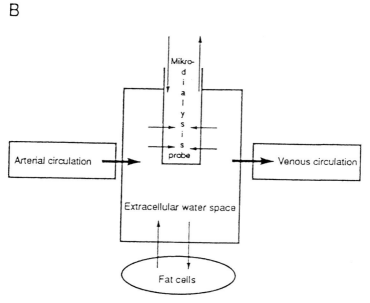

FIG. 1. Schematic presentation of a microdialysis probe (**A**) and the fluxes of compounds in the interstitial fluid of adipose tissue (**B**).

the dialysate leaves via the second cannula (26). The latter probe is not available in a ready-to-use form but has to be assembled in the laboratory. In both cases the system connects to a high-precision pump that can handle flow rates in the typical range of 0.1–10.0 µl/min. The perfusate solvents used have most commonly been saline or Ringers solution, either plain or with varying substances added to it. Usually membranes with a molecular mass cut-off point between 3,000 and 20,000 Daltons are used. Such membranes allow free permeability for small molecules such as glycerol, glucose, lactate, pyruvate, and ethanol, or small pharmacologic substances, such as adrenergic agents, prostaglandins, nicotine, and methylxantines. It is a tempting idea to dialyze larger molecules, such as proteins, by increasing the pore size of the membranes. This unfortunately alters the physical properties of the membranes and creates some problems with diffusion, volume recovery, and kinetics.

Under most circumstances the dialysate contains only a fraction of the concentration of a substance in the interstitial fluid. The degree of recovery depends on several factors, where the two most important are the area under the membrane in relation to the volume inside (i.e., the length of the membrane tubing) and the flow rate of the perfusate (determining the time allowed for equilibration over the membrane). The true interstitial concentration can be calculated indirectly in three different ways, but not by extrapolating from in vitro recovery to the in vivo situation because this has been shown to underestimate the interstitial concentrations. Measurement of the dialysate values from the start of perfusion until equilibrium is reached could be used with various mathematical models to predict the true concentrations (30,31). Specifically developed for adipose tissue is the so-called equilibrium technique (26). Increasing concentrations of the substance intended for measurement is added to the perfusate. The difference between perfusate and dialysate concentrations versus perfusate concentration are used in a linear regression analysis. The so-calculated perfusate concentration for which no difference exists should be equal to the interstitial concentration. The disadvantage of this method is that it is time consuming and also exposes the tissue to high concentrations of the substance. A third approach would be to make use of the fact that as long as the recovery is incomplete, any decrease in the flow rate should yield an increase in dialysate concentration. The flow rate is simply lowered stepwise until no further increase in dialysate concentration is seen, and then a situation with complete recovery is assumed. Thereby, the dialysate concentration should equal the concentration in the interstitial fluid. A situation with complete recovery is more easily achieved using longer probes (≥30 mm).

Microdialysis reflects the concentration of a particular substance in the interstitial fluid. This concentration is determined by the surrounding cells' release and uptake as well as by delivery and removal through the nutritive blood flow. Therefore, it is critical to monitor potential changes in local blood flow to be able to fully interpret microdialysis experiments. This is possible with a recently developed technique based on ethanol dilution in the interstitial fluid and will be discussed in more detail below.

REGIONAL DIFFERENCE IN VIVO

Studies of adipose tissue metabolism in humans with the microdialysis technique have focused on the abdominal and femorogluteal regions. It would of course be of interest to study even visceral fat in situ. Such studies would have to be conducted perioperatively and are thereby limited to a special metabolic situation. Microdialysis studies of visceral fat would furthermore raise some yet untried practical and ethical questions. Stored fat in other organs and tissues (e.g., muscle, liver, and bone marrow) should also be considered when discussing regional differences. A recent study (32) shows similarly high interstitial glycerol concentrations, as compared with plasma (approximately 35 times) in both adipose tissue and skeletal muscle. Even though this finding is at odds with previous reports (33–35) and is as yet unconfirmed, it still raises some interesting questions about triglyceride stores at sites other than adipose tissue. First, is this fat stored within other stromal cells or in interspersed adipocytes, and second, do these stores have a special function due to their proximity to myocytes or hepatocytes? The latter question could be seen as somewhat parallel to the question of the potential pathophysiologic significance of the metabolic and blood drainage differences between subcutaneous abdominal, femoro/gluteal, and visceral adipose depots. However, these three depots account for most of the stored triglycerides in the human body and must thus be considered of major importance from a quantitative point of view.

One disadvantage of microdialysis is its inability to discriminate between changes in cellular uptake or secretion on the one hand and changes in clearance or deposition by varying blood flow on the other in samples from the interstitial fluid. One way to overcome this problem is to monitor the local blood flow next to the microdialysis catheter. In order to make this possible, a technique was recently developed (36) where ethanol is added to the perfusate. Originally described for use in microdialysis of muscle, it was adapted for use in adipose tissue by our group. A prerequisite for a blood flow indicator is that it easily diffuses through the membrane and is metabolically inert in the tissue. Ethanol meets these criteria because it is readily diffusable and adipose tissue lacks alcohol dehydrogenase activity. In the concentrations used (50 mmol/L), ethanol does not seem to have any influence on lipid metabolism per se (37,38). Measurement of the ethanol concentrations in the perfusate and dialysate then allows for the construction of a ratio for ethanol in the dialysate to ethanol in the perfusate. This ratio is inversely correlated to changes in the blood flow because any increase in blood flow will increase ethanol disappearance, decrease ethanol concentration in the dialysate, and thereby decrease the ratio. The method has been evaluated in comparison with the ^{133}Xe clearance technique (39). A good intraindividual correlation (r = 0.78) and an excellent correlation (r = 0.90) with the ^{133}Xe clearance technique during thermoinduced variations in blood flow was seen (Fig. 2) (40). When using the ethanol disappearance technique, it is important to remember that the perfusion speed affects the absolute value of the ethanol ratio and thereby the suitability to detect either increases or decreases in blood flow. This can be illustrated with an in vitro experiment where perfusate (ethanol) and external (glycerol) (simulated interstitial fluid) are kept constant and perfusion flow rate is varied (Fig. 3). The wish to decrease the flow rate in order to maximize glycerol recovery must be weighed against the potential difficulty in detecting increases in blood flow if one starts with a very low ethanol ratio.

The simultaneous microdialysis measurement of lipolysis and blood flow has recently provided data on the adrenergic regulation of lipolysis and adipose tissue blood flow (37). In this study an apparent paradoxical lipolytic effect of the alpha-2 agonist clonidine (known from in vitro studies to have an antilipolytic effect through alpha$_2$-adrenoceptors) was shown when added to the perfusate. This effect was more pronounced in the gluteal area. This effect could be explained when local blood flow was taken into account. If a vasodilator was added to the perfusate, the lipolytic effect disappeared and a dose-dependent antilipolytic effect could be seen (Fig. 4). Secondly, it was shown via the ethanol

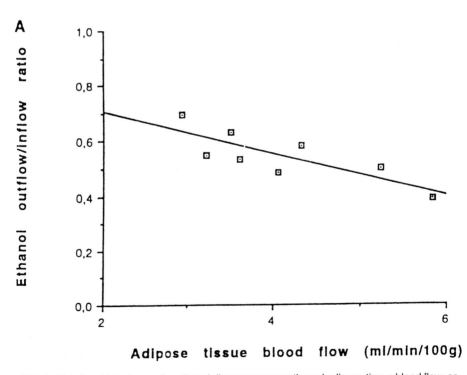

FIG. 2. Relationship between the ethanol disappearance ratio and adipose tissue blood flow, as determined with the ^{133}Xe clearance technique, in abdominal subcutaneous adipose tissue. Microdialysis probes (20 × 0.5 mm, 20,000 MW cut-off) were perfused with Ringer's solution supplemented with 50 mmol/L of ethanol at (**A**) 0.5 µl/min (n = 8) and (**B**) 1.5 µl/min (n = 5).

disappearance technique that clonidine yielded an increase in the ethanol ratio, indicative of a decrease in blood flow (Fig. 5). Thereby the increase in glycerol could be explained as an accumulation due to clonidine's microcirculatory effect rather than a dual effect on lipolysis. Other studies have shown significantly higher lipolytic activity in abdominal than in gluteal subcutaneous fat in response to short-term physical exercise (34). This difference was more pronounced in women than in men. It also has been demonstrated in both obese and nonobese individuals that lipid mobilization is more rapid from the subcutaneous abdominal than the subcutaneous peripheral adipose tissue regions during catecholamine stimulation, whereas there are no or minor differences in the basal rate of lipolysis between the regions (33,35).

In order to increase our understanding of adipose tissue metabolism, there is a need for in vivo studies. Arteriovenous cannulation techniques are most suitable for the quantitative estimation of substrate turnover. With the use of in situ microdialysis studies of adipose tissue, several new findings regarding adrenergic regulation of lipolysis have been made. Microdialysis is well suited for kinetic experiments as well as in situ manipulations of adipose tissue metabolism and blood flow in different subcutaneous regions.

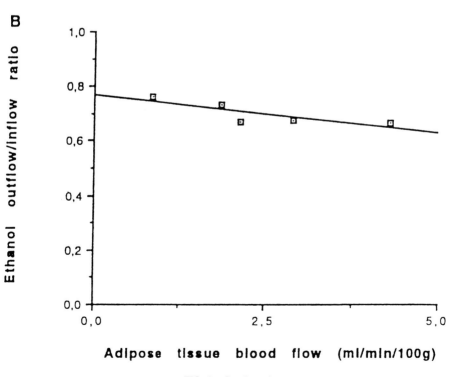

FIG. 2. *Continued.*

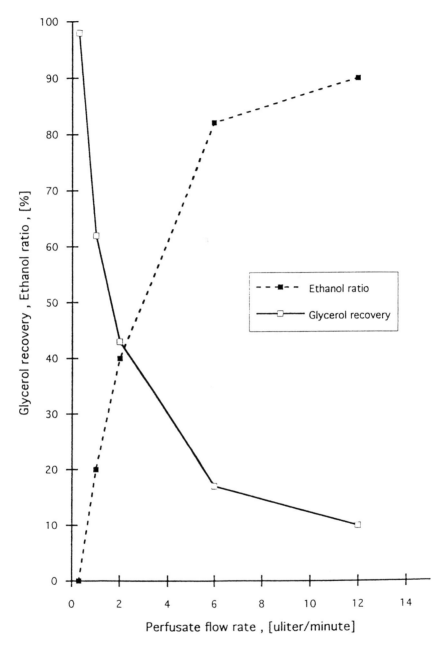

FIG. 3. Glycerol recovery and ethanol disappearence at varying flow rates in vitro. A microdialysis probe (10 × 0.5 mm, 20,000 MW cut-off) was submerged in Ringer's solution containing 86 (μmol/L glycerol and perfused with Ringer's solution supplemented with 48 mmol/L ethanol at 0.3, 1, 2, 6, and 12 μl/min. Results are expressed as the ethanol disappearance ratio (dialysate ethanol/perfusate ethanol) and relative glycerol recovery (dialysate glycerol/surrounding Ringer glycerol).

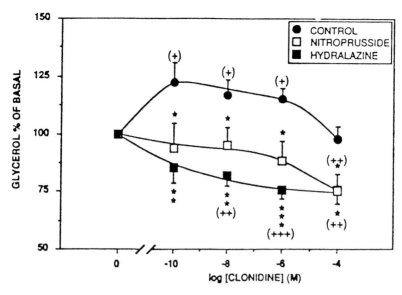

FIG. 4. Effect of direct-acting vasodilators on clonidine-induced changes in the glycerol level of gluteal subcutaneous adipose tissue. Three microdialysis probes were implanted in the gluteal area of each of eight healthy subjects. The three probes were perfused with either hydralazine (0.125 g/L) containing or nitroprusside (1.25 g/L) containing or plain Ringer's solution at 2.5 μl/min. Increasing concentrations of clonidine were added to the ingoing dialysis solvent at 30-min intervals. Values are mean ± SEM. +, values statistically different from basal values at $p < 0.05$ using paired t test; ++, $p < 0.01$; +++, $p < 0.001$. *, values statistically different from control values at $p < 0.05$ using paired t test; **, $p < 0.01$; ***, $p < 0.001$.

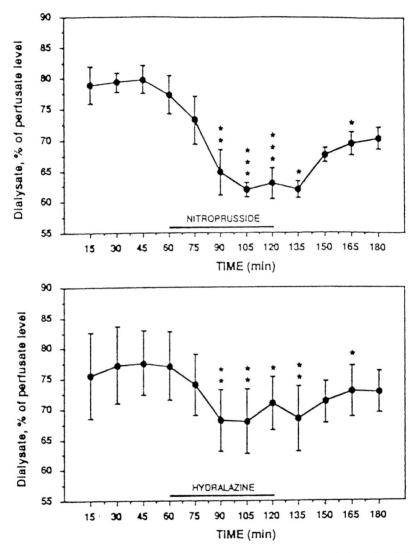

FIG. 5. Effect of vasoactive drugs on the ethanol disappearance ratio during microdialysis. Abdominal subcutaneous adipose tissue was microdialyzed with Ringer's solution containing 50 mmol/L of ethanol. Dialysate was collected at 15-min intervals and analyzed for ethanol. After 60 min, nitroprusside (1.25 g/L, upper graph, n = 6), hydralazine (0.125 g/L, middle graph, n = 4), or clonidine (0.1 nmol/L, lower graph, n = 4) were added during the next 60 min followed by a final 60-min period with plain Ringer-ethanol. The ratio of ethanol in dialysate over ethanol in perfusate was determined and expressed as a percentage value. Values are means ± SEM. *, values statistically different from control values at p < 0.05 using Students paired *t* test; **, p < 0.01; ***, p < 0.001.

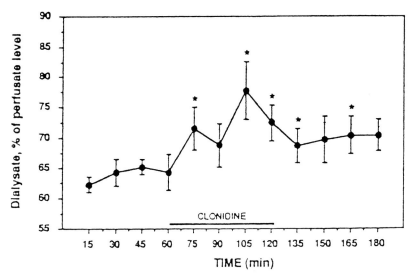

FIG. 5. *Continued.*

REFERENCES

1. Himms-Hagen J. Brown adipose tissue thermogenesis and obesity. *Prog Lipid Res* 1989;28:67–115.
2. Felig P, Wahren J. Fuel homeostasis in exercise. *N Engl J Med* 1975;293:1078–1084.
3. Nilsson-Ehle P, Garfinkel A, Schotz M. Lipolytic enzymes and plasma lipoprotein metabolism. *Ann Rev Biochem* 1980;49:667–693.
4. Hirsch J, Knittle JL. Cellularity of obese and nonobese human adipose tissue. *Fed Proc* 1970;29:1516–1521.
5. Pettersson P, Cigolini M, Sjöström L, Smith U, Björntorp P. Cells in human adipose tissue developing into adipocytes. *Acta Med Scand* 1984;215:447–451.
6. Vague J. La différenciation sexuelle-facteur déterminant des formes de l'obésité. *Presse Med* 1947;30:339–340.
7. Smith U. Regional differences in adipocyte metabolism and possible consequences in vivo. *Int J Obesity* 1985;9(suppl 1):145–148.
8. Björntorp P. Fat cell distribution and metabolism. *Ann N Y Acad Sci* 1987;499:66–72.
9. Davies J, Souness J. The mechanisms of hormone and drug action on fatty acid release from adipose tissue. *Rev Pure Appl Pharmacol Sci* 1981;2:1–112.
10. Honnor R, Dhillon G, Londos C. cAMP-dependent protein kinase and lipolysis rate in adipocytes. I. Cell preparation, manipulation and predictability in behaviour. *J Biol Chem* 1985;260:15122–15129.
11. Kather H, Bieger W, Michel G, Aktories K, Jakobs K. Human fat cell lipolysis is primarily regulated by inhibitory modulators acting through distinct mechanisms. *J Clin Invest* 1985;76:1559–1565.
12. Marcus C, Rhen H, Bolme P, Arner P. Regulation of lipolysis during the neonatal period: importance of thyrotropin. *J Clin Invest* 1988;82:1793–1797.
13. Fain J. Lipid mobilization in adipose tissue. In: Litwak G, ed. *Biochemical action of hormones.* New York: Academic; 1980:119–209.
14. Kahn C. The molecular mechanisms of insulin action. *Ann Rev Med* 1985;36:429–451.
15. Czech M. Insulin action. *Am J Med* 1981;70:142–150.
16. Larsson B, Bengtsson C, Björntorp P, et al. *Am J Epidemiol* 1992;135:266–273.
17. Björntorp P. "Portal" adipose tissue as a generator of risk factors for cardiovascular disease and diabetes. *Arteriosclerosis* 1990;10:493.

18. Bjorntorp P, Ottosson M, Rebuffé-Scrive M, et al. Regional obesity and steroid hormone interactions in human adipose tissue. In: Bray G, Ricquier D, Spiegelman B, eds. *Obesity: towards a molecular approach.* New York: Alan R Liss; 1990.
19. Svedberg J, Strömblad G, Wirth A, Smith U, Björntorp P. Fatty acids in the portal vein of the rat regulate hepatic insulin clearance. *J Clin Invest* 1991;88:2054.
20. Svedberg J, Björntorp P, Smith U, Lönnroth P. Free fatty acid inhibition of insulin binding, degradation and action in isolated rat hepatocytes. *Diabetes* 1990;39:570.
21. Leibel R, Edens N, Fried S. Physiologic basis for the control of body fat distribution in humans. *Annu Rev Nutr* 1989;9:417.
22. Wahrenberg H, Lönnqvist F, Arner P. Mechanisms underlying regional differences in lipolysis in human adipose tissue. *J Clin Invest* 1989;84:458–467.
23. Hellmér J, Marcus C, Sonnenfeldt T, Arner P. Mechanisms for differences in lipolysis between human subcutaneous and omental fat cells. *J Clin Endocrinol Metab* 1992;75:15–20.
24. Taouis M, Berlan M, Montastruc P, Lafontan M. Characterization of dog fat cell adrenoceptors: variations in alpha$_2$ and beta-adrenergic receptor distribution according to the extent of the fat deposits and anatomical location. *J Pharmacol Exp Ther* 1987;242:1041–1049.
25. Ungerstedt U. Measurements of neurotransmittor release by intracranial dialysis. In: Marsen C, ed. *Measurements of neurotransmittor release in vivo.* New York: Wiley; 1984:81–105.
26. Lönnroth P, Jansson PA, Smith U. A microdialysis method allowing characterization of the intercellular water space in humans. *Am J Physiol* 1987;253:E228–E231.
27. Arner P, Bolinder J, Eliasson A, Lundin A, Ungerstedt U. Microdialysis of adipose tissue and blood for in vivo lipolysis studies. *Am J Physiol* 1988;255:E737–E742.
28. Bolinder J, Ungerstedt U, Arner P. Long-term continuous glucose monitoring with microdialysis in ambulatory insulin-dependent diabetic patients. *Lancet* 1993;342:1080–1085.
29. Horal M, Ungerstedt U, Persson B, Westgren M, Marcus C. Metabolic adaptation in IUGR neonates determined with microdialysis—a pilot study. *Early Hum Dev* 1995;42:1–14.
30. Jacobsson I, Sandberg M, Hamberger A. Mass transfer in brain dialysis devices—a new method for the estimation of extracellular amino acids concentration. *J Neurosci Methods* 1985;15:263–268.
31. Lerma J, Herranz A, Herreras O, Abraira V, Martin Del Rio R. In vivo determination of extracellular concentration of amino acids in the rat hippocampus. A method based on brain dialysis and computerized analysis. *Brain Res* 1986;384:145–155.
32. Maggs D, Jacob R, Rife F, et al. Interstitial fluid concentrations of glycerol, glucose and amino acids in human quadricep muscle and adipose tissue. *J Clin Invest* 1995;96:370–377.
33. Jansson P, Smith U, Lönnroth U. Interstitial glycerol concentration measured by microdialysis in two subcutaneous regions in humans. *Am J Physiol* 1990;258:E918–E922.
34. Arner P, Kriegholm E, Engfeldt P, Bolinder J. Adrenergic regulation of lipolysis in situ at rest and during exercise. *J Clin Invest* 1990;85:893–898.
35. Jansson P, Larsson A, Smith U, Lönnroth P. Glycerol production in subcutaneous adipose tissue in lean and obese humans. *J Clin Invest* 1992;89:1610–1617.
36. Hickner R, Rosdahl H, Borg I, et al. Ethanol may be used with the microdialysis technique to monitor blood flow changes in skeletal muscle: dialysate glucose concentration is blood-flow-dependent. *Acta Physiol Scand* 1991;143:355–356.
37. Galitzky J, Lafontan M, Nordenström J, Arner P. Role of vascular alpha$_2$-adrenoceptors in regulating lipid mobilization from human adipose tissue. *J Clin Invest* 1993;91:1997–2003.
38. Fellönder G, Nordenström J, Tjäder I, Bolinder J, Arner P. Lipolysis during abdominal surgery. *J Clin Endocrinol Metab* 1994;78:150–155.
39. Larsen O, Lassen N, Quaade F. Blood flow through human adipose tissue determined with radioactive Xenon. *Acta Physiol Scand* 1966;66:337–345.
40. Felländer G, Linde B, Bolinder J. Evaluation of the microdialysis ethanol technique for monitoring of subcutaneous adipose tissue blood flow in humans. *Int J Obesity* 1996;20:220–226.

Physiology, Stress, and Malnutrition: Functional Correlates, Nutritional Intervention,
edited by J.M. Kinney and H.N. Tucker.
Lippincott–Raven Publishers © 1997.

Microdialysis in Normal and Injured Human Brain

*Urban Ungerstedt, *Tobias Bäckström, *Åse Hallström,
†Per Olof Grände, †Pekka Mellergård, and †Carl-Henrik Nordström

*Department of Physiology and Pharmacology, Karolinska Institute, S-171 77 Stockholm,
and †Department of Neurosurgery, Lund University Hospital, S-221 85 Lund, Sweden*

Online monitoring of chemical events in the human brain until recently has been largely impossible. Withdrawal of cerebrospinal fluid (CSF) from the ventricles or the spinal canal has provided some information but suffers from lack of anatomical resolution. Positron emission tomography and magnetic resonance imaging have provided anatomic resolution but a lack in time resolution and the number of chemical species that can be studied. None of the mentioned techniques are suited to continuous use in the neuro-intensive care unit (NICU).

A new technique, microdialysis, provides interesting possibilities. It was developed more than 20 years ago for monitoring chemical events in the animal brain (1,2) and has become a standard technique in neuroscience with well over 4,000 papers published. In the late 1980s we started to explore its possibilities for monitoring the human brain (3) and since then several studies have been published showing promising results (4–7). However, the lack of instruments suitable for routine use in the clinic, including bedside monitoring of relevant chemical compounds, have delayed the application of the technique.

In 1995, CMA Microdialysis (Stockholm, Sweden) introduced a sterile microdialysis catheter, a microdialysis pump, and a bedside analyzer, opening up the possibilities for monitoring human chemistry online. The instrumentation was intended for subcutaneous and intramuscular use, but with a slight modification of the catheter design it has been possible to use the catheter intracerebrally in humans. In this article we give an account of our first experience with the system applied to intracerebral monitoring in patients with severe brain trauma.

MICRODIALYSIS

The basic idea of microdialysis is to mimic the function of a blood vessel in the tissue by introducing a thin dialysis tube in the form of a microdialysis probe (for animals) or catheter (for humans). The microdialysis catheter (Fig. 1) consists of a thin dialysis tube that is fastened to the distal end of a plastic tube. A thin inner tube extends through the plastic tube all the way to the end of the dialysis tube. It attaches to the distal end of the dialysis tube in order to securely fix the membrane, preventing it from remaining in the body should it get damaged. An inlet tube connects the catheter to the microdialysis pump. Liquid flows along the inside of the dialysis membrane and enters the inner tube at its distal end through a tiny hole in its wall. The inner tube connects to the outlet tube, which ends in a microvial holder. The vial is designed to collect single microliters of fluid and minimize evaporation. It can be removed, replaced, and brought to the bedside chemical analyzer as often as every 10 min. However, for most occasions it is not necessary to monitor chemical events in the brain more often than once every hour.

The CMA/600 bedside analyzer monitors glucose, lactate, glycerol, urea, and, soon, pyruvate and glutamate. Each analysis takes about 1 minute, and the results are displayed as chemical trend curves showing changes over days or even weeks. The remaining liquid in the vial can be frozen, stored, and later analyzed for its content of e.g., amino acids, ions, purines, drugs, etc. This offline analysis is usually conducted using high-performance liquid chromatography techniques that allow for the analysis of nearly every compound of interest except neuropeptides. Here radioimmunoassay is usually the method of choice.

The CMA/60 catheter (Fig. 1) is designed for subcutaneous tissue and resting muscle. The catheter is perfused with a physiologic fluid (Ringer) at a very low

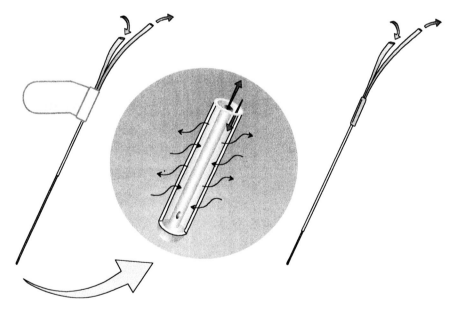

FIG. 1. Left: Flexible subcutaneous catheter with 30 mm membrane; middle: cross section of the catheter with the inner tube and the surrounding membrane; right: flexible intracerebral catheter with 10mm membrane.

flow rate (0.3 µl/min). In combination with a sufficiently long dialysis membrane (30 mm), it is possible to reach almost 100% recovery, i.e., the concentration of a particular substance in the perfusate is the same as the concentration in the extracellular fluid.

The intracerebral catheter has a similar design to the CMA/60 but it is more flexible (Fig. 1). The membrane is 10 mm long in order to cover the depth of the cortex when introduced at an oblique angle to the surface. The recovery is less than 100%, but we have found that it is possible to compare patients due to the similarity in recovery between different catheters.

Apart from the properties of the catheter, the recovery of substances from the brain parenchyma depends on their rate of production in the tissue, the diffusion coefficient, and the clearing from the tissue by capillary blood flow, or possibly by uptake into neurons or glia. In case substances are delivered to the tissue by the blood, their recovery also will be dependent on the concentration in the blood as well as the local blood flow at the time of dialysis. A change in the concentration of a particular substance, as measured by microdialysis, signals a change in its availability in the brain tissue. The relative change over time is often as important as the exact molar concentration of the substance.

INCLUSION CRITERIA AND SURGERY

At the Neurosurgery Clinic in Lund, patients with severe brain trauma are regularly implanted with ventricular catheters for pressure monitoring. Since mid-1995, all such patients have, in addition, been implanted with one or two microdialysis catheters. One catheter is implanted in the penumbra of the lesion, where blood and/or parenchyma has been removed during surgery, i.e., in tissue where survival is at risk. The other catheter is implanted in cortical tissue in the vicinity of the pressure catheter where brain tissue is considered to be the least damaged and where tissue survival is most probable. In cases where the damage is global, usually only one catheter is implanted. Obviously, this catheter placement strategy is to provide us with chemical information from sites representing tissue that is in the "best" as well as the "worst" condition. The goal of the therapy is then to improve the condition in the tissue at most risk while striving to preserve normal conditions in the best part of the parenchyma.

The surgical conditions usually vary between the two sites. In the best site the catheter can be introduced through a separate burr hole or in the same hole as the pressure catheter, whereas the worst site usually resides in the exposed brain surface uncovered by removal of a bone flap. In the best location the skull bone surrounding the drill hole offers some support to the catheter. In the worst location the catheter is usually only supported by the surrounding dura. However, we have found that this is of little consequence and that it is enough to firmly secure the inlet and outlet tubes of the catheters where they leave the scalp at the end of the tunnelation.

In the first study of microdialysis in the human brain (3), we noted that baseline concentrations of transmitters as well as metabolites were reached much faster than in animal brains. Our conclusion was that the larger mass of brain tissue gives away more easily, i.e., the trauma of the procedure is of less consequence. In the present study we have found little or no evidence of any appreciable trauma occurring as a consequence of the introduction of the microdialysis catheter into the brain tissue. The catheter in itself is much smaller in diameter than the pressure monitoring catheter, and in no instance did we cause any bleeding in the parenchyma at the site of introduction.

Upon arrival in the NICU, the patient is implanted with one subcutaneous reference catheter in the abdomen and often another subcutaneous catheter in the upper thorax or upper arm. The regular collection and analysis of samples can start within an hour after surgery. The catheters are left in place as long as they provide information of value for the treatment of the patient (usually 1–2 weeks). They are usually removed at the same time as the pressure catheter or immediately upon any malfunction such as an interruption in the flow of the perfusate.

THE ANALYTES AND THEIR SIGNIFICANCE

Glucose

The extracellular glucose concentration in subcutaneous tissue is considered by most investigators to be close to that in blood (8). The levels achieved in a microdialysis perfusate depend on a number of factors; most importantly, the perfusion flow and the length of the dialysis membrane. We are using a low perfusion flow (0.3μl) and a long membrane (30 mm), which gives close to 100% recovery under most circumstances. However, a lowering of local blood flow may cut down the delivery of glucose to the tissue to such an extent that the microdialysis exchange becomes supply dependent (9). This can be caused, for example, by a stress reaction redistributing blood from the skin to other organs or by a drug treatment contracting peripheral blood vessels.

Microdialysis glucose results differ between peripheral catheters and those implanted in the brain for the simple reason that the dialysis membrane length is 30 mm in the periphery but only 10 mm in the brain. At this stage of our development of the technique it is not possible to give a reliable figure for the brain/subcutaneous ratio for microdialysis glucose, but a reasonable estimate is that the concentration of glucose in the brain catheter is approximately 50–80% of the concentration in the brain.

Lactate and Pyruvate

Increased extracellular lactate in an organ usually signals insufficient oxygen supply. During normal glycolysis, glucose is converted to pyruvate, which is decarboxylated to acetyl-coenzyme A that enters the citric acid cycle. In case of insufficient oxygen supply, pyruvate is instead converted to lactate. In situations of severe trauma and increased intracerebral pressure, we find an increase in extracellular lactate concentrations in the brain. The magnitude of this change is dependent on the supply of glucose. During compression of the brain, the increasing lactate is abruptly reversed when extracellular glucose concentrations reach bottom values. In cases in which the substrate is limiting the formation of lactate, the lactate/pyruvate ratio gives a better measure of the ongoing changes in metabolism (5).

Glycerol

In previous studies (10) we have found that catecholamine-induced changes in subcutaneous glycerol are an indicator of physical as well as mental stress, making it a highly interesting variable in an intensive care situation. Glycerol is formed as the last metabolite during lipolysis. The subcutaneous catheter recovers glycerol at the very source, i.e., among the adipocytes. This means that any change in glycerol production is picked up by the subcutaneous catheter well before changes are visible in peripheral blood.

Lipolysis is under sympathetic control through catecholamine receptors on the adipocytes. The receptors are stimulated by circulating catecholamines as well as by local noradrenergic nerve endings. The relative contribution from humoral as compared with nervous catecholamines cannot be directly assessed in our experiments. However, the fact that we found situations in which lipolysis was strongly increased in, e.g., abdominal adipose tissue while there was no such change in upper arm tissue indicates that there are regional differences in lipolysis that can hardly be maintained unless lipolysis is under nervous control. In the brain, extracellular glycerol is not derived from metabolism of triacylglycerides as in subcutaneous fat. We assume that the increased glycerol we have seen in conjunction with trauma is due to a breakdown of glycerophospholipids. This is a new finding. In fact, the monitoring of extracellular glycerol in the brain may represent a new bedside method to evaluate the extent of cellular damage in the intensive care unit.

From a technical point of view it is necessary that the dialysis membrane of the catheter contain no glycerol. Most membranes made of cellulose, polycarbonate, or polysulfone are not glycerol free. These materials contaminate the perfusate and conceal any changes in endogenous glycerol. The membrane of the CMA/60 catheter, as well as the brain catheter, is made from dry, glycerol-free polyamide.

Urea

Urea is formed during protein metabolism and diffuses easily between different compartments of the body. Changes in urea concentrations take place over relatively long periods of time. We have found repeatedly that the levels

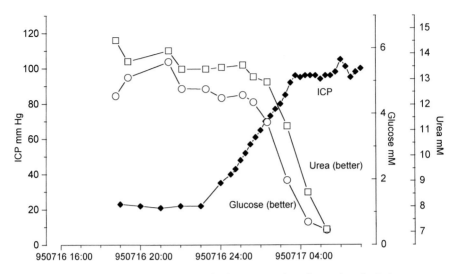

FIG. 2. Changes in urea levels during brain compression after serious brain trauma.

of urea are the same in blood, subcutaneous, muscular, and brain tissue. Our intention with measuring urea in the intensive care situation was to find an internal standard, i.e., a compound that can be expected to be at the same concentration wherever we measure it. Therefore, any differences in urea concentration should reflect differences in the recovery of the different catheters and might serve as a correction factor when comparing the different sites where microdialysis was performed. In addition, it seems conceivable that short-term changes in urea in one catheter might reflect local changes in blood flow and changes in the delivery of urea to the tissue. However, our data only partly support our hypothesis. We have found that urea levels are stable and often identical between catheters. However, the fact that urea diffuses easily from blood to tissue makes it difficult to assess the quantitative relationship between changes in extracellular urea and changes in nutritive capillary blood flow. It is possible that even large differences in local blood flow may result in relatively minor differences in urea concentration.

Despite uncertainty concerning how sensitively urea levels reflect changes in capillary blood flow, we were able to record directly parallel changes in urea and intracranial pressure (ICP) during the course of brain compression after serious brain trauma (Fig. 2).

Glutamate

Glutamate is an excitatory transmitter in the brain and seems to play an important role in the development of brain damage after trauma. The toxicity of glutamate relates to its ability to stimulate Ca^{2+} inflow into the neurons, which triggers a cascade of dysfunctional events in the cell such as phospholipid hydrolysis and the formation of free radicals.

Xanthine and Hypoxanthine

Brain trauma and ischemia leads to the breakdown of adenosine triphosphate (ATP) and the formation of xanthine and hypoxanthine, another important source of free radicals. We have found strong increases in hypoxanthine in both patients and experimental models of brain ischemia (5,11) and trauma (12).

CLINICAL FINDINGS

The use of microdialysis in monitoring the patient after severe trauma will be illustrated by a detailed analysis of a few cases where microdialysis has given unique information about the progressive change in brain and peripheral chemistry reflecting the developing clinical situation.

A 70-year-old man was admitted after a motorcycle accident. The computed tomography (CT) scan showed a large unilateral subdural hematoma and a pronounced deviation of the midline toward the contralateral hemisphere. The hematoma was removed via craniotomy, and an intraventricular pressure monitoring catheter was introduced into the contralateral ventricle. The first microdialysis catheter was introduced into the cortex contralateral to the hematoma. This side is referred to here as the "better" side. The second catheter was introduced into the cortex close to the bleeding in what may be referred to as a penumbra zone. This side is referred to here as the "worse" side. The third catheter is introduced subcutaneously in the abdomen.

A serious edema developed rapidly on the worse side. Over less than 24 hours the ICP increased to blood pressure levels. The case was of considerable interest because the situation was relatively well defined:

1. The worse side had, in all probability, a seriously damaged blood–brain barrier, and fluid entered from the blood to cause a massive swelling of the parenchyma.
2. The better side had, in all probability, an essentially intact blood–brain barrier. The gradually developing ischemia was due to swelling of the worse side and not to a process intrinsic to the better hemisphere.

A comparison of the events on the worse and better sides will therefore be a comparison of the chemistry developing in a severely traumatized parenchyma devoid of its blood–brain barrier with an essentially normal parenchyma with complete ischemia. In the ensuing figures, the chemical changes in the two hemispheres are displayed against the plot of the dramatically increasing ICP.

Signs of Ischemia

In the discussion above we explained our reasons for measuring urea in the brain. Figure 2 shows comparisons between the increase in ICP (♦) and the decrease in extracellular glucose (○) and urea (□) on the better side. We interpreted these events as due to the gradually developing ischemia decreasing the delivery of glucose as well as urea from the blood to the brain.

Glucose, Lactate, and Pyruvate

Figure 3 is a plot of glucose, lactate, and pyruvate for the two catheter placements in the brain. At the start of the ICP recording (♦), the glucose concentration of the better side (○) is normal, whereas it is extremely low on the worse side (⊗). Glucose decreases on both sides as ICP starts to increase as the blood supply to the brain gradually fails. Lactate is initially very high on the worse side (⊠)and well above normal on the better side (□). When ICP increases, lactate also increases on both sides. It reaches a peak on the better side and then starts to decrease, probably due to lack of substrate. This does not seem to happen on the worse side, where the damage occurred more than a day previously and where the injury is traumatic in nature in addition to the imposed ischemia.

Figure 4 depicts a comparison between the lactate concentrations [better (□), worse (⊠)] and the lactate/pyruvate ratios (⊗). It is striking how well the ratios reflect the increasing ICP as compared with lactate alone. This is typical of an ischemic situation. However, there are situations of increasing metabolism where the ratio may be constant while there is a strong increase in both lactate and pyruvate.

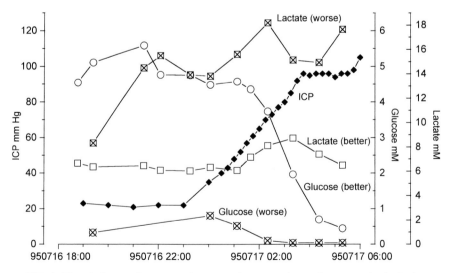

FIG. 3. Plot of glucose, lactate, and pyruvate for two catheter placements in the brain.

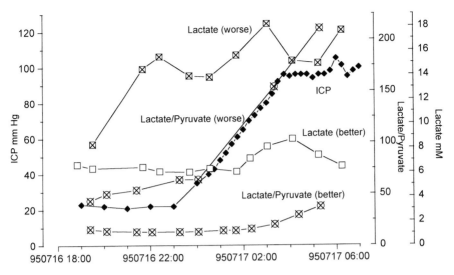

FIG. 4. Comparison between lactate concentrations and lactate pyruvate ratios in brain.

Cellular Damage

There is strong evidence linking cellular damage in the brain and increased glutamate release. Figure 5 demonstrates the relationship of glutamate concentration with increasing ICP (♦). Extracellular glutamate is already high in the worse side (⊠) at the onset of the ICP increase. It rapidly reaches a level that is out of range of the chemical assay. Interestingly, the glutamate increase on the better side (□) runs about 10 hours behind the worse side, emphasizing a possible difference between traumatic and ischemic damage. Glycerol concentrations are high on the worse side (⊗) several hours before the onset of ICP increase, and they increase even further on the worse side once the ICP has reached maximal levels. We believe that the increase in extracellular glycerol in connection with brain damage is an original finding that may prove important for the monitoring of brain trauma in an intensive care situation. The true cause of the increase in extracellular glycerol levels cannot be determined from our present findings. However, it seems probable that the hypoxia/anoxia caused calcium influx and activated phospholipases that split the fatty acids and the phosphate from the glycerol.

Xanthine and hypoxanthine (Fig. 6) are metabolites of ATP, and the increase on the worse side (⊗) is a sign of ATP breakdown after damage to the parenchyma. It seems reasonable to assume that this is an indication of free-radical formation in the damaged tissue.

The catastrophic developments on the worse side (Fig. 7) are also evident from the dramatic increase in extracellular potassium (⊗) in this hemisphere, signaling membrane depolarization and the inability to maintain chemical gradients between

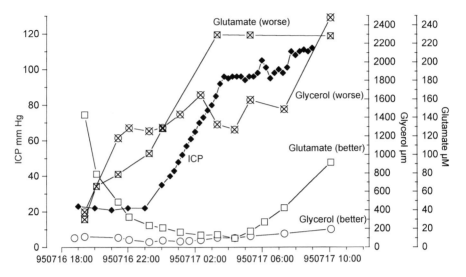

FIG. 5. Relationship of glucose concentration with increasing ICP.

the cell and the extracellular fluid. The immediate consequence is probably an influx of calcium and the subsequent activation of phospholipases (see above).

Regional Differences in Lipolysis

As discussed above, the monitoring of subcutaneous lipolysis may be a valuable tool for the assessment of sympathetic activity in an intensive care situa-

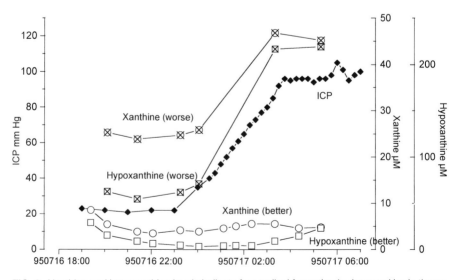

FIG. 6. Xanthine and hypoxanthine levels indicate free radical formation in damaged brain tissue.

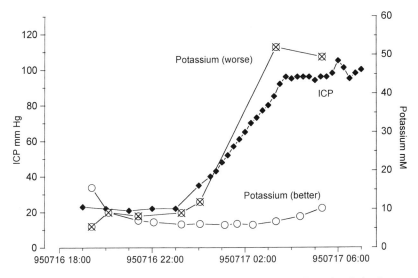

FIG. 7. Rising potassium levels after brain injury indicate cellular depolarization.

tion. In our experience, the control of lipolysis is highly regional and can signal events related to the spinal segment where the catheter is located. An interesting example of this is the strong increase in lipolysis about 40 hours after terminating barbiturates in brain trauma patients (Fig. 8). We initially believed that this was caused by decreased sedation and increased sympathetic stress.

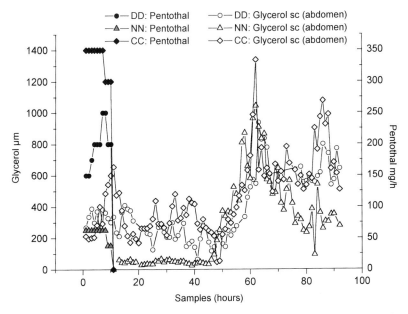

FIG. 8. Increase in lipolysis 40 hours after terminating barbiturates in brain trauma patients.

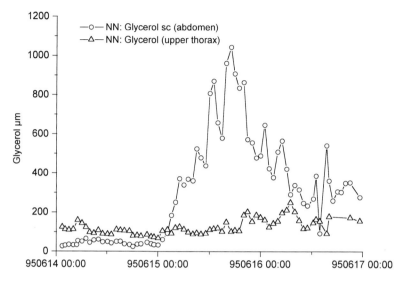

FIG. 9. Increased lipolysis was found in the abdominal catheter but not in the upper thorax catheter.

However, we found that the increased lipolysis only occurred in the abdominal catheter and not in the upper thorax catheter (Fig. 9). This seemed to exclude a general increase in sympathetic tone related to the level of sedation. We have tentatively explained our findings as being related to the pronounced increase in visceral activity starting at that time after the termination of barbiturate treatment.

GENERAL COMMENTS

The use of microdialysis in the human brain is still in its infancy. However, it seems to offer a unique possibility for monitoring chemical events in the injured brain. The lack of adequate clinical tools in this situation is disturbing, and the clinician is often forced to depend mainly on ICP and occasional CT scans. In this situation, microdialysis offers a direct link to the chemistry of the brain and the very process we are trying to influence with intensive care and drug treatments.

We have used a new strategy of systematically monitoring the better as well as the worse hemisphere whenever this is applicable to the clinical situation. This gives us an internal reference and an appreciation of the extremes that we must address. We can closely follow the response of the tissue at risk to our treatment and at the same time avoid any intervention that has a negative impact on the better tissue, where conditions still favor a positive outcome.

In this preliminary account of our work we have chosen to give a detailed analysis of a patient that deteriorated quickly and dramatically. Our purpose has not been to discuss treatment but instead to show the extreme chemical events occurring in the part of the brain that has been seriously damaged and compare those findings to a part of the same brain that has undergone a "clean" ischemia. The measurement of glucose shows how big the differences are between the two extremes. Although we are still uncertain regarding the interpretation of our findings, the most plausible explanation seems to be that the worse side has a decreased blood flow and an inadequate delivery of glucose.

An increase in lactate signals a decrease in aerobic glycolysis. However, the lactate/pyruvate ratio seems to make up for some of the shortcomings of the lactate variable, and the ratio is surprisingly well related to other clinical signs, such as ICP.

Increased levels of glutamate, xanthine, and hypoxanthine are strongly linked to ischemic and traumatic damage of the human brain, as well as experimental trauma in rats. We found greatly elevated levels in the hemisphere subjected to the trauma, whereas the hemisphere exposed to ischemia due to compression developed an increase in these compounds at a late stage.

The strong increase in glycerol after trauma and ischemia represents a new and original finding. The nature of this increase is different from the increase we find in subcutaneous catheters, where glycerol represents the end product in regular lipolysis. Such metabolism of triacylglycerides does not occur in the brain, and it seems more probable that the increase in glycerol originates from an enzymatic breakdown of glycerophospholipids in the cellular membranes. In fact, glycerol may represent an entirely new marker for the early stages of cellular damage, possibly even preceding any increase of excitatory transmitter release.

The subcutaneous glycerol change signals regular lipolysis and is an indirect measurement of sympathetic tone. Our experience is that this can represent highly regional events in the body related to the spinal segment projecting to the dermatoma, where microdialysis is performed. This variable may be of particular interest in assessing the state of sedation, pain, etc. in the intensive care situation.

In summary, we have presented a new concept and a new technique for online monitoring of chemical events in relevant sites of the human brain during intensive care. We found great differences in absolute levels and in the time course of chemical changes between the cortex of the worse and the better hemisphere.

REFERENCES

1. Ungerstedt U, Pycock CH. Functional correlates of dopamine neurotransmission. *Bull Schweiz Akad Med Wiss* 1974;1278:1–5.
2. Ungerstedt U. Microdialysis—principles and application for studies in animal and man. *J Intern Med* 1991;230:365–373.
3. Meyerson BA, Linderoth B, Karlsson H, Ungerstedt U. Extracellular measurements in the thalamus of parkinsonian patients. *Life Sci* 1990;46:301–308.

4. Hillered L, Persson L, PonténU, Ungerstedt U. Neurometabolic monitoring of the ischaemic human brain using microdialysis. *Acta Neurochir (Wien)* 1990;102:91–97.
5. Persson L, Hillered L. Chemical monitoring of neurosurgical intensive care patients using intracerebral microdialysis. *J Neurosurg* 1992;76:72–80.
6. During MJ, Fried I, Leone P, Katz A, Spencer DD. Direct measurement of extracellular lactate in the human hippocampus during spontaneous seizures. *J Neurochem* 1994;62:2356–2361.
7. Kanthan R, Shuaib A, Griebel R, Miyashita H. Intracerebral human microdialysis. In vivo study of an acute focal ischemic model of the human brain. *Stroke* 1995;26:870–873.
8. Bolinder J, Ungerstedt U, Arner P. Microdialysis measurement of the absolute glucose concentration in subcutaneous adipose tissue allowing glucose monitoring in diabetic patients. *Diabetologia* 1992;35:1177–1180.
9. Hickner RC, Rosdahl H, Borg I, Ungerstedt U, Jordfeldt L, Henriksson J. Ethanol may be used with the microdialysis technique to monitor blood flow changes in skeletal muscle: dialysate glucose concentration is blood-flow-dependent. *Acta Physiol Scand* 1991;143:355–356.
10. Hagström-Toft, Arner P, Wahrenberg H, Wennlund A, Ungerstedt U, Bolinder J. Adrenergic regulation of human tissue metabolism in situ during mental stress. *Endocrinol Metab* 1993;76:392–398.
11. Hillered L, Hallström Å, Segersvärd S, Persson L, Ungerstedt U. Dynamics of extracellular metabolites in the striatum after middle cerebral artery occlusion in the rat monitored by intracerebral microdialysis. *J Cereb Blood Flow Metab* 1989;9:607–616.
12. Nilsson P, Hillered L, Pontén L. Ungerstedt U. Changes in cortical extracellular levels of energy-related metabolites and amino acids following concussive brain injury in rats. *J Cereb Blood Flow Metab* 1990;10:631–637.

Physiology, Stress, and Malnutrition: Functional Correlates, Nutritional Intervention,
edited by J.M. Kinney and H.N. Tucker.
Lippincott–Raven Publishers © 1997.

Overview of Extracellular Metabolic Regulation

Jules Hirsch

Laboratory of Human Behavior and Metabolism, The Rockefeller University, New York, New York 10021–6399

Five excellent papers on various aspects of extracellular metabolic regulation are the subject of this discussion. The first, by Malaisse, addressed the sensing of glucose levels and alterations of the mechanism that occur during starvation. The work of Frayn and Hellmer discussed extracellular events in adipose tissue, particularly as affected by the circulation in this important storage tissue. The paper of Clark addressed similar regulations in muscle, and the work of Ungerstedt discussed the application of ingenious new technologies to the online study of changes in extracellular fluid.

It is no exaggeration to state that a revolution has occurred during the last quarter of this century that has made biologic science a more quantitative and orderly discipline than has been the case over hundreds of years of past investigations. The new understanding of intracellular events on a molecular level, known as molecular biology, and, finally, the unraveling of the nucleotide sequence that serves as the blueprint for cellular structure are occurrences unparalleled in the history of biology. In many respects this period is for biology what the early decades of the 20th century were for physics, when that science leapt forward into the modern period.

As the fruits of our biologic revolution are applied to understanding the nature of human health and disease, it is becoming obvious that the new biology will be restructured for different levels of integration. For example, structural biology has become of particular moment in recent years. We now want to have a picture of how molecular events occur within the cells. What do things really look like? We seek even higher levels of integration to understand how cells operate in concert and how they function in the context of an entire organ or the organism. This is the essence of physiology. Thus, once again, human physiology returns to the scene and becomes the vehicle whereby the intracellular studies so immensely productive in recent years are made useful for the understanding of health and disease. I know of no better call to action than that of Buchanan reviewing the lasting contributions of Sir James Paget: "Paget, I am certain, would have agreed with a conclusion of the International Congress of Physiological Sciences held in Glasgow in 1993 that although today's reductive sciences (molecular biology, cell biology, cell biophysiology) are important, the future lies with physiology, since the function of the whole organism is more than the sum of the functions of the individual parts; or as the Nobel Laureate of 1988, Sir James Black, commented, that the future lay in the progressive triumph of physiology over molecular biology" (1). These five chapters examining extracellular metabolic regulation are superb examples of the new physiology that is slated to become the cutting edge of biologic research in the next century.

I would like to discuss these five chapters by reference to work that has been done by colleagues in my laboratory at the Rockefeller University over many years, indicating the way in which our work is related to these new findings, with the hope that some of our observations will enrich and amplify this work.

The paper of Malaisse demonstrates clearly the special role of glucokinase in the pancreatic beta cell in the regulation of insulin release and the changes that occur during starvation. An important relationship between insulin release and total energy storage, which has been of interest to our group, relates the observations of Malaisse to the status of energy storage. Stern showed many years ago that there is an excellent correlation between human adipocyte size and insulin levels (2). Both in obese and in normal weight adults, a strong positive correlation was found between adipose cell size and the fasting level of immunoreactive insulin; correlations with fat cell size were stronger than correlations with total body fat or with body weight. In another study, Faust studied Osborne-Mendel rats known to be highly sensitive to a high-fat diet, by overeating, with rapid increase in body weight (3). This behavior was startlingly altered when lipectomy was performed early in life. The essentials of the experiment are as follows. A group of young Osborne-Mendel rats were subjected to extensive lipectomy of subcutaneous, inguinal, and epididymal fat. A control group received similar sham operations without fat removal. By this technique, about one third of the adipose depot was removed. Immediately thereafter, there was little effect on food intake or fat storage. Both control and lipectomized animals ate nearly the same, and hence the fat depots of both groups of animals enlarged. About 1 month after surgery, both groups had eaten the same amount of an ordinary chow diet (low in fat) and therefore had developed the same size fat depots. However, the lipectomized animals stored fat in fewer cells and hence cells were larger. A high-fat diet then was given ad libitum to both groups. The lipectomized animals initially were as hyperphagic as the sham group, but after a brief time the hyperphagia of the lipectomized group waned. The sham operated group continued to overeat to a much higher level of fat storage. At equilibrium, when both groups of animals achieved maximum weight, the lipectomized group and sham operated group had the same cell size, but the lipectomized group had eaten less and therefore had less total fat storage. Fat cell size seemed to be a restraining factor inducing satiety, an event that occurred earlier in animals with fewer cells.

Schneider (4) studied insulin levels in these animals. When cell size was different, but food intake and total fat storage the same, insulin levels were different. Higher levels were found when cells were larger; thus, independent of diet or total fat storage, fat cell size alone was correlated with differences in insulin levels. Lipectomized chow-fed animals had insulin levels that averaged 80.5 μU/ml as compared with sham chow-fed animals at 56.9 μU/ml. In contrast, when the animals were then fed the high-fat diet and the lipectomized animals plateaued body weight at 124.5 g versus 156.6 g in the sham-operated group fed the high-fat diet, insulin levels were the same. This is a startling reminder of the unusual and poorly understood direct relationship between fat cell size and pancreatic function.

Recently Hudgins (5) demonstrated that the eucaloric feeding of a low-fat diet rich in simple sugars leads in humans to de novo lipogenesis from carbohydrate. Diets with either 10% or 40% of calories as fat were fed, and the fatty acid composition of the diets was carefully matched to the adipose tissue fatty acid composition in each subject. In this circumstance, declines in very low density lipoprotein fatty acids that can be derived only from diets or from fat stores become an index of the degree of lipogenesis from carbohydrate. Evidence for lipogenesis was obtained, and the findings were corroborated by studies of the rate of ^{13}C incorporation into palmitic acid in low-density lipoproteins. With the increased use of low-fat diets, it will become increasingly important to analyze the likelihood and amount of de novo lipogenesis. This is undoubtedly a phenomenon that is at least in part insulin driven or insulin dependent. The relationships among insulin action, dietary carbohydrate, and fat storage then become of particular interest. Because the lipids newly synthesized from carbohydrate are of necessity saturated and there is a frequent occurrence of higher triglyceride levels in the plasma as well as lowering of high-density lipoprotein cholesterol, the indiscriminate use of a very low fat diet rich in simple sugars may not always be in the best behalf of the patient.

The fact that glucokinase is of such central importance in the regulation of the pancreatic response to starvation makes one wonder whether diseases that could have arisen by genetic selection as a defense against starvation would be related to this finding. The "thrifty" gene hypothesis so often mentioned in connection with adult-onset or non–insulin-dependent diabetes may be relevant because it is notable that one form of maturity-onset diabetes of the young has been shown in some kindreds to be due to mutations in the glucokinase gene (6). This ties the observations of Malaisse not only to the older observations of the relationship of fat cell size to pancreatic function, but also to those molecular genetic studies implicating glucokinase as a key enzyme in the causation of one type of adult-onset diabetes.

The papers addressing extracellular events in adipose tissue indicate the likely importance of adipose tissue blood flow in the total functioning of the adipose organ. The work of Edens (7), demonstrating that free fatty acids must leave the adipocyte before being available for re-esterification, is central to understanding why blood flow in adipose tissue may be of such importance. If, as suggested by the work of Frayn, there is an extracellular pool of free fatty acids that is sensitive to blood flow, then blood flow becomes an important determinant of the availability of free fatty acids for either re-esterification locally or for removal to more distant sites as an energy substrate.

The events occurring in humans at the termination of several days of fasting may be at last explained by the observations of Frayn. When a fast is abruptly ended by the administration of intravenous glucose and insulin, it is often observed that glycerol levels and hence lipolysis in adipose tissue continues for some hours and then slowly declines. In contrast, free fatty acid concentration in plasma may plummet to low levels within 30 minutes to 1 hour. It has been impossible to demonstrate a sudden change in the rate of re-esterification in adipose tissue occurring promptly after a fast, when tissues are removed and analyzed in vitro. However, it is more likely that extracellular circulatory events are a controlling element in this situation. If the blood flow to adipose tissue changes rapidly postfasting, then extracellular compartments of free-fatty acid as described by Frayn, could slow the washout of free fatty acids before lipolysis declines, leading to an increase in fatty acid substrate for adipose re-esterification. The techniques that have been described in the papers of Hellmer, Ungerstedt, and Frayn could provide an unambiguous determination of exactly how adipose function is altered when starvation ends.

It is interesting in this connection to speculate on the role of extracellular events and regional differences in the function of adipose tissue. It is usually assumed that the demonstration that abdominal or android obesity is particularly hazardous as a risk factor for diabetes and untoward cardiovascular events is related directly to differences in adipocyte function in abdominal as compared with gluteal areas. In fact, a good deal of important work on beta-1 and alpha-2 adrenoreceptors and their alterations in different sites has led to speculations on how fat cell differences in different regions could lead to different physiologic events. An alternate possibility, however, is that fundamental changes in blood flow patterns and changes in the regulatory systems of blood flow in different sites may lead both to different accumulations of fat as evidenced by the presence of a "pot belly" or the cosmetically disfiguring but less hazardous deposits of femoral gluteal fat, and at the same time could be a marker for other circulatory differences, important in the genesis of hypertension, strokes, or even diabetes. In short, is it possible that the fat accumulations are secondary markers, and the primary events, which relate to disease causation, may be more closely linked with differences in the control of vascular function, perhaps mediated by changes in autonomic function? Now the techniques are becoming available to examine this possibility.

The relationship of the autonomic nervous system and fat storage has become of particular interest in an analysis of how caloric expenditure varies as fat mass is changed. We studied the effects of fat storage on energy expenditure in humans (8). Both obese and nonobese subjects were studied first at their usual weight and then during plateau periods of weight maintenance 10% above initial weight, 10% below initial weight, and in the case of the obese, at even lower plateaus, 20% or 30% below usual body weight. In each of these study periods, caloric expenditure was measured by several techniques. Hydrodensitometry and other compartmental measures were made to assure that composition was not changing significantly during the weight plateaus.

It was found that usual weight is "defended," and when either obese or nonobese individuals are driven above or below their usual weight, significant changes in total caloric expenditure ensue. When 18 obese subjects and 23 nonobese subjects were examined in this way, a 10% reduction in body weight led, on average, to a reduction in total energy expenditure of roughly 6 kilocalories per kilogram of fat free mass per day. An increase of 10% above usual weight led to an increase in total energy expenditure of 9 kilocalories per kilogram of fat free mass per day. These total changes in energy expenditure are 10–15% above or below what would be predicted for individuals of such body composition when caloric expenditure is measured per unit of fat-free mass at usual weight. These unanticipated changes in caloric expenditure are most evident when individuals are free to walk about in an in-hospital study unit. During times of restricted activity, as occurs in a metabolic chamber, such changes in energy expenditure are diminished (9). It is likely, therefore, that our findings are related to physical activity. Studies of caloric expenditure during moderate levels of exercise are now underway and are confirming these observations.

In an effort to understand the underlying mechanisms of caloric expenditure as a function of fat storage, we have made estimates of autonomic function by the study of heart rate. There are sympathetic and parasympathetic inputs of different frequency to the sinoatrial node, which control heart rate and can be studied by spectral analysis. Initial studies showed that using a fast Fourier transform of heart rate variability over a brief interval, i.e., 256 seconds, permitted a reproducible spectral analysis between 0 and 2 Hz and a clear demonstration of one peak correlated with parasympathetic activity. This peak, at the frequency of respiratory rate, is the basis for sinus arrhythmia, and its power was used to estimate parasympathetic function (10), but sympathetic function occurring at lower frequencies was more difficult to evaluate. When individuals were changed above or below usual body weight, it was found that with upward weight change parasympathetic activity declined and sympathetic activity increased. With a decline in body weight, parasympathetic activity was enhanced. For more accurate analyses of parasympathetic and sympathetic control, another experimental approach has been used (11). Selective blockade of heart rate—with measures of heart period, beginning with a muscarinic blocker, atropine, and then by a beta-cardio-selective blocker, esmolol—altered heart periodicity, and the changes were considered as valid estimates of parasympathetic and sympathetic control. When weight was manipulated to 10% above or 10% below usual and maintained at this new plateau, there were systematic and highly significant changes in autonomic function. Increase in weight increased sympathetic and decreased parasympathetic control. Parasympathetic control played a larger role than sympathetic control. When weight declined, parasympathetic function increased to a greater degree than the sympathetic decline that occurred. These changes could play a role in the adjustment of energy output at different weight levels. In particular, one must consider whether altered autonomic output to skeletal muscle can direct changes in perfusion, so admirably described by Clark et al. Potential changes in red or white fiber activity have been considered as a cause for the altered energy state in muscle after changes in fat storage, but the variations in vascular perfusion described by Clark also must be considered. It is notable that insulin secretion that is altered by the state of fat storage also could be a significant actor in the control of skeletal muscle metabolism. This is made particularly attractive by the recent work of Baron relating insulin action to vasodilation in muscle (12).

Thus, all five chapters deal with interdependent phenomena. Vascular controls, insulin release, insulin action, the modulation of energy stores, and the sensing of the state of energy storage are central considerations in modern regulatory physiology. All future physiologic research, will assign meaningful roles to the findings of molecular genetics and molecular biology in human health and disease. These excellent papers are notable examples of what the new program of action will be for physiology in "postmodern" biology.

ACKNOWLEDGMENTS

I am indebted to the work of my colleagues at the Hospital of The Rockefeller University from 1960 to the present. They created the experimental findings that enabled me to compare our work with that of the authors of these five chapters. Work described in this chapter was funded in part by Grants DK30583 and GCRC RR00102 from the National Institutes of Health.

REFERENCES

1. Buchanan WW. Sir James Paget (1814–90): Surgical Osler? *Proc R Coll Phy Edinb* 1996;26:91–114.
2. Stern JS, Hollander N, Batchelor BR, et al. Adipose-cell size and immunoreactive insulin levels in obese and normal-weight adults. *Lancet* 1972;4:948–951.
3. Faust IM, Johnson PR, Hirsch J. Surgical removal of adipose tissue alters feeding behavior and the development of obesity in rats. *Science* 1977;197:393–396.
4. Schneider BS, Faust IM, Hemmes RB, Hirsch J. Effects of altered adipose tissue morphology on plasma insulin levels in the rat. *Am J Physiol* 1981;240:E358–E362.
5. Hudgins LC, Hellerstein M, Seidman C, et al. Human fatty acid synthesis is stimulated by a eucaloric low fat, high carbohydrate diet. *J Clin Invest* 1996;97:2081–2091.
6. Velho G, Froguel P, Clement K, et al. Primary pancreatic beta-cell secretory defect caused by mutations in glucokinase gene in kindreds of maturity onset diabetes of the young. *Lancet* 1992;340: 444–448.
7. Edens NK, Leibel RL, Hirsch J. Mechanism of free fatty acid re-esterification in human adipocytes in vitro. *J Lipid Res* 1990;31:1423–1431.
8. Leibel RL, Rosenbaum M, Hirsch J. Changes in energy expenditure resulting from altered body weight. *N Engl J Med* 1995;332:621–628.

9. Rosenbaum M, Ravussin E, Matthews DE, et al. A comparative study of different means of assessing long-term energy expenditure in humans. *Am J Physiol* 1996;270:R496–R504.
10. Hirsch J, Leibel RL, Mackintosh R, Aguirre A. Heart rate variability as a measure of autonomic function during weight change in humans. *Am J Physiol* 1991;261:R1418–R1423.
11. Aronne LJ, Mackintosh R, Rosenbaum M, et al. Autonomic nervous system activity in weight gain and weight loss. *Am J Physiol* 1995;269:R222–R225.
12. Baron AD. Hemodynamic actions of insulin. *Am J Physiol* 1994;267:E187–E202.

Physiology, Stress, and Malnutrition: Functional
Correlates, Nutritional Intervention,
edited by J.M. Kinney and H.N. Tucker.
Lippincott–Raven Publishers © 1997.

Tissue Distribution and Energetics in Weight Loss and Undernutrition

Marinos Elia

Medical Research Council Dunn Clinical Nutrition Centre,
Cambridge CB2 2DH, United Kingdom

THE APPARENT PARADOX OF RESTING ENERGY EXPENDITURE IN UNDERNUTRITION

The reduction in basal metabolic rate (BMR) that occurs in protein-energy undernutrition is probably largely due to loss of body mass or active metabolic tissue. However, a number of investigators have suggested that there are additional adaptive changes that reduce the metabolic rate of the remaining tissues. The seminal work of Keys et al. (1) strongly reinforced this concept through studies of healthy individuals who lost about a quarter of their initial body weight over a 6-month period of semi-starvation. During this period there was not only a reduction in the O_2 consumption of the whole body (-36%), but also a reduction in O_2 consumption per kilogram of body weight (-17%), per kilogram fat free mass (FFM) estimated by hydrodensitometry (-25%), and per kilogram of active tissue (body weight excluding fat, extracellular fluid, bone mineral estimated by standard weighing, hydrodensitometry, thiocyanate space, and x-rays, respectively). This concept of adaptive reductions in the metabolic rate is apparently supported by other studies in both adults (2) and children, especially in those with kwashiorkor (3,4). However, the reduction in BMR (BMR/kg body weight and BMR/kg FFM) in kwashiorkor is at least partly due to the presence of excessive fluid.

The effect of undernutrition on energy expenditure is far more complex than suggested above because several studies in undernourished young children (Fig. 1), older children (13), and adults (Fig. 2), as well as in animals (23), suggest that protein-energy malnutrition is associated with either little change or an increase in metabolic rate (per kg body weight and/or per kg fat free body weight). These results (Figs. 1 and 2) seem to be contrary to those that suggest that undernutrition produces adaptive reductions in metabolic rate. For example, McNeill et al. (19) studied a group of chronically undernourished men [mean body mass index (BMI) 16.6 ± 0.3 kg/m^2] and concluded that there was no evidence of adaptive reductions in resting energy expenditure because the BMR (per kg body weight, per kg$^{0.75}$, per kg FFM, and per m^2) was either normal or increased (Fig. 2).

In general, studies of undernourished animals suggest that the metabolic rate (per kg body weight or per kg FFM) is reduced (24), but this has not been an invariable finding. For example, in a classic study of a dog that was studied during progressive semi-starvation (9 weeks) until it lost 41% of its body weight (23), there was the expected overall reduction in BMR associated with a decrease in body size, but during the last 2 weeks of the study, BMR/kg body weight was 11–19% higher than at the start of the study.

Several explanations can be put forward to explain these apparently chaotic and discrepant results obtained from various human (Figs. 1 and 2) and animal studies.

Studies of malnutrition have included heterogeneous groups of subjects: individuals with dwarfism, marasmus, and kwashiorkor; undernourished individuals with and without edema; and normal subjects undergoing experimental total or partial starvation induced with a diet containing either all nutrients (1) or only some nutrients, e.g., carbohydrate (2).

Undernutrition has been studied while the nutritional status of the subjects was changing in different ways: deteriorating (weight losing), improving (weight gaining), and stable (weight stable) (or unspecified) (Fig. 1). Weight-losing situations in both children (12) and adults (1,2,22) seem to be associated with

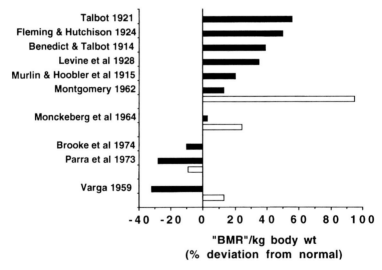

FIG. 1. Resting energy expenditure (kcal/kg body wt/day) in young undernourished children (predominantly of the marasmic type) expressed as a percentage of expected for age. In order to establish greater consistency in the types of patients used in the analysis (e.g., subjects without associated infections), some of the results reported by the original investigators were excluded. When values of appropriate weight for age were not reported by the original investigators (7), these were calculated. When studies did not include a control group and did not compare their results (5–7,11) with a stated reference value, it was assumed that values for resting energy expenditure were 53 kcal/kg/day.

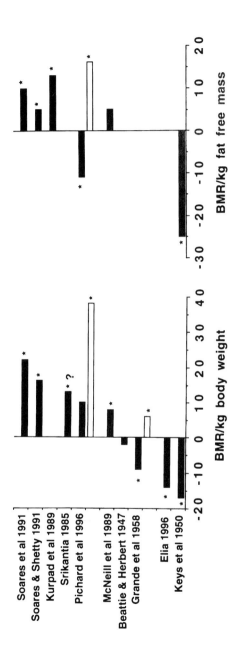

FIG. 2. Metabolic rate (per kg body weight and per kg fat free body) in undernourished adults expressed as a percentage of control values. The first five studies involved undernourished subjects with chronic protein energy malnutrition, who were weight stable. Each study had a control group of normally nourished subjects for comparison. In the remaining studies subjects acted as their own controls, mainly during experimental starvation or semi-starvation. Significant differences are indicated (*).

lower metabolic rates per kilogram body weight or per kilogram FFM than weight-gaining or weight-stable situations (Figs. 1 and 2). In contrast, during recovery from malnutrition, BMR/kg body weight in both children (3,4,10–12) and adults (1,2,21,22) increases and usually exceeds normal values (Fig. 3).

The conditions under which measurements of BMR have been made have varied, particularly in studies involving infants who become restless when they are not fed. Because restlessness increases metabolic rate, a number of workers have chosen to measure BMR during sleep, shortly after a drink of tea or ingestion of a light meal, or for variable periods of time after ingestion of a more substantial meal (ranging from 1.5 hours to 12 hours) (Fig. 1). However, meal ingestion increases thermogenesis to an extent that varies with time and depends on the amount of food ingested, and possibly the nutritional state of the subjects [e.g., Ashworth (25) has reported considerably greater diet-induced thermogenesis in undernourished children than in normal children].

Many of the high metabolic rates in marasmic children reported by early workers may be at least partly due to lack of attention to diet-induced thermogenesis (the feed has often been given shortly before the measurement; Fig. 1) and lack of attention to the phase of treatment (Figs. 1 and 3). Furthermore, some workers have attempted to reduce restlessness in children by administering sedatives (3,4,11,26), but the type and/or dose of sedative has varied or has not been specified. Furthermore, the same study has sometimes made measurements in both sedated and unsedated children (4), whereas other studies have made measurements during sleep that has not been induced by sedatives (8,9). Part of

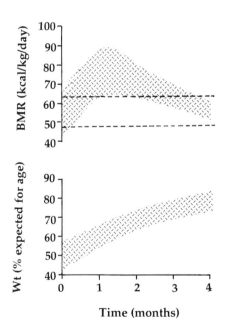

FIG. 3. Changes in BMR/kg body weight (upper), and changes in body weight (as a percentage of that expected for age, lower) in a marasmic child (9–12 months old) during recovery from undernutrition. The dotted lines on the upper graph represent the normal range.

the variability in results also may be due to differences in ambient temperature that has either not been specified or has varied substantially from study to study [e.g., 30–33°C (3), 21–22°C (12), or unspecified (5,7)].

Undernutrition has multiple causes, including malignant, infective, inflammatory, and traumatic diseases, all of which can affect metabolic rate measurements. In contrast, experimental starvation (1,2), anorexia nervosa (18,27–30), pyloric stenosis (12), and famine (10,20,21) may not be complicated by other diseases. Therefore, the presence or absence of underlying pathology can also help explain some of the variability in BMR, particularly in studies that include subjects with and without underlying pathology (7).

Differences in gross body composition (e.g., differences in percentage body fat) or differences in hydration status (e.g., overhydration in kwashiorkor or dehydration after diarrhea) can affect the results for obvious reasons. Several studies of adults and children with protein-energy malnutrition have been reported to produce much greater loss of adipose tissue than other tissues (e.g., cadaver analysis of malnourished children has frequently indicated <5% body fat (5,8,9). However, this is not invariable because autopsy studies in Jamaica suggest that children with marasmus or kwashiorkor often have 10–20% body fat (31,32), possibly because of "premature" death from infective diseases.

Differences between the proportion of tissues with a low metabolic rate (e.g., muscle, adipose tissue) and those with a high metabolic rate (organs) can vary considerably, especially in young infants. During the development of undernutrition, muscle (33,34) and adipose tissue (5,8,9,22) tend to be lost at faster rates than other tissues. This change tends to increase the values of metabolic rate per kilogram body weight or per kilogram FFM.

Apparently different conclusions about energy adaptation can be obtained by expressing BMR in different ways.

This chapter mainly addresses the latter three topics presented in the preceding paragraphs and attempts to show how some of the apparent discrepancies in the resting energy expenditure of undernourished individuals can be explained by variations in the size (± changes in the metabolic rate) of organs.

INADEQUACY OF MANY OF THE CONVENTIONAL INDICES OF BMR AND THE NEED TO CONSIDER ORGAN METABOLIC RATES

One of the most obvious ways to compare the BMR of individuals who differ in size is in relation to body weight (Table 1). Unfortunately, in both normal adults and normal older children, an increase in size (even when the percentage body fat remains constant) is associated with a decrease in the metabolic rate per kilogram body weight. This contrasts with infants (0–2 years of age), in whom the metabolic rate per kilogram body weight varies little.

An alternative way to express energy expenditure is in relation to the size of the FFM (Table 1), which is metabolically much more active than the fat mass

TABLE 1. *Different ways in which BMR has been expressed in malnourished individuals*

BMR in relation to	Reference
Whole body	1–3,5–9,15,16,35–37
Weight	1,3,5,8,10–12,19–21
Adjusted weight	14
Weight$^{0.75}$	3,15,19,38
Weight$^{0.73}$	2
Expected weight for age	6
FFM	14,16,19,39,40
FFM$^{0.75}$	3
Adjusted FFM	14,35
Surface area	2,3,5,8,12,13,17,20,21,41
Height	3,5,10,37
Sitting height	41
Body cell mass	1,2,20
Total body potassium$^{0.75}$	3
Fat-free soft tissue	[a]
Body solids (body weight; water)	4
Cell solids	35
Organ mass	[b],4
% of predicted value for normal individuals	
with the same height	
BMR	10,13
BMR/kg	13
with the same surface area	
BMR	13
BMR/m^2	13
of the same age	
BMR	4,13
BMR/kg	13
BMR/m^2	13
of the same height	
BMR	4,5

[a]Results obtained by dual-energy x-ray absorptiometry (Elia M, unpublished observations).
[b]Results from Elia M, this chapter.

(largely present in adipose tissue). Unfortunately, the metabolic rate per kilogram FFM in both adults and older children also becomes smaller as the size of FFM increases (42).

Kleiber (44,45) related metabolic rate to the weight of several mammalian species, ranging from small animals such as mice to large animals such as cattle, and suggested that BMR was proportional to weight$^{0.75}$. Although infants or children in the first 1–2 years of life were not included in Kleiber's analysis, several investigators have continued to express BMR of such children in relation to weight$^{0.75}$ (3,38). Some investigators have extended the concept further (3) by expressing BMR in relation to lean body mass$^{0.75}$ or total body potassium$^{0.75}$ (total body potassium in normal subjects reflects the size of the FFM, and more specifically the body cell mass). Unfortunately, these approaches have little scientific basis in infants (46–50). This is because the BMR of infants is approximately proportional to body weight (weight$^{1.0}$) rather than to weight$^{0.75}$. For example, the exponents of body weight were found to be 1.09 by Benedict and Talbot (46), 0.91 by Baer (47), 1.11 by Janet and Bochet (48), 0.92 by Karlberg (49), and 0.96 by Elia (unpublished observations). The use of total body potassium is subject to similar potential criticisms, but in addition, in the severely malnourished infant there may be substantial potassium depletion from several lean tissues (mmol/kg tissue or mmol/kg protein) so that total body potassium is no longer a good indicator of the size of the FFM. The extent of potassium depletion may be so large (31,32,51) that total body potassium may not even be a good indicator of body cell mass.

Other workers have expressed BMR in relation to surface area because Rubner's law (43) suggested that BMR is proportional to surface area (approximately 1,000 kcal/m^2). However, several investigators have found this law to be invalid in infants (46,50,52,53) because during the first year of life BMR/m^2 increases and then decreases substantially (53). However, in the absence of an ideal way of expressing BMR, various investigators have continued to express the results in relation to surface area, despite substantially different predictions of surface area by different formulae (43). The inaccuracy of the commonly used Dubois and Dubois formula for predicting the surface area of young normal infants (43) and the greater uncertainty about its accuracy in undernourished individuals makes this method of expressing results even less desirable.

Some investigators have expressed metabolic rate as a percentage of the predicted metabolic rate of normal individuals of the same weight, age, or height as the malnourished subjects (Table 1). However, some investigators have pointed out the inadequacies of using height, weight, and surface area for this purpose and have suggested alternative indices such as those involving sitting height (42). Topper and Muller (42) doubted the validity of the elevated BMR in underweight children, when it was expressed in relation to weight or surface area, and suggested that expressing results in relation to sitting height was far better. In their studies of 70 underweight children (5–15 years of age; 10–33% underweight) BMR/cm sitting height was within the normal range in 70% of children, but in the children who were more than 25% underweight, BMR/cm sitting height was reduced by ≥10%. However, although these investigators had some justification for criticizing the traditional methods of expressing results, they have not produced an adequate scientific justification for expressing BMR in relation to sitting height.

Montgomery (4) overcame the problems associated with the altered hydration status in kwashiorkor and marasmus by expressing metabolic rate in relation to body solids (body weight minus total body water, measured by isotopic dilution). He found that the most severely undernourished children (with only 20–35% of the normal mass of body solids) had values of resting energy expenditure per kilogram body solids that were two- to three-fold greater than the least undernourished infants (50–70% of normal body solids). This approach is unsatisfactory because body solids comprise a mixture of substances (fat, protein, glycogen, and mineral). As a consequence, high results may occur predominantly because of a low-fat mass rather than an increase in the metabolic rate of lean tissues. Other investigators have expressed BMR in relation to cell solids (36), but this requires measurement of body composition using multiple techniques, some of which rely on uncertain assumptions.

Realizing that there are difficulties in expressing the BMR of undernourished individuals in a single way, some investigators have expressed their results in multiple ways (2–4,13,14,19,20). However, even this approach is unsatisfactory, partly because of the lack of an adequate scientific basis for using many of the indices and partly because widely different results and conclusions may be obtained by expressing results in different ways. For example, in one study (4), marasmic infants (before treatment, n = 11) had a normal metabolic rate when it was expressed in relation to surface area (−3% of normal), but a slightly elevated value when expressed in relation to body weight (+13% of normal). In another study of undernourished infants [with (n = 8) and without edema (n = 10)], metabolic rates were lower than normal, but the extent varied with the method in which the results were expressed (−11% in relation to body weight of normal children; −22% in relation to total body potassium$^{0.75}$; and −43% in relation to height) (3). In contrast, the results of Blunt et al. (13) in undernourished children (8–12 years) suggested an increase in BMR to an extent (18–28%) that again depended on the way in which the results were expressed (e.g., in relation to children of the same age, same body weight, or same surface area). Even more complex are the data obtained by Garot (54) in undernourished children, which can be used to show either an increase or decrease in metabolic rate, depending on the way in which the results are expressed (+14% in relation to weight, 9% in relation to weight$^{0.75}$, −16% in relation to surface area, and −39% in relation to height).

Similar problems exist in adults. For example, Srikantia (17) found that when metabolic rate of undernourished adults (<70% weight for height) was expressed in relation to surface area it was 13% lower than in well-nourished subjects (>90% weight for height), but when it was expressed in relation to weight it was 8% higher than well-nourished controls. Beattie and Herbert (20) studied undernourished prisoners of war and found them to have a near normal metabolic rate when it was expressed in relation to body weight (−2%) or active cell mass [calculated using a similar model as that used by Keys et al. (1); +0.3%], but it was significantly reduced when expressed in relation to surface area (−16%). Soares and Shetty (15) reported that in a group of undernourished urban men the metabolic rate per kilogram body weight was 16% higher (p < 0.05) than in well-nourished individuals and 5% higher (p < 0.05) when the results were expressed in kcal/kg FFM. However, when the results were adjusted using a statistical approach to take into account the effect of size on BMR, the metabolic rate per kilogram body weight, and the metabolic rate per kilogram FFM, they became lower than in the control group of normally nourished subjects (−3% and −7%, respectively) and lower than in a separate group of underweight urban men (−6% and −7%; p < 0.05).

BMR in anorexia nervosa is usually low, when it is expressed in relation to the whole body, surface area, and as a percentage predicted from standard equations [e.g., Harris Benedict and Schofield equations (43) based on calculations by Elia using data provided by various investigators (27–30)]. However, BMR/kg body weight may not be significantly different from values obtained in normal subjects: −5% (29); −6% based on calculations by Elia using the ideal body weight of subjects and predicted BMR by the Schofield equation; and +1% (27) in patients with severe anorexia nervosa with a mean BMI of 13.3 kg/m^2 compared with repletion when there was a 25% increase in body weight. The last study also suggests no significant change in BMR/kg FFM (−7%), although other studies suggest a larger and significant reduction, e.g., −22% (30) on the basis of calculations by Elia using ideal or reference FFM (30) and BMR estimated using ideal body weight and the Schofield standards of BMR (28,43). Another study involving a group of nine patients with a mean BMI of 13.7 kg/m^2 (age 15–21 years) BMR/kg body weight (before treatment) was 10% higher than a control group of control subjects (NS), but BMR/kg FFM was reduced by 11%. After treatment, BMR/kg body weight and BMR/kg FFM increased significantly above the values obtained in the control subjects (up to +38% and +16%, respectively).

Further insights into the problems associated with expressing results in different ways can be obtained by inspecting Table 2. Some of the results in

TABLE 2. *Effect of expressing BMR in different ways in normally nourished and undernourished children with and without edema*

		Undernourished	
	Normally nourished	No edema (marasmus)	With edema (kwashiorkor)
Age (mo)	12	12	12
Weight (kg)	10	5	6
Height (cm)	76	67	67
Surface area (m^2)[a]	0.442	0.300	0.324
Assumed fat (% body weight)	20.0	10.0	10.0
FFM (kg)	8.0	4.5	5.4
Hydration of FFM (%)	78.0	79.0	84.0
BMR			
kcal/day	550	302.5 (−45.0%)	280.5 (−49.0%)
kcal/m^2/day	1,224	1,008 (−17.6%)	866 (−29.3%)
kcal/kg/day	55.0	60.5 (+10.0%)	46.75 (−15.0%)
kcal/kg$^{0.75}$/day	97.8	90.5 (−7.5%)	73.0 (−25.4%)
kcal/kg FFM/day	68.8	67.2 (−2.3%)	51.9 (−24.5%)
kcal/kg FFM$^{0.75}$/day	115.6	97.9 (−15.3%)	79.2 (−31.5%)
kcal/cm/day	7.24	4.51 (−37.6%)	4.19 (−42.2%)
BMR in relation to corrected hydration[b]			
kcal/kg $_{corr}$/day	55.0	63.1 (+14.7%)	62.0 (+12.7%)
kcal/kg $_{corr}^{0.75}$/day	97.8	93.4 (−4.5%)	90.4 (−7.6%)
kcal/kg FFM $_{corr}$/day	68.8	70.4 (+2.4%)	71.4 (+3.8%)
kcal/kg FFM $_{corr}^{0.75}$/day	115.6	101.4 (−12.3%)	100.5 (−13.0%)

[a]Calculated using the formula of Dubois and Dubois (43).
[b]BMR expressed in relation to body weight and FFM after correction to normal or reference hydration status (i.e., 78% of FFM). In the child with marasmus, the excess water is 0.205 kg so that the corrected body weight (body wt $_{corr}$) is 4.784 kg and the corrected FFM (FFM $_{corr}$) is 4.295 kg. In the child with kwashiorkor, the excess body water is 1.473 kg so that the body wt $_{corr}$ is 4.527 kg and FFM $_{corr}$ is 3.927 kg.

undernourished children are higher than those in normally nourished children, whereas others are lower. Differences in hydration status also can have major effects on the results. For example, the metabolic rate per kilogram body weight of the typical child with kwashiorkor (Table 2) is below normal (−15%), but when corrected for hydration it becomes higher than normal (+13%) and similar to that in the marasmic infant (Table 2).

It is obvious from the above discussion that it is difficult to draw definite conclusions about adaptations in resting energy metabolism in undernourished individuals. This is not too surprising because different tissues have widely different metabolic rates (54) (Fig. 4), and the relative proportions of these tissues can vary considerably in different clinical and nutritional circumstances. The additional potential variability in the metabolic rate of the same tissues (per kg tissue) under different circumstances also can help explain why the traditional methods of expressing results can be contradictory. In order to establish sound concepts about energy adaptation in undernutrition, it is necessary to have information about the size and metabolic rate of individual human tissues and the way they are affected by wasting conditions.

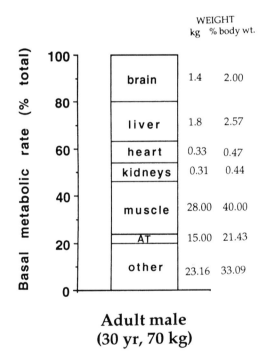

Adult male
(30 yr, 70 kg)

FIG. 4. Distribution of metabolic rate between the various tissues of reference man (30 years, 70 kg) with a BMR of 1,680 kcal/day and an infant (0.5 year, 7.5 kg) with a BMR of 390 kcal/day. AT, adipose tissue. The mass of tissues and their contribution to body weight are tabulated to the right of the bar charts.

ORGAN SIZE AND METABOLIC RATE IN HEALTH

Figure 4 shows the widely different metabolic rates of different tissues (53). In adult humans, four organs—liver, kidney, heart, and brain—that account for 5–6% of body weight are responsible for more than half of the BMR. It is believed that changes in the size of organs (± changes in organ-specific metabolic rate) largely account for the twofold reduction in metabolic rate (per kg body weight or per kg FFM) that occurs during growth and development. Indeed, the metabolic rate of the whole body when expressed in relation to the organ mass (Fig. 5) shows little change during growth and development. This is because the contribution of organ mass to body weight and FFM decreases during growth and development, although it is nearly constant in the first 2–3 years of life (Fig. 6). An analysis by Elia of cross-sectional data during growth (birth to adulthood) suggest that both BMR and organ weight are approximately proportional to weight$^{0.77}$. However, there is little direct information about changes in the metabolic rate of specific human tissues (in relation to their mass) during different stages of growth. The activity of specific metabolic processes such as protein turnover, which decreases as animals grow (even in the same tissue), tends to decrease the metabolic rate per kilogram of organ mass. In infancy and

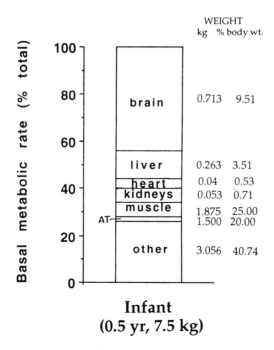

FIG. 4. *Continued.*

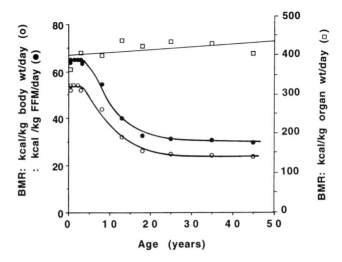

FIG. 5. Effect of age on BMR per kg body weight, per kg FFM, and per kg organ mass (liver + kidneys + heart + brains). Data for 0.5–45 years (0.5, 3, 8, 13, 18, 25, 35, and 45 years) were taken from Korenchevsky (55) and Elia (53). Data for 0–3 (years were taken from Copolletta et al., who provided values for organ mass and height). Values for height were used to establish the appropriate corresponding weight (50th percentile), which was then used to calculate FFM (assumed to be 80% body weight). The BMR corresponding to different weight was calculated using the Scofield equation. During the first 2 years of life BMR is approximately proportional to body weight. For 0–1 years BMR (kcal/day) = 45 body weight $^{1.10}$, r = 0.9998; and for 0–2 years BMR (kcal/day) = 46 body weight $^{1.09}$, r = 0.9998. For the age range 0–18 years (data for 0, 0.5, 3, 8, 13, and 18 years) BMR (kcal/day) = 79 body weight $^{0.77}$, r = 0.99; BMR (kcal/day) = 383 organ weight $^{1.08}$, r = 0.999; and organ weight (kg) = 0.24 body weight $^{0.71}$, r = 0.98).

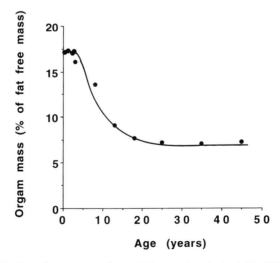

FIG. 6. The contribution of organ mass (liver + kidneys + heart + brain) to FFM. Values for body weight, FFM, and organ mass (liver + kidneys + heart + brains) are the same as those in Fig 5. During the first 2 years of life organ mass accounted for 12.9–13.9% body weight and 16.0–17.5% FFM. All the individual data points during this period are not shown.

early childhood, on the other hand, organs tend to be more hydrated and have a larger proportion of extracellular water than those of adults, and this tends to reduce the metabolic rate per kilogram of organ mass. Studies by Kennedy and Sokoloff (56) suggest no change in the O_2 consumption of the brain in children 3–11 years of age, although they tend to be slightly higher in children.

IMPORTANCE OF ORGAN SIZE IN DETERMINING BMR IN HEALTH

The twofold decrease in metabolic rate (per kg body weight and per kg FFM) between infancy and adulthood is paralleled by a decrease in the percentage contribution of organs (e.g., sum of brain, liver, kidney, and heart) to body weight. The result is that whole-body BMR/kg organ weight changes little during growth and development (Fig. 5). Using the cross-sectional data largely provided by Elia (53), it can be calculated that during growth and development (0, 0.5, 3, 8, 13, and 18 years), BMR is proportional to body weight$^{0.77}$ and to organ weight$^{1.08}$ (Fig. 5). From a cross-sectional analysis of a variety of mammals, Kleiber (44,45) concluded that body weight$^{0.75}$ represented the active metabolic mass (BMR ∞ weight$^{0.75}$). The observations by the present investigator (Elia) that the BMR of humans is approximately proportional to organ weight (liver, kidneys, heart, and brain) and that organ weight is proportional to body weight$^{0.71}$ (organ weight = 0.24 body weight$^{0.71}$; r = 0.98), are consistent with the view that much of Kleiber's active metabolic mass is represented by organ mass. However, in the first 1–2 years of human life, Kleiber's relationship between BMR and weight$^{0.75}$ does not apply (e.g., in the first year of life BMR (kcal/day) = 45 body weight$^{1.10}$, r = 0.999, and during the first 2 years of life, BMR (kcal/day) = 46 body weight$^{1.09}$, r = 0.999). During this period organ mass is approximately proportional to body weight (organ mass = 0.14 body weight$^{0.96}$, during the first year of life, r = 0.996; and organ wt = 0.13 body weight$^{1.0}$ during the first 2 years of life, r = 0.996; see Fig. 6). The result is that BMR remains approximately proportional to organ mass [BMR (kcal/day) = 416 organ weight$^{1.11}$ during the first year of life, and BMR (kcal/day) = 409 organ weight$^{1.06}$ during the first 2 years of life]. This is again consistent with the view that the size of organs largely reflect the extent of oxidative metabolism in the whole body.

The well-known reduction in BMR per kilogram body weight or per kilogram FFM that occurs with an increase in size, in both men and women of the same age (Fig. 5), causes obvious problems when comparing metabolic rates of individuals of different size. In an attempt to account for this problem, a number of investigators have introduced a size-dependent correction factor (43). However, there has been surprisingly little inquiry into the reason for the difference in metabolic rate (per kg body weight or per kg FFM) in individuals of different size, although a possible explanation (53) is that the contribution of organs to the body weight (or the FFM) of adults becomes smaller as the individual becomes larger. This not only appears to be the case between species (53), but also between healthy adults of different size (Fig. 7). Using

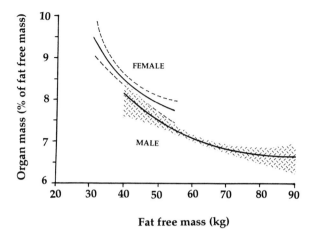

FIG. 7. The contribution of organ mass (liver + kidney + heart + brain) in 842 males and 390 females who were considered to be healthy up to the time of death. The shaded areas (male) and area between solid and dotted lines (female) indicate ±1 SEM. The graph was smoothed and redrawn from graphic data provided by Garby and Lammert (57).

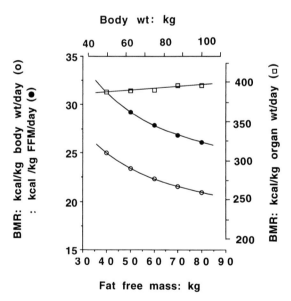

FIG. 8. The effect of increasing body weight and FFM in male adults on the metabolic rate (whole body) per kg body weight, per kg FFM, and per kg organ mass (liver + kidney + heart + brain). BMR was calculated using the following equation: BMR (kcal/day) = 21.01 FFM + 410.5 (see text). The contribution of organ mass to FFM was estimated from the graphical data of Garby and Lammert (57). The graph relating to body weight (lowest graph) assumed that FFM accounted for 80% of body weight.

the information shown in Fig. 7 and a prediction formula to estimate BMR from FFM

$$\text{FFM (kcal/day)} = 21.01 \text{ FFM (kg)} + 410.5 \text{ [mean of 10 equations reported by}$$
$$\text{Elia (43); SD for FFM} = 0.93 \text{ and SD for constant} = 104],$$

it is possible to illustrate diagramatically that there is no decrease (in fact a small increase) in BMR/kg organ weight as the size of the FFM increases (Fig. 8).

ORGAN SIZE IN UNDERNUTRITION

Table 3 summarizes the percentage loss of different organs in undernourished adults. The data for children are shown in Table 4 (which does not include muscle) and Table 5 (which includes muscle). In undernutrition, abdominal and tho-

TABLE 3. *Percentage loss of body and organ weights in autopsies of emaciated bodies*[a]

	Cachexia	Tumor	Chronic infections	Tuberculosis
Body weight	−38.8 (11)	−38.0 (27)	−43.9 (31)	−43.0 (40)
Heart	−34.7 (11)	−33.2 (25)	−30.7 (31)	−31.9 (39)
Liver	−42.1 (10)	−32.8 (21)	−28.0 (15)	−27.7 (29)
Kidneys	−36.0 (11)	−27.5 (25)	−15.5 (31)	−17.6 (39)
Spleen	−46.6 (8)	−27.6 (22)		
Brain	−4.6 (10)	−3.4 (19)	−2.8 (23)	−4.0 (25)
Pancreas		−33.0 (6)	−30.5 (26)	−38.6 (17)
Thyroid		−20.6 (10)	−32.3 (23)	−35.8 (25)
Adrenals		−21.5 (9)	+23.2 (23)	+6.6 (24)
Testes		−28.7 (12)	−40.4 (24)	−39.4 (27)

[a]Data from Krieger (58). Values in parentheses indicate the number of subjects. Negative values indicate loss of weight; positive values indicate gain in weight.

TABLE 4. *Whole body and organ weights of malnourished infants who were victims of famines (n = 30–50 for each organ)*

Organ	Final body weight	Maximum body weight during life[a]	Body length	Age
Whole body	0.0	−20.9	−31.6	−51.5
Brain	+25.9	+1.5	−7.7	−12.3
Kidneys	+20.5	−5.7	−1.0	−19.4
Lungs	+24.5	−4.5	−20.6	−21.2
Spleen	+9.5	−14.9	−20.5	−31.3
Heart	−0.9	−20.9	−14.9	−28.0
Liver	−6.3	−33.0	−23.2	−27.1
Suprarenals	−43.3	−60.5	−56.9	−38.5
Thymus	−71.8	−80.7	−80.6	−82.6

Values are the average percentage differences when the observed weight is compared with the (estimated) normal for each of the categories listed as column headings.
[a]Based on subset of infants in whom the maximum weight in life was known. Data from Jackson (59).

TABLE 5. *Body composition of atrophic infants*

	Percentage of normal
Whole body	52
Brain	90
Kidneys	80
Heart	60
Fat	5
Skeleton	85
Muscle	30
Surface area	70

Data from Kerpel-Fronius and Frank (34).

racic organ weight is lost more readily than that of the brain, which loses virtually no weight. Muscle and adipose tissue tend to be lost to a greater extent than
in other tissues (33,34) (Table 5), whereas the brain and skeleton (22) are preserved more than are other tissues. The characteristic appearance of the malnourished marasmic infant with a large head and a wasted body reflects this situation.
Indeed, it is possible for the brain to continue to grow even while other organs lose
weight (59). The brain has a special role in explaining the overall metabolic rate
of the young child because of the large contribution of the brain to BMR [>40%
of the BMR of the newborn is due to the brain, compared with 20% in the adult
(53)]. Furthermore, because the brain probably plays an even more important role
in explaining the BMR of the undernourished child, it is important to undertake
a detailed assessment of brain size and composition in undernutrition. Figure 9

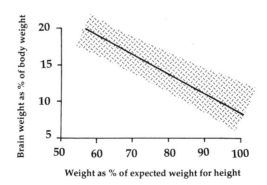

FIG. 9. The effect of undernutrition (expressed as weight as percentage expected (weight for
height) in children (n = 45) on the contribution of the brain to body weight). In the most severely
undernourished children the brain accounts for about a fifth of body weight, which is about
twofold greater than in normal children of the same age. The large variability indicated by the
shaded area (approximately 95% confidence interval) is partly the result of differences in age
(e.g., in a subgroup of children for which individual data are available the age ranged from 6 to
16 months) and partly to variation in body composition. The graph was redrawn and modified
using data provided by Alleyne et al. (51); $y = -0.27x + 35$; $p < 0.005$.

TABLE 6. *Size and composition of the whole body, brain, and liver of malnourished children with and without edema*[a]

	Malnourished children without edema, n=5 (3F, 2M;12 ± 2 mo)	Malnourished children with edema, n=5 (4F, 1M; 12 ± 4 mo)	Reference children (12 mo)[b]
Whole body			
Weight (kg)	5.8 ± 1.7[a]	6.1+1.3[a]	10
Weight (% expected for age)	60 ± 15[a]	62 ± 7	100
Water (% of fat-free body)	78.9 ± 1.4	84.1 ± 1.2	78
Brain			
Brain weight (% body weight)	14.5 ± 3.1[a]	11.8 ± 2.2[a]	9
Brain weight	93 ± 7	81 ± 8	100
% Water	84.4 ± 2.6	86.0 ± 1.4	87
% Fat	5.2 ± 1.2	8.0 ± 1.1	5.3
% Protein	9.5 ± 2.4	8.1 ± 0.6	7.3
Liver			
Weight (% body weight)	3.7 ± 1.1	5.9 ± 2.3	3
Weight (% expected for age)	86.2 ± 1.1[a]	119 ± 35.7	100
Fat-free weight (% expected for age)	60.0 ± 9.5	82.8 ± 10.5	100
% Fat	13.2 ± 13.2	30.9 ± 16.4	5
% Protein	15.2 ± 4.9	9.2 ± 3.5	16
% Water	70.8 ± 10.1	59.0 ± 13.0	76
% Water in fat-free liver	81.7 ± 3.7	85.5 ± 2.1	80

[a]Most children died with infections, e.g., chest and ear infections. Results calculated by Elia using information provided by Garrow et al. (31) and Halliday et al. (32).
[b]Based on Snyder et al. (62), Garrow et al. (31), and Widdowson and Dickerson (63).

shows that as the severity of undernutrition increases, the contribution of the brain to body weight also increases (up to twofold in the most severe cases). Some studies (e.g., studies based on computerized tomography), suggest that during and after undernutrition there is some atrophy of the brain (60,61), with the result that brain tissue is replaced by cerebrospinal fluid (CSF). Because CSF has a density (about 1.006 g/ml) similar to that of brain tissue (about 1.04 g/ml) (62), the overall weight of the brain may change little even if there is cerebral atrophy. However, this atrophy is generally not marked, and therefore the hydration and gross composition of the brain in severe undernutrition is similar to that of normal children of the same age (64) (Table 6). The same approximate conclusion applies to a variety of other organs (31), with the exception of the liver, which may show a large infiltration with fat (especially in kwashiorkor, where up to half of the body fat may be in the liver). The result is a reduction in the proportion of other components within the liver (water and protein) (Table 6).

ORGAN METABOLIC RATE IN UNDERNUTRITION

The rate of O_2 consumption (by the whole body and by individual tissues) has been widely used as an approximate index of energy expenditure. This is because the energy equivalents of 1 L O_2 (Eeq O_2) varies little between fuels, even if they are partially combusted. For example, the Eeq O_2 for glycogen is 21.12 kJ/L, glucose 20.89 kJ/L, triacylglycerol 19.6 kJ/L, acetoacetic acid 19.80 kJ/L, and 3 hydroxybutyric acid 19.89 kJ/L.

However, there have been few attempts to relate organ metabolic rate to their masses (kcal/kg organ/day) in undernutrition, but positron emission tomography (PET) has demonstrated no significant change in the overall O_2 consumption of the brain (or of its component regions) during 3 weeks of total starvation in obese individuals (65) (Table 7). Therefore the reduction in BMR in this situation is due to a loss in the mass of other tissues, either with or without an associated reduction in their metabolic rate (per gram tissue). The O_2 consumption of forearm tissues (per 100 ml tissue) also shows no change during 5 weeks of starvation (67) (Table 7). This might lead to the conclusion that the energy expenditure of limb tissues decreases because of a reduction in their mass, rather than in the O_2 consumption per gram of forearm tissue. However, the full interpretation of the result is more complex (68) because the forearm comprises different tissues (skin, adipose tissue, bone, muscle) whose relative masses and blood flow may change during starvation. Indeed there is evidence that adipose tissue is lost at a greater rate than lean tissues during prolonged starvation (22) and that blood flow to adipose tissue increases almost twofold during starvation (at least after 4 days of starvation in the obese) (69).

Although there is little direct information to indicate whether the energy expenditure of other human tissues (per kg weight organ) changes during starvation, semi-starvation, or chronic stable protein-energy undernutrition, it is possible to draw some important conclusions about energy metabolism in young undernourished children (e.g., with marasmus) by taking into account the size of

TABLE 7. *Oxygen consumption by the human brain and forearm during total starvation in obese individuals*

	Weight (kg)	BMI (kg/m^2)	O_2 consumption [ml/100 g/min (1); ml/100 ml/min (2)]
Brain			
PET (n = 4) (65)			
Before starvation	107.5 ± 9.3	36.2 ± 4.1	3.45 ± 0.27 (1)
After 3 weeks of starvation	95.0 ± 9.8	32.0 ± 4.2	3.70 ± 0.49 (1)
Arteriovenous Exchange (n = 3) (66)			
Before starvation	133.1 ± 9.9	43.2 ± 2.7	—
After 5–6 weeks of starvation	110.9 ± 2.7	36.0 ± 3.7	3.3 ± 0.4 (1)[a]
Forearm			
Arteriovenous exchange (n = 8) (67)			
Before starvation	125.6 ± 24.8	44.5 ± 9.7	0.22 ± 0.03 (2)
After 3 days of starvation	—	—	0.24 ± 0.06 (2)
After 24 days of starvation	110.2 ± 21.8	39.0 ± 8.0	0.27 ± 0.04 (2)

[a]The blood flow in two of the subjects was exactly the same (45 ml/100 g/min). The same blood flow was assumed to occur in the third subject.

TABLE 8. Energy expenditure of the whole body, FFM brain, and FFM (FFM – brain) other than brain of a normal child and a marasmic child before nutritional therapy and at peak hypermetabolism during recovery[a]

	Weight				Metabolic rate					
					Body		Brain		FFM – brain	
	Body	FFM	Brain	FFM – brain	kcal/day	kcal/kg/day	kcal/kg/day	kcal/day [7] • (3)	kcal/day [(5) – (8)]	kcal/kg/day [(9) ÷ (4)]
Normal (12 months)	10+	8	0.9	7.1	550	55	225	202.5	347.5	48.9
Marasmus (before treatment) (12 months)	5++	4.5	0.8	3.7	302.5 (−45%)	60.5 (+10%)	225 (0%) 202.5 (−10%) 180 (−20%)	180 (−11%) 162 (−20%) 144 (−29%)	122.5 (−65%) 140.5 (−60%) 158.5 (−54%)	33.1 (−32%) 38.0 (−22%) 42.8 (−12%)
Marasmus (during treatment at peak hypermetabolism) (12 months)	6+++	5.25	0.8	4.45	450 (−18%)	75.0 (+36%)	225 (0%) 270 (+30%)	180 (−11%) 216 (+7%)	270 (−22%) 234 (−33%)	60.7 (+24%) 52.6 (+8%)

These calculations assume that FFM is responsible for all the metabolic rate of the body, which is not entirely true, partly because adipose tissue makes a small contribution to BMR (probably ~3% in children) and partly because some fat is present in organs such as the brain. Similar trends exist even if correlations are made for minor changes in hydration status (see text and Table 2).

[a]The calculations assume that the metabolic rate of normal brain is 225 kcal/kg/day. A range of values are assumed for the marasmic infants. +, 20% fat; ++, 10% fat; +++, 12.5% fat.

the brain size relative to body weight (Table 8). Even if the metabolic rate of the brain of a 12-month-old marasmic child (kcal/kg brain/day) is 0–20% below normal, it can be calculated that the brain is likely to contribute ≥50% BMR. Using published data of BMR, it also can be calculated that the metabolic rate of the remaining fat-free tissues is reduced. Therefore, the apparent paradox of an increased BMR observed in some marasmic infants (BMR per kg FFM) can be explained by an increase in the proportion of oxidatively active tissues (e.g., brain) relative to less active lean tissues (56,70). The results (Table 8) are compatible with reduction in the oxidative metabolism of lean tissues other than the brain (and possibly a reduction in the O_2 consumption of the brain itself).

Some of the paradoxical data of energy expenditure in adults also can be explained by a change in the proportion of tissues with different oxidative metabolic activity. For example, Soares et al. (14) found that the BMR/kg FFM was elevated in undernourished individuals. However, using urinary creatinine as an index of muscle mass and skinfold thickness as an index of percentage body fat, the investigators concluded that in chronic protein-energy malnutrition the proportion of muscular tissues (with a low resting energy expenditure) to nonmuscular lean tissues (with a higher resting energy expenditure) was decreased (0.95 vs. 1.43 in control subjects). This is in keeping with previous reports by Barac-Nieto et al. (71) (muscle cell to visceral cell ratio = 2.49 in mild undernutrition compared with 1.14 in severe undernutrition). Both of these studies have used body composition techniques that may not be entirely valid in undernutrition. However, the reported differences in the composition of the FFM are large and could provide an explanation for the increase in BMR/kg FFM reported in some studies (14,10). For example, if the metabolic rate of muscle in the undernourished subjects studied by Soares et al. (14) was either 13 kcal/kg muscle/min (54) or even 10% lower (11.7 kcal/kg/day), it can be calculated that the metabolic rate (kcal/kg/day) of nonmuscular tissues is reduced by 4% and 2%, respectively. This again suggests possible adaptation, although the observed increase in BMR/kg FFM (+10%; $p < 0.05$) (14) might suggest the reverse. Some investigators have had no difficulty in concluding that the metabolic rate (per kg) of the lean tissues of undernourished subjects is decreased because their results indicate a decrease in BMR, irrespective of whether they are expressed in relation to body weight (1,3), FFM (1,3), or total body potassium (3).

The evidence presented above suggests that untreated undernutrition is associated with adaptive reductions in metabolic rate (per kg) of lean tissues that may be partly due to reduced core temperature. However, in two situations the reverse may be true: wasting conditions associated with inflammatory disease (especially acute inflammatory disease) and during recovery from undernutrition. Both of these situations may be associated with either a normal or increased body temperature and metabolic rate.

During recovery from undernutrition, organ size increases, but the increase in BMR/kg fat-free body can be so large that there may be an increase in the metabolic rate of individual lean tissues (per kg tissue) (Table 7). The cause for the increase in metabolic rate is almost certainly due to multiple causes, including an increase in protein synthesis, an increase in body temperature, an increase in cardiac output, and possibly persistence of diet-induced thermogenesis after a large meal (especially when BMR is measured ≤4 hours after a large meal in young hyperphagic children recovering from undernutrition).

Systemic disease also leads to wasting, but its effects on relative organ size and on the metabolic rate of individual tissues may be different from undernutrition uncomplicated by disease. For example, there is abundant evidence from animal studies that injury (e.g., from aseptic abscess or endotoxin administration) increases the size of central organs, whereas other more peripheral tissues (muscle, skin) lose both mass and protein content (71–74). The tensile strength of the skin (e.g., after surgical wounds) is also reduced (72). An example of the changes induced by aseptic abscesses in normal and protein malnourished animals are shown in Table 9. Protein malnutrition not only attenuates the acute-phase protein response (72) but also the changes in tissue mass and protein content (Table 9). Some of the changes in the size of organs can be reproduced by administering cytokines such as tumor necrosis factor (75) or hormones such as corticosteroids (76).

In humans, chronic conditions such as tuberculosis and malignancy also tend to preferentially preserve central organs, as suggested by Krieger's autopsy studies (Table 3). Modern scanning techniques (e.g., computerized axial tomography) have been used in real life to confirm that central organs are preserved in malignancy. For example, Jebb et al. (39) reported that the volume of central abdominal organs in malignant disease (carcinoma of the lung) that was unresponsive to treatment was up to 30% greater than in malignant disease that responded to treatment, but the variability was large and the differences were statistically not significant. The BMR of patients who did not respond to treatment (mean weight 60 kg, BMI

TABLE 9. *Effect of aseptic abcesses (2 days after turpentine injection) and pair feeding on tissue protein content (g/100 g body weight) of normally nourished and protein-deprived rats*

	Fed ad libitum (saline controls)	Pair-fed	Fed ad libitum (turpentine)
Normally nourished			
Liver	0.882	0.780	1.029***†††
Heart	0.059	0.056	0.073*
Kidney	0.138	0.128	0.170***††
Lung	0.101	0.090	0.134*
Protein malnourished			
Liver	0.706	0.7171	0.809**††
Heart	0.089	0.082	0.086
Kidney	0.166	0.168	0.180**
Lung	0.141	0.123	0.145*

*p < 0.05; **p < 0.01; ***p < 0.001 compared with saline control group. †p < 0.05; ††p < 0.01; †††p < 0.001 compared with saline control group pair fed controls.
Data from Jennings and Elia (72).

24.6 kg/m^2) was significantly higher than that of patients who responded to treatment (mean weight 63 kg; BMI 24.4 kg/m^2)—by 8% in relation to predicted BMR; by +13% in relation to body weight; and by +10% in relation to FFM.

Heymsfield and McManus (77) used computerized tomography to undertake a more extensive analysis of organ size in patients with malignant disease and made measurements in three patients with anorexia nervosa. However, they did not measure BMR or oxygen consumption. Organ size (liver + kidney + spleen + heart) was greater than normal in patients with nonmetastatic malignancy and considerably less than normal in anorexia nervosa. Muscle mass was considerably reduced in both patients with malignancy (about 40%) and anorexia nervosa (about 50%). These observations suggest that the low BMR in anorexia nervosa [as a percentage of that predicted by the Harris-Benedict or Schofield equations (42)] is due to a decrease in organ mass, although additional reductions in the metabolic rate per kilogram organ mass are also possible. In malignancy the increased metabolic rate is probably at least partly due to a greater contribution of organ mass (plus malignant tissue) to the FFM, although the development of edema, pleural effusions, and ascites complicates interpretation of results.

Although there is little information in humans about the effect of acute traumatic and infective conditions on tissue size and metabolic rate, the large increase in metabolic rate in some conditions (e.g., in up to twofold in severely burned patients), which occurs in the absence of obvious clinical visceromegaly (and absence of gross visceromegaly on radiographs), suggests that there is likely to be an increase in metabolic rate per kilogram of organ mass. Direct measurements of O_2 consumption by individual tissues after burns and sepsis suggest an increase in the energy expenditure of multiple organs (78). Head injury has a variable effect on the energy expenditure of the brain, although it is frequently unaltered (79), whereas the energy expenditure of other tissues increases and contributes to the increase in BMR, which may be more than 35–50% above normal (80).

POSSIBLE SIGNIFICANCE OF CHANGES IN ORGAN SIZE IN DISEASE

The reason for the preferential preservation of central organs after injury or inflammatory conditions is uncertain, although tissues that "work" harder, mechanically or metabolically, might be expected to enlarge, whereas tissues that become less active might be expected to atrophy (e.g., muscle wasting during immobility or reduced physical activity). The preferential sparing of the heart in systemic disease is associated with a high resting cardiac output in the flow phase of injury, and the sparing of the lung is associated with increased resting ventilation. The enlarged liver is associated with increased gluconeogenesis and increased protein synthesis, which is at least partly due to the increased production of secretory proteins such as acute phase proteins. The reticuloendothelial system, which is found predominantly in the liver and to a lesser extent other tissues such as the lung, becomes functionally more active in inflammatory conditions (e.g., to help remove toxins). The relative sparing of the kidney is associated with excretion of more nitrogenous end products, especially during the flow phase of injury.

Pyrexia, common in many diseases, probably also increases the metabolic rate of multiple tissues.

BODY TEMPERATURE, THERMOREGULATION, AND ORGAN METABOLIC RATES

A large body of evidence suggests that energy expenditure (O_2 consumption of human and nonhuman cell preparations, biopsies, and isolated perfused organs) is affected by the temperature of the medium in which they are bathed and the composition of the medium that is used to perfuse them. The same might be expected to occur in vivo, particularly in situations where the set point for body temperature is altered.

As early as the 1st century A.D., a link was made between undernutrition and cold. Although a near normal body temperature has been reported in experimental studies of human starvation undertaken in controlled environments, a wealth of clinical records from the 19th and 20th centuries suggest that famine is associated with a low body temperature (80). Low body temperature also has been reported in kwashiorkor and in many types of undernourished animals. The relationship between BMR and body temperature is complex, but a significant positive relationship has been established between them in both health and undernutrition (adults and children) (81–83). However, it is difficult to come to conclusions about cause and effect, although it is well known that clinical hypothermia produces a low BMR, which increases when the subject is heated artificially. Talbot's report in 1921 (5) suggest that clinicians at that time were well aware of the predisposition of undernourished children to hypothermia and the common clinical difficulties associated with elevating the body temperature of malnourished children. They were also aware that when the metabolic rate is not sufficiently high to equal energy expenditure, body temperature decreases, but this may be reversed by artificial insulation or heating. In these situations, infants resemble poikilotherms (cold-blooded animals), whose metabolism is determined by the ambient temperature. McCance and Widdowson (84) showed that hypothermia could be brought about more quickly in starving newborn piglets compared with fed piglets, and Baric (86) reported that the young rat (2–4 days) behaved like a homeotherm when well fed, and like a poikilotherm when starved. Brooke et al. (86) reported a similar phenomenon in malnourished infants. The core temperature of the malnourished infant (about 1°C lower than control subjects), responded to diurnal variations in ambient temperature, whereas in the normal or recovered infant it did not. Earlier work by Kerpel-Fronius et al. (83) had shown that the rectal temperature of malnourished children exposed to a controlled cool ambient temperature decreases more rapidly than that of normal children. The pronounced decrease in body temperature that can occur in the sleeping malnourished child (or adult), especially in climates with low nocturnal temperatures, is well known. During recovery many of these abnormalities disappear (86).

Other studies suggest that undernutrition, whether it be in elderly subjects (87) or young children (88), is associated with failure to adequately increase heat production in response to cooling. For example, in a group of malnourished Jamaican children 4–16 months of age (49% of expected weight for age and 77% of expected weight for height), cooling the environmental air from an ambient temperature of about 32–33°C to 24–25°C did not produce an increase in heat production, and as a consequence rectal temperature decreased at a rate of 1°C/hour (88). In contrast, after substantial recovery (70% weight for age, and 103% weight for height), lowering the ambient temperature to 24–25°C produced a 20% increase in heat production, which was of the nonshivering type. The result was that rectal temperature in these children decreased to a much smaller extent than in the severely malnourished infants (88). The Jewish physicians of the Warsaw ghetto (89) (Poland 1940) not only noted the low body temperature of malnourished subjects (~1.3°C lower than normal) but also that it often remained low during typhus infection, which is usually characterized by high fever (89). However, other studies suggest that a substantial fever response can be mounted in malnourished children with acute infections (83).

ORGAN METABOLIC RATE AND BMR IN RELATION TO WHOLE-BODY TOTAL ENERGY EXPENDITURE

In health the most variable component of total energy expenditure is physical activity. Therefore, it is possible that undernutrition, with or without associated disease, may markedly affect energy balance by influencing physical activity.

Using data from the Minnesota study of experimental semi-starvation (1), Taylor and Keys (90) concluded that more energy was saved by reduced physical activity (energy cost of 1,567 kcal/day before semi-starvation vs. 451 kcal/day after 25% loss of body weight) than by the decrease in BMR (1,576 kcal/day vs. 962 kcal/day). The 35% reduction in BMR is considered to be due to loss of metabolizing mass (65%) and a reduction in the metabolic rate per kilogram of this mass (35%). A number of other investigators (1) also have concluded that undernutrition reduces muscle strength, produces early fatigue, and reduces spontaneous physical activity. The data with respect to spontaneous activity in adults have not always been consistent [e.g., increased energy expenditure due to physical activity has been reported in anorexia nervosa (91)] and are confounded by behavioral and social pressures, such as the pressure to work and earn money. In some studies the incentive to work has been encouraged by administering financial or other forms of rewards for the work done (92,93). In one study of undernourished individuals who were ingesting fixed amounts of food, rewards for extra work done resulted in increased productivity at the expense of body weight, which decreased (92). In another study dietary supplements to malnourished Gambian men produced no improvement in work output, possibly because of the confounding effects of the financial rewards, which were given to both the supplemented and unsupplemented group of men (93). Studies of malnourished children during school hours also have their limitations because of the large component of compulsory activities that occurs in this setting. For example, Spurr and Reina (94) reported that the total energy expenditure [assessed by a combination of indirect calorimetry (BMR) and heart rate monitoring using individual calibration procedures] in a group of marginally undernourished boys (n = 19; <95% weight for height) was not different from a control group of children (>95% weight for height) during school days (1,826 vs. 2,008 kcal/day, respectively). However, during summer camp where supervised sports and play activities were encouraged, total energy expenditure was significantly lower in the undernourished (1,979 vs. 2,452 kcal/day). Perhaps a better human model for studying the effects of undernutrition on spontaneous physical activity is the preschool child, because a child of this age is influenced less by some of the social pressures that affect older children and adults. Torun (95) reviewed (short-term and long-term) studies that have documented the time spent by undernourished children in different activities and concluded that dietary restriction results in important early reductions in physical activity. For example, in a small group of boys 1.5–4.5 years of age, changes in activity patterns were found to occur within a few days of restricting dietary intake from 120–150 kcal and 3–4 g protein/kg/day, to 90 kcal and 1.8–2.0 g protein/kg/day (96). In a longer term study of boys 25–40 months of age, the energy content of the diet was reduced twice at 40-day intervals from a mean of 90 ± 3 to 82 ± 4 kcal/day and then to 71 ± 4 kcal/kg/day (97). The first reduction did not affect weight gain, and therefore the children presumably continued to grow at the expense of reduced physical activity (energy expenditure was calculated from BMR and heart rate monitoring, which was calibrated against O_2 consumption). The second reduction in dietary intake not only reduced total energy expenditure further, but essentially abolished growth. Although some studies have included only a small number of subjects, the overall information in preschool children suggests that dietary restriction may have important consequences on physical activity (95). Furthermore, although under famine conditions adults sometimes undertake considerable physical activity in the hope of finding food (1), descriptions of lethargy are plentiful (1,98), and the terminal apathy and inactivity of severe or preterminal malnutrition are characteristic. The reduction in spontaneous physical activity is even more marked when disease either precipitates or complicates undernutrition.

CLINICAL IMPLICATIONS

In chronic protein-energy malnutrition, the major cause of reduced energy expenditure is a reduction in body weight and its constituent tissues. However, in undernutrition, with or without underlying disease, changes in the overall BMR also may occur from the disproportionate loss of tissues with widely different metabolic rates, as well as from changes in tissue-specific metabolic rates, which are probably influenced by reduced body temperature that frequently accompanies moderate to severe undernutrition. Although undernutrition is associated with reduced insulation and a large body weight/surface area (which tends to reduce body temperature), the observations on thermoregulation have led to the proposition that there is resetting of the hypothalamic thermostat to a lower level (3). This may not only contribute to the reduction in BMR, but also reduced glucose use and reduced risk of hypoglycemia, which may complicate malnutrition. Although under appropriate conditions such a change conserves energy and prolongs survival, in colder conditions it increases the risk of hypothermia. Therefore, the response appears to have a double edge because it may produce a favorable or adaptive outcome in some circumstances (conservation of energy stores) and possible detrimental effects in cold environmental conditions (hypothermia and death).

Similarly, reductions in physical activity can be regarded as important behavioral adaptations that conserve energy. However, if these effects are prolonged, reductions in exploratory behavior and in physical and psychologic interaction with other subjects may result in impaired social and cognitive development. Therefore, although reductions in physical activity may be regarded as adaptive in the short-term (conservation of energy stores), the long-term consequences of such compensatory responses may have potentially important detrimental developmental consequences.

REFERENCES

1. Keys A, Brozek J, Henschel A, et al. *The biology of human starvation.* Vol. 1. St. Paul, MN: University Minnesota Press, North Central Publishing; 1950:303–339.
2. Grande F, Anderson T, Keys A. Changes in basal metabolic rate in man in semistarvation and refeeding. *J Appl Physiol* 1958;12:230–238.
3. Brooke OG, Cocks T, March Y. Resting metabolic rate in malnourished babies in relation to total body potassium. *Acta Paediatr Scand* 1974;63:817–825.
4. Montgomery RD. Changes in the basal metabolic rate of the malnourished infant and their relation to body composition. *J Clin Invest* 1962;41:1653–1663.
5. Talbot FB. Severe infantile malnutrition. *Arch Dis Child* 1921;22:358–370.
6. Fleming GB, Hutchison HS. A study of the metabolism of the undernourished infant. *Q J Med* 1924; 17:339–357.
7. Benedict FG, Talbot FB. Studies in the respiratory exchange of infants. *Am J Dis Child* 1914;8:1–49.
8. Levine SZ, Wilson JR, Gottschall G. The respiratory metabolism in infancy and childhood VIII. The respiratory exchange in marasmus: basal metabolism. *Am J Dis Child* 1928;35:615–630.
9. Murlin JR, Hoobler R. The energy metabolism of ten hospital children. *Am J Dis Child* 1915;9: 81–119.

10. Mönckeberg F, Beas F, Horwitz I, et al. Oxygen consumption in infant malnutrition. *Pediatrics* 1964; 33:554–561.
11. Parra A, Garza C, Garza Y, et al. Changes in growth hormone, insulin, and thyroxine values, in energy metabolism of marasmus infants. *J Pediatr* 1973;82:133–142.
12. Varga F. The respective effects of starvation and changed body composition on energy metabolism in malnourished infants. *Pediatrics* 1959;23:1085–1090.
13. Blunt K, Nelson A, Oleson HC. The basal metabolism of underweight children. *J Biol Chem* 1929; 49:247–262.
14. Soares MJ, Piers LS, Shetty PS, et al. Basal metabolic rate, body composition and whole-body protein turnover in Indian men with different nutritional status. *Clin Sci* 1991;81:419–425.
15. Soares MJ, Shetty PS. Basal metabolic rates and metabolic economy in chronic undernutrition. *Eur J Clin Nutr* 1991;45:363–373.
16. Kurpad AV, Kulkarni RN, Sheela ML, Shetty PS. Thermogenic responses to graded doses of noradrenaline in undernourished Indian male subjects. *Br J Nutr* 1989;61:201–208.
17. Srikantia SG. Nutritional adaptation in man. *Proc Nutr Soc Ind* 1985;31:1–16
18. Pichard C, Kyle UG, Slosman DO, Penalosa B. Energy expenditure in anorexia nervosa: can fat free mass as measured by bioelectrical impedance predict energy expenditure in hospitalized patients? *Clin Nutr* 1996;15:109–114.
19. McNeill G, Rivers JPW, Payne PR, et al. Basal metabolic rate of Indian men: noevidence of metabolic adaptation to a low plane of nutrition. *Hum Nutr Clin Nutr* 1987;41C:473–483.
20. Beattie J, Herbert PA. The estimation of the metabolic rate in the fasted state. *Br J Nutr* 1947;1: 185–191.
21. Beattie J, Herbert P. Basal metabolism from severe under nutrition. *Br J Nutr* 1947;1:192–202.
22. Elia M. Effect of starvation and very low calorie diets on protein energy interrelationships in lean and obese subjects. In: Scrimshaw NS, SchürchB, eds. *Protein:energy interactions.* Lausanne, Switzerland: IDECG Nestlé Foundation; 1992:249–284.
23. Morgulis S. *Fasting and undernutrition.* New York: Dutton; 1923.
24. Rutihauser IHE, McCance RA. Calorie requirements for growth after severe undernutrition. *Arch Dis Child* 1968;43:252–256.
25. Ashworth A. Metabolic rates during recovery from protein-calorie malnutrition: the need for a new concept of specific dynamic action. *Nature* 1969;223:407–409.
26. Brooke, OG, Harris M, Salrosa CB. The response of malnourished babies to cold. *J Physiol* 1973;233:75–95.
27. Melchior JC, Rigand D, Rozen R, et al. Energy expenditure economy induced by decrease in lean body mass in anorexia nervosa. *Eur J Clin Nutr* 1989;43:793–799.
28. Vaisman N, Rossi MF, Goldberg E, et al. Energy expenditure and body composition in patients with anorexia nervosa. *J Pediatr* 1988;113:919–924.
29. Stordy J, Marks MA, Kalucy RS, Crisp AH. Weight gain, thermic effect of glucose and resting metabolic rate during recovery from anorexia nervosa. *Am J Clin Nutr* 1977;30:138–146.
30. Forbes GB, Kreipe RE, Lipinski BA, Hodgman CH. Body composition changes during recovery from anorexia nervosa. *Am J Clin Nutr* 1984;40:1137–1145.
31. Garrow JS, Fletcher K, Halliday D. Body composition in severe infantile malnutrition. *J Clin Invest* 1965;44:417–425.
32. Halliday D. Chemical composition of the whole body and individual tissues of two Jamaican children whose death resulted primarily from malnutrition. *Clin Sci* 1967;33:365–370.
33. Reeds PJ, Jackson AA, Picon D, Poulter N. Muscle mass and composition in malnourished infants and children and changes seen after recovery. *Pediatr Res* 1978;12:613–618.
34. Kerpel-Fronius E, Frank K. Einige besonder-heilen der korperzusammensetzung und wasserverteilung bei der sanglingsatrophiei. *Ann Paediatr* 1949;173:321–330.
35. Piers LS, Soares MJ, Kulkarnia RN, Shetty PS. Thermic effect of a meal. Effect of dietary supplementation in chronically undernourished human subjects. *Br J Nutr* 1992;67:187–194.
36. Venkatachalam S, Srikantia SG, Copalan C. Basal metabolism in nutritional edema. *Metabolism* 1954;3:138–141.
37. Wang CC, Kern R, Frank M, Hays BB. Metabolism of undernourished children. II. Basal metabolism. *Am J Dis Child* 1926;32:350–359.
38. Ablett JG, McCance RA. Energy expenditure in children with kwashiorkor. *Lancet* 1971;2:517–519.
39. Jebb SA, Osborne RJ, Dixon AK, et al. Measurement of resting energy expenditure and body composition. before and after treatment of small cell lung cancer. *Ann Oncol* 1994;5:915–919.

40. Walker JM, Bond SA, Voss LD, et al. Treatment of short normal children with growth hormone—a cautionary tale. *Lancet* 1990;336:1331–1334.
41. Shetty PS. Adaptive changes in basal metabolic rate and lean body mass in chronic undernutrition. *Hum Nutr Clin Nutr* 1984;38C:443–451.
42. Topper A, Mulier H. Basal metabolism in children of abnormal body weight II underweight children. *Am J Dis Child* 1929;38:299–309.
43. Elia M. Energy expenditure in the whole body. In: *Energy metabolism tissue determinants and cellular corollaries.* Kinney JM, Tucker HN, eds. New York: Raven; 1992:19–59.
44. Kleiber M. Energy metabolism. *Ann Rev Physiol* 1956;18:35–52.
45. Kleiber M. *The fire of life.* New York: Wiley; 1961.
46. Benedict FG, Talbot FB. *Metabolism and growth from birth to puberty.* Washington, DC: Carnegie Institute of Washington; 1921.
47. Baer H. Zur technik der ruhe-nüchtern-umsatz-bestimmung beim säugling. J Beeinflusst Somnifen diesen Umsatz? *Kinderheilkd* 1929;47:226.
48. Janet Bochet HM. Sur le métabolisme basal du nourrisson. *Bull Soc Pediatr Paris* 1933;31:359–368.
49. Karlberg P. Determinations of standard energy metabolism (basal metabolism) in normal infants. *Acta Paediatr* 1952;41(suppl 49).
50. Benedict FG, Talbot FB. *The gaseous metabolism of infants.* Washington, DC: Carnegie Institute of Washington; 1914.
51. Alleyne GAO, Halliday D, Waterlow JC, Nichols BL. Chemical composition of children who die of malnutrition. *Br J Nutr* 1969;23:783–790.
52. Sinclair JC, Scopes JW, Silverman WA. Metabolic reference standards for the neonate. *Pediatrics* 1967;39:724–732.
53. Elia, M. Organ and tissue contribution to metabolic rate. In: Energy metabolism: tissue determinants and cellular ccorollaries. Kinney JM, Tucker HA, eds. New York: Raven; 1992:61–79.
54. Garot L. Contribution à l'étude des troubles du métabolism chimique dans la dénutrition grave du nourisson. Excrétion créatinique et métabolism basal. *Rev Fr Pediatr* 1933;9;273–312.
55. Korenchevsky V. *Physiological and pathological ageing.* New York: Karger; 1961:38–47.
56. Kenedy C, Sokoloff L. An adaptation of the nitrous oxide method to the study of the cerebral circulation of children: normal values for cerebral blood flow and cerebral metabolic rate in children. *J Clin Invest* 1957;36:1130–1137.
57. Garby L, Lammert O. An explanation for the nonlinearity of the relation between energy expenditure and fat free mass. *Eur J Clin Nutr* 1992;46:235–236.
58. von Kreiger M. Uber die atrophie der menschlichen organ bei inanition. *Leitschrift Angewandte-Anatomie Konstutional* 1921;7:78–131.
59. Jackson CM. *The effects of inanition upon growth and structure.* London: J&A Churchill; 1925.
60. Househam KC, De Villiers JFK. Computed tomography in severe protein energy malnutrition. *Arch Dis Child* 1987;62:589–590.
61. Handler LC, Stock MB, Smythe PM. CT brain scans: part of a body development study following gross undernutrition in infancy. *Br J Radiol* 1981;54:953–954.
62. Snyder WS, Cook MJ, Nassett ES, et al. *Report of the task group on reference man.* International commission on radiological protection. No. 23. Oxford, England: Pergan; 1975.
63. Widdowson EM, Dickerson JWT. Chemical composition of the body. In: Comar CL, Bronner F, eds. *Mineral metabolism.* Vol. II. New York: Academic; 1964:1–247.
64. Winick M, Rosso P, Waterlow JW. Cellular growth of cerebrum, cerebellum, and brain stem in normal and marasmic children. *Exp Neurol* 1970;26:393–400.
65. Redies C, Hoffer J, Beil C, et al. Generalized decrease in brain glucose metabolism during fasting in humans studied by PET. *Am J Physiol* 1989;256:E805–E810.
66. Owen OE, Morgan AP, Kemp HG, et al. Brain metabolism during fasting. *J Clin Invest* 1967;46:1589–1595.
67. Owen OE, Reichard A. Human forearm metabolism during progressive starvation. *J Clin invest* 1971;50:1536–1545.
68. Elia M, Kurpad A. What is the blood flow to resting human muscle? *Clin Sci* 1993;84:559–563.
69. Neilsen SL, Bitsch V, Larsen OA, et al. Blood flow through human adipose tissue during lipolysis. *Scand J Clin Lab Invest* 1968;22:124–130.
70. Waterlow JC. Energy sparing mechanisms: reductions in body mass, BMR and activities: their relative importance and priority in undernourished infants and children. In: Schurch B, Scrimshaw NS, eds. *Activity, energy expenditure, and energy requirements of infants and children.* Lausanne, Switzerland: IDECG Nestlé Foundation; 1990:239–252.

71. Barac-Nieto M, Spurr GB, Loreto H, Maksud MG. Body composition in undernutrition. *Am J Clin Nutr* 1978;31:23–40.
72. Jennings G, Elia M. Changes in protein distribution in normal and protein deficient rat during an acute phase "injury" response. *Br J Nutr* 1996;76:123–132.
73. Wusterman M, Elia M. Protein metabolism after injury with turpentine: a rat model clinical trauma. *Am J Physiol* 1990;259:E763–E769.
74. Wusterman M, Hayes A, Stirling D, Elia M. Changes in protein distribution in the rat during prolonged systemic injury. *J Surg Res* 1994;56:331–337.
75. Hoshino E, Pichard C, Greenwood CE, et al. Body composition and metabolic rate in rat during continuous infusion of cachectin. *Am J Physiol* 1991;23:E27–E36.
76. Lunn PG, Whitehead RG, Austin S. The effect of corticosterone acetate on the course of development of experimental protein-energy malnutrition in rats. *Br J Nutr* 1976;36:537–550.
77. Heymsfield SB, McManus CB. Tissue components of weight loss in cancer patient. *Cancer* 1985;55:238–249.
78. Wilmore DW, Aulick LH. Metabolic changes in burned patients. *Surg Clin North Am* 1978;58:1173–1178.
79. Weekes E, Elia M. Observations on the patterns of 24h energy expenditure changes in body composition and gastric emptying in head-injured patients receiving inasogastric tube feeding. *J Parenter Enter Nutr* 1996;20:31–32.
80. McCance RA, Mount LE. Severe undernutrition in growing adult animals. *Br J Nutr* 1960;14:509–518.
81. Barnes B. Basal temperature versus basal metabolism. *JAMA* 1942;119:1072–1074.
82. Rising R, Keys A, Ravussin E, Bogandus C. Concomitant interindividual variation in body temperature and metabolic rate. *Am J Physiol* 1992;263:E730–E734.
83. von Kerpel-Fronius E, Varga F, Kun K. Pathogenese der decomposition II. *An Pediatr* 1954;183:1–28.
84. McCance RA, Widdowson EM. The effect of lowering the ambient temperature on the metabolism of the new-born pig. *J Physiol* 1959;147:124–134.
85. Baric I. Contribution a la conaissance de l'intogenese du metabolism de base. *Bull Acad Sci Math Nat* 1953;12:77–83.
86. Brooke OG. Influence of malnutrition on the body temperature of children. *Br Med J* 1972;331–333.
87. Fellows IW, Macdonald IA, et al. The effect of undernutrition in thermoregulation in the elderly. *Clin Sci* 1985;69:525–532.
88. Brooke OG, Harris M, Salvosa CB. The response of malnourished babies to cold. *J Physiol* 1973;233 75–91.
89. Winick M, ed. Hunger diseases: studies by the Jewish physicians in the Warsaw Ghetto. New York: Wile; 1979.
90. Taylor HL, Keys A. Adaptation to caloric restriction. *Science* 1950;112:215–218.
91. Casper RC, Schoeller DA, Kushner R, et al. Total daily energy expenditure and activity level in anorexia nervosa. *Am J Clin Nutr* 1991;53:1143–1150.
92. Kraut AA, Muller EA. Caloric intake and industrial output. *Science* 1946;104:495–497.
93. Diaz E, Goldberg GR, Taylor M. Effect of dietary supplementation on work performance in Gambian Labourers. *Am J Clin Nutr* 1991;53:803–811.
94. Spurr GB, Reina JC. Influence of dietary intervention on artificially increased activity in marginally malnourished Colombian boys. *Eur J Clin Nutr* 1988;819–834.
95. Torun B. Short and long term effects of low or restricted energy intakes on the activity of infants and children. In: Schürch B, Scrimshaw NS, eds. *Activity, energy expenditure and energy requirements of infants and children.* Lausanne, Switzerland: IDECG Nestlé Foundation; 1990:335–360.
96. Viteri FE, Torun B. Nutrition, physical activity and growth. In: Ritzen M, Aperia A, Hall K, et al., eds. *The biology of normal growth.* New York: Raven; 1981:265–273.
97. Torun B, Viteri FE. Energy requirements of pre-school children and effects of varying energy intakes on protein metabolism. United Nations University. *Food Nutr Bull* 1981;5(suppl):229–241.
98. Leyton GB. The effects of slow starvation. *Lancet* 1946;2:73–79.

Physiology, Stress, and Malnutrition: Functional Correlates, Nutritional Intervention,
edited by J.M. Kinney and H.N. Tucker.
Lippincott–Raven Publishers © 1997.

Effects of Bed Rest with or without Stress

Arny A. Ferrando and *Robert R. Wolfe

*Department of Surgery/Metabolism, and *Departments of Surgery, Anesthesiology, and Biochemistry, University of Texas Medical Branch, Galveston, Texas 77550*

Bed rest is an integral aspect of illness and medical care. Indeed, certain metabolic alterations of critical illness can be attributed to bed rest alone. The inactivity associated with bed rest alters the body's physiology apart from the medical pathology. However, despite the hormonal alterations that distinguish critical illness or injury from inactivity, both paradigms result in the same deleterious loss of lean body mass (LBM). Because this loss of LBM due to bed rest alone potentially affects patient recovery and mobility, it is important to understand the underlying metabolic alterations.

The effects of bed rest and immobilization on metabolic functions have long been noted (1). Considerable research has been conducted on healthy volunteers to study the effects of inactivity on various physiologic parameters. Bed rest studies have taken different forms according to the desired physiologic disturbance. For example, studies designed to investigate the effects of inactivity on muscle function, strength, or metabolism have used a strict bed rest model. Most of the work in this area has focused on bed rest as a ground-based model for the perturbations of space flight. In this light, head-down bed rest, or the placing of subjects in a 6–10° head-down position, has been used to mimic the shift of body fluid to the head that accompanies space flight. However, the head-down tilt does not present a unique response of muscle or whole-body macronutrient metabolism. Therefore, for the purpose of this discussion on the effects of inactivity/bed rest on whole-body and muscle metabolism, the results of horizontal bed rest and head-down bed rest will be consolidated.

The loss of LBM has been consistently documented in bed rest (2–6). A loss of postural and locomotive muscle mass is evident within 7 days of bed rest and continues throughout 35 days (Table 1). It is important to note that this loss of LBM does not appear to plateau after 35 days. Indirect evidence suggests that the loss of LBM may continue with longer periods of bed rest. Zorbas et al. (7) noted a 30% increase in total and amino nitrogen excretion after 100 days of bed rest. Thus, it is likely that the body does not readily adapt to preserve LBM with longer periods of bed rest. This may become clinically relevant to the chronically bed-ridden patient. However, because long periods of bed rest are not associated with mortality from loss of LBM, adaptation must eventually occur.

TABLE 1. *Decreases in LBM with bed rest*

Study	Duration of Bed Rest (d)	Methodology	Site and LBM Decrease
Shangraw et al., 1988 {Shangraw1988}	7	MRI	Calf 1% Thigh 1.6%
Ferrando et al., 1995 {Ferrando1995}	7	MRI	Paraspinal 4.2% Thigh 3%
Suzuki et al., 1994 {Suzuki1994}	20	DEXA	Leg 4.3%
Convertino et al., 1989 {Convertino1989}	30	CT	Calf 4.8% Thigh 8.1%
LaBlanc et al., 1988	35	MRI	Calf 12%

MRI, magnetic resonance imaging; DEXA, dual-energy x-ray absorptiometry; CT, computed tomography.

Even though studies on long-term adaptation have not been conducted, the reason for short-term loss of LBM has been determined. A primary determinant for the loss of LBM with bed rest is an alteration in protein metabolism. Although the nature and cause of this alteration vary with inactivity and stress, the clinical result remains the same.

PROTEIN METABOLISM

Net protein breakdown, and the subsequent losses of LBM, is characteristic of both inactivity and stress. Loss of nitrogen has been documented in bed rest through increased urea excretion (3,7) and negative nitrogen balance (3,5). Major trauma, burns, and sepsis also result in an increased urea production (8,9). Although the loss of nitrogen can be ameliorated in bed rest by increased dietary protein (3,10), this intervention is less effective in the stressed patient (11). In healthy subjects in bed for 7 days, a protein intake of 1.0 g/kg body weight/day was shown to alleviate the negative nitrogen balance associated with a lower protein intake (10). However, when a similar diet (1.1 g/kg body weight/day) was given to subjects bed-rested for 2 weeks, it was again found that nitrogen balance was not significantly lower during the first week. Negative nitrogen balance was evident during the second week (3). Thus, increasing protein intake appears to provide only a short-term solution to the negative nitrogen balance of bed rest. Likewise, protein intakes as high as 3.7 g/kg body weight/day may still result in a net protein catabolism in the burned patient (9).

Whole-body protein turnover (WBPT) measures represent an amalgamation of various tissue measures. The body's metabolic state determines the extent to which these measures reflect specific tissue metabolism. During periods of stress, hepatic synthesis of acute-phase proteins and proteins involved in wound repair may account for a larger proportion of the whole-body measure (12). However, during inactivity without stress, changes in WBPT largely reflect muscle protein turnover (3). WBPT decreases with inactivity in as little as 9 hours of bed rest (13). After 7 and 14 days of bed rest, WBPT decreases primarily as a result of decreased muscle protein synthesis (3). Figure 1 depicts 24-hour WBPT in the fed state. WBPT decreases by ~15% during bed rest as a result of decreased protein synthesis, whereas whole-body protein breakdown does not change (3). The result is a net catabolism of body protein and prior loss of LBM. For comparison, WBPT in the burned and septic patients are included in Fig. 1. These data indicate that WBPT in the stressed patient can be two- to fourfold higher than that of ambulation or inactivity. In the burned patient, WBPT may indicate a net balance between synthesis and breakdown in the fed state (14); however, the synthesis of acute-phase proteins and proteins involved in the immune response and wound repair may be largely responsible (15). There is a net catabolism of skeletal muscle in the burned patient, even in the fed state (16). Similarly, sepsis causes a net catabolism of body protein that cannot be ameliorated with feeding (17) (Fig. 1). Thus, whereas bed rest alone causes an apparent depletion of body nitrogen, the mechanisms involved are different from injury or sepsis.

The relationship of activity and stress to WBPT remains intact when skeletal muscle protein turnover is investigated. Bed rest has been shown to decrease muscle protein turnover (3), whereas the opposite holds true for serious illness or injury (11). This relationship is demonstrated in Fig. 2, which depicts skeletal muscle protein turnover by arteriovenous balance of labeled phenylalanine (15). Muscle protein synthesis decreases from ambulation to bed rest in fasted patients, without a change in protein breakdown (3). The lack of change in protein break-

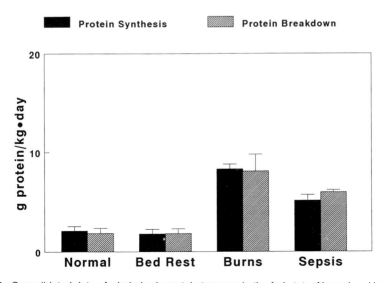

FIG. 1. Consolidated data of whole-body protein turnover in the fed state. Normal and bed rest data are derived from Ferrrando et al. (3); burn data from Wolfe et al. (14); and septic data from Shaw et al. (17).

down with bed rest also has been reported by Stuart et al. (17). The chronic result of this decrease in skeletal muscle protein synthesis is the loss of LBM in an otherwise healthy subject (3,5).

In contrast to the situation of bed rest alone, activity causes an increase in muscle protein turnover (18). Furthermore, there is a net muscle protein balance after exercise in the absence of food intake (18), whereas muscle net balance in the postabsorptive state is negative with inactivity alone (3). The absence of muscular activity more prominently contributes to the demonstrated effects of bed rest alone, whereas the stress response predominates the effects of inactivity. The magnitude of response of protein metabolism in critically ill patients is far greater than that of exercise, and negative muscle balance is pronounced (19).

Comparative evaluation of skeletal muscle protein turnover in the postabsorptive burned patient (20) (Fig. 2) shows that the synthetic rate is over twofold higher than that of inactivity alone, whereas the breakdown rate is almost threefold higher. The increased turnover of muscle protein is reflected in a net outward transport of amino acids. Transmembrane amino acid transport rates are depicted in Fig. 3 for each paradigm. It can be seen that inactivity produces minor alterations in transmembrane transport rates. However, in the burned patient there is a dramatic imbalance of amino acid transport that results in a net loss of amino acids from the muscle. The same pattern as shown in Fig. 3 applies for other amino acids, especially alanine. Alanine is a precursor of importance for gluconeogenesis, which is stimulated in stress (19), and the enhanced release of alanine makes it more readily available for gluconeogenesis. The modest alterations

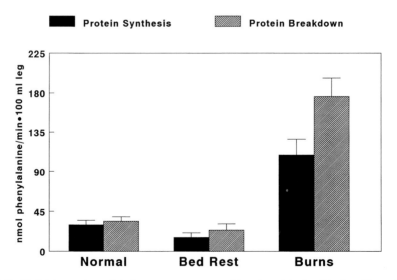

FIG. 2. Skeletal muscle protein turnover as measured by phenylalanine kinetics. Normal and bed rest data from Ferrando et al. (3); burn data from Biolo et al. (20).

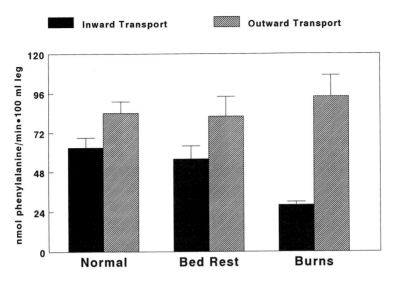

FIG. 3. Skeletal muscle transport of phenylalanine based on the model of Biolo et al. (65). Normal and bed rest data from Ferrando et al. (3); burn data from Biolo et al. (20).

in amino acid transport after bed rest alone correspond to both the less pronounced catabolic response of muscle, and the absence of a gluconeogenic response (3). The impaired inward transport in burn injury may be the mechanism responsible for the decreased efficiency of nutritional support in maintaining muscle mass in critical illness (16). In contrast, the lack of an impairment in transmembrane transport with bed rest is consistent with the responsiveness, at least in the short term, of muscle to an increased protein intake (10).

Clearly, from this discussion the bed rest component is partly responsible for the loss of body nitrogen and LBM in stressed patients. Skeletal muscle protein metabolism is altered with inactivity such that protein synthesis is insufficient to counter protein breakdown. The decrease in protein synthesis is accompanied by a concomitant outward transport of amino acids from the muscle. On the other hand, the magnitude of the response to bed rest is modest compared with the catabolic response to burn injury or sepsis. It is unclear the extent to which the bed rest component contributes to the response in burned or septic patients because the effect of inactivity in stressed patients has never been evaluated.

CARBOHYDRATE METABOLISM

Carbohydrate metabolism is also altered by both stress and inactivity. Hyperinsulinemia and insulin insensitivity are present in both bed rest and critical illness. Furthermore, the nature of the change in the hypoglycemic action of insulin in bed rest and stress (e.g., burn injury) is comparable. The most

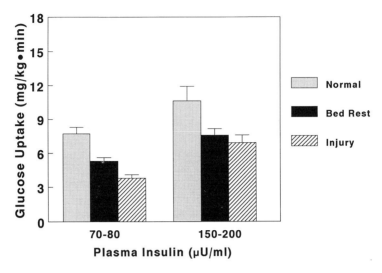

FIG. 4. Whole-body glucose uptake at physiologic plasma insulin concentrations with euglycemic clamp. Normal and injury data from Black et al. (21); bed rest data from Stuart et al. (24).

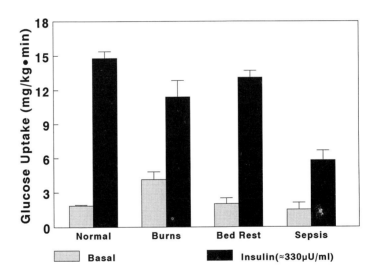

FIG. 5. Whole-body glucose uptake with hyperinsulinemic euglycemic clamp. Normal and bed rest data derived from Stuart et al. (24); burns and sepsis data from Shangraw et al. (22).

prominent derangement in each case is a shift to the right of the insulin dose-response curve for whole-body glucose utilization, with a less prominent effect on the maximal glucose utilization rate. Thus, physiologic concentrations of insulin are much less effective than normal in stimulating glucose uptake, whereas the maximal effectiveness of a pharmacologic amount of insulin is not as markedly affected in either burn injury or bed rest (Figs. 4 and 5). This is reflected by the half-maximally effective insulin concentration, which was increased from the normal value of 45 ± 3 to 78 ± 8 µU/ml after 7 days of bed rest. Burn injury results in similar but somewhat higher values (21). In addition to an altered insulin effectiveness after burn injury, the clearance of infused insulin is also affected. Insulin must be infused at approximately twice the rate in a burn patient as in a normal volunteer in order to increase the plasma insulin concentration an equivalent amount (22,23). The clearance of infused insulin is not significantly affected by bed rest (24).

INSULIN AND PROTEIN METABOLISM

Whereas alterations in the hypoglycemic action of insulin have been widely studied, the effect of insulin on protein metabolism is potentially more important in determining the changes in LBM that occur with bed rest. Insulin is an important anabolic hormone. Under normal conditions it directly stimulates muscle protein synthesis and inhibits protein breakdown in splanchnic tissues (25). The modest increase in insulin concentration after a meal is sufficient to have a significant anabolic effect, particularly in muscle (25). At the whole body level, the predominant effect of insulin infusion is a suppression of protein breakdown, which causes a decrease in blood amino acid concentration (26). When the effect of infusing insulin at various rates was assessed in normal volunteers before and after 7 days of bed rest, no deficiency in the action of insulin was seen at any insulin infusion rate (5). Concentrations of insulin ranging from 10 to almost 1,000 µU/ml were produced by the various insulin infusions. At all concentrations tested, the suppressive effect of insulin on whole-body protein breakdown, as reflected by the rate of appearance of leucine, was suppressed to the same extent before and after bed rest. Similarly, the response of protein breakdown to insulin infusion in the fasted state appears to remain intact in burn injury and in sepsis. In each clinical situation, the rate of protein breakdown (R_a leucine) was markedly elevated in the basal state, but maximal hyperinsulinemia (>750 µU/ml) suppressed R_a leucine in both sepsis and burn injury at least as much as in normal subjects. On the other hand, R_a leucine was still approximately double the normal value during maximal hyperinsulinemia in burns and sepsis (Fig. 6).

The responsiveness to insulin has classically been investigated in the fasting state. The primary reason for this is that the rate of glucose uptake can only be quantified precisely in the absence of glucose absorption. However, the fasting state is not a physiologically relevant circumstance with regard to the effect of

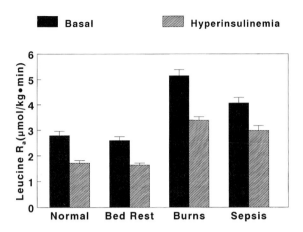

FIG. 6. Leucine R_a, a measure of whole-body proteolysis, during hyperinsulinemic euglycemic clamp. Normal and bed rest data taken from Shangraw et al. (5); burn and sepsis data from Jahoor et al. (8).

insulin on protein metabolism. Insulin is normally only elevated after a meal, at which time amino acid availability is also increased. In contrast, the availability of both blood and intracellular amino acids decreases markedly during a hyperinsulinemic clamp procedure conducted during the fasting state (27). If intravenous amino acids are provided concurrently with glucose infusion during the hyperinsulinemic clamp, the decrease in whole-body protein synthesis that occurs in the absence of the amino acid infusion is prevented (26). The difference in the response to insulin in the fasting and fed states in patients with burn injury is dramatic. In contrast to the insulin-induced suppression of both whole-body protein synthesis and breakdown seen in the fasted state, in the fed state a pharmacologic amount of insulin (>500 µU/ml) actually increases protein turnover. In muscle, both synthesis and breakdown are significantly increased by high-dose insulin in the fed state in burn patients (16). The response of muscle protein metabolism to insulin has not been assessed in normal subjects during bed rest in either the fasted or fed state. However, WBPT studies suggest that the derangement in protein metabolism is more prominent in the fed versus postabsorptive state (3,5).

RELATIONSHIP BETWEEN ALTERED GLUCOSE AND PROTEIN KINETICS

The extent to which the hypoglycemic action of insulin is diminished in either bed rest or critical illness is not likely to directly affect the rate of muscle loss. A direct effect of altered glucose kinetics on protein metabolism could potentially occur only if there is a relationship between the intracellular oxidation of glucose and the rate of protein synthesis or breakdown. However, this does not appear to be the case. This was assessed in patients by increasing glucose oxidation with the administration of dichloroacetate (DCA), which stimulates the activity of pyruvate dehydrogenase. Pyruvate dehydrogenase is the enzyme necessary for pyruvate, the end-product of glycolysis, to enter the tricarboxylic acid (TCA) cycle. DCA was administered to patients in whom the concentrations of both glucose and insulin were held constant by means of the euglycemic–hyperinsulinemic clamp technique. In this setting, DCA caused a significant increase in glucose oxidation, yet this resulted in no change in the rate of either protein breakdown or leucine oxidation (8). Thus, it appears that the rate of glucose oxidation does not directly influence the rate of protein breakdown or amino acid oxidation. Furthermore, in both the insulin-resistant states after bed rest and after burn injury, there is no evidence that the actual rate of glucose uptake is altered, only that higher concentrations of glucose and insulin are required to clear a given amount of ingested glucose. Therefore, the alterations in protein metabolism with inactivity and stress cannot be attributed to insulin insensitivity.

ENERGY METABOLISM

A link between energy metabolism and protein kinetics has long been recognized. For any given protein intake, nitrogen balance is improved by increased energy intake (28). Consequently, alterations in energy metabolism are potentially important in all catabolic states. Energy metabolism is affected by many factors during bed rest and stress. Resting energy expenditure (REE) normally accounts for approximately 65% of the total energy expenditure (TEE), so a change in basal metabolic rate (BMR) has a profound effect on TEE. In turn, BMR is determined by hormonal status, the quantity of active metabolic tissue, muscular activity, and dietary intake (29). Several older studies and those of the former Soviet Bloc have reported that BMR decreases during inactivity. These studies have been thoroughly reviewed by Greenleaf and indicate that BMR has been found to remain unchanged or to decrease by as much as 2–22% over 7–70 days of bed rest (29). Greenleaf appropriately points out that the variability in findings may be due to the lack of standardization of basal measurement conditions. Two recent studies are particularly noteworthy. Basal energy expenditure (BEE) measures were conducted on resting subjects upon awakening, 12 hours postabsorptive, and within a thermoneutral environment. Gretebeck et al. (30) noted that BEE did not change throughout a 10-day bed rest period. In addition, it was reported that resting energy expenditure was also unchanged. As expected, TEE (determined by dilution of doubly labeled water) decreased during bed rest (30). The results suggest that the reduction in TEE is not due to a decrease in BMR or resting energy, but instead the result of decreased physical activity.

In contrast to these findings, Harauna et al. (31) also used indirect calorimetry to determine REE over 20 days of bed rest. Decreases of 13% and 21% were noted in males (n = 9) and females (n = 5), respectively. Although the quantitative effect of inactivity on BMR remains equivocal, it is important to note that qualitatively, BMR either decreases or remains unchanged with inactivity in healthy subjects.

The decreased contribution of activity to TEE during bed rest is to be expected. The extent to which this decrease reduces caloric requirements (below normal) depends on the activity of the individual before bed rest. Representative results shown in Fig. 7 illustrate the wide range of TEE in relation to REE possible in normal subjects (30,32,33). Normal activity for an individual that does not include any specific exercise routine may elevate TEE only modestly above that during bed rest. On the other hand, training for competition in endurance sports, such as swimming, requires almost a doubling of caloric intake to maintain energy balance. In any case, loss of muscle mass with bed rest is clearly not related to altered energy expenditure. Only a negative energy balance would be expected to contribute to loss of muscle mass, and matching the caloric requirements during bed rest should not be a problem. To the contrary, the reduction in TEE with bed rest leads to accumulation of fat if normal food intake is not reduced.

In contrast to the inactivity of bed rest, hypermetabolism, or an increase in REE, has long been considered to be the quintessential metabolic response to stress. Catecholamines have been considered to be involved in mediating this response (34), although this classical observation has not been supported by more recent findings (35). Despite the increase in REE above that predicted for a normal person of comparable age and weight, however, caloric requirements

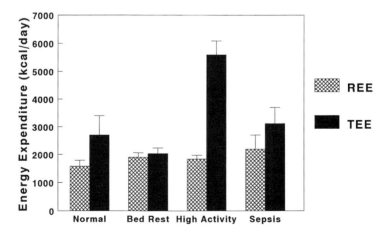

FIG. 7. Measured total and resting energy expenditure. Normal data from the research of Carpenter et al. (32); bed rest data from Gretebeck et al. (30). High activity represents elite swimmers of Trappe et al. (33); sepsis data from Koea et al. (66).

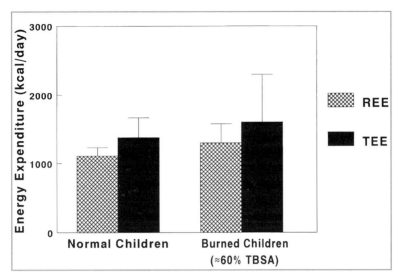

FIG. 8. Comparative ratio of resting energy expenditure to total energy expenditure in normal and burned children. Data from Goran et al. (36,37).

are not markedly different for patients and for normal volunteers. This is because the reduction in activity in patients decreases the ratio of TEE/REE below normal (36,37) (Fig. 8). Consequently, with modern alimentation techniques, it is not difficult to supply adequate calories to meet the requirements of TEE in patients. Therefore, as in bed rest, changes in REE and TEE cannot explain the catabolism of the LBM in stressed patients. Rather, the primary nutritional concern in each circumstance involves the potentially detrimental effects of excess calories.

LIPID METABOLISM

Investigations concerning the relationship between inactivity and lipid metabolism are limited. Alterations in fatty acid concentrations are not evident with bed rest (38); however, fatty acid metabolism has not been investigated. The alterations in lipoprotein metabolism with inactivity may provide indirect evidence of possible changes in fat metabolism. In healthy subjects, Yanagibori et al. (38) reported that 20 days of bed rest resulted in a decrease of apolipoprotein AI (Apo-AI) and high density lipoprotein-2 (HDL_2) cholesterol fractions, although total cholesterol and triglyceride (TG) concentrations were unchanged. The most widespread effect of inactivity on lipid metabolism appears to be the decrease in high-density lipoprotein (HDL) cholesterol. This finding is present in surgical (39), critically ill (39), trauma (40), and quadriplegic (41) patients.

Thus, it is thought that long-term inactivity presents an increased risk for coronary heart disease (CHD) (42).

Most notably, the HDL_2 fraction has been shown to decrease with inactivity (38,41). HDL_2 is responsible for the transport of cholesterol from body tissues to the liver (42). HDL_2 concentrations are also directly related to lipoprotein lipase activity and inversely related to the incidence of CHD (42). Other aspects of the lipoprotein profile that accompany inactivity suggest a higher risk for CHD. LDL-TG (triglyceride) levels increase with trauma (40) and critical illness (39). Furthermore, although LDL concentrations may increase (39) or remain unchanged (40), the ratio of total cholesterol/HDL or LDL/HDL is increased. Thus, inactivity results in a lipoprotein profile known to increase the risk of CHD.

Taken together, the inverse changes in LDL-TG and HDL_2 suggest an alteration in lipoprotein metabolism that may indicate an altered fatty acid metabolism. These changes oppose those induced by exercise. HDL_2 has been shown to increase within 2 weeks of starting exercise (43). In fact, higher HDL_2 concentrations have been consistently demonstrated in exercising subjects (44,45). Fatty acid utilization also has been repeatedly shown to increase with training (46). Therefore, as with HDL_2, it is likely that a converse alteration in fatty acid metabolism is induced by prolonged inactivity. This analogy also may provide evidence that changes in lipid metabolism with bed rest are related to reduced muscular activity and not a function of the inherent stress of illness.

Increased lipolysis is characteristic of the stressed patient (47). This would appear to be unrelated to bed rest because β-adrenergic blockade suppresses the lipolytic response to a normal basal rate (47), and increased sympathetic activity does not accompany bed rest. Increased availability of free fatty acids provides ample substrate for oxidative metabolism (47). The high rate of lipolysis in stress is not readily suppressed because even during high-dose glucose feedings it has been found that plasma free fatty acids (rather than de novo synthesized fatty acids) are the primary precursor for hepatic triglyceride synthesis (48). This would suggest that the body's fat stores are more than capable of meeting its energy requirements. Thus, it is unlikely that alterations in lipid metabolism are related to the catabolism of body protein in either the stressed or inactive patient. Furthermore, the alteration of the lipoprotein profile may only be clinically relevant to the chronically immobile patient.

HORMONAL RESPONSES

The hormonal environment often dictates the metabolic response, and differences in the hormonal response to bed rest and to critical illness are the most likely explanation for the often divergent metabolic responses. Hormones such as insulin (25), growth hormone (49), testosterone (50), and insulinlike growth factor (IGF) (51) have been shown to provide an anabolic affect on macronutrient metabolism. In contrast, cortisol (51) and glucagon (52) can cause catabolic actions on these macronutrients. Thus, the responses of cortisol, insulin, and glucagon to bed rest and critical illness have been widely studied for their established effects on energy and macronutrient metabolism. In general, trauma and critical illness induce a profound alteration in many hormones. By contrast, bed rest and inactivity in an otherwise healthy individual result in minimal disturbances of hormonal regulation. The primary exception is that insulin sensitivity is altered comparably with both inactivity and critical illness.

The hypothalamopituitary axis responds to trauma with pronounced increases in adrenocorticotropic hormone (ACTH) (53) and cortisol (54,55). Thermal injury results in a rapid and sustained increase in blood cortisol concentrations that may be elevated for weeks after injury (54). Furthermore, cortisol concentrations are related to the severity of the injury (53,54). Blood cortisol concentrations can increase two- to fourfold during injury or critical illness (9,56).

Bed rest, however, induces little or no alteration in cortisol concentrations. Seven (5,24) or 14 days (3,57) of strict bed rest did not change fasting cortisol levels. Considerable evidence confirms this absence of a stress response during bed rest. Growth hormone, which is known to increase after trauma (3,58,59), remains at normal levels throughout bed rest (24). The sympathoadrenal response is one of normal or decreased production of catecholamines (60) with clearance unchanged (24). Cytokines, such as tumor necrosis factor-α or interleukin-1, are known to change acutely with the stress of critical illness (61), but 20 days of bed rest did not change these serum concentrations (62). Further evidence of the stable hormonal environment of bed rest is provided by the lack of change in steroidal and growth factor hormones. Typically, the gonadal hormones decrease after injury in both men and women (55). On the other hand, neither 7 nor 14 days of bed rest changed total or free testosterone concentrations in men (3). Another related measure, IGF-1, is known to increase in the blood (49) and intracellular (50) constituents with elevated blood concentrations of growth hormone and testosterone. However, 7 and 14 days of bed rest did not cause a change in circulating IGF-1 concentrations (3), providing additional evidence of bed rest's inability to alter the hormonal environment.

Thus, except for an insulin resistance that is common to critical illness or injury and inactivity, the hormonal responses are disparate. It is tempting to speculate that high levels of the classic "catabolic" hormones in the stressed patient are related to the catabolism of body protein. The concomitant decreases in testosterone also may serve to alter the anabolic/catabolic hormone ratio and further impede muscle anabolism. The infusion of stress hormones in healthy subjects has resulted in increased proteolysis (52,63,64). Testosterone normalization in hypogonadal men has been shown to increase skeletal muscle protein synthesis and strength (50). However, the effects of blocking cortisol production or its action have not been investigated in the patient population. Neither has the restoration of testosterone levels in critically ill patients been investigated. The only available information is the relationship of various stressors to blood hormone concentrations. Given the actions of each hormone, the resultant change in blood values is often extrapolated to physiologic endpoints. Therefore, it is important to understand that these proposed mechanisms are purely speculative.

CLINICAL IMPLICATIONS

The loss of muscle mass is common to both bed rest and critical illness. Thus, a component of the muscle loss of critical illness or injury is related to the effects of bed rest. However, the loss of muscle in the two circumstances occurs by different mechanisms. Bed rest results in a decrease in muscle protein synthesis, whereas protein breakdown is unaltered. In contrast, critical illness and injury increase both the rate of muscle protein breakdown and the rate of synthesis; however, the rate of synthesis is not increased sufficiently to match the accelerated rate of breakdown. Elevations in the classical "stress" hormones in the catabolic patients, but not during bed rest in normal subjects, may be an explanation for the disparate metabolic responses. Importantly, the magnitude of the catabolic response in bed rest is minimal as compared with the response in critical illness, and thus we might conclude that the inactivity component of critical illness or injury is not of major concern. However, this conclusion would be overstepping the limits of available data because the effects of activity on protein metabolism have not been assessed in critically ill patients. It may be possible, for example, that the stress hormones would exert a more potent effect on muscle during bed rest than under normal circumstances. In any case, the mediator(s) of the catabolic response in stress is the primary factor responsible for the loss of LBM rather than the bed rest per se. Consequently, treatment in these patients is focused appropriately on blocking the mediators of the catabolic response, rather than on the lack of exercise.

The losses in muscle with short-term (7–14 days) bed rest, although statistically significant, are not physiologically important. It is likely that much longer periods of bed rest are necessary to cause a clinically consequential deterioration in muscle mass and strength. Also, physiologic effects of changes in energy metabolism, insulin responsiveness, and lipid metabolism would presumably require months or even years to become fully manifested. However, no data are available to clarify the long- term response to bed rest. It is likely that the abnormalities documented to occur in the first few weeks of bed rest are ameliorated as adaptation to inactivity occurs. Otherwise, total depletion of LBM would occur in a matter of months. However, individuals remain in bed for years without losing all of their LBM. The time period over which adaptation to bed rest occurs is unclear, as is the mechanism(s) of adaptation. Adaptive responses not withstanding, however, it is likely that the physiologic importance of bed rest in individuals who cannot physically get out of bed, particularly in the elderly, is greater than indicated by short-term studies of bed rest in healthy volunteers.

ACKNOWLEDGMENT

The authors wish to acknowledge the support of Shriners Hospital Grant 15849 and National Institute of Health Grant DK33952 in the preparation of this manuscript.

REFERENCES

1. Deitrick JE, Whendon GD, Shorr E. Effects of immobilization upon various metabolic and physiologic functions of normal men. *Am J Med* 1948;4:3–36.
2. Convertino VA, Doerr DF, Mathes KL, Stein SL, Buchanan P. Changes in volume, muscle compartment and compliance of the lower extremeties in man following 30 days of exposure to simulated microgravity. *Aviat Space Environ Med* 1989;60:653–658.
3. Ferrando AA, Lane HW, Stuart CA, Wolfe RR. Prolonged bed rest decreases skeletal muscle and whole-body protein synthesis. *Am J Physiol* 1995;270.
4. LeBlanc A, Gogia P, Schneider V, Krebs J, Schonfeld E, Evans H. Calf Muscle area and strength changes after five weeks of horizontal bed rest. *Am J Sports Med* 1988;16:624–629.
5. Shangraw RE, Stuart CA, Prince MJ, et al. Insulin responsiveness of protein metabolism in vivo following bedrest in humans. *Am J Physiol* 1988;255:E548–E558.
6. Suzuki Y, Murakami T, Haruna Y, et al. Effects of 10 and 20 days bed rest on leg muscle mass and strength in young subjects. *Acta Physiol Scand* 1994;616:5–18.
7. Zorbas YG, Merkov AB, Nobahar AN. Metabolic changes in man under hypokinesia and physical exercise. *J Environ Pathol Toxicol Oncol* 1989;9:361–370.
8. Jahoor F, Shangraw RE, Miyoshi H, et al. Role of insulin and glucose oxidation in mediating the protein catabolism of burns and sepsis. *Am J Physiol* 1989;20:323–331.
9. Jahoor F, Desai M, Herndon DN, Wolfe RR. Dymanics of the protein metabolic resonse to burn injury. *Metabolism* 1988;37:330–337.
10. Stuart CA, Shangraw RE, Peters EJ, Wolfe RR. Effect of dietary protein on bed-rest-related changes in whole-body-protein synthesis. *Am J Clin Nutr* 1990;52:509–514.
11. Wolfe RR. Metabolic response to burn injury: nutritional implications. *Keio J Med* 1993;42:1–8.
12. Carraro F, Hartl WH, Stuart CA, et al. Whole body and plasma protein synthesis in exercise and recovery in human subjects. *Am J Physiol* 1990;258:E821–E831.
13. Bettany GE, Ang BC, Georgiannos SN, et al. Bed rest decreases whole-body protein turnover in post-absorptive man. *Clin Sci* 1996;90:73–75.
14. Wolfe RR, Goodenough RD, Burke JF, Wolfe MH. Responses of protein and urea kinetics in burn patients to different levels of protein intake. *Ann Surg* 1983;197:163–171.
15. Harries RH, Phillips LG. Hematologic and acute phase response. In: Herndon DN ed. *Total burn care.* Philadelphia, PA: WB Saunders; 1996:293–301.
16. Sakurai Y, Aarsland A, Herndon DN, et al. Stimulation of muscle protein synthesis by long-term insulin infusion in severely burned patients. *Ann Surg* 1995;222:283–297.
17. Shaw JH, Wildbore M, Wolfe RR. Whole body protein kinetics in severely septic patients. *Ann Surg* 1987;205:288–294.
18. Biolo G, Maggi SP, Williams BD, et al. Increased rates of muscle protein turnover and amino acid transport following resistance exercise in humans. *Am J Physiol* 1995;268:E514–E520.
19. Gore DC, Jahoor F, Hibbert J, DeMaria EJ. Except for alanine, muscle protein catabolism is not influenced by alterations in glucose metabolism during sepsis. *Arch Surg* 1995;130:1171–1177.
20. Biolo G, Maggi SP, Fleming RYD, Herndon DN, Wolfe RR. Relationship between tansmembrane amino acid transport and protein kinetics in muscle tissue of severely burned patients [Abstract]. *Am J Clin Nutr* 12(suppl 2):1993.
21. Black PR, Brooks DC, Bessey PQ, et al. Mechanisms of insulin resistance following injury. *Ann Surg* 1982;196:420–433.
22. Shangraw RE, Jahoor F, Miyoshi H, et al. Differentiation between septic and postburn insulin resistance. *Metabolism* 1989;38:983–989.
23. Wolfe RR, O'Donnell TF, Stone MD, et al. Investigation of factors determining the optimal glucose infusion rate in total partenteral nutrition. *Metabolism* 1980;29:892–900.

24. Stuart CA, Shangraw RE, Prince MJ, et al. Bed-rest-induced insulin resistance occurs primarily in the muscle. *Metabolism* 1988;37:802–806.
25. Biolo G, Fleming RYD, Wolfe RR. Physiologic hyperinsulinemia stimulates protein synthesis and enhances transport of selected amino acids in human skeletal muscle. *J Clin Invest* 1987;79: 1062–1069.
26. Tessari P, Inchiostro S, Biolo G, et al. Differential effects of hyperinsulinemia and hyper-aminoacidemia on leucine-carbon metabolism in vivo. *J Clin Invest* 1987;80:1784–1793.
27. Castellino P, Luzi L, Simonson DC, et al. Effect of insulin and plasma amino acid concentrations on leucine metabolism in man. *J Clin Invest* 1987;80:1784–1793.
28. Butterfield GE. Whole-body protein utilization in humans. *Med Sci Sports Exerc* 1987;19: S157–S165.
29. Greenleaf JE, Bernauer EM, Ertl AC, et al. Work capacity during 30 days of bed rest with isotonic and isokinetic exercise training. *J Appl Physiol* 1989;67:1820–1826.
30. Gretebeck RJ, Schoeller DA, Gibson EK, Lane HW. Energy expenditure during antiorthostatic bed rest (simulated microgravity). *J Appl Physiol* 1995;78:2207–2211.
31. Haruna Y, Suzuki Y, Kawakubo K, et al. Decremental reset in basal metabolism during 20-days bed rest. *Acta Physiol Scand* 1994;(suppl 43–49).
32. Carpenter WH, Poehlman ET, O'Connell M, Goran MI. Influence of body composition and resting metabolic rate on variation in total enegy expenditure: a meta-analysis. *Amer J Clin Nutr* 1995;61: 4–10.
33. Trappe TA, Gastaldelli A, Jozsi AC, Troup JP, Wolfe RR. Energy expenditure of elite female swimmers during high volume training by the doubly labeled water method. *Med Sci Sports Exerc* 1997 (in press).
34. Wilmore DW, Long JM, Mason AD. Catecholamines: mediator of hypermetabolic response to thermal injury. *Ann Surg* 1974;180:653–668.
35. Caldwell FT, Bowser BH, Crabtree JH. The effect of occlusion dressing on the energy metabolism of severely burned children. *Ann Surg* 1981;193:579–591.
36. Goran MI, Carpenter WH, McGloin A, Johnson R, Hardin JM, Weinsier RL. Energy expenditure in children of lean and obese parents. *Amer J Phys* 1995;268:E917–E924.
37. Goran MI, Peters EJ, Herndon DN, Wolfe RR. Total energy expenditure in burned children using the doubly labeled water technique. *Am J Physiol* 1990;259:E576–E585.
38. Yanagibori R, Suzuki Y, Kawakubo K, et al. Carbohydrate and lipid metabolism after 20 days of bed rest. *Acta Physiol Scand* 1994;(suppl 51–57).
39. Lindholm M, Eklund J, Rossner S. Pronounced dislipoproteinemia in intensive care patients. *J Parenter Enter Nutr* 1982;6:432–438.
40. Nikkila EA, Kuusi T, Myllynen P. High density lipoprotein and apolipoprotein A-I during physical inactivity. *Atherosclerosis* 1980;37:457–462.
41. Shetty KR, Sutton CH, Rudman IW, Rudman D. Lipid and liproprotein abnormalities in young quadraplegic men. *Am J Med Sci* 1992;303:457–462.
42. Mayes PA. Cholesterol systhesis, transport, and excretion. In: Anonymous, ed. *Harper's biochemistry.* Norwalk, CT: Appleton & Lange; 1988:241–252.
43. Nye E, Carlson K, Kirsten P, Rossner S. Changes in HDL subfractions and other lipoproteins induced by exercise. *Clin Chem Acta* 1981;113:51–57.
44. Williams PT, Krauss RM, Wood PD, et al. Lipoprotein subfractions of runners and sedentary men. *Metabolism* 1986;35:45–52.
45. Wood PD, Haskel WL. The effect of exercise on plasma high density liproproteins. *Lipids* 1979;14: 417–427.
46. Coggan AR, Williams BD. Metabolic adaptations to endurance training: substrate metabolism during exercise. In: Hargraves M, ed. Champaign, IL: Human Dinetics; 1995:177–210.
47. Wolfe RR, Herndon DN, Jahoor F, et al. Effect of severe burn injury on substrate cycling by glucose and fatty acids. *N Engl J Med* 1987;317:403–408.
48. Aarsland A, Chinkes D, Wolfe RR, et al. Beta-blockade lowers peripheral lipolysis in burned patients receiving growth hormone: rate of hepatic VLDL triglyceride secretion remains unchanged. *Ann Surg* 1996;223(6):777–789.
49. Fleming RD, Rutan RL, Jahoor F. Effect of recombinant growth hormone on catabolic hormones and free fatty acids following thermal injusy. *J Trauma* 1992;32:698–703.
50. Urban RJ, Bodenburg YH, Gilkison C, et al. Testosterone administration to elderly men increases skeletal muscle strength and protein synthesis. *Am J Physiol* 1995;269:E820–E826.

51. Fryburg DA, Jahn LA, Hill SA, et al. Insulin and insulin-like growth factor-I enhance human skeletal muscle protein anabolism during hyperaminoacidemia by different mechanisms. *J Clin Invest* 1995;96:1722–1729.
52. Gelfand RA, Matthews DE, Bier DM, Sherwin RE. Role of counterregulatory hormones in the catabolic response. *J Clin Invest* 1984;74:2238–2248.
53. Barton RN, Stoner HB, Watson SM. Relationship among plasma cortisol, adrenocorticotrophin, and severity of injury in recently injured patients. *J Trauma* 1987;27:384–392.
54. Wise L, Margraf HW, Ballinger WF. Adrenal cortical function in severe burns. *Arch Surg* 1972;105: 213–220.
55. Woolf PD. Hormonal responses to trauma. *Crit Care Med* 1992;20:216–226.
56. Jeevanandam M, Peterson SR, Shamos RF. Protein and glucose fuel kinetics and hormonal changes in elderly trauma patients. *Metabolism* 1993;42:1255–1262.
57. Lipman RL, Schnure JJ, Bradley EM, Lecocq FR. Impairment of peripheral glucose utilization in normal subjects by prolonged bed rest. *J Lab Clin Med* 1970;76:221–230.
58. Chiolero R, LeMarchand T, Schutz Y, et al. Plasma pituitary hormone levels in severe trauma with or without head injury. *J Trauma* 1988;28:1368–1374.
59. Ross RJ, Miell JP, Holly JM. Levels of growth hormone, insulin-like growth factor binding proteins, insulin, blood glucose and cortisol in intensive care patients. *Clin Endocr* 1991;35:361–367.
60. Gharib C, Gauquelin G, Pequignot JM, et al. Early hormonal effects of head-down tilt (−10 degrees) in humans. *Aviat Space Environ Med* 1988;59:624–629.
61. Mariano MA, Moldawer LL, Fong Y, et al. Cachectin/TNF production in experimental burns and pseudomonas infection. *Arch Surg* 1988;123:1383–1388.
62. Fukuoka H, Kiriyama M, Nishimura Y, et al. Metabolic turnover of bone and peripheral monocyte release of cytokines during short-term bed rest. *Acta Physiol Scand* 1994;(suppl 37–41).
63. Brillon DJ, Zheng B, Campbell RG, Matthews DE. Effect of cortisol on energy expenditure and amino acid metabolism in humans. *Am J Physiol* 1995;268:E501–E513.
64. Simmons PS, Miles JM, Gerich JE, Haymond MW. Increased proteolysis: an effect of increases in plasma cortisol within the physiologic range. *J Clin Invest* 1984;73:412–420.
65. Biolo G, Fleming DY, Maggi SP, Wolfe RR. Transmembrane transport and intracellular kinetics of amino acids in human skeletal muscle. *Am J Physiol* 1995;268:E75–E84.
66. Koea JB, Wolfe RR, Shaw JHF. Total energy expenditure during total parenteral nutrition: ambulatory patients at home versus septic patients in surgical intensive care. *Surgery* 1995;118:54–62.

Physiology, Stress, and Malnutrition: Functional
Correlates, Nutritional Intervention,
edited by J.M. Kinney and H.N. Tucker.
Lippincott–Raven Publishers © 1997.

Variability of Fat and Lean Tissue Loss during Physical Exertion with Energy Deficit

Karl E. Friedl

Army Operational Medicine Research Program, U.S. Army Medical Research and Material Command, Fort Detrick, Frederick, Maryland 21702-5012

The nature of the linkage between lean and fat is important to our understanding of adaptive responses to environmental stressors. Although lean and fat behave as true companions in many situations (1), there is a common perception that physical exercise shifts the balance to enhance fat loss and preserve lean tissue. At one extreme, in physical training programs with energy balance, fat loss can occur in the fattest individuals even while lean mass is increasing. For example, young female soldiers in 8 weeks of basic training gained an average of 2 kg of lean mass, regardless of initial adiposity, while losing 1 kg fat mass for every 5% body fat over 25% body fat (2). These changes occurred in response to increased levels of physical exercise, with an average energy expenditure of 2,800 kcal/day (3). Similar results have been obtained from training studies involving men (4). At another extreme, in settings of high energy deficit, anabolic influences are likely to be suppressed. This leads to the very interesting question of whether physical exertion can still exert a protective effect on the lean mass, at least attenuating the loss of lean tissue to the preferential utilization of fat stores. This is also an important question, because in a severely undernourished population, the consequences to health and performance depend largely on the extent of lean tissue loss. Most of the experimental studies in this area have involved research using sedentary obese patients on very low calorie diets (VLCDs) or hospitalized patients who are catabolic as a result of intercurrent illness. These responses may not be the same as those observed in soldiers operating away from their supply lines, refugee populations in flight from their homes, or athletes such as wrestlers reducing weight in preparation for their competitive season. In each of these circumstances, the energy deficit produced by a restricted intake is accompanied by a high energy flux produced by continued work.

This chapter reviews the influence of strenuous exercise on change in body composition with energy deficit. The emphasis here is on natural experiments using military training, which offers a view of data on physiologic extremes not readily available from investigator-planned laboratory paradigms. This will draw heavily on studies of U.S. Army Ranger students, performed in 1991 and 1992, when energy deficits were satisfied by mobilization of a majority of the available fat stores. The observed rates of weight loss were even higher than those in the 1950 Minnesota Starvation study (5), although the final weight losses achieved were roughly half those observed in that study because of the shorter duration of the Ranger course. The focus of this chapter is on the variability of lean mass loss, the endocrine markers and determinants of lean mass changes, and the functional consequences.

SEMI-STARVATION STUDIES

In the Minnesota Starvation study (5), Ancel Keys and his colleagues demonstrated large proportions of lean tissue loss in healthy young men performing physical work while semi-starved. Dietary restriction was customized so that each man would lose 25% of his initial body weight within 24 weeks. At the midpoint of this weight loss, at 12 weeks, most of the men had achieved the lowest levels of body fat, and at least half of the weight loss was from lean tissue; at the end of 24 weeks, 57% of the total weight loss was lean tissue. This illustrates an extreme level of weight loss in which most available fat stores were depleted before the end of the study and increasing amounts of lean tissue were necessarily catabolized to fuel the individuals. Even if there was an exercise-induced preservation of lean mass in the earlier stages of this semi-starvation, it is unlikely that this could continue in the face of such a profound deficit. Although protein catabolism declined over time in the Minnesota Study, this remained a high proportion of the total catabolism even though total energy requirements diminished due to other responses to this extreme of weight loss (e.g., reduction in protein turnover rates, an overall reduction in metabolism, and increased behavioral efficiencies (6,7)).

We have examined similar relationships in young men exposed to a multistressor environment with a high level of energy deficit and concurrently high level of physical exertion. However, in these studies, we discovered a semi-starvation paradigm that just bordered on the depletion of fat stores for the average participant. Our model was the U.S. Army Ranger training school in which deliberate food restriction was one of several stressors encountered by students in the physically demanding course (Table 1). This represented titration to the lower limit of fat stores without substantial losses of fat-free mass for most of the men. This appeared to be the threshold of tolerated weight loss, at which the leanest men began to be eliminated for food violations.

In the Ranger studies, there were four phases of training that expose the soldiers to different types of environments. In each of these 2-week phases, soldiers alternate between semi-starvation and partial repletion. Each phase begins with a few days of adequate feeding while soldiers are being taught new skills and is then followed by 7–10 days with one meal per day during realistic small unit tactical operations typically involving 8- to 12-km patrols with loaded rucksacks in hostile terrain. At the end of the course, students were carrying an average weight of 33 kg on patrolling exercises.

TABLE 1. *Principal environmental stressors encountered in summer Ranger training*

Stressor (ref.)	Description and method
Food restriction (8)	Deficit = 1,000 kcal/day for 8 wk, from body composition change
Physical exertion (10)	Energy expenditure = 4,000 kcal/day, up to 6,000 kcal/day, from $^2H_2^{18}O$
Sleep restriction (9)	Sleep = 3.6 h/day for 8 wk, from 24-h wrist activity monitors
Thermal strain (11)	Average daily maximum temperature = 30°C; relative humidity = ~80%
Medical problems (12)	Blisters, insect bites, sprains and strains, cellulitis and respiratory infections
Evaluation anxiety	(unquantified)

The consequences of this regimen are a high rate of weight loss, averaging 16% of initial body weight in the first (Ranger I) of two connected studies (8). In the second Ranger study (Ranger II), the course training remained the same and average sleep (3.6 h/day) did not change (9). However, in response to the findings of the first study (Ranger I), subsequent classes received 400 kcal/day more food in a mixed diet (caloric content was divided into approximately 50% carbohydrate, 35% fat, 15% protein). Thus, the Ranger II study represents the object of a feeding intervention study that could not be ethically compared in a side-by-side study. The seemingly small attenuation of the deficit to 1,000 kcal/day produced some marked benefits.

A different model of semi-starvation is represented by very short term military operations that may require extremely high energy expenditure. Studies of physically elite soldiers engaged in such realistic military training inevitably report weight loss even when adequate calories are provided (Table 2). The important factor driving observed weight losses in acute studies with high-intensity physical exertion can usually be traced to energy deficit due to inadequate intakes (20). [This may not be as true for women, based on studies demonstrating that women are more likely to increase energy intake to maintain weight during physical training (21)]. In most of the acute military studies (all involving only male soldiers), the fat loss represents a large portion of the body composition change, although it may be partially masked by changes in hydration (Table 2). In a controlled laboratory study, Taylor et al. (22,23) reported that weight loss during starvation with work was more than twice as large as the weight loss typically reported in studies without work, but after 4 days the rates began to coincide, and energy deficit, not physical exertion itself, determined the rates.

NEAR-DEPLETION OF FAT ENERGY STORES

Most of the men in the Ranger I study had achieved a near depletion of body fat by the end of the 8 weeks and could only have continued this deficient energy intake by transitioning to a substantial reliance on lean tissue for energy (8). There was also a large variability in individual responses to the energy deprivation, with

TABLE 2. *Published models of physically intensive direct action (acute) missions*

Authors	Study subjects	Scenario/key stressors	Energy intake	Weight changes
Consolazio et al., 1979 (13)	U.S. soldiers during jungle training exercise (n = 38 heat–acclimated men)	10 days combat maneuvers in Panamanian jungle during the rainy season	1–600 kcal/day 2–1,000 kcal/day 3–1,500 kcal/day 4–3,500 kcal/day	-2.6 kg (-0.4 kg TBW) -3.7 kg (-1.5 kg TBW) -2.9 kg (-1.8 kg TBW) 0 (-0.2 kg TBW)
Rognum et al., 1982 (14)	Norwegian military academy cadets during Ranger training (n = 12)	4.5 days continuous combat activities (~1 h sleep total)	1,500 kcal/day	-3.4 ± 1.3 kg (-2.7 ± 1.5 kg fat)
Rognum et al., 1986 (15)	Norwegian military academy cadets during Ranger training (n = 24)	4.5 days continuous combat (~1–2 h sleep total)	1–1,500 kcal/day 2–6,400 kcal/day	-3.6 ± 1.6 kg -0.6 ± 0.6 kg
Kosano et al., 1986 (16)	Japanese Rangers during field training exercise (n = 23)	4 days continuous operations, including 50 km walking with 35–kg loads (3 h/day sleep)	600 kcal/day	[only reported muscle isoenzymes and serum myosin light chains]
Jacobs et al., 1989 (17)	Canadian Forces commandos during field training (n = 30)	4.5 days, winter war games, including 16–km marches and combat activities	1–2,570 kcal/day 2–3,220 kcal/day	-1.9 kg -1.1 kg
Singh et al. 1991 (18)	U.S. Navy SEAL trainees in initial "hell week" (n = 47)	5 days of combat exercises, swimming, and boat races (1 h/day sleep)	Intakes increased from 4,600 ± 150 (pre) to 5,850 ± 550 kcal/day (trng)	+2.3 ± 0.3 kg (plasma volume +7.2 ± 0.6%)
Guezzenec et al., 1994 (19)	French special operations soldiers in commando training in the Pyrenees (n = 27)	4 days, walking 30 km/day with 11–kg loads (3–4 h sleep/day)	1–1,800 kcal/day 2–3,200 kcal/day 3–4,200 kcal/day	-2.9 ± 0.7 kg (SE) -1.9 kg -1.5 kg

mean initial body weights in most studies = 70–80 kg.
TBW, total body water (deuterium dilution).

two of the initially leanest men changing to opposite extremes of lean mass loss within the group. One of these men lost 23% of his body weight within the 8-week period; six other men lost at least 20%, and all of the 55 men lost ~10% or more of their initial body weight. These high rates of weight loss reduced most of the men to 4–6% body fat (Fig. 1).

The modest increase in caloric intake in the second study attenuated the loss of body fat. The energy deficit declined from 1,200 kcal/day in Ranger I to 1,000 kcal/day in this second study. This time, only one of the 50 soldiers achieved the lowest level of body fat by the end of the course (Fig. 1).

These extraordinarily low levels of body fat are interesting in view of the relatively small losses of fat-free mass of most of the men. These losses averaged 7% of initial fat-free mass in the first study and 6% in the second. Some animals indigenous to cold regions retain body fat even in the face of starvation (e.g., gray seal and emperor penguin), presumably because of the higher priority in survival for protection from the cold. At the other extreme, hibernating bears recycle nitrogen and preserve lean mass to the almost exclusive use of fat for energy during the fasting months (24). The adaptive response in humans appears to be to use most available fat before severe decimation of lean mass stores; however, a maladaptive response, for example, in patients with acquired immunodeficiency syndrome, results in the apparently inappropriate preservation of fat over lean tissue (25). In our sample, the men followed a general two-thirds fat of total weight loss relationship (Fig. 2). This held true for body fat estimated by two quite different methods [dual-energy x-ray absorptiometry (DEXA) or skinfold measurement using the Durnin and Wormersley equation] (26). It also held true even as the men approached the lowest level of body fat, with measurements at 8 weeks. This latter observation is counterintuitive because many men had already achieved very low fat levels by 6 weeks, and it would be expected that the contribution to the deficit would increase from the lean tissue component; however, the rate of total weight loss diminished in this final period as well, suggesting increased metabolic efficiencies that reduced the demand for body energy stores.

The changes in this study are also interesting because of the individual variability. The average proportion of fat loss of the total weight loss was 0.60 ± 0.18 for this group, as demonstrated by the regression lines in Fig. 2; however, the proportion ranged from 0.14 to 1.07 (gain in fat-free mass) for individuals. This variation is better explained in terms of initial adiposity (Fig. 3). This is consistent with the findings of higher proportions of fat loss in obese patients, where almost no lean tissue may be lost (27). In the Minnesota Starvation study, the energy density of the weight loss was lower by nearly half of that predicted from obese patients in a clinical setting (6), again suggesting the effect of leanness of the subjects rather than any consistent effect of the inclusion of physical exertion.

The location of fat stores may also be important to their availability for mobilization. A study by Rognum et al. (14) demonstrated that there is a regional fat site hierarchy in the mobilization of triglyceride from fat cells in

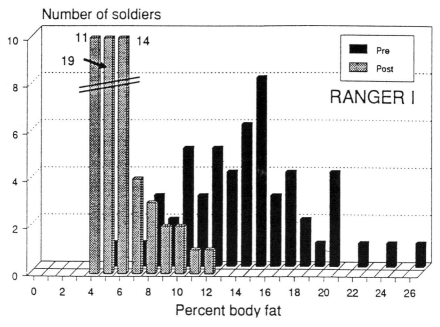

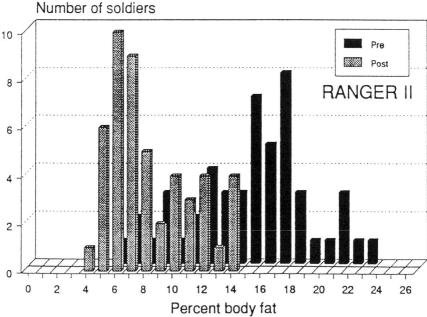

FIG. 1. Distribution of soldiers according to adiposity at the start and at the end of 8 weeks of Ranger training. The top graph illustrates the distribution in the first Ranger study with an average energy deficit of 1,200 kcal/day. Comparison of the bottom graph with this shows the effect of a small decrease in energy deficit, to 1,000 kcal/day, with fewer individuals pushed to a lower limit of fatness at the end of the course.

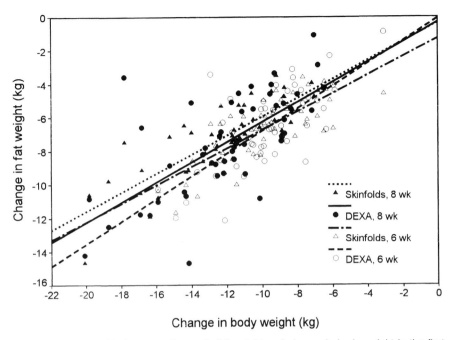

FIG. 2. The relationship between change in fat weight and change in body weight in the first Ranger study demonstrates an average two-thirds contribution from fat. There was no difference in the relationship between 6 and 8 weeks of semi-starvation, or based on the method of fat estimation [skinfolds, using the equation of Durnin and Womersely, or dual-energy x-ray absorptiometry (DEXA)].

lean young soldiers. In fat biopsy specimens from abdominal, gluteal, and femoral sites before and after a 4.5-day intensive military training course, the gluteal and abdominal sites were diminished, whereas no significant changes were noted in the femoral site. The gluteal adipocyte size at the end of the course provided the only correlation with circulating fatty acids and glycerol, leading to speculation about the metabolic importance of gluteal fat, even over abdominal stores. This is consistent with our regional DEXA changes, which indicate similar group average changes in arm and leg fat (28). When sorted by adiposity, however, those with the greatest reserves had more fat in the arms and mobilized this fat before decreasing the leg fat (29). The fat mobilized by Rognum's subjects represented nearly 80% of the total weight loss. This is probably typical of the weight loss observed in most studies of direct action type (short-term) military missions and is readily sustainable from fat stores. Even at the highest rates of energy expenditure, such as the estimated 10,000 kcal/24 h requirement in the Norwegian model, most men have the 4–5 kg of storage fat necessary to sustain this level of deficit (Table 2). In our more prolonged energy deficit studies, with averages of approximately 8 kg of fat, some

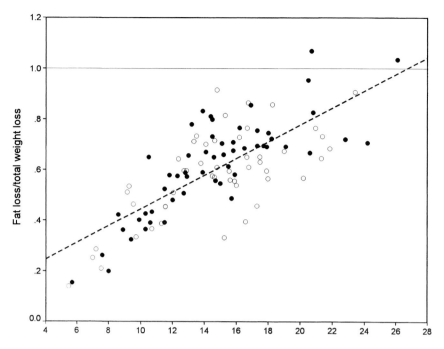

FIG. 3. The contribution of fat to total weight loss in relation to initial adiposity (r = 0.65). Data are shown for 105 lean men (14.7 ± 4.2% body fat) from two separate Ranger studies (open vs. filled circles).

of the leanest individuals must be fat depleted before the end of the course unless a higher proportion of lean tissue is catabolized.

LEAN MASS MEASUREMENT ARTIFACTS INTRODUCED BY HYDRATIONAL CHANGES

An analysis of the lean mass loss should be reflected by declines in body cell mass [including an appropriate proportion of water (~73%)], roughly in a one-third proportion to the total weight loss to complement the observed fat changes. However, changes in the fat-free mass are complicated by large alterations in hydration. If the methodologic issues are not carefully considered, one can easily be led to an inappropriate conclusion about smaller than actual losses of lean tissue. This may not be a problem limited to situations of energy deficit with high work levels.

If assessed by a body composition assessment method that relies on body water, it would appear that there was no decline in fat-free mass in our Ranger students. Bioelectrical impedance, for example, demonstrated no significant change in resistance values before and after Ranger training. If this had been the only method of body composition used in the study, we could have drawn the astounding conclusion that some combination of factors in Ranger training led to a protein-sparing effect, with fat-free mass largely preserved, or even increased, in the face of massive weight loss (Fig. 4). Similarly, the DEXA analysis suggested that there was no loss of lean mass, at the same time that a measurement artifact indicated the presence of more tissue (+2.8 kg) than the floor scales measured (8). These findings with the DEXA analysis were duplicated in the Ranger II study, suggesting an error in the assessment of the fat-free mass from the attenuation of the energy beam in tissue that has an abnormally high level of hydration. To produce a more realistic estimate of fat-free mass change, the percentage body fat value obtained from DEXA was combined with gravimetrically assessed body weights (as plotted in Fig. 4); the values for fat mass obtained in this way closely matched the fat mass detected by DEXA in the soft-tissue mass and were similar to estimates obtained from skinfolds (Table 3).

Using body water measurements, we were able to verify an increased hydration of the fat-free mass in a small subset of men in both of the Ranger studies. Based on stable isotope dilutions performed for free-ranging energy expenditure measurements, we estimated an increased hydration of the fat-free mass in excess of 80% by the mid-point of the course (8). Using bioelectrical impedance to predict total body water, a method proven to be reliable in our studies of

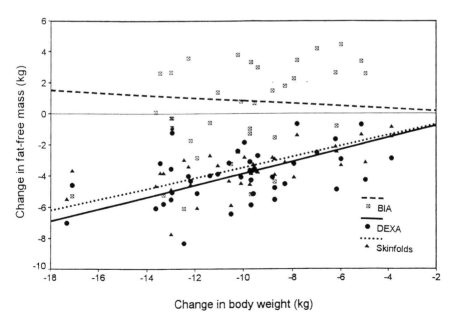

FIG. 4. The relationship between change in fat-free mass and change in body weight, with fat-free mass estimated by bioelectric impedance analysis (BIA), DEXA, and skinfolds (using the Durnin and Womersely equation).

TABLE 3. *Changes in body composition during 8 weeks of U.S. Army Ranger training*

Component	Initial measure	Final measure	Change
Body weight	78.4 ± 8.7	68.4 ± 7.0	−10.0 ± 2.8
Fat weight			
DEXA	11.7 ± 3.9	5.8 ± 2.2	−6.0 ± 2.6
Skinfolds	14.1 ± 3.7	7.5 ± 2.0	−6.6 ± 2.5
Fat–free mass			
DEXA	66.7 ± 6.3	62.6 ± 6.1	−4.0 ± 1.7
Skinfolds	64.6 ± 6.0	61.1 ± 5.5	−3.5 ± 1.4
Total body water[a]	50.1 ± 4.8	49.4 ± 5.4	−0.7 ± 2.6

n = 50 male soldiers. Values are mean kg ±1 SD.
[a]Estimated from bioelectrical impedance at 50 kHZ; the values shown here are a subset of the fat-free mass values shown.

weight-stable subjects (30), we measured body water at the start and end of the Ranger II study.

The results suggested only a small decrease in total body water (Table 3); in other words, a disproportionately small reduction in body water in relation to loss of fat-free mass. Dr. Francis Moore had noted this effect in chronically ill patients, in association with energy deficit and loss of muscle mass (31). He measured coefficients as high as 0.82–0.85 hydration of the fat-free mass.

A similar problem of increased hydration of the fat-free mass was reported by Keys et al., and by the end of the 24-week Minnesota Starvation study (32), some of the men had clinically evident edema of the lower extremities. The correction of the lean mass density for the increased proportion of water was offset by the increasing proportion of bone mineral, which did not diminish with the soft-tissue catabolism. Deurenberg et al. (33) examined the changes produced by dietary restriction in a group of obese women losing 10 kg of weight in 8 weeks (the same average weight loss and rate of weight loss achieved by our lean Ranger students). On the basis of hydrostatic weighing, they concluded that there was some loss of fat-free mass (23% of the total weight loss); however, resistance values from bio-electrical impedance did not change, suggesting that there was no reduction in body water. As with the Ranger studies, if body composition changes were inter-preted solely on the basis of bioelectrical impedance, one would draw the unlikely conclusion that there was no reduction in lean mass.

One possible explanation for this increased hydration of semi-starved lean tissue is the retention of electrolytes and water. This could be associated with well-established changes in growth hormone during starvation. This class of hor-mones has known osmoregulatory roles (34), which may all figure prominently in volume expansion during heat and exercise exposures and may involve stim-ulation of mineralocorticoids (35). It also may involve stress-stimulated increases in vasopressin. In order to increase the solute load, some intake is nec-essary; thus, in studies involving complete starvation, there is no water retention effect (22).

Most of the acute military training scenarios result in a prompt decline in body weight, indicating less of a fluid derangement. However, studies of U.S. Navy SEAL trainees demonstrate a prominent fluid retention, which results in a net weight gain within 1 week of training, attributed to the increased dietary salt intake (18,36).

BIOCHEMICAL MARKERS OR DETERMINANTS OF LEAN MASS LOSS

Instead of preserving lean mass, there is a possibility that high-intensity training, especially in conjunction with energy deficit, produces an overtraining-like effect that results in both direct and indirect muscle catabolic influences. These effects could be produced through inflammatory damage to muscle cells and through a reduction in the anabolic hormones, such as circulating androgens.

A study of Japanese Rangers considered the question of muscle tissue breakdown in young men participating in a grueling 93-hour military training exercise. Although they found elevated levels of muscle enzymes including creatine kinase and lactate dehydrogenase isoenzymes typical of marathon runners (37), serum levels of myosin light chain were relatively low. The levels were far lower than those observed in patients with myopathies and suggested minimal muscle damage (16). Similar work with French commandos demonstrated relatively modest increases in myoglobin (16). Serum glycerol and fatty acids remained elevated at the end of the Ranger course (11), which may be important in preserving lean mass by preventing a breakdown of myofibrillar protein (38). Endurance exercise reduces the rate of degradation of contractile proteins, even though there may be a net breakdown of body protein (39).

Another effect of elevated fatty acids is the continued suppression of catabolic hormones such as cortisol. Cortisol did not increase significantly until the second half of the course, as fat stores and fatty acid availability diminished. Similar elevations of cortisol have been reported in anorexic patients (40). It is clear that the pituitary-adrenal axis does not remain activated in response to chronic military stressors (41). In a 4.5-day Norwegian Ranger training course with no food or sleep, cortisol increases briefly and then recovers before the end of the training (42), although this is not always consistent between studies. This response to a metabolic need, rather than as a generalized stress response, was clearly apparent in our Ranger studies. The highest concentration of cortisol was measured at the end of one of the courses in the individual with 23% loss of weight. Fat-free mass loss represented nearly 80% of the total weight loss in this individual, and although triiodothyronine levels were typical of the low values of most other individuals, other mediators of metabolism were markedly suppressed; for example, interleukin-6 (IL-6) concentrations in the serum of this individual were the lowest measured. One can only speculate on the severity of the loss of lean mass that may have occurred in this individual if the hypermetabolic effects of cytokines such as IL-6 (43) were not suppressed by the high levels of cortisol.

Few studies relate endogenous hormone stimulation by exercise to the preservation of lean mass during weight loss produced by energy deficit. A relationship between training responses and endogenous anabolic hormones is implied from observations of gender differences in the response to weight loss (21). In studies without weight loss, resistance exercise stimulation of growth hormone and testosterone has been suggested to explain lean mass increases produced by high-intensity training with short rest intervals (44). These anabolic influences appear to be negated even at moderate levels of energy deficit. Without energy deficit, even the highest levels of physical exertion do not result in reduced circulating levels of anabolic hormones; thus, physical training during energy restriction would not be predicted to specifically increase the loss of lean mass, but it is also unlikely to preserve lean mass on the basis of observed endocrine changes (Table 4).

The correlation between serum testosterone levels and changes in body weight or lean mass (absolute or relative to total weight loss) is weak in the Ranger students (Fig. 5). Even the few individuals who did not demonstrate a substantial decline in mean testosterone concentrations in the Ranger course were unremarkable for their ability to preserve lean mass. Although there is a general correspondence between mean weight loss and mean serum hormone changes, simple correlations are inadequate to relate these effects of energy deficit with hormone levels changing acutely and body weight (and lean mass) changing over a more sustained period.

These points can be illustrated by comparison of the results from two different elite Army training courses, the 21-day Special Forces Assessment and Selection (SFAS) course (45) and the mid-point of the Ranger course, at 4 weeks. Although the energy expenditure measured using the doubly-labeled water technique was higher in the SFAS course, the net weight loss of 4% of body weight was less than half that observed for Ranger students by the mid-point (−9.2%), reflecting a smaller energy deficit. Serum testosterone levels declined by 15% in this group, compared with a 69% decline in Ranger students, whereas cortisol was not significantly elevated in the SFAS study but increased

TABLE 4. *Summary of typical endocrine responses to acute and chronic energy deficit and exercise stressors*

Hormone	Energy deficit		Exercise	
	Acute	Chronic	Acute	Chronic
Cortisol	↑ or normal	↑	↑	Normal
Testosterone	↓[a]	↓↓[a]	↑ or ↓	Normal
IGF1	↓	↓↓	Normal	?
Growth hormone	↑	↑↑	↑ or normal	Normal
Triiodothyronine	↓[a]	↓↓[a]	↓	Normal

Large acute energy deficit can produce large hormone changes.
[a]Binding proteins increase, further reducing bioavailable hormone.

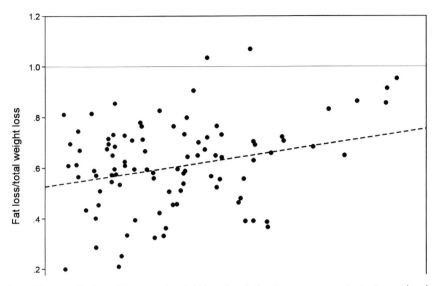

FIG. 5. The contribution of fat to total weight loss in relation to mean serum testosterone levels from three morning blood samples drawn during the second half of the Ranger course. There is a significant but weak correlation (n=0.31).

by 25% in Ranger students. In acute studies, Opstad et al. demonstrated that testosterone declined into the hypogonadal range within the first 24 hours of stressful high-intensity training without energy intake (46). Guezennec et al. (19) found a 20–25% decline in serum testosterone with deficits of 1,500 kcal/day and a 50% decline with deficits in excess of 3,000 kcal/day. The elevation of sex hormone–binding globulin in both the acute (47) and chronic studies (11) further decreases bioavailability of the hormone. This decrease in testosterone in response to energy deficit permits an increased availability of amino acids (48), and this may be critically important as glutamine and other amino acid levels decline with exertion (49). Changes in the pituitary–gonadal axis do not explain the reduction in bone mass that has been reported in male long distance runners (50), and no reduction in bone mass was noted within the relatively short 8-week Ranger course.

An overabundance of published studies on serum testosterone and cortisol changes with respect to exercise level reiterate the observation that lasting changes are not produced by high-energy expenditure or exercise intensity. The only consistently reported change is an acute elevation testosterone and cortisol induced by alterations in hormone clearance and/or reflecting measurement artifacts caused by fluid shifts that affect the concentration of protein-bound steroids in the intravascular space. Declines in testosterone in long-term studies are consistently explained by energy deficit rather than any influence of physical exertion.

Two metabolic hormones that are relatively unaffected by chronic exercise were acutely sensitive to energy deficit status. Insulin-like growth factor-1

(IGF-1) and triiodothyronine demonstrated a progressive decline over the training course with fat loss and demonstrated a prompt recovery during refeeding both within a training phase as well as within the first week after the training course. More importantly, concentrations of both of these hormones were better sustained in the second Ranger study with increased energy intake. There was a slight attenuation of the loss of lean mass (~15% difference), paralleling the 15% increase in the daily energy intakes. The remarkable benefits of this modest increase in energy appear to be related to keeping the soldiers just below the threshold for marked muscle catabolism, which would occur as fat stores approach depletion. This resulted in a mean triiodothyronine level in the Ranger II study that remained within the normal limits, as compared with the Ranger I study, where levels decreased well below the lower limit of normal. This has potentially important metabolic consequences, including rates of cellular metabolism, thermogenesis, and selective muscle fiber type preservation (51–53).

One can suggest some interesting consequences of an exercise overlay on these relationships. Growth hormone is well stimulated by intensive exercise, particularly anaerobic resistance training routines (44). When recombinant human growth hormone was administered to obese patients on a low-calorie diet and exercise regimen, triiodothyronine was maintained at normal levels while decreasing in the placebo controls (54). Although our Ranger students demonstrated very large pulsatile surges of growth hormone, they differed from these patients with recombinant human growth hormone treatment by demonstrating a decrease in IGF-1 from baseline values. We can only surmise that IGF-1 may have declined to still lower levels in the absence of the endogenous growth hormone surges. From the controlled Ranger studies of Opstad et al. (42,55), we know more about the stressors involved in the growth hormone responses. There is an immediate increase in mean growth hormone concentrations, even in single samples, within 24 hours of starting into a course with no food and no organized sleep. Groups receiving 3 hours of sleep per night maintained elevated growth hormone levels better than those deprived of all sleep (42). Cadets receiving 6,400 kcal/day, compared with those receiving 1,500 kcal/day, demonstrated lower levels of growth hormone (55). Thus, U.S. Army Ranger students, receiving 3.6 h/day sleep and maintaining a high energy deficit, are primed for high growth hormone secretion rates, as we consistently observe. In the absence of exercise controls and careful high-frequency blood samples to quantitatively define the growth hormone release, we can only guess if exercise may further stimulate growth hormone release.

When divided by quartiles of weight loss, the largest men lost the smallest proportion of weight. They also retained the highest circulating levels of IGF-1 at the end of the course (there were no differences between groups at the start), indicating that these larger fatter men had a better metabolic status after 8 weeks of a relatively fixed energy deficit. Other measured hormones, including testosterone and triiodothyronine, demonstrated no differences with respect to the extent of weight loss (Fig. 5). A prompt and profound decline in each of these hormones after the start of the Ranger course correspond to the high energy deficit (56,57). Opstad has demonstrated that these changes occur within the first day of the physically intensive Norwegian ranger training course (46,58). Thus, the same changes are accelerated in the 5-day Norwegian Ranger course, where little or no food is offered and energy expenditure is estimated to be in excess of 10,000 kcal/day, over the changes that occur at a slower rate in U.S. Army Ranger students, where average energy deficit is 1,000 kcal/day.

FUNCTIONAL CONSEQUENCES OF WEIGHT LOSS IN RANGER STUDENTS

Some of the key consequences that have been described in Ranger training are summarized in Table 5. Immune status, physical strength, and lean mass outcomes are interrelated. Reduction in fat-free mass did not directly correlate with any of the indices of immune function status in the Ranger studies; however, immune status is a sensitive endpoint of nutritional status (64). Changes in immune function result in and from changes in the cytokine environment, and these cytokines, in turn, play a critical role in the alterations in body composition. Sarcopenia, the loss of muscle mass frequently associated with aging, exemplifies how cytokines have been implicated. IL-1 and IL-6 are examples of cytokines that cause hypermetabolism and loss of nitrogen and lean mass (43,65). On the basis of the responses of IL-2 and IL-6 in our Ranger studies, it appears that semi-starvation helps to suppress these potentially maladaptive responses (63).

Immunologic function has been primarily assessed in Ranger students using in vitro proliferative activity of lymphocytes. No consistent results were obtained using delayed hypersensitivity tine tests with antigens to seven microorganisms.

TABLE 5. *Physiologic/functional consequences of multistressor exposure in summer Ranger training*

Function (ref.)	Description and indicators
Energy metabolism (11)	↓ fasting glucose (−20%) and insulin (−40%) ↓ metabolic rate (↓T3) ↑ counter-regulatory hormones (hGH and cortisol)
Protein status	↑ protein catabolism (−6% of total FFM) without protein deficiency (↓ prealbumin, ↔ total proteins, ↑ RBP)
Physical (59,60)	↓ maximum aerobic capacity (−14%) ↓ maximum lift strength and vertical jump (−20%)
Cognitive (61,62)	↓ decoding speed (−33%) ↓ pattern analysis speed (−15%) ↓ reasoning speed (−20%)
Immunologic (63)	↓T- and B-lymphocyte proliferation response in vitro ↓ IL-2, IL-2 receptor, IL-6

However, phytohemagglutinin-stimulated T-lymphocyte activity demonstrated marked and reproducible declines in both Ranger studies, with the largest attenuation in response associated with periods of highest energy expenditure and deficit. IL-2 receptor and IL-2 secretion from stimulated lymphocytes demonstrates recoveries before the end of the course and in advance of recovery of the T-lymphocyte proliferative activity (11).

Ranger students are more susceptible to infectious diseases, including problems with cellulitis, uncommon in other soldiers (12). Another problem that is uncommon in healthy adults, streptococcal pneumonia, has been a significant problem for winter Ranger students. A limited trial was made with administration of prophylactic bicillin to entire classes in an effort to reduce the infectious disease problems (12). A modest increase in food intake appears to attenuate both the infection rate and some of the observed decrements in in vitro immune function measures. Treated infections decreased from 25% in the second half of the Ranger course to negligible levels in the Ranger II study. Whether this reduced illness rate is actually related to metabolic status and energy deficit remains to be determined. We have been unable to demonstrate a statistical relationship between immune function outcomes and any aspect of body composition status; however, reductions in immune function are reported to parallel loss of lean mass (65).

Change in immune status is in turn reported to affect body composition and may explain some of the individual variability in loss of lean mass. Cytokines IL-1β and tumor necrosis factor α may be involved in increased protein turnover rates (65), and their release is enhanced by exercise in individuals with normal energy balance.

Physical performance is affected by lean tissue loss, but only at levels exceeding at least 10% of body weight. In an earlier study of Ranger students, Dr. Herman Johnson demonstrated a decline in maximal aerobic capacity, based on treadmill tests (59). This decremented capacity or test performance persisted even after several days of rest and refeedings. In a sampling of military field studies with aerobic capacity, substantive declines in aerobic capacity emerge only for groups losing >10% of initial body weight (66). One concern with high rates of weight loss is the effect on cardiac muscle. In the earlier Ranger study, Herman Johnson included electrocardiographic studies before and after the course and found no abnormalities. An interesting study with rodents supports the suggestion that exercise helps to substantially preserve heart muscle mass, whereas dietary restriction without exercise leads to substantial losses (67). This protective effect of exercise occurred even at severe levels of energy restriction in rats when skeletal muscle was no longer protected in comparison with the dietary restriction only group.

Maximal strength performance, like aerobic capacity, is difficult to test in a consistent manner, and different tests yield different results. A maximal strength test in the Ranger studies (a clean lift) demonstrated reductions of approximately 20%, a difference of about 40 pounds in lift capacity between the start and end of the course. In the Ranger I study, this was shown to be a progressive decline, with additional reductions in lift capacity observed between 6 and 8 weeks (60). The individual reductions in strength correlated reasonably well with the individual losses of fat-free mass (60).

Maximal lift strength reflects a measure of overall body strength, involving many large muscle groups. A more specific strength test, the grip strength, which reflects only hand and forearm strength, yielded different results in the Ranger I study. Despite high rates of weight loss and approximately 7% reduction in fat-free mass, including a reduction of nearly 1 kg (12%) of arm muscle mass (28), there was no decline in grip strength or grip endurance time across five measurement periods spread across the course (60). This was true even for the subject with the most extreme weight loss. Grip strength declines only when much higher levels of fat-free mass loss occur (>10%), as demonstrated in the Minnesota study. The explanation for this may be related to the gripping action required during most of the 8-week course because soldiers carry their weapons. This suggests either that this exercise preserved specific muscle function in these soldiers or that the arms are better protected against catabolic influences of energy deficit than are other muscle groups.

CONCLUSIONS

The majority of healthy young soldiers participating in high-intensity training adapt appropriately to energy restriction, sacrificing fat mass with some smaller portion of lean mass. The range of individual responses is large and corresponds in part to the total available fat stores. There is a relatively small loss of lean tissue, with an average loss of approximately one third of the mass from lean tissues. The catabolic environment in more protracted or severe energy deficit includes a reduction in testosterone and IGF-1 and an increase in cortisol; however, other potentially catabolic activity is reduced through suppression of key hormones such as triiodothyronine and cytokines such as IL-6, reducing metabolic demands, and preserving tissue energy stores. The specific role of exercise on these relationships remains poorly defined and speculative, but may contribute no more than an additional energy requirement in extreme conditions. The methods to assess body composition may be seriously confounded by alterations in hydration produced by semi-starvation, and this complicates interpretation of the results of many studies.

ACKNOWLEDGMENTS

The opinions or assertions expressed in this chapter are the private views of the author and are not to be construed as reflecting the official views of the Department of the Army.

Portions of this chapter were previously presented at the Beltsville Agricultural Research Center Symposium, "Advances in human energy metabolism:

balancing energy requirements and energy intake," May 8–11, 1994, and at a NATO workshop on "Recovery from exhaustive military exercises," April 2–5, 1995, Oslo, Norway.

Some new analyses of data from the Ranger I and Ranger II studies are reported in this chapter. These studies were conducted in accordance with the principles of the Declaration of Helsinki and the explicit directives of Army Regulation 70-25, "Use of Volunteers as Subjects of Research," including approval by an Institutional Review Board at the U.S. Army Research Institute of Environmental Medicine, Natick, Massachusetts, and by the Human Use Review Office, Office of the Surgeon General, Department of the Army.

REFERENCES

1. Forbes GB. The companionship of lean and fat. In: Ellis KJ, Eastman JD, eds. *Human body composition.* New York: Plenum; 1993:1–14.
2. Westphal KA, Friedl KE, Sharp MA, et al. Health, performance, and nutritional status of U.S. Army women during basic combat training. Technical Report No. T96-2, USARIEM, AD-A32042. Natick, MA, May 1995:161.
3. Friedl KE, Westphal KA, Marchitelli LJ. Reproductive status and menstrual cyclicity of premenopausal women in Army basic combat training (BCT) [Abstract]. *FASEB J* 1995;9:292.
4. Krzywicki HJ, Consolazio CF, Johnson HL, Witt NF. Effects of exercise and dietary protein levels on body composition in humans. Technical Report No. 62, Letterman Army Institute of Research, Presidio of San Francisco, CA, July 1978:19.
5. Keys A, Brozek J, Henschel A, Mickelsen O, Taylor HL. *The biology of human starvation.* Minneapolis: University of Minnesota Press, 1950.
6. Alpert SS. The energy density of weight loss in semistarvation. *Int J Obes* 1988;12:533–542.
7. Grande F, Anderson JT, Keys A. Changes in basal metabolic rate in man in semistarvation and refeeding. *J Appl Physiol* 1958;12:230–238.
8. Friedl KE, Moore RJ, Martinez-Lopez LE, et al. Lower limit of body fat in healthy active men. *J Appl Physiol* 1994;77:933–940.
9. Popp KA, Redmond DP. Duration and patterns of sleep, In: RL Shippee, KE Friedl, MZ Mays, et al. Nutritional and immunological assessment of Ranger students with increased caloric intake. Technical Report No. T1-95, USARIEM, Natick, MA. December 1994:6.1–6.10,
10. Hoyt RW, Moore RJ, DeLany JP, Friedl KE, Askew EW. Energy balance during 62 days of rigorous physical activity and caloric restriction [Abstract]. *FASEB J* 1993;7:726.
11. Moore RJ, Friedl KE, Martinez-Lopez LE, et al. Changes in soldier nutritional status and immune function during the Ranger training course. Technical Report No. T13-92, USARIEM, AD-A257 437. Natick, MA, September 1992:162.
12. Martinez-Lopez LE, Friedl KE, Moore RJ, Kramer TR. A prospective epidemiological study of infection rates and injuries of Ranger students. *Milit Med* 1993;58:433–437.
13. Consolazio CF, Johnson HL, Nelson RA, et al. The relationship of diet to the performance of the combat soldier minimal calorie intake during combat patrols in a hot humid environment (Panama). Technical Report No. 76, Letterman Army Institute of Research, Presidio of San Francisco, CA. October 1979:65.
14. Rognum TO, Rodahl K, Opstad PK. Regional differences in the lipolytic response of the subcutaneous fat depots to prolonged exercise and severe energy deficiency. *Eur J Appl Physiol* 1982;49:401–408.
15. Rognum TO, Vartdal F, Rodahl K, et al. Physical and mental performance of soldiers on high and low energy diets during prolonged heavy exercise combined with sleep deprivation. *Ergonomics* 1986;29: 859-67.
16. Kosano H, Kinoshita T, Nagata N, et al. Change in concentrations of myogenic components of serum during 93 h of strenuous physical exercise. *Clin Chem* 1986;32:346–348.
17. Jacobs I, Anderberg A, Schele R, Lithell H. Muscle glycogen in soldiers on different diets during military field manoeuvres. *Aviat Space Environ Med* 1983;54:898–900.

18. Singh A, Smoak BL, Patterson KY, et al. Biochemical indices of selected trace minerals in men: effect of stress. *Am J Clin Nutr* 1991;53:126–131.
19. Guezennec CY, Satabin P, Legrand H, Bigard AX. Physical performance and metabolic changes induced by combined prolonged exercise and different energy intakes in humans. *Eur J Appl Physiol* 1994;68:525–530.
20. Marriott BM. *Not eating enough—overcoming underconsumption of military operational rations.* Washington DC: National Academy Press; 1995.
21. Andersson B, Xu X, Rebuffe-Scrive M, Terning K, Krotkiewski M, Bjorntorp P. The effects of exercise training on body composition and metabolism in men and women. *Int J Obes* 1991;15:75–81.
22. Taylor HL, Henschel A, Mickelsen O, Keys A. Some effects of acute starvation with hard work on body weight, body fluids and metabolism. *J Appl Physiol* 1954;6:613–623.
23. Brozek J, Grande F, Taylor HL, Anderson JT, Buskirk ER, Keys A. Changes in body weight and body dimensions in men performing work on a low calorie carbohydrate diet. *J Appl Physiol* 1957;10: 412–420.
24. Nelson RA, Jones JD, Wahner HW, McGill DB, Code CF. Nitrogen metabolism in bears: urea metabolism in summer starvation and in winter sleep and role of urinary bladder in water and nitrogen conservation. *Mayo Clin Proc* 1975;50:141–146.
25. Kotler DP, Wang J, Pierson RN Jr. Body composition studies in patients with the acquired immunodeficiency syndrome. *Am J Clin Nutr* 1985;42:1255–1265.
26. Durnin JVGA, Womersley J. Body fat assessed from total body density and its estimation from skinfold thickness: measurements on 481 men and women aged from 16 to 72 years. *Br J Nutr* 1974;32: 77–97.
27. Hammer RL, Barrier CA, Roundy ES, Bradford JM, Fisher AG. Calorie-restricted low-fat diet and exercise in obese women. *Am J Clin Nutr* 1989;49:77–85.
28. Friedl KE, Vogel JA, Marchitelli LJ, Kubel SL. Assessment of regional body composition changes by dual-energy x-ray absorptiometry. In: Ellis KJ, Eastman JD, eds. *Human body composition.* New York: Plenum; 1993:99–103.
29. Nindl BC, Friedl KE, Marchitelli LJ, et al. Regional fat placement in physically fit males and regional changes with weight loss. *Med Sci Sports Exerc* 1996;28:786–793.
30. Friedl KE, DeLuca JP, Marchitelli LJ, Vogel JA. Reliability of body-fat estimations from a four-compartment model using density, body water, and bone mineral measurements. *Am J Clin Nutr* 1992;55: 764–770.
31. Moore FD. Energy stores as revealed by body compositional study. In: Morgan AP, ed. *Energy metabolism and body fuel utilization, with particular reference to starvation and injury. Proceedings of the Committee on Metabolism in Trauma of the U.S. Army Research and Development Command.* Cambridge, MA: Harvard University Printing Office; 1966:110–118.
32. Keys A, Taylor HL, Mickelsen O, Henschel A. Famine edema and the mechanism of its formation. *Science* 1946;103:669–670.
33. Deurenberg P, Weststrate JA, Hautvast JGAJ. Changes in fat-free mass during weight loss measured by bioelectrical impedance and by densitometry. *Am J Clin Nutr* 1989;49:33–36.
34. Pratt JH, Peacock M, Henry DP. Effect of recombinant human growth hormone on adrenocortical function, and on sodium and potassium homeostasis. *Pharmacology* 1993;47:36–42.
35. Opstad PK, Oktedalen O, Aakvaag A, Fonnum F, Lund PK. Plasma renin and serum aldosterone during prolonged physical strain. *Eur J Appl Physiol* 1985;54:1–6.
36. Smoak BL, Singh A, Day BA, et al. Changes in nutrient intakes of conditioned men during a 5-day period of increased physical activity and other stresses. *Eur J Appl Physiol* 1988;58:245–251.
37. Apple FS, McGue MK. Serum enzyme changes during marathon training. *Am J Clin Pathol* 1983;79: 716–719.
38. Lowell BB, Goodman MN. Protein sparing in skeletal muscle during prolonged starvation: dependence on lipid fuel availability. *Diabetes* 1987;36:14–19.
39. Dohm GL, Tapscott EB, Kasperek GJ. Protein degradation during endurance exercise and recovery. *Med Sci Sports Exerc* 1987;19(suppl):166–171.
40. Smith SR, Bledsoe T, Chhetri MK. Cortisol metabolism and the pituitary-adrenal axis in adults with protein-calorie malnutrition. *J Clin Endocrinol Metab* 1975;40:43–52.
41. Mason JW. Specificity in the organization of neuroendocrine response profiles. In: Seeman P, Brown G, eds. *Frontiers in neurology and neuroscience research.* Toronto: University of Toronto; 1974:68–80.
42. Opstad PK, Aakvaag A. The effect of sleep deprivation on the plasma levels of hormones during prolonged physical strain and calorie deficiency. *Eur J Appl Physiol* 1983;51:97–107.

43. Stouthard JML, Romijn JA, van der Poll T, et al. Endocrinologic and metabolic effects of interleukin-6 in humans. *Am J Physiol* 1995;268:E813–819.
44. Kraemer WJ, Gordon SE, Fleck SJ, et al. Endogenous anabolic hormonal and growth factor responses to heavy resistance exercise in males and females. *Int J Sports Med* 1991;12:228–235.
45. Fairbrother B, Askew EW, Mays MZ, et al. Nutritional assessment of the special forces assessment and selection course. Technical report (in preparation).
46. Opstad PK. Androgenic hormones during prolonged physical stress, sleep, and energy deficiency. *J Clin Endocrinol Metab* 1992;74:1176–1183.
47. Aakvaag A, Sand T, Opstad PK, Fonnum F. Hormonal changes in young men during prolonged physical strain. *Eur J Appl Physiol* 1978;39:283–291.
48. Guezennec CY, Serrurier B, Aymonod M, Merion D, Pesquies PC. Metabolic and hormonal response to short term fasting after endurance training in the rat. *Horm Metab Res* 1984;16:572–575.
49. Rowbottom DG, Keast D, Goodman C, Morton AR. The haematological, biochemical and immunological profile of athletes suffering from the overtraining syndrome. *Eur J Appl Physiol* 1995;70:502–509.
50. Hetland ML, Haarbo J, Christiansen C. Low bone mass and high bone turnover in male long distance runners. *J Clin Endocrinol Metab* 1993;77:770–775.
51. Schantz P, Henriksson J, Jansson E. Adaptation of human skeletal muscle to endurance training of long duration. *Clin Physiol* 1983;3:141–151.
52. Russell DM, Walker PM, Leiter LA, et al. Metabolic and structural changes in skeletal muscle during hypocaloric dieting. *Am J Clin Nutr* 1984;39:503.
53. Caizzo VJ, Herrick RE, Baldwin KM. Response of slow and fast muscle to hypothyroidism: maximal shortening velocity and myosin isoforms. *Am J Physiol* 1992;C86:263.
54. Drent ML, Wever LD, Ader HJ, van der Veen EA. Growth hormone administration in addition to a very low calorie diet and an exercise program in obese subjects. *Eur J Endocrinol* 1995;132:565–572.
55. Opstad PK, Aakvaag A. The effect of a high calory diet on hormonal changes in young men during prolonged physical strain and sleep deprivation. *Eur J Appl Physiol* 198146:31–39.
56. Kyung NH, Barkan A, Klibanski A, et al. Effect of carbohydrate supplementation on reproductive hormones during fasting in men. *J Clin Endocrinol Metab* 1985;60:827–835.
57. Minuto F, et al. Insulin-like growth factor-I in human malnutrition: relationship with some body composition and nutritional parameters. *J Parenter Enter Nutr* 1989;13:392–396.
58. Opstad PK, Falch D, Oktedalen O, Fonnum F, Wergeland R. The thyroid function in young men during prolonged exercise and the effect of energy and sleep deprivation. *Clin Endocrinol* 1984;20:657–669.
59. Johnson HL, Krzywicki, HJ, Canham JE, et al. Evaluation of calorie requirements for Ranger training at Fort Benning, Georgia. Technical report No. 34, Letterman Army Institute of Research, Presidio of San Francisco, CA, 1976.
60. Johnson MJ, Friedl KE, Frykman PN, Moore RJ. Loss of muscle mass is poorly reflected in grip strength performance in healthy young men. *Med Sci Sports Exerc* 1994;26:235–240.
61. Pleban RJ, Valentine PJ, Penetar DM, Redmond DP, Belenky GL. Characterization of sleep and body composition changes during Ranger training. *Milit Psychol* 1990;2:145–156.
62. Friedl KE, Mays MZ, Kramer TR. Acute recovery of physiological and cognitive function in U.S. Army Ranger students in a multistressor field environment. In: NATO AC/243 panel VIII. Workshop on the effect of prolonged exhaustive military activities on man— physiological and psychological changes—possible means of rapid recuperation. April 1995.
63. Kramer TR, Moore RJ, Shippee RL, et al. Influences of energy intake and expenditure on expressed T-lymphocyte activation. *Int J Sports Med* 1997 (in press).
64. Sauberlich HE. Implications of nutritional status on human biochemistry, physiology and health. *Clin Biochem* 1984;17:132–142.
65. Roubenoff R. Hormones, cytokines and body composition: can lessons from illness be applied to aging? *J Nutr* 1993;123:469–473.
66. Friedl KE. When does energy deficit affect soldier physical performance? In: Marriott BM, ed. *Not eating enough.* Washington, DC: National Academy Press; 1995:253–283.
67. Ballor DL, Tommerup LJ, Smith DB, Thomas DP. Body composition, muscle and fat pad changes following two levels of dietary restriction and/or exercise training in male rats. *Int J Obes* 1990;14:711–722.

Physiology, Stress, and Malnutrition: Functional Correlates, Nutritional Intervention,
edited by J.M. Kinney and H.N. Tucker.
Lippincott–Raven Publishers © 1997.

Limits of Human Endurance: Lessons from the Tour de France

Wim H.M. Saris

Nutrition Research Institute "NUTRIM", University of Maastricht, Maastricht 6200 MD, The Netherlands

A classical nutrition article appeared in the *New England Journal of Medicine* in 1935 from Edwards, Thorndike, and Dill (1). They discussed the energy requirements during strenuous muscular exercise by Harvard football players and challenged the reader with descriptions of exercise-related energy metabolism. Today there continues a growing interest by a wide segment of the population in understanding the limits of human performance even though mechanization of most occupations has reduced everyday physical labor demands drastically. Now people try to reach the limits of human endurance just to prove that ability. These efforts have even become part of accepted recreational activities. Swimmers who swim the English Channel do double crossings, runners run 100 or more miles, and climbers attack Mount Everest without benefit of supplementary oxygen. However, few sports are as varied and physiologically challenging as professional competitive cycling. The Tour de France is the ultimate test of the peak of human performance. During the Tour de France a cyclist must pedal about 4,000 km over a period of 22 days with only one day allowed for rest.

The capacity of an individual to do hard muscular exercise day after day has a definite limit. The classical study of sustained muscular effort was conducted with lumber workers from Maine in 1904. The study relied on the measurement of energy intake to estimate energy expenditure. Wood and Mainsfield concluded that the study participants expended regularly up to 33 MJ/day (2). In contrast, energy expenditures during the Tour de France have been measured up to 38 MJ/day using the more precise doubly-labeled water techniques (3). It is interesting to note also that the work challenges during the Tour de France vary much more than most of the classical studies on endurance. The daily workload varies from the resting day to racing days with extremely long work duration (up to 8–9 hours of cycling per day). Additionally, extremes in intensity vary when cycling over five to six mountain passes per day at altitudes of over 2,000 m. Other days consist of short speed trials with 30 minutes of high-intensity work. The human physiologic demands resulting from these variations in intensity make the Tour de France cyclist an attractive model on which to base the study the regulatory mechanisms that must come into play to maintain energy balance under extraordinary conditions. Further investigation of these subjects also provides insight regarding metabolic processes that lead to physical exhaustion and depletion. Because these subjects are without the underlying disease that is often the case in hospitalized malnourished patients, the data are not complicated by the concomitant disease process.

The purpose of this chapter is to describe the physiologic effects on professional cyclists during the 3 weeks of the Tour de France and to draw attention to physiologic lessons learned from these observations that might be relevant to the physiologic stress and to malnutrition, and with functional correlates of nutritional intervention that might provide some insight into the future clinical care of hospitalized patients.

METHODOLOGY

Eight male subjects, all members of a leading professional cycling team, were recruited to participate in this study. Five of the eight were willing to record their daily food intake and nutritional supplement consumption during the race. One cyclist had an accident on the fifth day of the race and was forced to withdraw; however, one of the other cyclists was willing to provide nutrient consumption information for the last 2 weeks to replace the data of the injured cyclist.

Independent of the collection of nutrient intake data, the four remaining cyclists also participated in the detailed measurement of energy expenditure using the doubly-labeled water technique over the three 1-week periods. Fasting blood samples were taken from all eight cyclists before the tour, at the last day of each week, and at the end of the tour. Samples were analyzed for hematologic parameters, vitamins, minerals, and individual amino acid concentrations. Energy expenditure also was calculated from a diary of daily activities based on equations from the literature. Data on body composition was gathered within 1 week before and within 1 week after the tour. The percentage body fat was estimated using the sum of four skinfold thickness measurements according to the method of Durnin and Womersley (4). Maximum aerobic power of each subject was measured before the race using continuously increasing stress test (25 Watt/min) by means of an electronically braked cycle ergometer, and oxygen consumption was monitored using an automatic metabolic analyzer.

The study results of energy expenditure measured by doubly-labeled water technique (3), aspects of food intake (5), and adequacy of vitamin and mineral supply (6) have been reported previously. This chapter focuses on the effect of the tour on the cyclists' energy balance and amino acid metabolism.

TABLE 1. *Cyclists' characteristics*

Subject	Height (m)	Aerobic power (VO$_2$ ml/ kg/min)	Weight (kg) Before	After	Body fat (%) Before	After
1	1.81	75.2	71.6	71.6	13.2	13.2
2	1.80	79.0	75.2	74.0	11.1	10.6
3	1.69	80.8	61.4	61.9	9.8	10.0
4	1.81	82.4	68.7	68.3	12.1	11.8
Mean (n = 4 subjects)	1.78	79.4	69.2	68.9	11.6	11.4
Mean ± SD (n = 7 subjects)	1.79 ± 0.06	80.3 ± 3.6	69.5 ± 4.5	69.3 ± 4.7	11.2 ± 1.6	11.1 ± 1.6

CHARACTERISTICS OF THE CYCLISTS

Table 1 provides information for each of the four cyclists with respect to aerobic power and body composition and the mean results for the group of seven finishing cyclists before and after the race.

In 1935 and 1955, data for eight internationally famous distance runners and six cross-country skiers were published under the heading "New Records in Human Power" (7,8). The maximal aerobic power published for these men ranged from about 70 ml O$_2$/kg/min to a maximum of 81.7 ml O$_2$/kg/min. Except for some outstanding individual reports (9), it appears that values between 75 and 85 ml O$_2$/kg/min represent the top of the aerobic power for today's elite endurance athletes as represented by the cyclists in our study group. To our knowledge, a mean aerobic power of 80.3 ml O$_2$ kg/min is the highest recorded value for a group of athletes. It is interesting to note that these values have not changed since the 1930s despite the more advanced training methods that have evolved over the years. The second important observation is the consistency and balance in body weight with respect to body fat over the entire 3-week period of the Tour de France. It is obvious that these athletes were able to maintain their energy balance in the face of enormous challenges remarkably well.

ENERGY EXPENDITURE

The energy expenditure of four Tour de France cyclists was calculated through the 22 days of the race using the following procedure:

Actual sleeping time was recorded and a value of 0.074 kJ min/kg was used to calculate sleeping energy expenditure.

Activities during nonracing, nonsleeping times were kept to a minimum by the cyclists so that they could rest, eat, and recover for the next day. Our subjects kept no diary of these activities; we assumed nonracing energy expenditure at 1.5 times the sleeping level.

For the race itself, detailed information was available about the length of each day's tour, differences in altitude over the course, road paving, length of ascents and descents, and finishing times.

Energy output was calculated according to the following equations (10,11):

$$E_{cycl} = (K_1 V^3 + K_2 V) \times T + K_3 H \qquad [1]$$

where E_{cycl} is the energy output (kJ), V is the cycling speed (m/s), T is the cycling time (s), and H is the change in altitude (m); K_1, K_2, and K_3 are factors of air resistance, rolling resistance, and weight, respectively.

$$K_1 = 1 \times <m135>^3 m \times p \times s \times e^{-0.000125\ H} \qquad [2]$$

where l is subject height (length) in meters, m is subject weight or mass in kilograms, p is posture (for vertical posture, p = 1.15; for race posture, p = 1), s is shielding (for maximal shielding, s = 0.7), and H is altitude (m). Shielding is the reduced air resistance cyclists seek by riding closely behind another cyclist. The rolling resistance value K_2 is a function of weight of the subject (m_s) and of the bike (m_b) and of road paving (r).

$$K_2 = (m_s + m_b) \times r \qquad [3]$$

The factor K_3 is calculated from Eq. 4

$$K_3 = (m_s + m_b) \times 9.82 \qquad [4]$$

Because it was impossible to record the cycling posture and shielding, we decided to calculate energy output based on assumptions that were as close to the race situation as possible. For the flat course, we calculated K_1-based shielding 90% of the time and a vertical posture. For the hilly courses, 50% shielding and 50% vertical posture was used, and in the mountainous courses we assumed that there was a vertical position and no shielding. Cycling against or with the wind (V) was not included in the equation because over a period of 22 days it is reasonable to assume that this factor is zero. For mechanical efficiency a value of 22% was chosen.

Energy intake was measured from food records with the cyclists noting their daily food intake in a diary. A nutritionist made weekly checks of the diary and cross-checked the information recorded with the record of food supplied during the race. The information recorded also included beverages because carbohydrate-rich energy drinks made up a substantial part of the daily energy intake. The data were converted to energy intake using a computerized nutrient data bank.

The cycling course of the Tour de France can be segmented into periods of different exercise intensity. The first 9 days of the tour, the terrain was essentially flat. A second period followed on day 10 with a 227-km course over six mountain passes. The terrain became hilly through day 14. Day 15 was a resting day. During the last week, the course again took the cyclists over several mountain passes.

Table 2 shows the results of the calculated energy intake and energy expenditure over the 3-week period, including the highest mean daily expenditure and intake levels. Relative percentage contribution of macronutrients to energy intake also is given. Energy expenditure varied over the days from 12.9 MJ during the resting day to a mean 32.7 MJ on the most taxing day (day 10). Days 8 and 21 required a long-distance ride of over 300 km. During these days a high-energy expenditure was predicted that was comparable with that of the mountain-climbing days (days 10, 17, 18, and 19), on which the distances were shorter (151–227 km) but more taxing. The results from the measurements with the doubly-labeled water technique showed even higher values of 32 MJ per day, up to 39 MJ on day 10 (3). The energy expenditures of these cyclists are the highest that have been reported for periods of longer than seven days.

A question often posed to exercise physiologists, and to the athletes themselves, is to what extent can existing endurance records be exceeded. In other words, is there an energy expenditure ceiling? When comparing different energy expenditures by species, including *Homo sapiens*, comparable ratios are shown when 24-hour energy expenditure divided by resting metabolic rate. Animal activity indexes ranged from 1.0 to 6.9, whereas the human activity index ranged from low levels of 1.0–1.2 up to 5.6 for the professional cyclists. Only four species have higher reported values than the athletes in our study—a small Australian possum reached 5.7; a macaroni penguin reached 5.8; and the gannet (a large seabird) and a small Australian marsupial mouse both reached the highest recorded value of 6.9. Based on data from a wide range of homeotherms under energy-demanding conditions such as rapid growth, heavy lactation, hard work, and living in a cold environment, Kirkwood suggested that there is an interspecies limit for endurance capacity of about five times basal metabolic rate (BMR) (12). In particular, experiments with lactating animals and nesting birds feeding young have shown that metabolic rate does not exceed five to six times BMR. Even after adopting extra pups, the metabolic rate of this apparent maximum is not exceeded. With further increase of litter size, the mother begins to refuse some pups.

What factors are that might impose an upper limit on work performance is an intriguing question. Although beyond the scope of this chapter, it is of interest

TABLE 2. *Mean energy expenditure and energy intake (±SD) and means of the lowest and highest values of energy expenditure and intake (±SD)*

	Energy expenditure	Multiple of BMR[a]	Energy intake
Mean MJ/day	25.4 ± 1.4	3.4	24.7 ± 2.4
Lowest MJ/day	12.9 ± 0.9	1.7	16.1 ± 3.9
Highest MJ/day	32.7 ± 1.6	4.4	32.4 ± 4.4
Relative contribution to total energy intake	Protein	Fat	Carbohydrate
Energy %	15.4 ± 2.4	22.4 ± 1.3	60.6 ± 2.9

[a]Multiple of BMR was calculated from calculated sleeping expenditure and total expenditure.

to comment briefly on the role of the ability of the intestine to absorb nutrients in limiting energy intake. The data from Brener et al. (13) describing the gastric emptying characteristics for glucose are provided in most gastroenterology text-books as the standard for regulating of nutrient energy release to the duodenum. The result obtained from healthy (but most likely not very active subjects) was 2.13 kcal/min. We have measured gastric emptying of glucose in highly trained endurance athletes over the years and always found values higher than 4.0 kcal/min (14).

In 1975 Crane published (15) the first quantitative comparison of intestinal nutrient absorptive capacities and nutrient intake. He calculated that the small intestine can absorb quantities of sugar equivalent to over 50,000 kcal/day. This is far beyond the energy requirements in relation to the maximal endurance capacity. Based on a review of experimental animal work, Karasov and Daimond (16) came to the conclusion that there are many examples of adaptive responses that increase the intestinal capacity to absorb nutrients. However, in contrast to those previous beliefs, the small intestine possesses only a modest excess of nutrient absorptive capacity over nutrient intake.

In recent years it has become clear that this enormous excess in absorption capacity does not exist. Animal studies using new and more precise luminal glu-cose concentration measurements suggest an absorptive capacity of only about 10,000 kcal for carbohydrates. From these data, derived from luminal glucose concentrations ranging up to 50 mmol, it has been calculated that the absorptive capacity exceeds intake by a factor of approximately two (16). Although the intestine possesses some excess capacity sufficient to handle an unexpected increase in carbohydrate load, these reports suggest that there is not an enormous excess capacity and that an enormous excess capacity that might waste energy on carbohydrate transporters that will not be used does not occur.

In a simulation study in the respiration chambers with a carbohydrate intake of 1,282 g/day, the carbohydrate oxidation rate did not exceed 950 g/day. During the 3-week Tour de France study period the mean carbohydrate intake was 851 g/day (3,400 kcal). The total energy expenditure measured during the two cycling days in the chambers was 5,590 kcal/day (17). These data underline the impression that an energetic ceiling of human endurance capacity was reached during the 22-day cycling race.

ENERGY BALANCE

The day-to-day energy balance under these extreme conditions is of special physiologic interest. Previously, several studies have addressed the topic of energy balance by a detailed analysis of daily energy intake and energy expenditure in subjects, primarily military cadets in training camps (18). Data from 1,076 man-days representing a total of 57 subjects did not show any relationship between daily intake and daily expenditure. Also, daily weight changes and energy balance on a day-to-day basis showed no relationship. Over a period of 1 week, however, there was a highly significant correlation between weight changes and energy balance. Similarly, mean weekly intake and expenditure were considered there was a significant correlation. It was suggested in some of the studies that intake follows expenditure with a 2-day interval, although this lag is not confirmed by others. To study this phenomenon in our athletes, we calculated the moving average for energy expenditure and for energy intake over 2–5 days and determined the individual relationships between intake and expenditure over the periods from day 1 to day 5. In Table 3 it is clearly shown that the correlation became more apparent comparing day 1 with day 3. Further extension of the period did not yield further relationship changes between either variable.

The close relationship between intake and expenditure over a 3-day period is demonstrated in Fig. 1. It is clear that intake closely follows expenditure. During days on which there were sharp increases or decreases in expenditure (days 7–9, 13–15, and 16–18), intake at first lagged, then changed and achieved balance. Over the 22 days there was an overall deficit of only 3,000 kcal representing only about 2% of the total energy expenditure for the period. The observed 3-day period is interesting and indicates that the 2-day lag period suggested by Edholm (18) seems to represent a physiologic phenomenon under the conditions of hard physical work. Many of the compensating mechanisms previously suggested—body temperature, blood lipid, glucose or insulin concentrations—might well come into play on a short-term basis, but it is difficult to understand how these mechanisms might work over an extended 2- to 3-day period. The recently cloned appetite and energy expenditure regulatory hormone, leptin, produced by the adipose tissue in vivo, could play an important role (19). However, if this is the case, we need to reformulate concepts concerning the metabolic capacity of the fat cell under these conditions. Besides the physiologic explanations for this remarkable capacity to keep energy balance in line under such conditions, we have to include the possibility of behavioral aspects. These highly experienced cyclists have learned how to eat an enormous amount of food during hard physical work. We calculated that only about a 50% of total food intake (approximately 3,000 kcal) was ingested during the race per se (5). Because the digestive capacity is limited, it is clear that it would be difficult to compensate for the resulting negative energy balance from one day during the next day. To compete successfully, the professional cyclist learns to

TABLE 3. *Individual Pierson correlation coefficients of the moving average of energy expenditure and energy intake over 1–5 days*

	Cyclists			
	1	2	3	4
1 day	0.75	0.79	0.80	0.82
2 days	0.81	0.88	0.84	0.91
3 days	0.91	0.95	0.93	0.96
4 days	0.93	0.95	0.95	0.96
5 days	0.93	0.95	0.94	0.97

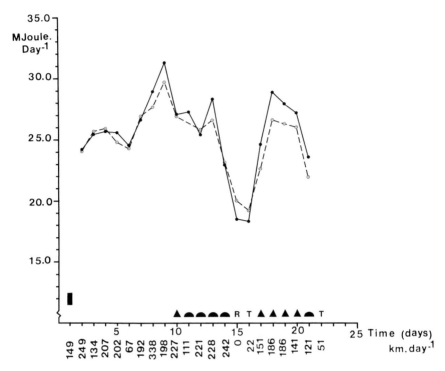

FIG. 1. Three-day moving average of the mean values per day of four subjects for calculated energy expenditure (●—●) (MJ/day) and energy intake (⊙----⊙) (MJ/day) during the 22-day cycling race of the Tour de France. Characteristics of the race are plotted on the x-axis: ▲, mountain circuit, ◭ hill circuit; R, resting day; T, time trial race over short distance. Each day's cycling distance is given in km. For comparison, the recommended energy intake for young adults doing light work is 9.6–13.0 MJ/day with a mean intake of about 12 MJ/day (hatched bar on y-axis).

attempt to maintain energy balance on a day-to-day basis. This knowledge could also be an important driving force in the energy intake habits in these elite athletes.

PROTEIN INTAKE AND PLASMA AMINO ACID CONCENTRATION DURING ENDURANCE EXERCISE

Each racing day induces an acute disturbance of homeostasis in cells and organs that is related to fatigue. During the recovery phase, homeostasis must be reestablished. However, even under these extreme circumstances recovery must take place within 16 hours because another demanding exercise bout is scheduled the next day. Little is known about metabolism during the day-to-day exercise and recovery phases. We demonstrated for the first time that glycogen resynthesis can be achieved within 16 hours after exhausting exercise if a high-level carbohydrate intake is maintained (17). To date, information about protein metabolism during recovery is lacking. Because amino acids are the key elements for the contracting muscle cell, changes in plasma amino acid concentration over time during exercise is of interest. Although individual amino acid concentrations do not necessarily reflect turnover rate of amino acids or proteins, decreases or increases in the fasting resting plasma amino acids could perhaps give some indication of changes in the metabolic process resulting from extreme exercise. Table 4 lists the most important amino acids and their metabolites. Values were obtained from venous blood samples drawn early in the morning, just after waking up, and before having breakfast. Samples were taken on day 0, day 7 (after 1 week), day 15 (after 2 weeks), day 16 (after resting 1 day), and at the end of day 22.

Urea is the major product of protein metabolism in humans. The increased concentration of urea after the first week suggests that under these conditions protein turnover is high. In general, endurance exercise promotes a decrease in protein synthesis with perhaps an increase in protein breakdown (20). Previous exercise studies have concentrated primarily on the amino acid leucine and indicate a substantial increase in leucine oxidation that approaches daily leucine requirements. Although the relative protein to energy intake is within the normal range (approximately 15% of total energy), the amount of protein ingested daily by these cyclists is extremely high. In absolute terms, mean

TABLE 4. *Resting plasma amino acid concentrations in seven cyclists at days 0, 7, 15, 16, and 22 of the race*

Amino acid	Day 0	Day 7	Day 15	Day 16	Day 22	p
Urea 10^3	7.6 ± 0.7	9.1 ± 1.2	8.3 ± 1.1	7.0 ± 1.1	7.8 ± 0.5[b]	
Taurine	68 ± 13	59 ± 11	50 ± 10	51 ± 8	42 ± 11[a,b]	
Threonine	109 ± 24	113 ± 23	106 ± 20	116 ± 25	122 ± 25	
Serine	1.04 ± 22	80 ± 24	79 ± 13	76 ± 15	81 ± 16[a,b]	
Aspartic acid	56 ± 13	60 ± 32	67 ± 9	43 ± 12	71 ± 11[a,c]	
Glutamic acid	29 ± 15	43 ± 23	45 ± 5	58 ± 27	32 ± 8	
Glutamine	568 ± 56	523 ± 48	503 ± 51	510 ± 45	479 ± 65[a,b]	
Glycine	251 ± 67	195 ± 29	221 ± 25	241 ± 36	222 ± 44	
Alanine	382 ± 72	349 ± 46	336 ± 47	406 ± 62	336 ± 62	
Citrulline	76 ± 18	41 ± 7	33 ± 7	32 ± 7	34 ± 12[a,b]	
Valine	282 ± 54	312 ± 57	296 ± 10	251 ± 32	342 ± 81[a,b]	
Methionine	28 ± 4	34 ± 7	29 ± 4	29 ± 4	32 ± 4	
Leucine	142 ± 14	168 ± 38	155 ± 7	157 ± 13	177 ± 37[a]	
Isoleucine	76 ± 9	88 ± 20	80 ± 5	68 ± 7	97 ± 22[a,b]	
Tyrosine	59 ± 14	65 ± 10	61 ± 6	61 ± 10	71 ± 12[a]	
Phenylalanine	52 ± 5.6	61 ± 9	61 ± 4	57 ± 5	60 ± 16[b]	
Ornithine	74 ± 16	81 ± 17	81 ± 17	90 ± 23	101 ± 18[a]	
Lysine	201 ± 27	230 ± 20	240 ± 21	230 ± 24	251 ± 25[a,b,c]	
Histidine	74 ± 15	77 ± 10	73 ± 5	77 ± 5	86 ± 10	
Arginine	80 ± 28	75 ± 20	68 ± 21	76 ± 11	86 ± 17	

Values are mean μmol/L ± SD.
[a]$p < 0.05$;ANOVA over days 0, 7, 15, and 22.
[b]$p < 0.05$;paired *t* test day 0 vs. 7.
[c]$p < 0.05$;paired *t* test day 15 vs. 16.

daily intake was 3.9 g protein/kg body weight. Therefore, amino acid intake was abundant compared with daily requirements. Whether the significant increase in plasma leucine was a reflection of this increased intake during the race is not known. Exercise does not increase the oxidation of all amino acids (21). Therefore, endurance exercise may cause negative nitrogen balance and increased urea production due to an increased requirement for a specific amino acid. Although a relatively large number of the amino acids did increase or decrease significantly over time, it is difficult to interpret these changes.

The most remarkable changes occurred during the first week of cycling, indicating a relatively higher exercise stress during that period. This was confirmed by the changes in plasma cortisol and testosterone concentrations. Cortisol increased by 62% over baseline levels, whereas testosterone decreased by 13%. The cortisol/testosterone ratio nearly doubled in this first week (from 27.4 to 50.7). It has been suggested that the cortisol/testosterone ratio is indicative of signs associated with fatigue (22). The cyclists themselves indicated that this period was the most demanding. In weeks 2 and 3 the ratio returned to pre-race levels (34.4 and 28.6, respectively). This was in contrast to the degree of exercise stress that increased over the weeks. Based on the information from the athletes, it is suggested that the start of this type of exercise causes much greater stress on a day-to-day basis on the human body than an extreme level of exercise after the body has adapted to high-intensity exercise.

The nature of this study does not allow speculation about the metabolic change of each amino acid in relation to endurance exercise stress. But the results in Table 4 clearly show that the repeated bouts of exercise have an impact on amino acid metabolism. The recovery periods seem to be too short to restore homeostasis despite adequate intake of protein. Although total amino acid concentration does not change significantly (20), there are changes in specific amino acids: an increase in lysine, ornithine, and the branched chain amino acids (valine leucine and isoleucine) and a decrease in taurine, serine, citrulline, and glutamine. Detailed stable isotope studies with the specific amino acids should reveal the metabolic importance of the observed shifts over time (23).

CLINICAL IMPLICATIONS

The observation of the physiologic changes in healthy subjects during extreme endurance exercise over long periods could be of importance to provide better insights regarding the metabolic processes during the malnutrition and catabolism associated with the hospitalized patient. A number of physiologic variables have been described in a group of professional cyclists during the world's most demanding sporting event, the Tour de France. These cyclists must have extremely well-developed endurance capacity in order to cope with the high level of endurance exercise. Individual energy expenditure reached 9,500 kcal (40 MJ)/day. The mean expenditure over the 3-week period was 6,070 kcal (25.4

MJ)/day. The data are consistent with an energy expenditure ceiling in humans as has been described in various other species. Energy intake followed expenditure closely with a maximal time lag of 2 days. Again the lag seems logical from a physiologic point of view. Without the 2-day lag, the food intake required to compensate for immediate energy needs would quickly exceed intestinal absorption capacity. Because the energy turnover is extremely high, energy stores such as adipose tissue, intramuscular triglycerides, and glycogen in liver and muscle are of minor importance. As a consequence, these cyclists maintain energy balance remarkably well on a day-to-day basis. It can be concluded that they were able to recover within 16 hours with respect to carbohydrate and probably fat stores.

The resting total concentration of plasma amino acids did not change during the race. However, individual amino acids significantly decreased or increased, indicating that the recovery periods are too short to restore amino acid homeostasis despite the fact that protein intake was very high (>3 g/kg/day). Indicators of endurance exercise stress such as the cortisol/testosterone ratio showed an increase only in the first week. The importance of exercise stress on amino acid metabolism is indicated by the changes in resting plasma amino acids concentration that were pronounced in this early period. However, the limited data from this study do not allow speculation on the nature of the metabolic changes.

REFERENCES

1. Edwards HT, Thorndike AA, Dill DB. The energy requirement in strenuous muscular exercise. *N Engl J Med* 1935;213:532–535.
2. Wood CD, Mansfield ER. *Studies of the food of Maine lumbermen.* Bull no. 149. Washington, DC: U.S. Department of Agriculture; 1904.
3. Westerterp KR, Saris WHM, Es van M, Hooten F. Use of doubly labeled water technique in humans during heavy sustained exercise. *J Appl Physiol* 1986;61:2162–2167.
4. Durnin JVGA, Womersley J. Body fat assessed from local body density and its estimation from skinfold thickness: measurements of 481 men and women aged from 16 to 72 years. *Br J Nutr* 1974;32:77–97.
5. Saris WHM, Erp-Baart van MA, Brouns F, Westerterp KR, Hoorten F. Study on food intake and energy expenditure during extreme sustained exercise: the Tour de France. *Int J Sport Med* 1989;10(suppl 1): 26–31.
6. Saris WHM, Schrijver J, Erp-Baart van MA, Brouns F. Adequacy of vitamin supply under maximal sustained work loads: the Tour de France. *Int J Vit Nutr Res* 1989;59:205–212.
7. Robinson S, Edwards HT, Dill DB. New records in human power. *Science* 1937;85:409–410.
8. Astrand PO. New records in human power. *Nature* 1955;176:922–923.
9. Astrand PO, Rodahl K. *Textbook of work physiology.* New York: McGraw-Hill; 1977.
10. Faria IE, Cavanaugh PR. *The physiology and biomechanics of cycling.* New York: Wiley; 1978.
11. Whitt FR, Wilson DG. *Bicycling science.* Cambridge, MA: MIT Press; 1974.
12. Kirkwood JK. A limit to metabolisable energy intake in mammals and birds. *Comp Biochem Physiol [A]* 1983;75:1–3.
13. Brener W, Hendrix TR, McHugh PR Regulation of the gastric emptying of glucose. *Gastroenterology* 1983;85:76–82.
14. Brouns F, Senden J, Beckers EJ, Saris WHM. Osmolarity does not affect the gastric emptying rate of oral rehydration solutions. *J Parenter Enter Nutr* 1995;19:403–406.
15. Crane RK. The physiology of the intestine absorption of sugars. In: Hodges JA, ed. *Physiological effect of food carbohydrates.* Washington, DC: American Chemical Society; 1975:1–19.
16. Karasov WH, Daimond JM. Adaptive regulation of sugar and amino acid transport by vertebrate intestine. *Am J Physiol* 1983;245:G443–G462.

17. Brouns F, Saris WHM, Beckers EJ, et al. Metabolic changes induced by sustained exhaustive cycling and diet manipulation. Int J Sport Med 1989;10(suppl 1):49–62.
18. Edholm OG. Energy balance in man. *J Hum Nutr* 1977;31:413–431.
19. Considine RV, Sinha MK, Heiman ML, et al. Serum immunoreactive-leptin concentrations in normal weight and obese humans. *N Engl J Med* 1996;334:292–295.
20. Lemon PWR. Does exercise alter dietary protein requirements? In: Brouns F, Newsholm EA, Saris WHM, eds. *Advances in nutrition and top sport.* Basel, Switzerland: Karger; 1996:15–37.
21. Wolfe RR, Wolfe MA, Nadel ER, Shaw JHF. Isotopic determination of amino acids-urea interactions in exercise in humans. *J Appl Physiol* 1984;54:458–466.
22. Fry RW, Morton R, Keast D. Overtraining in athletes: an update. *Sport Med* 1991;12:32–65.
23. Wolfe RR. *Radioactive and stable isotope tracers in biomedicine.* New York: Wiley-Liss; 1992.

Physiology, Stress, and Malnutrition: Functional Correlates, Nutritional Intervention, edited by J.M. Kinney and H.N. Tucker. Lippincott–Raven Publishers © 1997.

Biochemical Aspects of Muscle Fatigue

Paul L. Greenhaff, Anna Casey, D. Constantin-Teodosiu, Allison L. Green, E. Hultman, K. Soderlund, and James A. Timmons

Department of Physiology and Pharmacology, University Medical School, Queen's Medical Centre, Nottingham N67 2UH, United Kingdom

Exercise rapidly increases the energy demand of skeletal muscle, and because the store of adenosine triphosphate (ATP) in skeletal muscle is limited [24 mmol/kg dry matter (dm)], this necessitates an equivalent increase in the rate of ATP resynthesis for contraction to continue. During submaximal exercise, rapid anaerobic ATP resynthesis from phosphocreatine (PCr) and glycogen hydrolysis occurs at the onset of exercise until a steady-state condition is achieved and oxidative phosphorylation becomes the major contributor. However, during maximal exercise, when the energy demand of contraction can be very high (e.g., 11 mmol/kg dm/s) and fatigue occurs rapidly, anaerobic energy provision can account for the majority of the total ATP demand of contraction. By way of example, Bangsbo et al. (1) reported that during 192 seconds of exercise at a workload equivalent to 130% of maximal consumption, anaerobic ATP resynthesis during the initial 30 seconds of exercise contributed approximately 80% of the total ATP demand. This then declined to 45% from 60 to 90 seconds and to 30% after 120 seconds of exercise. These investigators also presented data to indicate that the remainder of the ATP demand was met by a parallel increase in oxidative phosphorylation.

The present chapter will be concerned principally with the biochemistry of intense muscular contraction, and therefore the majority of the studies described relate to exercise intensities of a considerably higher intensity than those described above, i.e., situations in which the anaerobic contribution to ATP production is greater than 80% and fatigue development occurs in less than 30 s.

ANAEROBIC ENERGY PROVISION DURING INTENSE MUSCLE CONTRACTION

Margaria et al. (2) reported in the 1960s that during maximal exercise of 10–15 seconds duration the total energy demand of contraction could be met by hydrolysis of muscle ATP and PCr stores. These investigators postulated that only when the muscle PCr store was depleted would ATP resynthesis occur via glycogen hydrolysis to lactate. This belief arose as a consequence of PCr being stored in the cytosol in close proximity to the sites of energy utilization and because PCr hydrolysis does not depend on oxygen availability or necessitate the completion of several metabolic reactions before energy is liberated to fuel ATP resynthesis. However, this hypothesis is now less well accepted because several groups have demonstrated that PCr hydrolysis and lactate production do not occur in isolation (3–6). For example, Bergstrom et al. (3) demonstrated that the muscle PCr concentration had declined by 20% and the lactate concentration had increased by 15 mmol/kg dm within 6.6 seconds of isometric contraction.

With the introduction of percutaneous electrical stimulation (7), it became possible to investigate muscle metabolism and fatigue under conditions where complications relating to subject motivation were avoided and under which it was possible to study muscle metabolism in a closed compartment. The use of electrical stimulation also enabled muscle biopsy samples to be obtained during isometric contraction, which is obviously not possible during dynamic exercise. Using this technique, it was demonstrated that as little as 1.3 seconds of stimulation was sufficient to degrade PCr by 11 mmol/kg dm and increase lactate accumulation by 2 mmol/kg dm (8). This study clearly demonstrated that PCr and lactate production occurred simultaneously at the onset of contraction.

Although it is now accepted that anaerobic degradation of glycogen to lactate also makes a significant contribution to ATP resynthesis during the initial seconds of intense exercise, the importance of PCr hydrolysis lies in the extremely rapid rates at which it can resynthesize ATP. This is especially true of maximal short-duration exercise. For example, Fig. 1 shows the rate of muscle ATP resynthesis from PCr hydrolysis during 30 seconds of maximal electrically evoked isometric contraction (9). PCr hydrolysis was at its highest within 2 seconds of the initiation of contraction. It is likely that the momentary increase in adenosine diphosphate (ADP) concentration at the onset of contraction was the primary stimulus for this hydrolysis. After only 2.6 seconds of contraction, however, the rate of ATP production from PCr had declined by about 15%, and after 10 seconds of contraction it was reduced by more than 50%. The contribution of PCr to ATP resynthesis in the last 10 seconds of a 30-second exercise bout was small, amounting to only 2% of the initial yield. The mechanisms responsible for the almost instantaneous decline in the rate of PCr utilization during maximal exercise are at present unknown but may be related to a local myofibrillar decline in its availability. Considering the high-energy demand of maximal exercise, it is possible that the rapid rate of PCr utilization at the onset of contraction could be responsible for a rapid depletion of stores at the sites of rapid energy translocation (actomyosin cross-bridges). Certainly, this seems plausible because when intense exercise is continued for more than 20 seconds, the cellular store of PCr becomes almost depleted, which is likely to be a consequence of mitochondrial ATP production being unable to match the rate of PCr hydrolysis.

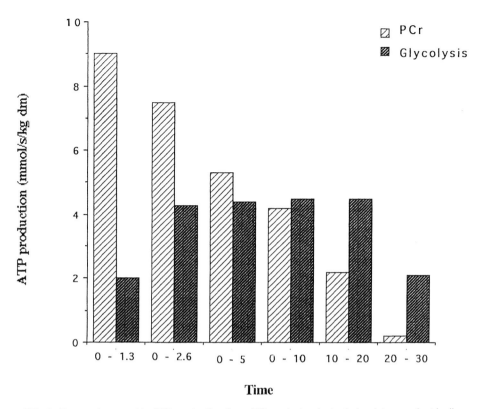

FIG. 1. Rates of anaerobic ATP production from PCr and glycolysis during intense electrically evoked muscle contraction in humans.

Although glycogen hydrolysis to lactate is now known to proceed almost instantaneously from the onset of contraction, it is clear from the rate of decline in the rate of PCr hydrolysis in Fig. 1 that if maximal exercise is to continue beyond only a few seconds, glycogenolysis and glycolysis must begin to proceed at rapid rates within a few seconds of the initiation of contraction. The integrative nature of energy metabolism ensures that the activation of muscle contraction by Ca^{2+} and the accumulation of the products of ATP and PCr hydrolysis [ADP, adenosine monophosphate (AMP), inosine monophosphate (IMP), ammonia (NH_3^+), and inorganic phosphate (Pi)] act as stimulators of glycogenolysis and glycolysis and in this way guarantee that anaerobic ATP production is maintained, at least in the short term.

The control of glycogenolysis during muscle contraction is a highly complex mechanism that can no longer be considered to center around the degree of transformation of less active glycogen phosphorylase *b* to the more active *a* form (10). For some time it has been known that glycogenolysis can proceed at a negligible rate, despite almost total transformation of phosphorylase to the *a* form (11). Conversely, an increase in glycogenolytic rate has been observed during circulatory occlusion, despite a relatively low mole fraction of the phosphorylase *a* form (10). From this and other related work, it was concluded that Pi accumulation arising from ATP and PCr hydrolysis played a key role in the regulation of the glycogenolytic activity of phosphorylase *a,* and by doing so served as a link between the energy demand of the contraction and the rate of substrate utilization. However, the findings that glycogenolysis can occur within 2 seconds of the onset of muscle contraction without any significant increase in Pi (12), and more recently that glycogenolysis can proceed at a low rate despite a high phosphorylase *a* form and Pi concentration (13), suggests that factors other than the degree of phosphorylase transformation and Pi availability are involved in the regulation of glycogenolysis. More recent evidence suggests that both IMP and AMP are more important regulators of glycogenolysis during exercise (14,15). IMP is thought to exert its effect by increasing the activity of phosphorylase *b* during contraction [apparent Km of phosphorylase *b* for IMP ~1.2 mmol/L intracellular water (16,17)]. AMP also has been shown to increase the activity of phosphorylase *b,* but it is thought to require an unphysiologic accumulation of free AMP to do so [apparent Km of phosphorylase *b* for AMP ~1.0 mmol/L intracellular water (16,17)]. Furthermore, because 90% or more of the total cell content of AMP has been suggested to be bound to cell proteins in vivo (18), it has in the past been questioned whether the increase in free AMP during contraction is of a sufficient magnitude to affect the kinetics of phosphorylase *a* (14). However, more recent work has demonstrated that a small increase in AMP concentration (10 μmol/L) can markedly increase the in vitro activity of phosphorylase *a* (14). Furthermore, in vivo evidence demonstrating a close relationship between muscle ATP turnover and glycogen utilization suggests that an exercise-induced increase in free AMP and inorganic phosphate may be the key regulators of glycogen degradation during muscle contraction (14,15).

Anaerobic glycolysis involves several more steps than PCr hydrolysis but compared with oxidative phosphorylation is still rapid. As Fig. 1 shows, ATP resynthesis from glycolysis during 30 seconds of maximal electrically evoked contraction begins to occur almost immediately at the onset of exercise. Furthermore, unlike PCr hydrolysis, ATP production from glycolysis does not reach its maximal rate until after 5 seconds of contraction and is maintained at this high rate for several seconds, such that over 30 seconds of exercise, the contribution from anaerobic glycolysis to ATP resynthesis is nearly double that from PCr. This is reflected by the high muscle lactate concentrations (>100 mmol/kg dm) achieved during maximal exercise lasting 30 seconds or more. Ultimately, it is clear that ATP resynthesis via glycolysis cannot be maintained indefinitely. The mechanisms responsible for the decline in glycolysis observed during maximal exercise are unclear but are unlikely to be related to a depletion (local or otherwise) of muscle glycogen stores because levels are still high at the end of maximal exercise (19,20). Indeed, it is unlikely that glycogen availability will limit maximal exercise performance until the preexercise concentration decreases below 100 mmol/kg dm (21,22). A pH-mediated decrease in the activity of phosphorylase and phosphofructokinase (PFK) has been suggested as a possible mechanism that may be responsible for the decrease in glycolysis. However, it is now generally accepted that any potential for a pH-mediated inhibition of glycolysis during maximal exercise is overcome in the in vivo situation by the accumulation of the activators of PFK [e.g., AMP and ammonia (23)]. As stated earlier, both AMP and IMP have been associated with the regulation of glycogen degradation during exercise. It has been suggested that once the rate of glycogen utilization has reached its peak, a decrease in the sarcoplasmic concentration of free AMP (as a consequence of a decrease in the rate of ADP formation and/or a pH-induced increase in the activity of AMP deaminase, the enzyme which catalyses the deamination of AMP to IMP) will result in a diminished activation of phosphorylase *a* and thereby may be responsible for the decline in the rate of glycogenolysis and glycolysis during maximal exercise (9).

SINGLE FIBER RESPONSES DURING INTENSE CONTRACTION

The quadriceps muscle group in humans is known to be composed of at least two fibers that are diametrically opposite in their metabolic and physiologic characteristics (24–27). Type I fibers are characterized as being slow contracting, highly oxidative, and fatigue resistant. Conversely, type II fibers are fast contracting, highly glycolytic and fatigue rapidly. As might be expected, therefore, the two fiber types differ in their maximal rates of ATP utilization and abilities to generate and sustain power output (28). However, it should be appreciated that it is likely that a natural continuum exists between type I and II fibers, and the present classification systems are there principally for convenience sake. The majority of studies aimed at investigating the biochemical and physiologic differences between muscle fiber types have been performed using animal skeletal muscle composed of predominantly a single fiber type. These studies have demonstrated that fast contracting muscle has a relatively high initial power output, which is accompanied by a high rate of anaerobic ATP utilization, but cannot be sustained for more than several seconds. Conversely, muscle composed of predominantly type I fibers has a relatively low initial power output and ATP utilization rate, both of which are maintained during contraction (24–27).

As previously stated, the quadriceps muscle group in humans is not homogeneous, and it is therefore not unreasonable to suggest that the analysis of mixed-fiber muscle biopsy samples will not truly reflect the metabolic and physiologic responses that occur in human skeletal muscle during exercise. We have attempted to relate energy metabolism of type I and II muscle fibers to the development of fatigue during electrically evoked contraction. In one study (29), muscle biopsy samples were obtained from the vastus lateralis at rest and after 10 and 20 seconds of intermittent electrical stimulation (1.6 seconds stimulation,

1.6 seconds rest, at a frequency of 50 Hz) with muscle blood flow intact. The concentrations ATP and PCr were then measured in type I and II muscle fibers dissected from each biopsy sample and are depicted in Fig. 2. During the initial 10 seconds of contraction, the rate of PCr degradation was 60% greater in type II fibers. However, during the remaining 10 seconds of contraction, PCr degradation decreased in type II fibers by 60%, such that there was no difference between fiber types in the rate of PCr degradation. At the end of contraction the PCr concentration in type II fibers was very low.

We have also investigated glycogenolysis in different muscle fiber types during contraction in humans under a variety of experimental conditions, e.g., electrical stimulation (1.6 seconds stimulation, 1.6 seconds rest for 30 seconds) with open circulation (30), electrical stimulation with open circulation and adrenaline infusion (30), electrical stimulation with occluded circulation (31), and during maximal sprint exercise (32). The results are depicted in Fig.

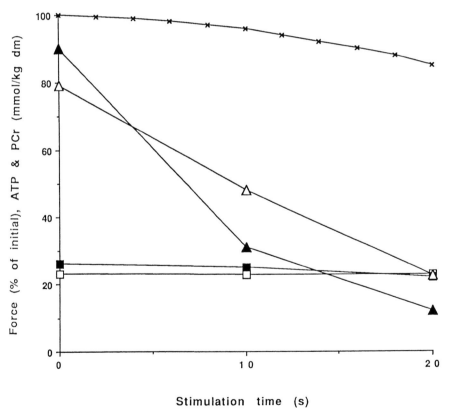

FIG. 2. Muscle isometric force production (× and ATP (□) and PCr (Δ) concentrations in type I (open symbols) and type II (closed symbols) muscle fibers during 20 s of intense electrical stimulation (1.6 s stimulation, 1.6 s rest; 50 Hz) in humans.

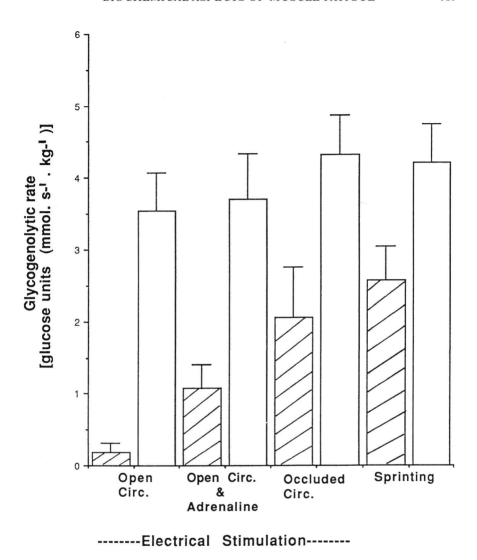

FIG. 3. Glycogenolytic rates in type I (hatched bars) and type II (open bars) fibers during 30 s of intermittent electrical stimulation at 50 Hz with open circulation (circ), open circulation with adrenaline infusion, occluded circulation, and during 30 s of maximal sprint running in humans.

3. In short, it would appear that during intense contraction with circulation intact, glycogenolysis was already occurring maximally in type II fibers, such that when attempts were made to stimulate glycogenolysis further using adrenaline infusion and circulatory occlusion, no increase in glycogenolysis was observed. This suggestion is supported by the finding that the rates of glycogenolysis observed were close to the maximal reaction velocity of phosphorylase measured in type II fibers (33). Glycogenolysis was negligible in

type I fibers during electrically evoked contraction with blood flow intact. This was probably attributable to the comparatively low anaerobic ATP turnover rate of this fiber type during contraction and the oxidative resynthesis of ADP during each 1.6 seconds of recovery between each contraction. This latter suggestion has recently been confirmed by an experiment in which the interval between each contraction was reduced to 0.8 seconds, which resulted in a rapid increase in type I fiber glycogenolysis, i.e., the oxidative rephosphorylation of ADP between each contraction was reduced, resulting in AMP accumulation and the activation of glycogen phosphorylase (Field et al., unpublished observation). Similarly, when blood flow was occluded or when sprint exercise was performed, glycogenolysis was also dramatically increased in type I fibers (Fig. 3), presumably by the same mechanism. This conclusion is supported by the dramatic decline in type I fiber ATP concentrations in the latter studies (31,32) and in the study of Field et al. It is logical that the increase in glycogenolysis in type I fibers after adrenaline infusion occurred as a direct consequence of the activation of phosphorylase by adrenaline (30).

FATIGUE DEVELOPMENT

Can the biochemical changes observed in the above series of studies offer any explanation for the development of fatigue during intense contraction? It is highly likely that fatigue development is a multi-factorial process. However, the findings presented above suggest that during near maximal intensity exercise, ATP is supplied initially by maximal rates of PCr degradation and glycogenolysis, particularly in type II muscle fibers. As exercise progresses, it would appear that the rate of anaerobic ATP turnover declines due to lack of availability of PCr and reduced rate of glycogenolysis. In short, therefore, an imbalance between the rate of ATP demand and ATP provision occurs that could be the mechanism responsible for the development of fatigue. Support for this suggestion comes in part from experiments where repeated bouts of maximal exercise have been performed with short recovery periods between exercise bouts (34,35). These studies have shown that a significant relationship exists between the extent of PCr resynthesis between exercise bouts and subsequent exercise performance. Indeed, we have recently demonstrated that when two bouts of 30 seconds maximal, isokinetic cycling exercise were performed, separated by 4 minutes of recovery, the extent of PCr resynthesis during recovery was positively correlated with work output during the second bout of exercise ($r = 0.8$, $n = 9$, $p < 0.05$) (35). Furthermore, in agreement with the suggestion that the depletion of PCr specifically in type II muscle fibers may be primarily responsible for fatigue, it was demonstrated that the rate of PCr hydrolysis during the first bout of exercise was 35% greater in type II fibers compared with type I fibers. However, during the second bout of exercise the rate of PCr hydrolysis declined by 33% in type II fibers (Fig. 4), which was attributable to incomplete resynthesis of PCr in this

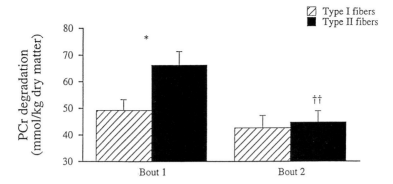

FIG. 4. Changes in PCr in type I and type II muscle fibers during two bouts of 30 s maximal intensity, isokinetic cycling exercise in humans. Each bout of exercise was performed at 80 rev/min and separated by 4 min of passive recovery. *, significant differences between fiber types ($p < 0.05$); ††, significantly different from exercise bout 1 ($p < 0.01$).

fiber type during recovery. Conversely, PCr resynthesis was almost complete in type I fibers during recovery from exercise bout 1, and PCr utilization was unchanged in this fiber type during exercise bout 2 (Fig. 4). This led us to conclude that the reduction in work output during the second bout of exercise may have been related to a slower resynthesis and consequently a reduced availability of PCr in type II muscle fibers (35).

The importance of PCr availability to muscle force production is confirmed by recent experiments demonstrating that dietary creatine (Cr) supplementation can markedly influence muscle Cr uptake and subsequent maximal exercise performance in humans.

CREATINE SUPPLEMENTATION AND FATIGUE

Creatine Biosynthesis and Storage

Creatine, or methyl guanidine-acetic acid, is a naturally occurring compound and in healthy individuals the total body Cr pool is approximately 120 g, 95% of which is found in skeletal muscle. This pool is replenished at a rate of approximately 2 g/day by endogenous Cr synthesis and/or dietary Cr intake, e.g., meat and fish. Oral ingestion of Cr has been demonstrated to suppress biosynthesis, but this response is abolished upon cessation of supplementation (36).

Endogenous Cr synthesis proceeds via two successive reactions involving two enzymes. The first reaction is catalyzed by glycine transamidinase and results in an amidine group being reversibly transferred from arginine to glycine, forming guanidinoacetic acid. The second reaction involves the irreversible transfer of a methyl group from S-adenosylmethionine (SAM) catalyzed by guanidinoacetate methyltransferase, resulting in the methylation of guanidinoacetate and the formation of Cr. The distribution of the two enzymes across tissues varies between mammalian species. In humans, the liver is the major site of de novo Cr synthesis. Because little Cr is found in the major sites of synthesis, it is logical to assume that transport of Cr from its sites of synthesis to storage must occur, thus allowing a separation of biosynthesis from utilization (36).

Muscle Cr uptake occurs actively against a concentration gradient, possibly involving Cr interacting with a specific membrane site that recognizes the amidine group (37). A specific Cr transporter was identified recently in skeletal muscle, heart, and brain (38). About 60% of muscle total Cr store exists in the form of PCr, which, due to its phosphorylated state, is unable to pass through membranes, thus trapping Cr. This entrapment results in the generation of a concentration gradient. However, phosphorylation is not the sole mechanism of cellular Cr retention. For example, the binding of Cr to intracellular components and the existence of restrictive cellular membranes have been proposed as mechanisms that facilitate muscle Cr retention (36).

Creatinine has been established as the sole end product of Cr degradation being formed nonenzymatically in an irreversible reaction (38,39). Because skeletal muscle is the major store of the body Cr pool, this is the major site of creatinine production. The daily renal creatinine excretion is relatively constant in an individual but can vary between individuals, being dependent on the total muscle mass in healthy individuals (38,40).

Effect of Creatine Ingestion on Muscle Cr Concentration in Humans

Studies earlier this century demonstrated that Cr administration resulted in a small increase in urinary creatinine excretion (38–40). However, there was no increase in excretion until a significant amount of the administered Cr had been retained. It was also noted that Cr retention was greatest during the initial stages of administration. In general, urinary creatinine excretion increased slowly during prolonged Cr administration and, upon cessation, around 5 weeks elapsed before a significant decrease in creatinine excretion was observed.

These studies invariably involved periods of chronic Cr ingestion. However, with the application of the muscle biopsy technique, it has become apparent that the ingestion of 20 g of Cr each day in solution for 5 days (4 × 5 g doses) can lead to an average increase in muscle total Cr concentration of about 20%, of which approximately 30% is in the form of PCr (41,42). In agreement with earlier urinary excretion studies, it appears that the majority of muscle Cr retention occurs during the initial days of supplementation, e.g., about 30% of the administered dose is retained during the initial 2 days of supplementation, compared with 15% from days 2–4 (41). The natural time-course of muscle Cr decay after 5 days of 20 g/day ingestion occurs over the course of several weeks rather than days (43) (Fig. 5A).

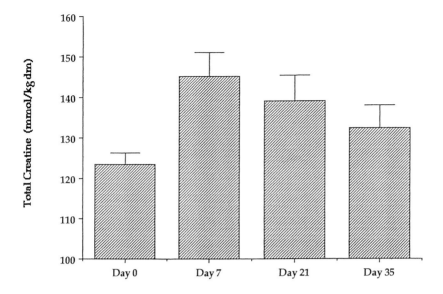

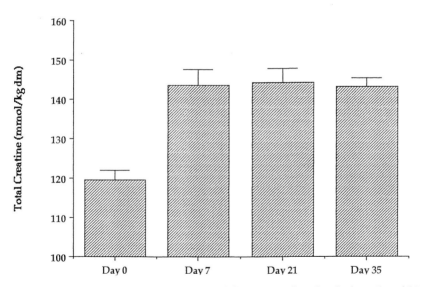

FIG. 5. The upper figure represents muscle total Cr concentration after the ingestion of 20 g of Cr for 6 consecutive days. Muscle biopsy samples were obtained before ingestion (day 0) and on days 7, 21, and 35. The lower figure represents muscle total Cr concentration after the ingestion of 20 g of Cr for 6 consecutive days and thereafter at a rate of 2 g/day for the next 28 days. Muscle biopsy samples were taken before ingestion (day 0) and on days 7, 21, and 35.

As might be expected, lower dose Cr supplementation (e.g., 3 g/day for 2 weeks) is slower at increasing muscle Cr concentration compared with a 5-day regimen of 20 g/day (43). However, after 4 weeks of supplementation at this lower dose, muscle Cr accumulation is no different when comparing regimens (43). It also appears that muscle Cr stores remain elevated for several weeks when the supplementation regimen of 20 g/day for 5 days is followed by lower dose supplementation (2 g/day; Fig. 5B) (12), which seems to agree with the earlier suggestion that Cr is "trapped" within skeletal muscle once absorbed and that muscle Cr degradation to creatinine occurs at a rate of about 2 g/day.

Effect of Creatine Ingestion on Exercise Performance

Despite the important roles for Cr and PCr during muscle contraction, little has been published relating to Cr ingestion and exercise performance. In 1981, Sipila et al. (44) reported that in a group of patients receiving 1 g Cr/day as a treatment for gyrate atrophy, there was a comment from some patients of a sensation of strength gain after a 1-year period of supplementation. Indeed, Cr ingestion was shown to reverse the type II muscle fiber atrophy associated with this disease, and one athlete in the group of patients improved his personal best record for the 100-m sprint by 2 seconds.

Based on more recently published work, it would appear that the ingestion of 4×5 g Cr/day for 5 days significantly increases exercise performance in healthy male volunteers during repeated bouts of fatiguing short-lasting maximal exercise, e.g., maximal isokinetic knee extensor exercise, maximal dynamic cycling exercise, maximal isokinetic cycling exercise, and controlled "track" running experiments (45–48). The consistent finding from these studies is that Cr ingestion significantly increased exercise performance by 5–7% by sustaining force or work output during exercise. Some studies also have reported an increase in maximal strength or torque at the onset of contraction (46). More recently, however, results from our laboratory indicate that approximately 30% of subjects who have ingested Cr in an attempt to increase muscle Cr concentration have failed to retain substantial quantities of Cr (42,49). These results also have shown that any improvement in exercise performance as a consequence of Cr supplementation is clearly associated with the extent of muscle Cr retention during supplementation, i.e., those individuals who experienced the highest muscle Cr accumulation during supplementation were those that demonstrated the better improvements in exercise performance (Fig. 6) (49). Therefore, it would appear that the extent of muscle Cr retention during supplementation is critical to subsequent exercise performance. In support of this conclusion, further results from our laboratory have shown that those individuals who experienced more than a 25% increase in muscle total Cr concentration after 5 days of Cr ingestion also showed an accelerated rate of PCr resynthesis during 2 minutes of recovery from intense fatiguing muscular contraction. Conversely, those individuals who

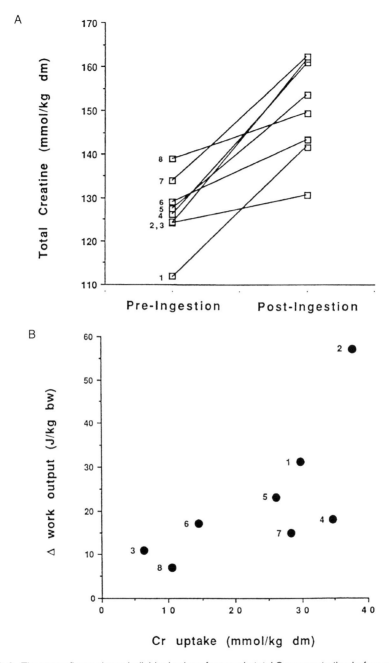

FIG. 6. The upper figure shows individual values for muscle total Cr concentration before and after 5 days of Cr ingestion (20 g/day). Subjects have been numbered 1–8 based on initial muscle total Cr concentration. The lower figure shows individual increases in muscle total Cr for the same group of subjects, plotted against the change in work production during 2 × 30 s bouts of maximal isokinetic cycling after Cr ingestion. Values on the y-axis were calculated by subtracting total work output during exercise before Cr ingestion from the corresponding value after Cr ingestion.

experienced no or little Cr accumulation during ingestion (on average an 8% increase) showed no measurable change in PCr resynthesis during recovery (42).

Creatine's Mechanism of Action

The exact mechanism by which Cr ingestion improves performance during maximal exercise is not yet clear. The available data indicate that it may be related to the stimulatory effect that Cr has on pre-exercise PCr availability (49) and on PCr resynthesis during exercise and recovery (42). Given that PCr availability is generally thought to limit exercise performance during maximal exercise, both of these effects would increase muscle contractile capability by maintaining ATP turnover during exercise. This suggestion is supported by reports showing that the accumulation of plasma ammonia and hypoxanthine (accepted markers of skeletal muscle adenine nucleotide loss) are reduced during maximal exercise after Cr ingestion, despite a higher work output being achieved (45–47). More convincing evidence comes from a recent study showing that Cr supplementation can reduce the extent of muscle ATP degradation by 30% during maximal isokinetic cycling exercise while at the same time increasing work output (49) (Fig. 7). Furthermore, the latter study also demonstrated that the increase in resting PCr in type II muscle fibers after Cr supplementation was positively correlated with PCr degradation in this fiber type during subsequent exercise (r = 0.78, n = 8, p < 0.05) and with the increase in work production observed during

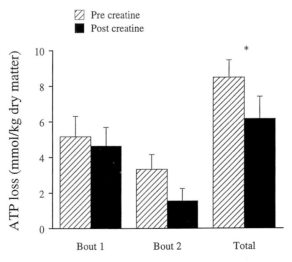

FIG. 7. The decline in muscle ATP concentration during 2 bouts of a 30 s maximal intensity, isokinetic cycling exercise. Each bout of exercise was performed at 80 rev/min and separated by 4 min of passive recovery. Total decline in ATP refers to the sum of the decline during bouts 1 and 2. Significant difference pre and post creatine supplementation is donated by * (p<0.05).

exercise (r = 0.66, n = 8, p < 0.05). No corresponding correlations were observed with respect to type I muscle fibers. These observations led us to suggest that the improvements in exercise performance resulted from the increased pre-exercise PCr concentration in type II muscle fibers after Cr ingestion, which increased ATP resynthesis during exercise.

Research has shown that the extent of muscle Cr accumulation during supplementation varies greatly between individuals (41,42,49). As outlined above, the improvements in maximal exercise performance and PCr resynthesis during recovery from exercise appear to be critically dependent on the extent of muscle Cr accumulation during Cr supplementation; therefore, future work should focus on elucidating the principal factors regulating muscle Cr transport in humans. In this respect, we have recently demonstrated that Cr ingested in conjunction with carbohydrate can increase muscle Cr uptake by ~60% in humans and appears to be insulin mediated (50,51).

OXIDATIVE ENERGY PRODUCTION DURING INTENSE CONTRACTION

At the onset of intense muscle contraction, a rapid and substantial accumulation of lactate occurs. However, if exercise is repeated over several exercise bouts, interspersed by short rest periods, the rate of muscle lactate accumulation substantially declines (52,53). It has been suggested that this response occurs because of feedback inhibition of glycolysis caused by the accumulation of end-products such as hydrogen, lactate, and phosphate ions (8). However, data are available to demonstrate that the accumulation of several positive modulators of glycolysis also occurs during exercise (23); therefore, this cannot completely explain the decline in lactate production seen during repeated bouts of contraction. Furthermore, data are available to show that if the recovery interval between exercise bouts is extended, such that muscle metabolite concentrations are substantially diminished, there is still a reduction in lactate accumulation during subsequent exercise (54). Recent studies also have demonstrated that the reduction in work production during repeated bouts of maximal exercise is less than the reduction observed in anaerobic energy provision (34,55). For example, the former study demonstrated that despite a 40% reduction in anaerobic energy production during a second bout of 30 seconds maximal exercise, total work declined by only 17%. This led the investigators to suggest that the observed decline in anaerobic energy production may have been offset by the 16% increase in oxygen consumption observed. Therefore, it would appear that the contribution of oxidative phosphorylation to total ATP production during maximal exercise has perhaps been underplayed.

This being the case, what might be the mechanism by which the contribution from oxidative phosphorylation is increased during maximal exercise? Recent data suggest that there is a progressive increase in flux through the pyruvate dehydrogense complex (PDC) over the course of several bouts of exercise, which may be responsible for this observed decline in lactate accumulation and increase in oxygen consumption (56). The investigators calculated that the contribution of pyruvate flux through PDC to total ATP production during three bouts of 30 seconds maximal exercise interspersed by 4 min of recovery accounted for 29%, 33%, and 63% of total energy production. We have recently tested this hypothesis more closely by pharmacologically activating PDC before intense contraction using dichloroacetate (DCA), which activated PDC by inhibiting the PDC kinase (57). In short, we found that pretreatment of resting canine gracilis muscle with DCA resulted in an increase in oxidative ATP production, a substantial reduction in anaerobic ATP production, and a marked improvement in muscle isometric force production during 20 minutes of subsequent ischemic contraction (25% of normal exercise-induced flow). This led us to conclude that PDC activation and acetyl group availability, and not oxygen availability, were the primary limiting factors to oxidative ATP production under these conditions. Furthermore, we went on to hypothesize that it may be the rate of PDC activation and, therefore, acetyl group availability at the onset of contraction (i.e., during rest to steady-state transition period) that may regulate the contribution made by oxidative phosphorylation and anaerobic ATP production during intense exercise. Recent data from our laboratory, again using an ischemic canine gracilis muscle model, indicate that this is the case (58). Table 1 shows muscle tension development and metabolite concentrations at rest and after 1 and 6 minutes of ischemic contraction after pretreatment with DCA and saline (control). Note that acetylcarnitine and acetyl group availability was maximal at rest and remained elevated during contraction after DCA administration. This finding was associated with a marked reduction in muscle lactate accumulation and PCr hydrolysis after both 1 and 6 minutes of contraction and an improvement in muscle tension development at 6 minutes. These data enabled us to conclude that the improvement in ischemic muscle function occurred as a

TABLE 1. *Muscle tension and ATP, PCr, lactate (Lac) and acetylcarnitine (Ac) concentrations at rest and following 1 and 6 min of ischemic contraction in canine gracilis muscle pre-treated with DCA and saline (control)*

	Rest		1 min		6 min	
	Control	DCA	Control	DCA	Control	DCA
Tension	300	300	4,605±306	4,626±154	2,288±209	3,117±176[a]
ATP	262 ±0.7	25.0±0.6	25.5±0.6	24.6±0.8	22.7±0.9	24.5±0.7
PCr	80.3±2.9	78.9±2.1	43.9±3.9	54.7±3.6[a]	21.5±5.9	47.5±7.9[a]
Lac	5.1±1.4	1.0±0.3[a]	23.9±3.8	13.5±3.7[a]	60.7±8.7	24.5±9.3[b]
Ac	3.3±0.7	22.2±0.4[b]	5.1±1.0	20.2±1.3[b]	13.0±1.6	20.6±0.6[b]

Values are means ±1 SEM and data are expressed as mmol/kg dry muscle with the exception of tension, which is g/100 g muscle. Statistical differences between corresponding control and DCA-treated muscles are indicated as follows: [a] $p < 0.05$; [b] $p < 0.01$ (repeated measures analysis of variance and Tukey post-hoc test).

result of a faster onset of oxidative ATP production and decline in anaerobic metabolism. This work points to an important role for acetyl group availability, rather than oxygen availability, in dictating the relative contributions made by anaerobic and oxidative metabolism during the rest to steady-state period of muscle contraction.

CONCLUSION

The findings drawn together here suggest that during intense muscular contraction ATP is supplied at near maximal rates by PCr degradation and glycolysis. As exercise progresses, it would appear that anaerobic ATP turnover is reduced due to the depletion of PCr and a reduction in the rate of glycogenolysis resulting in a reduction in force and power. More recent studies have implicated the depletion of PCr, specifically in type II muscle fibers, with the development of fatigue during intense exercise. The importance of PCr availability to muscle function has been confirmed by studies demonstrating that Cr supplementation can increase muscle PCr concentration at rest, improve exercise performance, and facilitate PCr resynthesis during recovery from exercise. Finally, recent studies have demonstrated that the reduction in work production during repeated bouts of maximal exercise is less than the reduction observed in anaerobic energy provision. This has led to the suggestion that the contribution of oxidative phosphorylation to total ATP production during intense muscle contraction may have been underestimated, especially during repeated bouts of maximal exercise. This suggestion has been substantiated by recent work pointing to an important role for acetyl group availability rather than oxygen availability, in dictating the relative contributions made by anaerobic and oxidative metabolism during the rest to steady-state period of muscle contraction.

ACKNOWLEDGMENTS

We thank the Wellcome Trust (036554/Z/92/MP/jf), Smithkline Beecham, Zeneca Pharmaceuticals and The Defense Research Agency for their support of the experiments described in this chapter.

REFERENCES

1. Bangsbo J, Gollnick PD, Graham TE, et al. Anaerobic energy production and O_2 deficit-debt relationship during exhaustive exercise in humans. *J Physiol* 1990;42:539–559.
2. Margaria R, Oliva D, Di Prampero PE, Cerretelli P. Energy utilization in intermittant exercise of supramaximal intensity. *J Appl Physiol* 1969;26:752–756.
3. Bergstrom J, Harris RC, Hultman E, Nordesjo L-O. Energy rich phosphagens in dynamic and static work. *Adv Exp Med Biol* 1971;11:341–355.
4. Boobis L, Williams C, Wootton SA. Human muscle metabolism during brief maximal exercise. *J Physiol* 1982;338:21–22.

5. Jacobs I, Tesch P, Bar-Or O, et al. Lactate in human skeletal muscle after 10 and 30 s of supramaximal exercise. *J Appl Physiol* 1983;55:365–367.
6. Jones NL, McCartney N, Graham T, et al. Muscle performance and metabolism in maximal isokinetic cycling at slow and fast speeds. *J Appl Physiol* 1985;59;132–136.
7. Hultman E, Sjoholm I, Jaderholm EK, Krynicki J. Evaluation of methods for electrical stimulation of human muscle in situ. *Pflugers Arch* 1983;398:139–141.
8. Hultman E, Sjoholm H. Substrate availability. In: Knuttgen HG, Vogel HG, Poortmans JA, eds. *Biochemistry of exercise*. Champaign, IL: Human Kinetics Publishers; 1983:63–75.
9. Hultman E, Greenhaff PL, Ren J-M, Soderlund K. Energy metabolism and fatigue during intense muscle contraction. *Biochem Soc Trans* 1991;19:347–353.
10. Cori GT. The effect of stimulation and recovery on the phosphorylase a content of muscle. *J Biol Chem* 1945;158:333–339.
11. Chasiotis D, Sahlin K, Hultman E. Regulation of glycogenolysis in human muscle in response to epinephrine infusion. *J Appl Physiol* 1983;54:45–50.
12. Hultman E, Sjöholm H. Energy metabolism and contraction force of human skeletal muscle in situ during electrical stimulation. *J Physiol* 1983;345:525–532.
13. Ren J-M, Hultman E. Regulation of glycogenolysis in human skeletal muscle. *J Appl Physiol* 1989; 67:2243–2248.
14. Ren J-M, Hultman E. Regulation of phosphorylase a activity in human skeletal muscle. *J Appl Physiol* 1990;69:919–923.
15. Sahlin K, Gorski J, Edstrom L. Influence of ATP turnover and metabolite changes on IMP formation and glycolysis in rat skeletal muscle. *Am J Physiol* 1990;259:C409–C412.
16. Cori GT, Colowick SP, Cori CF. The action of nucleotides in the disruptive phosphorylation of glycogen. *J Biol Chem* 1938;123:381–389.
17. Lowry OH, Schulz DW, Passoneau JV. Effects of adenylic acid on the kinetics of muscle phosphorylase *a*. *J Biol Chem* 1964;239:1947–1953.
18. Sols A, Marco R. Concentrations of metabolites and binding sites. Implications in metabolic regulation. *Curr Top Cell Regul* 1970;2:227–273.
19. Symons JD, Jacobs I. High intensity exercise performance is not impaired by low intramuscular glycogen. *Med Sci Sports Exerc* 1989;21:550–557.
20. Ren J-M, Broberg S, Sahlin K, Hultman E. Influence of reduced glycogen level on glycogenolysis during short term stimulation in man. *Acta Physiol Scand* 1990;139:427–474.
21. Jacobs I, Kaijser P, Tesch P. Muscle strength and fatigue after selective glycogen depletion in human skeletal muscle fibers. *Eur J Appl Physiol* 1981;46:47–53.
22. Casey A, Short AH, Curtis S, Greenhaff PL. The effect of glycogen availability on power output and the metabolic response to repeated bouts of maximal isokinetic exercise in man. *Eur J Appl Physiol* 1996;72:249–255.
23. Spriet LL, Soderlund K, Bergstrom M, Hultman E. *J Appl Physiol* 1987;62:611–615.
24. Barany M. ATPase activity of myosin correlated with speed of muscle shortening. *J Gen Physiol* 1967;50 :197–218.
25. Burke RE, Levine DN, Zajac FE III, et al. Mammalian motor units: physiological-histochemical correlation in three types of cat gastrocnemius. *Science* 1971;174:709–712.
26. Hintz CS, Chi MM-Y, Fell RD, et al. Metabolite changes in individual rat muscle fibers during stimulation. *Am J Physiol* 1982;242:C218–C228.
27. Faulkner JA, Claflin DR, McCully KK. Power output of fast and slow fibers from human skeletal muscles. In: Jones NL, McCartney N, McComas AJ, eds. *Human muscle power*. Champaign, IL: Human Kinetics Publishers; 1986:81–89.
28. Green HJ. Muscle power: fiber type recruitment, metabolism and fatigue. In: Jones NL, McCartney N, McComas AJ, eds. *Human muscle power.* Champaign, IL: Human Kinetics Publishers; 1986:65–79.
29. Soderlund K, Greenhaff PL, Hultman E. Energy metabolism in type I and type II human muscle fibers during short term electrical stimulation at different frequencies. *Acta Physiol Scand* 1992;144:15–22.
30. Greenhaff PL, Ren J-M, Soderlund K, Hultman E. Energy metabolism in single human muscle fibers during contraction without and with epinephrine infusion. *Am J Physiol* 1991;260:E713–E718.
31. Greenhaff P L, Soderlund K, Ren J-M, Hultman E. Energy metabolism in single human muscle fibers during intermittent contraction with occluded circulation. *J Physiol* 1993;460:443–453.
32. Greenhaff PL, Nevill ME, Soderlund K, et al. The metabolic responses of human type I and II muscle fibers during maximal treadmill sprinting. *J Physiol* 1994;478:149–155.
33. Harris RC, Essen B, Hultman E. Glycogen phosphorylase in biopsy samples and single muscle fibers of musculus quadriceps femoris of man at rest. *Scand J Clin Lab Invest* 1976;36:521–526.

34. Bogdanis GC, Nevill ME, Boobis LH, Lakomy HKA. Contribution of phosphocreatine and aerobic metabolism to energy supply during repeated sprint exercise. *J Appl Physiol* 1996;80:876–884.
35. Casey A, Constantin-Teodosiu D, Howell S, et al. The metabolic response of type I and II muscle fibers during repeated bouts of maximal exercise in humans. *Am J Physiol* 1996;271:E38–E43.
36. Walker JB. Creatine: biosynthesis, regulation and function. *Adv Enzymol Relat Areas Mol Med* 1979; 50:177–242.
37. Fitch CD, Lucy DD, Bornhofen JH, Dalrymple GV. Creatine metabolism in skeletal muscle. *Neurology* 1968;18:32–39.
38. Schloss P, Mayser W, Betz H. The putative rat choline transporter chot1 transports creatine and is highly expressed in neural and muscle-rich tissues. *Biochem Biophys Res Commun* 1994;198: 637–645.
38. Bloch K, Schoenheimer R. The metabolic relation of creatine and creatinine studied with isotopic notrogen. *J Biol Chem* 1939;131:111–121.
39. Hunter A. The physiology of creatine and creatinine. *Physiol Rev* 1922;2:586–599.
40. Chanutin A. The fate of creatine when administered to man. *J Biol Chem* 1926;67:29–37.
41. Harris RC, Soderlund K, Hultman E. Elevation of creatine in resting and exercised muscle of normal subjects by creatine supplementation. *Clin Sci* 1992;83:367–374.
42. Greenhaff PL, Bodin K, Soderlund K, Hultman E. The effect of oral creatine supplementation on skeletal muscle phosphocreatine resynthesis. *Am J Physiol* 1994;266:E725–E730.
43. Hultman E, Soderlund K, Timmons J, et al. Muscle creatine loading in man. *J Appl Physiol* 1996;81:232–237.
44. Sipila I, Rapola J, Simell O, Vannas A. Supplementary creatine as a treatment for gyrate atrophy of the choroid and retina. *N Engl J Med* 1981;304:867–870.
45. Greenhaff PL, Casey A, Short AH, Harris RC, Soderlund K, Hultman E. Influence of oral creatine supplementation on muscle torque during repeated bouts of maximal voluntary exercise in man. *Clin Sci* 1993;84:565–571.
46. Birch R, Noble D, Greenhaff PL. The influence of dietary creatine supplementation on performance during repeated bouts of maximal isokinetic cycling in man. *Eur J Appl Physiol* 1994;69:268–270.
47. Balsom PD, Ekblom B, Soderlund K, et al. Creatine supplementation and dynamic high-intensity intermittent exercise. *Scand J Med Sci Sports* 1993;3:143–149.
48. Harris RC, Viru M, Greenhaff PL, Hultman E. The effect of oral creatine supplementation on running performance during maximal short term exercise in man. *J Physiol* 1993;467:74.
49. Casey A, Constantin-Teodosiu D, Howell S, et al. Creatine supplementation favourably affects performance and muscle metabolism during maximal intensity exercise in humans. *Am J Physiol* 1996;271:E31–E37.
50. Green AL, Simpson EJ, Littlewood JJ, et al. Carbohydrate ingestion augments creatine retention during creatine feeding in man. *Acta Physiol Scand* 1996;158:195–202.
51. Green AL, Sewell DA, Simpson EJ, et al. Carbohydrate ingestion stimulates creatine uptake in human skeletal muscle. *J Physiol* 1995;489:27.
52. McCartney N, Spreit LL, Heigenhauser GJF, et al. Muscle power and metabolism in maximal intermittent exercise. *J Appl Physiol* 1986;60:1164–1169.
53. Gaitanos GC, Williams C, Boobis LH, Brooks S. Human muscle metabolism during intermittent maximal exercise. *J Appl Physiol* 1993;75:712–719.
54. Bangsbo J, Graham TE, Kiens B, Saltin B. Elevated muscle glycogen and anaerobic energy production during exhaustive exercise in man. *J Physiol* 1992;451:205–227.
55. Medbo JI, Tabata I. Relative importance of aerobic and anaerobic energy release during short-lasting exhausting bicycle exercise. *J Appl Physiol* 1989;67:1881–1886.
56. Putman CT, Jones NL, Lands LC, et al. Skeletal muscle pyruvate dehydrogenase activity during maximal exercise in humans. *Am J Physiol* 1995;269:E458–E468.
57. Timmons JA, Poucher SM, Constantin-Teodosiu D, et al. Increased acetyl group availability enhances contractile function of canine skeletal muscle during ischemia. *J Clin Invest* 1996;97:879–883.
58. Timmons JA, Poucher SM, Constantin-Teodosiu D, et al. Dichloroacetate decreases anaerobic ATP regeneration during the rest to steady-state period of contracting canine muscle. *J Physiol* 1996;491.p.62.

Physiology, Stress, and Malnutrition: Functional Correlates, Nutritional Intervention, edited by J.M. Kinney and H.N. Tucker. Lippincott–Raven Publishers © 1997.

Overview of Weight Loss, Muscle Activity, and Fitness

John M. Kinney

The Hirsch-Leibel Laboratories, The Rockefeller University, New York, New York 10021

This overview combines information from chapters in this Horizons volume devoted to muscle activity as well as related issues discussed in other chapters. There are a variety of ways in which muscle is related to malnutrition. The term "malnutrition" is widely used in the medical community, yet there is no concise definition that is widely accepted. Of the various factors involved, most doctors mention weight loss before any of the other variables. Muscle loss is assumed to be part of weight loss, particularly because weakness and fatigue are common symptoms. A negative nitrogen balance nearly always accompanies weight loss and is consistent with loss of muscle. However, it is not the loss of muscle mass per se that is important but rather the loss of muscle function. Unfortunately, our information on the correlation between loss of body weight and loss of muscle function is extremely limited. Such knowledge is needed both to evaluate changes during the catabolic phase of disease and injury and to assess the progress of anabolism during convalescence.

Information about muscle metabolism was greatly enlarged during the 1960s and 1970s by the use of arteriovenous catheterization, isotopic tracers, and chemical analysis of muscle biopsy samples (1). Behavior of skeletal muscle in whole-body exercise has been extended to the examination of individual fiber types and even to work performance of isolated fibers (2). Sports medicine has given new impetus to measurements of muscle strength and endurance. The growth of nutritional support has reduced the incidence of hospital malnutrition and thereby reduced the erosion of muscle mass in patients with inadequate intake. Subsequently, the techniques of cellular and molecular biology have been applied to the study of muscle (3).

Muscle is a curious tissue, capable of the abrupt onset and cessation of high levels of energy conversion in exercise yet playing a key role at rest in the metabolic integration with other organs and tissues. Regular exercise training appears to offers metabolic benefits to other organs and tissues beyond muscle (4). Further understanding of muscle behavior is needed to provide perspective for its role as a target tissue in acute disease and injury.

It is well established that muscle can enlarge and function at high levels of energy expenditure in elite exercise where everything from blood flow to substrates move to the muscle preferentially over resting normal values. This is opposite to acute catabolic conditions where muscle breakdown occurs with supply of amino acids and other substrates to support functions elsewhere in the body. However, more information is needed on how muscle can serve in the one instance as "giver" and in the other instance as "taker" of metabolic resources which are normally shared in some sort of metabolic balance which is between these extreme conditions.

MUSCLE FUELS AND ENERGY METABOLISM

There is significant variation in energy expenditure among people, independent of body size and composition. Because of its relatively low resting energy metabolism, skeletal muscle often has been neglected when investigators have tried to explain such interindividual differences in metabolic rate. Zurlo et al. (5) studied the possibility that skeletal muscle may be a major determinant in this variability by comparing the 24-hour energy expenditure in a chamber with resting oxygen uptake in the forearm. Their data indicate that skeletal muscle may be important in explaining the variability in energy expenditure and that persons with a low metabolic rate appear to be at increased risk for gaining weight. The suggestion that exercise is followed by an increase in the resting energy expenditure for the following 1 to 2 days has been offered as the rationale for stressing exercise in weight loss programs. However, a well-controlled, long-term study has demonstrated that there is no change in basal, overnight, or sleeping metabolic rate after 9 weeks of exercise training (6).

New opportunities for studying energy metabolism in muscle have been provided by phosphorus-31 nuclear magnetic resonance (NMR spectroscopy), which has made it possible to perform noninvasive determinations of high-energy compounds in resting and exercising muscle. Despite the tremendous promise of NMR spectroscopy, various investigators have questioned how the findings of this new method compare with chemical measurements, particularly when muscle activity is involved. A recent study of one-legged exercise in normal men was performed with NMR spectroscopy and muscle biopsies at three different exercise levels (7). A good agreement was found between the measurements for adenosine triphosphate (ATP) and creatine phosphate, but the adenosine diphosphate content was higher when measured via NMR spectroscopy in association with an increase in muscle inosine phosphate.

The substrate oxidized in muscle is determined by the availability of glucose from the liver and fatty acids from adipose tissue. In the reverse direction, muscle contributes to the liver in the form of 3-carbon intermediates such as lactate and alanine for gluconeogenesis. Skeletal muscle is a major tissue that contributes to systemic glucose disposal, becoming increasingly important as the insulin concentration increases. However, the effects of an increase in plasma glucose alone on skeletal muscle have not been as well characterized in humans. Mandarino et al. (8), combining clamp techniques with leg balance studies, concluded that at basal insulin levels, hyperglycemia increases muscle glucose storage and glycolysis, whereas glucose oxidation is increased by activation of the pyruvate dehydrogenase complex. During hyperinsulinemia, additional increases in substrate availability further activate glycogen synthase and preferentially stimulate glycogen synthesis.

The branched-chain amino acids undergo minimal degradation in the liver but undergo transamination in peripheral tissues such as muscle. Muscle releases large amounts of alanine and glutamine for gluconeogenesis and nitrogen transport. A positive relationship has been demonstrated between glutamine and protein synthesis in rat muscle; a relationship that is present in starvation, protein deficiency, or endotoxemia (9). The release of glutamine has been proposed as the primary role whereby muscle serves as the source of critical intermediates for immune cells, intestinal mucosa, and other cells with rapid rates of turnover (10). However, during exercise the major fuels are carbohydrate and fatty acids, and protein does not become a significant fuel in previously well fed individuals.

The major adaptation in muscle during starvation is to use free fatty acids (FFAs) from elevated plasma levels and later to use ketones from synthesis in the liver associated with increasing glucagon levels. Muscle proteolysis decreases in starvation with a corresponding decrease in release of muscle amino acids. Leucine in plasma increases as muscle uptake decreases, although plasma levels later return toward normal.

VASCULAR AND ENDOCRINE REGULATION IN MUSCLE

The vascular effects of pharmacologic agents were initially studied independently of metabolic effects. The history of muscle physiology includes numerous studies of hindlimb animal preparations. During the past decade the results of hindlimb studies began to be compared with studies of incubated muscle preparations (11). More recently, Clark et al. (12) have summarized the vasoconstrictor agents that increase and those that decrease oxygen consumption in the perfused rat hindlimb. The vasoconstrictor-induced increases in oxygen consumption were found to be associated with increased muscle output of lactate and glycerol. The mechanism by which site-specific vasoconstriction leads to changes in metabolism and thermogenesis remains unknown.

Muscle blood flow often has been measured using xenon-133 clearance, which involves interpretation of of a decay curve over time with certain associated assumptions. The technique of microdialysis offers new possibilities for measuring the kinetic behavior of small molecules such as glucose or glycerol in the interstitial space, but it is very sensitive to changes in local blood flow. Low concentrations of ethanol in the dialysis medium offer the possibility of detecting changes in local blood flow while conducting metabolic studies with microdialysis. Hickner et al. (13) have reported the comparison of blood flow measurements by xenon-133 with the ethanol technique during intermittent exercise and found that the latter technique provided valid measurements of changes in local muscle perfusion.

In many diseases, the metabolic behavior is dominated by what happens to insulin action. There can be inadequate amounts (diabetes), excess amounts in the circulation (cirrhosis), or insulin resistance (renal failure or sepsis). Insulin is the important common factor in regulating flow of metabolites in respect to both energy and amino acids after feeding and fasting.

Possible explanations by which vasomodulating agents affect muscle contractility include the idea that muscle blood flow is divided into nutritional and non-nutritional portions and that the balance of these two parts of the muscle circulation can be altered by nervous or pharmacologic means. On the basis of hindlimb studies, Rattigan et al. (14) proposed a hemodynamic basis for insulin resistance in skeletal muscle. This idea is based on having a high proportion of functional vascular shunting occurring early in the development of insulin resistance. This might occur as a result of hypertension-associated site-specific vasoconstriction in the skeletal muscle vasculature, which would reduce access for glucose, insulin, and other nutrients and hormones. As this condition persists, the impaired access would lead to permanent changes in both the vasculature and muscle fibers characteristic of long-term insulin resistance. This presupposes the presence within muscle of functional vascular shunts of small diameter, which are different from the large anatomical arteriovenous shunts of other tissues.

The major muscle adaptation in exercise is an increase in alanine release. In fasting, the muscle receives increased amounts of branched chain amino acids from viscera and oxidizes increased amounts of leucine. Elevated levels of insulin and glucose in sepsis inhibit the flow of FFAs from adipose tissue. Thus, in starvation with ketosis, the onset of sepsis causes the ketosis to disappear. The secretion of insulin accelerates the muscle uptake of the branched chain amino acids and increases the release of alanine and glutamine, allowing increased gluconeogenesis and higher blood glucose levels. The capacity to make these metabolic responses in sepsis is less in infants due to the smaller muscle mass.

HEMODYNAMIC ROLE OF INSULIN AND INSULIN RESISTANCE

Immobilization leads to insulin resistance in rodent skeletal muscle, whereas bed rest in humans leads to impaired insulin action and limb glucose uptake (15). Conversely, exercise training increases insulin action on muscle glucose uptake (16). Clamp studies after one-leg immobilization (17) demonstrated that 7 days of immobilization is followed by a local decrease in insulin action on glucose uptake and net protein degradation.

Physical training in humans has been shown to enhance insulin-stimulated glucose uptake in all three of insulin's target tissues (muscle, liver, and adipose tissue) (4). The human interaction of exercise and insulin on fat, carbohydrate, and protein metabolism has been studied during rest, exercise, and recovery (18). Exercise and insulin were found to act synergistically in stimulating total glucose utilization and carbohydrate oxidation. Most of the exercise-induced increase in these variables was independent of insulin action. Exercise also increased the suppressive effect of fatty acid concentrations and fat oxidation, but had no influence on the insulin antiproteolytic action. The effect is that of training in contrast to the result of brief bouts of acute exercise (16). Training was found to increase the insulin action of glucose uptake, due to the local mechanisms of contractile activity during training. Glycolysis is enhanced in proportion to glycogen synthesis. Insulin clearance in muscle is not influenced by training.

The responsiveness of insulin has classically been investigated in the fasting state. The chapter by Ferrando and Wolfe has noted that the fasting state is not a physiologically relevant circumstance with regard to the effect of insulin on protein metabolism. Insulin is normally only elevated after a meal, at which time the amino acid availability is also increased. If intravenous amino acids are provided together with the glucose infusion during the hyperinsulinemic clamp, the decrease in whole-body protein synthesis rate is prevented. In contrast to the insulin-induced suppression of both whole-body protein synthesis and breakdown seen in the fasted state, in the fed state a pharmacologic amount of insulin actually increases protein turnover. In muscle, both synthesis and breakdown are significantly increased by high-dose insulin when burn patients are fed. Although comparable studies during bed rest have not been reported, results of the whole-body protein turnover (WBPT) studies suggest that the derangement in protein metabolism is more prominent in the fed versus the postabsorptive state.

Studies in which glucose oxidation was stimulated by administering dichloroacetate showed no change in the rate of either protein breakdown or leucine oxidation (19). This was considered evidence that the alterations in protein metabolism with inactivity and stress were not due to insulin insensitivity.

Considerable evidence has accumulated to suggest an association between hyperinsulinemia and hypertension, independent of obesity. Baron and Brechtel (20) measured systemic and leg vascular resistance and whole-body and leg glucose uptake in lean (insulin-sensitive) and obese (insulin-resistant) subjects by varying insulin concentrations while maintaining euglycemia using the glucose clamp technique. These investigators concluded that (a) insulin decreases vascular resistance more in the leg than in the whole body, thus directing blood flow to the leg; (b) this effect is blunted in obesity; and (c) insulin decreases mean arterial pressure and vascular resistance more effectively in insulin-sensitive than in insulin-resistant tissues. Therefore, insulin resistance rather than hyperinsulinemia appeared to be the predisposing factor in the development of hypertension. Insulin's ability to decrease skeletal muscle resistance was recognized as important in its overall action to stimulate glucose uptake. These investigators proposed that insulin might be a vasoactive peptide, perhaps by a local action on endothelium to increase nitric oxide synthesis followed by vasodilatation.

Laakso et al. (21) showed that whole-body glucose uptake is correlated with both cardiac output and leg blood flow over a wide range of insulin concentrations. These findings led to the proposal that insulin augmentation of muscle perfusion enhances glucose uptake via recruitment of previously underperfused muscle tissue available to participate in insulin-mediated glucose metabolism.

Steinberg et al. (22) demonstrated that insulin-mediated vasodilation in muscle is nitric oxide dependent because it could be completely abrogated by the infusion of N-monomethyl-l-arginine, a specific inhibitor of nitric oxide synthase. This technique was then applied to measure the effect of perfusion rate on the time course of insulin-mediated skeletal muscle glucose uptake. Baron et al. (23) demonstrated that insulin-mediated vasodilation has a modest effect in slowing the time course of which insulin stimulates glucose uptake but has a marked effect in augmenting the maximal rate of glucose uptake in muscle.

High insulin concentrations stimulate limb blood flow in humans, but it is not known whether there is an associated increase in muscle blood volume that might reflect capillary recruitment. Raitkari et al. (24) have used 15-O CO and positron emission tomography to demonstrate that increased insulin concentrations are associated with an increased muscle blood volume. This is further evidence that insulin in a true vasodilator in muscle.

MUSCLE METABOLISM IN BED REST VERSUS CRITICAL ILLNESS

"The question is frequently asked whether a medical examination is advisable before commencing a training program. Certainly anyone who is doubtful about his state of health should consult a physician. In principle, however, there is less risk in activity than in continuous inactivity. In a nutshell, our opinion is that it is more advisable to pass a careful medical examination if one intends to be sedentary in order to establish whether one's state of health is good enough to stand the inactivity" (25).

The metabolic changes associated with bed rest have been largely overlooked, although bed rest is an essential part of normal life and an integral part of medical care. Both bed rest and acute disease or injury result in the loss of lean body mass (LBM), yet the underlying mechanisms and functional significant of such changes require further examination.

Studies of long-term metabolic adaptation to bed rest are not available, but mechanisms underlying short-term loss of LBM (3 weeks or less) have been investigated. Extensive research in both bed rest and critical illness has come from the laboratories of Wolfe et al. (11,26), and much of the following material is based on the work of this group.

The chapter by Ferrando and Wolfe emphasizes that many of the metabolic changes of bed rest are diametric to those of critical illness. However, hyperinsulinemia and insulin insensitivity occur in both bed rest and critical illness. There is a shift to the right of the insulin dose-response curve for whole-body glucose utilization, with a less prominent effect on the maximal glucose utilization rate. Thus, physiologic concentrations of insulin are less effective than normal in stimulating glucose uptake, whereas the maximal effectiveness of a pharmacologic amount of insulin is not as markedly affected in either burn injury or bed rest. In addition, insulin must be infused at approximately twice the rate in a burn patient as in a normal volunteer to increase the plasma insulin an equivalent amount.

Alterations in energy metabolism are potentially important in all catabolic states. For any given protein intake, nitrogen balance is improved by increasing the energy intake. The basal metabolic rate (BMR) may remain unchanged or decrease somewhat when normally fed subjects have up to 10 days of bed rest. Thus, any loss of muscle mass during this situation is not related to increased energy expenditure. Changes in resting and total energy expenditure cannot be explained during either bed rest or acute catabolism on the basis of breakdown of lean tissue. Ironically, there is now an increasing attention to the detrimental effects of excessive rather than inadequate calories during nutritional support.

The most widespread effect of bed rest on lipid metabolism appears to be the decrease in high-density lipoprotein cholesterol. This finding has been noted in various forms of critical illness. Therefore, inactivity results in a lipoprotein profile known to increase the risk of coronary heart disease. These changes are the opposite of those induced by exercise. Increased lipolysis is characteristic of the stressed patient. This high rate of lipolysis is not readily suppressed because even high-dose glucose feedings are associated with de novo synthesis of fatty acids in the liver, largely from plasma fatty acids. Thus, it is unlikely that altered lipid metabolism contributes to the catabolism of body protein in either the stressed or inactive patient.

Bed rest in a healthy individual induces minimal disturbance of hormonal regulation. This is in contrast to the increase in counter-regulatory hormones, which characterizes the stress state. However, insulin sensitivity does seem to be altered comparably in both inactivity and critical illness. Cytokines are known to change acutely with stress but do not change with bed rest. The increased catabolic hormones in stress seem to be related primarily to body protein, whereas decreased testosterone also may impede protein anabolism.

The negative nitrogen balance of bed rest can be offset by dietary protein; however, this is less effective in acute illness and injury, roughly in proportion to the severity of the stress. During inactivity without stress, changes in WBPT largely reflects muscle protein turnover. This is in contrast to periods of stress, where hepatic synthesis of acute-phase proteins and proteins of wound repair may account for a significant proportion of WBPT. After 7 to 14 days of bed rest, WBPT decreases primarily as a result of decreased muscle protein synthesis. The result is a net catabolism of body protein and decreased LBM. In the burned or septic patient, the WBPT can be two- to fourfold higher than inactivity. Although the WBPT may indicate a balance between synthesis and breakdown with ample dietary intake, the synthesis of acute-phase proteins and those involved in the immune response and wound repair may be largely responsible. There is a net catabolism of skeletal muscle in the burned patient or septic patient, even in the fed state. Skeletal muscle protein synthesis decreases from bed rest in fasted patients, with no change in protein breakdown. Activity causes an increase in muscle protein turnover, which remains in balance, in contrast to bed rest alone, where the balance is negative. The magnitude of change in protein metabolism with overall negative nitrogen balance is far greater in critically ill patients than during exercise, and negative balance in muscle is pronounced. Muscle protein turnover in the postabsorptive burn patient indicates that synthesis rates are twofold higher than inactivity, whereas breakdown rates are threefold higher. Inactivity produces minor alterations in transmembrane transport of muscle amino acids, whereas there is a marked increase in amino acids crossing the membrane of muscle in burned patients. The impaired inward transport in burn injury may be the mechanism responsible for the decreased efficiency of nutritional support in maintaining muscle mass in critical illness.

The data concerning metabolic changes in bed rest versus stress states suggest that the appropriate focus of treatment should be on the blocking of mediators of the catabolic response rather than on the lack of exercise. However, there is an important lack of data on the long-term effects in both bed rest and stress, particularly in regard to the type of metabolic adaptation that may occur in muscle at times beyond that seen in the current short-term studies.

ENERGETICS AND SUBSTRATES IN EXERCISE

"Exercise physiology is an area of applied physiology that concerns itself primarily with the mechanisms related to organ system integration and adaptations that occur during acute and chronic exercise such that there is minimal homeostatic disruption of a cell's milieu interieur" (3).

In healthy, well-nourished individuals, skeletal muscle uses little glucose at rest, deriving up to 90% of its energy from FFAs and most of the remainder from glucose. At the onset of exercise, energy needs abruptly increase, and there is rapid mobilization of both carbohydrate and lipid stores within muscle tissue as well as the more gradual increase in uptake of glucose and FFA from the circulation. Muscle glycogen is the major fuel for brief strenuous exercise. For periods of up to 2 hours, circulating substrates account for about 90% of the increased tissue fuel. The rate of glucose uptake is sharply increased above the resting state, and whole-body glucose turnover may be increased several fold (27). During prolonged exercise, muscle glycogen is used rapidly, and the onset of fatigue is associated with glycogen depletion. Thus, endurance is correlated with the initial muscle glycogen and its rate of decrease during exercise.

It was postulated by Randle et al. (28) in the 1960s that enhanced fat oxidation downregulated carbohydrate metabolism due to inhibition of phosphofructokinase and pyruvate dehydrogenase. Although this concept has been supported by the results of in vitro studies, there has been controversy regarding the existence of the glucose–fatty acid cycle in human skeletal muscle during exercise. Dyck et al. (29) studied men receiving either saline or Intralipid (Pharmacia, Stockholm) infusion at rest and for 15 minutes of cycling at 85% VO_2max followed by muscle biopsy. The results were consistent with regulation of glycogenolysis at the level of muscle glycogen phosphorylase rather then the classic glucose–fatty acid cycle.

High-energy phosphates have been analyzed in type I and type II muscle fibers in male subjects in association with electrical stimulation both with and without epinephrine stimulation (2). It was shown that during short-term maximal muscle contraction, rapid muscle glycogenolysis occurs predominantly in type II fibers even though both types I and II are recruited and epinephrine stimulation of glycogenolysis is predominantly limited to type I fibers.

Carbohydrate is the major fuel for exercise at work loads over 50% of Vmax. However, carbohydrate stores are limited in muscle and liver and can be depleted during prolonged exercise. A depletion of carbohydrate stores limits the rate of ATP resynthesis and thus decreases the work capacity to the level that can be sustained by fat oxidation (approximately 50% of Vmax). A depletion of liver glycogen results in decreased blood glucose content, limiting glucose uptake and utilization both by working muscle and by the central nervous system. Either effect can cause fatigue (30).

As exercise is continued beyond 2 hours, glucose utilization decreases and FFA becomes the dominant substrate. This is associated with increased release of FFA from lipolysis in adipose tissue and increasing blood levels of FFA. The sympathetic nervous system is activated with the release of norepinephrine, whereas insulin declines. There is an increase in the counter-regulatory hormones. However, the hormone balance in two organs is critical: insulin and glucagon in the liver to regulate glucose output and the regulation of lipolysis in adipose tissue by the balance of insulin and norepinephrine. The recovery period after exercise is one of transition from the acute catabolic responses of exercise to the anabolic responses associated with restoration of glycogen stores in muscle and liver, as well as lipid stores and perhaps continued release of increased quantities of alanine and lactate for an much as 2 hours after exercise. This may represent a means of directing carbon to hepatic gluconeogenesis and increased muscle uptake for glycogen restoration.

The maintenance of body protein is critical to health and survival, yet a negative nitrogen balance is the hallmark of most disease and injury. This negative balance has been shown to be the result of a decrease in protein synthesis in starvation, whereas synthesis is increased in acute catabolic conditions at a time when breakdown rates are increased even more. The specific measurement of the rates of synthesis and breakdown of muscle protein has challenged investigators for the past two decades (31). Muscle comprises approximately 80% of total body protein. However, protein synthesis in muscle makes up only about one quarter of WBPT. The rapid turnover of visceral protein prevents muscle from being the predominant contributor to the flux of amino acid nitrogen in the normal body.

The rate of incorporation of labeled leucine into muscle has been measured before, during, and after aerobic exercise in men (32). It was shown that exercise may stimulate muscle protein breakdown, yet the stimulus to protein synthesis in recovery can result in no change of total muscle protein.

ELITE OR HIGH-LEVEL EXERCISE

Sir Roger Bannister (33) noted that "in the last 50 years, we have seen a massive new awareness of connections between sport and health, but it has so far been imperfectly translated into action." New records are continually being set in elite sports, where there has been tremendous growth and sophistication in sports medicine. Recreational sports are involving larger segments of the population and raise fundamental questions regarding its link to health. Does it lower the risk of common diseases in the exercising individual and if so, how much exercise is required to produce the benefit? One also may ask if there is information from elite or recreational sport that can offer guidance toward better concepts for the preservation of muscle function in association with illness or injury.

This Horizons volume has included chapters regarding three different forms of sustained, severe exercise: (a) the Tour de France, which is carefully programmed to provide high-level exercise with adequate nutrition for energy balance (Saris); (b) the field training of the U.S. Army Rangers, which is programmed to combine heavy exercise with periods of malnutrition and sleep deprivation (Friedl); and (c) a nonprogrammed trip on foot across the Antarctic with heavy exercise combined with malnutrition and severe environmental thermal challenges (Stroud).

At least three possible limitations to sustained VO_2 were considered: (a) the absorptive capacity for energy fuel when high-energy intake is required in a fixed period of time; (b) the ability of human thermoregulation to function at high levels of energy flux, particularly in the presence of malnutrition; and (c) the metabolic factors that cause fatigue and the time needed to correct those factors.

Can exercise conserve lean tissue during times of inadequate nutrition or stress? Dengel et al. (34) studied the effects of weight loss by diet alone or combined with aerobic exercise on body composition in older men. The addition of exercise to the hypocaloric diet did not attenuate the loss of lean tissue. Donnelly et al. (35) examined muscle hypertrophy with resistance training added to major weight loss in obese females. The cross-sectional area of slow-twitch and fast-twitch fibers remained unchanged in the sedentary group but was significantly increased in the resistance training group. Heavy exercise in highly motivated Ranger trainees appeared to protect the LBM, whereas large proportions of their body fat were lost.

Fong et al. (36) studied the effect of adding exercise to total parenteral nutrition after 10 days of bed rest and starvation in normal subjects. The exercise did not improve nitrogen balance, resting energy expenditure, or extremity amino acid flux. Is lack of exercise in the hospitalized patient a major contributor to the loss of muscle mass and function, particularly in an older population? If so, can some different form of exercise or muscle stimulation be applied in the hospital to reduce the loss of lean tissue, which is such a consistent finding in patients requiring bed rest?

Endurance exercise in young adult subjects has been shown to produce adaptations in skeletal muscle that result in a decreased reliance on carbohydrate and thereby an increased endurance during submaximal exercise. Coggan et al. (37) investigated whether the same adaptations could occur in older people. They demonstrated that after 9 to 12 months of endurance exercise training, changes were present in fiber subtype distribution, fiber size, capillarization, and glycolytic and mitochondrial enzyme activities similar to those of younger subjects. It was suggested that prior reports indicating that such changes did not occur in older individuals were probably related to inadequate length of time for the exercise stimulus.

MUSCLE METABOLISM AND FATIGUE

It was hypothesized over 30 years ago that after the muscle phosphocreatine (PCr) stores were depleted, ATP resynthesis would occur via glycogen breakdown to lactate (38). Subsequent evidence showed that PCr depletion and glycogen breakdown could occur simultaneously. With the introduction of percutaneous electrical stimulation, it became possible to investigate muscle metabolism and fatigue under conditions where complications relating to subject motivation are avoided and muscle biopsies could be obtained during isometric contraction. Studies with this technique emphasized that the importance of PCr hydrolysis was related to the extremely rapid rates at which it could provide the resynthesis of ATP. The chapter by Greenhaff et al. suggests that the rapid rate of PCr utlization at the onset of contraction could be responsible for a rapid depletion of stores at the sites of rapid energy translocation (actomyosin cross-bridges). The stimulus of glycogenolysis was formerly thought to be the transformation of phosphorylase and the availability of inorganic phosphate. More recently, evidence suggests that both inosine monophosphate (IMP) and adenosine monophosphate (AMP) are more important regulators of glycogenolysis.

Human muscle research often involves muscle biopsies, and the most frequent site of such biopsies is the quadriceps femoris. This muscle group in humans is composed of two fibers that are diametric in their metabolic and physiologic characteristics. Type I fibers are slow contracting, highly oxidative, and fatigue resistant. Conversely, type II fibers are fast contracting, highly glycolytic, and fatigue rapidly. Therefore, the two types differ in their maximal rates of ATP utilization and ability to generate and sustain power generation. Type II fibers have a relatively high initial power output, which is accompanied by a high rate of anaerobic ATP utilization but cannot be sustained for more than several seconds. This is in contrast to type I fibers, which have a relatively low initial power output and ATP utilization rate, both of which are maintained during contraction. Glycogenolysis is negligible after electrical stimulation in type I fibers, whereas during intense contraction glycogenolysis occurs maximally in type II fibers. Such studies suggest that during near maximal intensity exercise ATP is supplied initially by maximal rates of PCr degradation and glycogenolysis, particularly in type II fibers. As exercise progresses, the rate of anaerobic ATP turnover declines due to the lack of availability of PCr and the reduced rate of glycogenolysis. Therefore, an imbalance occurs between the rate of ATP demand and ATP supply, which could underlie the development of fatigue.

Birch et al. (39) found that ingestion of 20 g of Cr daily for 5 days led to an average increase in muscle total Cr of about 20%, of which 30% was PCr. This dose was shown to increase exercise performance by 5% to 7%. However, approximately one third of the subjects receiving this dose did not increase their muscle Cr stores, and they showed no increase in exercise performance. A recent study has indicated that a dietary supplement with Cr can reduce the extent of ATP degradation by 25% during maximal isokinetic cycling exercise while at the same time increasing work output. Ferrando et al. suggested that the improvements in exercise performance with dietary Cr supplementation result from the increase in preexercise PCr concentration in type II muscle fibers, which increase ATP resynthesis during exercise.

Fatigue has been defined as the decrease in muscle force-generating capacity resulting from physical activity. However, this definition is not readily applied to conventional dynamic leg exercise, such as treadmill or cycle ergometry, where gradually increasing fatigue during a constant work rate cannot be observed. Fulco et al. (40) have summarized the problems of studying fatigue with conventional ergometry and proposed using the dynamic knee extension isolated to the quadriceps femoris for the study of fatigue. This allows progressive muscle fatigue to serve as a framework to study both mechanisms and the effect of intervention.

The use of phosphorus-31 magnetic resonance spectroscopy allows the noninvasive separation of phases of metabolism that occur during the transition from rest to fatigue in an isometrically exercising muscle. Kent-Braun et al. (41) described the assessment of "oxidative potential" and three phases of metabolism in this transition where a steady state is present at the beginning and is gradually lost.

The chapter by Kehlet and Rosenberg reviews postoperative fatigue, which is defined as a nonpsychological but somatically precipitated event of multifactorial origin. They review the role of stress reduction, pain relief, early mobilization, and oral nutrition, emphasizing that treating one factor alone is not effective in reducing postoperative fatigue.

Intensive care and nutritional support both were developed during the turbulent 1960s. However intensive care has had its major focus on resuscitation and support of vital organs. There was the unspoken assumption that muscle tissue was expendable and therefore less important in patient care. Nutritional support in the hospital had a major focus on improving nitrogen balance and therefore conserving body protein. However, the extent to which an improved nitrogen balance represents conserving muscle mass and muscle function has not been well established. Weakness and easy fatigue continue to be important features of anyone who has undergone a severe catabolic response. The shortening of the length of hospital stay and more importantly, reducing the time required for complete convalescence, should involve patient management based on a better understanding of muscle metabolism and function.

REFERENCES

1. Munro HN. Metabolic integration of organs in health and disease. *JPEN* 1982;6:271–279.
2. Greenhaff PL, Ren J-M, Soderlund K, et al. Energy metabolism in single human muscle fibers during contraction without and with epinephrine infusion. *Am J Physiol* 1991;260:E713–E718.
3. Booth FW. Perspectives on molecular and cellular exercise physiology. *J Appl Physiol* 1988;65: 1461–1471.
4. Rodnick KJ, Haskell WL, Swislocki ALM, et al. Improved insulin action in muscle, liver, and adipose tissue in physically trained human subjects. *Am J Physiol* 1987;253:E489–E495.
5. Zurio F, Larson K, Bogardus C, et al. Skeletal muscle metabolism is a major determinant of resting energy expenditure. *J Clin Invest* 1990;86:1423–1427.
6. Bingham SA, Goldberg GR, Coward WA, et al. The effect of exercise and improved physical fitness on basal metabolic rate. *Br J Nutr* 1989;61:155–173.
7. Bangsbo J, Johansen L, Quistorff B, et al. NMR and analytic biochemical evaluation of CrP and nucleotides in the human calf during muscle contraction. *J Appl Physiol* 1993;74:2034–2039.
8. Mandarino LJ, Consoli A, Jain A, et al. Differential regulation of intracellular glucose metabolism by glucose and insulin in human muscle. *Am J Physiol* 1993;265:E898–E905.
9. Jepson MM, Bates PC, Broadbent P, et al. Relationship between glutamine concentration and protein synthesis in rat skeletal muscle. *Am J Physiol* 1988;255:E166–E172.
10. Newsholme EA, Newsholme P, Curi R, et al. A role for muscle in the immune system and its importance in surgery, trauma, sepsis and burns. *Nutrition* 1988;4:261–268.
11. Bonen A, Clark MG, Henriksen EJ. Experimental approaches in muscle metabolism: hindlimb perfusion and isolated muscle incubations. *Am J Physiol* 1994;266:E1–E16.
12. Clark MG, Colquhoun EQ, Rattigan S, et al. Vascular and endocrine control of muscle metabolism. *Am J Physiol* 1995;268:E797–E812.
13. Hickner RC, Bone D, Ungerstedt U, et al. Muscle blood flow during intermittent exercise: comparison of the microdialysis ethanol technique and 133-Xe clearance. *Clin Sci* 1994;86:15–25.
14. Rattigan S, Dora KA, Colquhoun EQ, et al. An α-adrenergic vascular effect of norepinephrine to inhibit insulin-mediated glucose uptake in the perfused rat hindlimb. *Am J Physiol* 1995;268: E305–E311.
15. Stuart CA, Shangraw RE, Prince MJ, et al. Bed-rest–induced insulin resistance occurs primarily in muscle. *Metabolism* 1988;37:802–806.
16. Wasserman DH, Geer RJ, Rice DE, et al. Interaction of exercise and insulin actin in humans. *Am J Physiol* 1991;260:E37–E45.
17. Richter EA, Keins B, Mizuno M, et al. Insulin action in human thighs after one-legged immobilization. *J Appl Physiol* 1989;67:19–23.

18. Dela F, Mikines KJ, von Linstow M, et al. Effect of training on insulin-mediated glucose uptake in human muscle. *Am J Physiol* 1992;263:E1134–E1143.
19. Jahoor F, Shangraw RE, Miyoshi H, et al. Role of insulin and glucose oxidation in mediating the protein catabolism of burns and sepsis. *Am J Physiol* 1989;20:E323–E331.
20. Baron AD, Brechtel G. Insulin differentially regulates systemic and skeletal muscle vascular resistance. *Am J Physiol* 1993;265:E61–E67.
21. Laakso M, Edelman SV, Brechtel G, et al. Decreased effect of insulin to stimulate skeletal muscle blood flow in obese man: a novel mechanism for insulin resistance. *J Clin Invest* 1990;85:1844–1852.
22. Steinberg HO, Brechtel G, Johnson A, et al. Insulin-mediated skeletal muscle vasodilation is nitric oxide dependent. *J Clin Invest* 1994;94:1172–1179.
23. Baron AD, Brechtel-Hook G, Johnson A, et al. Effect of perfusion rate on the time course of insulin-mediated skeletal muscle glucose uptake. *Am J Physiol* 1996;271:E1067–E1072.
24. Raitakari M, Juhani Knuuti M, Ruotsalainen U, et al. Insulin increases blood volume in human skeletal muscle: studies using [15-0]CO and positron emission tomography. *Am J Physiol* 1995;269:E1000–E1005.
25. Astrand PO, Rodahl K. *Textbook of work physiology.* 1st ed. New York: McGraw-Hill; 1970:608.
26. Ferrando AA, Lane HW, Stuart CA, et al. Prolonged bed rest decreases skelegal muscle and whole-body protein synthesis. *Am J Physiol* 1996;270:E627–E633.
27. Horton ES. Metabolic fuels, utilization and exercise. *Am J Clin Nutr* 1989;49:931–937.
28. Garland PB, Randle PJ. Control of pyruvate dehydrogenase in the perfused rat heart by the intracellular concentration of acetyl-coenzyme A. *Biochem J* 1964;91:6c–7c.
29. Dyck DJ, Putman CT, Heigenhauser JF, et al. Regulation of fat-carbohydrate interaction in skeletal muscle during intense aerobic cycling. *Am J Physiol* 1993;265:E852–E859.
30. Hultman E. Nutritional effects on work performance. *Am J Clin Nutr* 1989;49:949–957.
31. Measuring human muscle protein systhesis. *Nutr Rev* 1989;47:77–79.
32. Carraro F, Stuart CA, Hartl WH, et al. Effect of exercise and recovery on muscle protein synthesis in human subjects. *Am J Physiol* 1990;259:E470–E476.
33. Bannister R. Special presentation. Health, fitness, and sport. *Am J Clin Nutr* 1989;49:927–930.
34. Dengel DR, Hagberg JM, Coon PJ, et al. Effects of weight loss by diet alone or combined with aerobic exercise on body composition in older obese men. *Metabolism* 1994;43:867–871.
35. Donnelly JE, Sharp T, Houmard J, et al. Muscle hypertrophy with large-scale weight loss and resistance training. *Am J Clin Nutr* 1993;58:561–565.
36. Fong Y, Hesse DG, Tracey KJ, et al. Submaximal exercise during intravenous hyperalimentation of depleted subjects. *Ann Surg* 1988;March:297–304.
37. Coggan AR, Spina RJ, King DS, et al. Skeletal muscle adaptations to endurance training in 60- to 70-yr-old men and women. *J Appl Physiol* 1992;72:1780–1786.
38. Margaria R, Oliva D, Di Prampero PE, et al. Energy utilization in intermittent exercise of supramaximal intensity. *J Appl Physiol* 1969;26:752–756.
39. Birch R, Nobel D, Greenhaff PL. The influence of dietary creatine supplementation on performance during repeated bouts of maximal isokinetic cycling in man. *Eur J Appl Physiol* 1994;69:268–270.
40. Fulco CS, Lewis SF, Frykman PN, et al. Quantitation of progressive muscle fatigue during dynamic leg exercise in humans. *J Appl Physiol* 1995;79:2154–2162.
41. Kent-Braun JA, Miller RG, Weiner MW. Phases of metabolism during progressive exercise to fatigue in human skeletal muscle. *J Appl Physiol* 1993;75:573–580.

Physiology, Stress, and Malnutrition: Functional Correlates, Nutritional Intervention, edited by J.M. Kinney and H.N. Tucker. Lippincott–Raven Publishers © 1997.

Thermoregulation in the Neutral Zone

George L. Brengelmann and Margaret V. Savage

Department of Physiology and Biophysics, University of Washington, Seattle, Washington 98195

That body temperature regulation has a "neutral zone" is a concept we hold intuitively. It is connected with the concepts of normal body temperature and the "set point" of thermoregulation.

NORMAL BODY TEMPERATURE AND THE NEUTRAL ZONE

We think of normal body temperature with implicit constraints regarding the circumstances under which it can be discerned. We would not expect to read normal body temperature in a person sweating vigorously in a hot environment, nor in one shivering in the cold, nor in someone exercising. For example, a man might run at a marathon pace in a warm environment for hours with a stable body temperature of 39°C, thanks to evaporation of two liters of sweat secreted per hour (1). Although his high temperature is perfectly normal, it is not what we mean by his normal body temperature.

We look for normal body temperature in neutral thermal conditions: a limited range of environments that impose no thermal stress that would displace body temperature from normal in an inactive person. This zone of neutrality is wide, in terms of environmental temperature. Antarctic weather could be neutral for an adequately clothed person. What thermally neutral individuals in extremely different environments have in common is similar thermal conditions in the immediate vicinity of the body surface. These are the net result of environmental temperatures, wind speed, etc.; thermal properties of clothing; and the rate at which heat is delivered from the body core to the body surface. That thermal balance is reflected in skin temperature.

The neutral zone, specified as a range of skin temperatures compatible with thermal neutrality, is narrow—only a few degrees.

DEFINITION OF THE NEUTRAL ZONE

Technical

To specify the neutral zone in terms of skin temperatures in an operationally meaningful way, we need measures of what we mean by core temperature, Tc, and skin temperature, Tsk. Definition of either poses problems because temperatures vary throughout the body interior and over the body surface. The concept of body thermal compartments in relation to Tc is discussed briefly near the end of this chapter; for a critical review of measures of Tc, see the text of Brengelmann (2). For the moment, take any of the sites that closely track temperature in the major arteries, e.g., pulmonary artery, distal esophagus, tympanum, as representative of Tc. Also, for simplicity, take Tsk as represented by an area-weighted average of temperatures of representative areas of the body surface (3,4). The single number defined as Tsk by the various schemes for averaging do not differ appreciably because surface temperatures are relatively uniform in neutral conditions. The issue can be further simplified in experimental situations by forcing skin temperature to be uniform.

One way of specifying the neutral range is the range of Tsk perceived as neutral. If temperature over the body surface is uniform, this range is centered near 34°C and not much more than 2°C wide (5).

The alternative is a physical definition—the range of skin temperatures compatible with a thermal steady state accomplished without resort to either sweating or shivering. The temperature range may be the same as the perceived range of thermal neutrality, near 33–35°C in young adults.

Historical Definition and Association with Peripheral Vasomotor State

The neutral zone was discovered when physiologists in the era just before the Second World War studied thermal balance in human subjects over a wide range of environments by means of whole-body calorimeters (6–8). They found that rectal temperature remained constant without activation of sweating or shivering within a skin temperature range of approximately 33–35°C (6).

These findings were interpreted as evidence that the insulation of the body was changing because the difference between the temperatures of the body core and surface varied, but the total heat loss remained equal to the fixed, baseline rate of heat production. It was clear that this was the consequence of altered convective transport of heat from the body interior to the body surface by peripheral blood flow and that what controlled peripheral blood flow was neural modulation of vascular tone. Early on, therefore, the terms "neutral zone" and "vasomotor zone" came into use interchangeably.

Although the terms have been in common use ever since and part of the usual textbook treatment of body temperature regulation (9), this zone of human thermoregulation has received little experimental attention. Physiologists who studied temperature regulation were more interested in the dramatic effector responses on either side of the neutral zone.

MORE RECENT STUDIES OF TEMPERATURE REGULATION IN THE NEUTRAL ZONE

One study that more or less incidentally included monitoring of Tc at neutral levels of Tsk was the work of Craig and Dvorak in 1966 (10). They recorded metabolic rate and both rectal and tympanic membrane temperatures during 60-minute periods of controlled Tsk, set at particular levels that included 32, 34, 35, and 36°C, by means of immersing the subjects in a well-stirred temperature-controlled water bath. According to their concept of the neutral zone, only the range of Tsk that resulted in no disturbance of Tc from baseline qualified as neutral. They reported that range as only 35–35.5°C. This stringent criterion overlooks the fact (discussed below) that a range of stable Tc linked with the range of neutral Tsk is to be expected within the neutral zone.

Other studies conducted in relatively recent years have appeared to relate to the issue of temperature regulation in the neutral zone but actually address questions about thresholds in the adjoining zones (11,12). These focused on identifying the level of Tc at which sweating ceased during a downward trend and the Tc level at which shivering began during continued Tc decline. They sought to identify how widely these thresholds are separated and likened the separation, if any, to a "dead zone" in temperature regulation. However, it was necessary to hold Tsk fixed in order to avoid confusion in interpretation (thresholds differ at different levels of Tsk). Also necessary was the use of a Tsk level low enough to bring Tc down to levels at which shivering would result. Therefore, these studies were performed with Tsk outside of the neutral zone and do not answer questions about control within that zone.

Finally, practical questions about suitable environments have motivated studies of thermal balance in infants (13,14)

NEUTRAL ZONE AND SKIN BLOOD FLOW

One thing has become more clear since the days of whole-body calorimeters. That is, it seems almost certain that the vasomotor control that alters the heat transport from the body interior to the surface is limited to the cutaneous vasculature. The only other possible participant is the vasculature of skeletal muscle. However, muscle blood flow has been shown to be affected neither by temperature changes within the muscle itself in the range below 40°C (15) nor under conditions of systemic hyperthermia (16). Admittedly, these studies were concerned with the zone of temperatures above the neutral zone. To infer that this indifference of the vasculature of skeletal muscle to temperature stimuli would include the narrow range encountered in the neutral zone is an extrapolation, but all the evidence available indicates that this vasculature is not on the efferent side of thermoregulatory reflexes. That evidence does include constant muscle blood flow monitored during the initial temperature increase in the prehyperthermic phase of the experiments of Detry et al. (16).

WHY STUDY THE NEUTRAL ZONE TODAY?

In the above material, the neutral zone is treated as if delimited by constants that could be defined by the Bureau of Standards. More likely, the boundaries of the zone differ for each individual and vary in a given individual from time to time.

For practical reasons, comparison of neutral zone boundaries in particular groups relative to, for example, young men and women, would be valuable; e.g., in the aged, in heart failure patients, in patients with peripheral neuropathies.

There is also an absolutely basic reason to investigate temperature regulation in the neutral zone: to discover the characteristics of control. Until recently (17), no research has been devoted to the question of how skin blood flow is regulated in the neutral range of skin temperatures. As a fundamental physiologic mechanism, the control process is interesting in itself. Besides that, understanding of the control process and development of effective ways to evaluate parameters of control are a necessary foundation for addressing the kinds of questions that arise when people want to know if thermoregulation has been altered in various situations.

The experimental context for research on control of skin blood flow in regulation of Tc includes terminology and concepts such as set points, thresholds, and so forth, which are briefly reviewed below.

SET POINT OF BODY TEMPERATURE AND THE NEUTRAL ZONE

Set Point Concept in Human Thermoregulation

The concept that body temperature is regulated with respect to a set point is widely held but usually only vaguely defined. The usage is natural because the temperature regulation systems we encounter in everyday life have set points obvious from numbers on dials or digital displays. By analogy, we assume that normal temperature under neutral conditions reflects a Tc set point.

Students are taught that fever is a manifestation of an elevated set point; indeed, febrile body temperature seems to be actively regulated at a higher level than would otherwise be observed in the same environment. Counteracting physiologic responses occur if attempts are made to change body temperature in a febrile person (18,19).

The marathon runner also has stable Tc (1). The elevated Tc of exercise appears to be maintained against the influences of changes in the environment and has long been interpreted as evidence that the set point of temperature regulation, Tset, is altered by exercise (20). The logic and the nature of the experimental evidence are quite similar to the support for the idea that Tset is elevated in fever. However, the conclusion is disputed by others who have noted that (a) the high rate of heat production during exercise constitutes a load imposed on the thermoregulatory system, (b) the elevated temperature is a necessary "load error," and (c) the stability of the elevated temperature, despite altered environmental conditions, is the characteristic behavior of the class of temperature regulation systems in which effector output is adjusted in proportion to load error (21). Those with this point of view reject the idea that the set point of thermoregulation is elevated in exercise, but they retain the idea of set point, at least implicitly, because a load error is a deviation relative to a fixed reference.

To escape the complication of load error, one could limit one's concern with Tset to neutral zone thermoregulation in a nonexercising person. Isn't Tset simply the level at which Tc equilibrates? How do we find Tset experimentally?

Practical Problem of Determining the Set Point of a System

The common approach, for a nonfebrile, nonexercising person, is to describe as Tset the temperature at which Tc stabilizes in a nonexercising, nonfebrile person in the neutral zone. For example, the circadian changes in Tc are described as reflecting changes in the set point of thermoregulation. Someone goes to sleep and the temperature decreases to a lower level in fixed, neutral, thermal conditions; ergo, the set point has decreased.

It seems reasonable, intuitively, to say that we can at least identify a change in stable Tc as the consequence of an equal change in Tset. That interpretation would indeed be reasonable for certain simple kinds of temperature regulation systems. But it could be wrong for systems that approach the level of complexity of thermoregulation in humans. A change in stable Tc could be the consequence of an altered sensitivity in the response of skin blood flow to Tc or Tsk. Other likely influences on stable Tc include posture and variations in Tsk within the neutral zone. Below, these points are expanded upon and related terms are defined with the aid of simple models of systems that regulate temperature.

SET POINTS AND OTHER PROPERTIES OF SIMPLE THERMOREGULATORY SYSTEMS

Thermostatic Control

The characteristics of a simple thermostatic system are illustrated in Fig. 1. Control issues from a thermostatic device that is basically a switch that changes state at a particular temperature, which can be defined unequivocally as Tset. Below Tset, the switch is in the state that activates heating. Temperature in the controlled medium, Tmed, will increase. When temperature at the thermostat passes Tset, the switch toggles to the state that activates cooling, forcing Tmed down; or merely shuts off the heater, allowing Tmed to decrease passively.

The regulatory behavior of such a system is characterized by oscillation. The heater must necessarily be powerful enough to bring Tmed up above Tset. When it is activated, it is at 100% power, so Tmed will increase. When it is switched off, Tmed will decrease. Tmed is always doing one or the other. But, notwithstanding the oscillation, such systems can produce satisfactory constancy of average Tmed. A thermostatically controlled water bath can be designed to hold Tmed constant within 0.01°C in a room in which air temperature does not fluctuate more than a few degrees.

Experimental identification of Tset in a thermostatic system is easy, in principle, given means for recording Tmed and observing the behavior of the effectors. Simply note Tmed at the point that the change in effector state occurs. Accuracy of the determination is limited only by the accuracy of the Tmed instrumentation, possible differences between Tmed at the site of measurement and Tmed at the thermostat, and confusion introduced by lag time between the change in state of the thermostat and the observed activity of the effectors.

However, even in this simplest of thermoregulatory systems, a practical problem intrudes because real thermostatic systems are slightly more complicated,

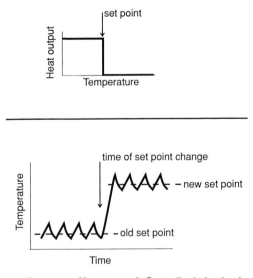

FIG. 1. Simple thermostatic system. **Upper panel:** Controller behavior. In a system limited to a heater and a thermostatic switch, the heater is switched on when temperature at the thermostat decreases below the set point. **Lower panel:** System behavior. In such systems, temperature cycles continually because the heater needs to be powerful enough to raise the temperature of the system under all ambient conditions. The temperature increases when the heater is on. When the system temperature reaches the set point, the heater switches off, but the temperature usually continues to increase briefly as stored heat in the heater equilibrates. Then the temperature decreases passively. After it passes the set point, the cycle repeats. The pattern of response to an altered set point is shown. After the set point is adjusted to a higher temperature, the system temperature cycles around the new set point. Experimentally, the set point level can be estimated from the average level of the equilibrium cycling pattern.

particularly if effectors are used both for cooling and heating rather than allowing one state to be passive. That is, a "dead band" separates the temperatures at which transitions occur. Consequently, the system exhibits hysteresis: each effector turns on at a temperature different from the one at which it turns off. This keeps the cooler from turning on the instant the heater turned off and allows them both to remain in the off state within the range of Tmed within the dead band. Temperature coasts, so to speak, within the dead band, affected by the passive heat exchange with the environment and dynamic factors such as heat stored at elevated temperature within the deactivated heating element.

Consequently, the experimental definition of Tset identifies the points of transition in the hysteresis behavior, the margins of the dead band. But the meanings of the experimentally determined parameters are clear, and a change in Tset could be assessed quantitatively in terms of the altered position of the dead band.

Proportional Control

In the next stage in sophistication of design of temperature control systems, effector output is controlled in proportion to changes in Tmed (Figs. 2 and 3 compare a proportional heater control system with the thermostatic system of Fig. 1). The system is connected in a negative feedback loop. A reference input, which we can define as Tset, is compared with Tmed. The difference, the error signal, is the control signal that sets the level of effector output. If the equipment that accomplishes the conversion is linear, the ratio of output level to error signal is a constant. This parameter is called the open loop gain of the system.

Potentially, such systems are free of the inevitable oscillation of a simple thermostatic system. Temperature seeks an equilibrium in which the error signal (Tmed − Tset) causes exactly the level of effector activity that balances the passive heat exchange with the environment. If environmental temperature changes, then a new level of effector activity will be necessary to match the new conditions for passive heat exchange; Tmed will change until the new error signal again results in effector activity that balances the new conditions.

The higher the open loop gain in such systems, the better the regulation. To accommodate a change in thermal load on the system, the error signal must change in order to produce the matching effector output. With high open loop

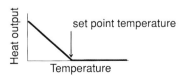

FIG. 2. Controller behavior in a simple proportional control system. In proportional control of a heater, heater output increases in proportion to the difference between system temperature, Tmed, and a reference, or set point temperature, Tset. In a heater control system, the slope is negative, resulting in positive effector output when Tmed is below Tset.

gain, only a small deviation from a previous equilibrium level suffices to elicit the necessary change. The ratio of the deviations in equilibrium Tmed to deviations in environmental temperature is the closed loop gain. The higher the open loop gain, the lower the closed loop gain, with a theoretical minimum of zero where infinitesimal changes in Tmed produce instantaneous corrections in effector output to match large changes in environmental temperature. Given the dynamics of real systems, however, high open loop gain results in overshoots in corrections, i.e., oscillations, so practical compromises require levels of open loop gain that result in tolerably small deviations of Tmed for the expected range of environmental conditions.

How is Tset determined experimentally for such a system? Particularly, how can a change in Tset be identified?

For example, consider a system for evaporative cooling somewhat analogous in properties to the physiologic system that controls sweating. The response, fluid

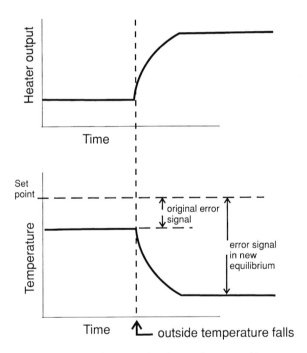

FIG. 3. System behavior in a simple proportional control system. Heater output and system temperature for a simple system for proportional control of a heater are plotted on the same time scale. The initial equilibrium temperature is below Tset, resulting in an error signal that produces sufficient heat for thermal balance in the original environment. After a decline in outside temperature, system temperature decreases because of increased heat loss. Heater output increases in proportion to the decline until a new equilibrium is reached. Neither steady temperature indicates the set point temperature because both are associated with error signals necessary to elicit the appropriate heater response.

secretion rate (SR), would be regulated in proportion to temperature increase relative to a reference. The response is inherently nonlinear in that SR cannot take on negative values (and also is subject to a finite limit). SR is elicited only above some threshold temperature. Below that temperature, SR is zero. That zero response temperature point can be unequivocally defined as Tset. SR, then, is proportional to (Tmed − Tset), except zero when Tmed < Tset, with a constant of proportionality (a) the open loop gain.

With freedom to manipulate the environmental temperature, Tamb, it is easy to determine Tset, given means of measurement of Tmed and SR. Make Tamb low enough to bring Tmed below the point at which SR is zero. Make a note of the value of Tmed at which SR reached zero. Elevate Tamb sufficiently to make Tmed increase. Note the value of Tmed at which SR can first be observed. This is exactly Tset, except for possible lag in SR onset dynamics and discrepancies between Tmed where measured and where sensed. (Some idea of the contribution of dynamics can be gained from any difference between this data point and the value of Tmed when SR touched zero during the time of low Tamb.) By recording subsequent concomitant SR and Tmed increases, the open loop gain also can be determined. As a practical matter, regression analysis of the latter data can be used to determine the intercept of the SR:Tmed response with zero, for refinement of the determination of Tset.

However, where environmental conditions result in equilibrium levels of Tmed and SR, and where the freedom to manipulate Tmed is limited, it is not so easy to determine the parameters of the SR:Tmed relationship. Certainly, equilibrium Tmed associated with an equilibrium elevated SR level should not be confused with Tset. That would be the same fallacy as interpreting the stable elevated Tc of exercise as evidence of an elevated set point; if Tmed were at Tset, error signal would be zero and effector activity would be nil.

Can we determine Tset in this kind of situation, i.e., where some peculiarity such as a transition to zero level of the effector cannot be obtained? That depends on whether a reasonable range of Tmed and response level (R) can be spanned. If the Tmed:R data pairs trace out a sloped line with a satisfactory confidence interval, then extrapolation to zero response level would be justifiable if the extrapolation were modest.

Can we take it as evidence that Tset has changed if we observe an altered equilibrium Tmed in a fixed environment? That question implies the possibility that the parameters of the control relationship are variable. If Tset can be a variable, why not the slope of the R:Tmed relationship (open loop gain)? A change in either alters the level of Tmed that activates the equilibrium level of R. Once we admit the possibility that R is a function of more than one variable, the simple observation of altered equilibrium Tmed can no longer be interpreted as a set point change.

Of course, actual physiologic temperature regulation systems are complex and everyone recognizes that no effector is controlled as a simple function of one variable. Nonetheless, the set point concept persists. Does it have any meaning in more complex systems?

Control Relative to Dual Inputs: System Properties Comparable with Actual Thermoregulation

The difficulties with the set point concept in more complex systems can be illustrated by adding a second input variable to the simple proportional control system described above.

In design of temperature regulation systems, improved stability of Tmed can often be obtained by modifying effector behavior, R, according to additional information. If the objective is to control Tmed within a system to minimize changes due to altered thermal conditions in the surrounding environment, it might even be possible to use information about the environmental conditions to compute the precise level of R necessary to achieve thermal equilibrium. In such feedforward systems, Tmed stability can be as perfect as the knowledge of the parameters that determine heat exchange between the controlled system and its environment. Imperfect knowledge of those parameters can be compensated by including a negative feedback loop through which R is adjusted in relation to deviations of Tmed from a reference level.

Another way of using information about the outside environment is to use it in a second negative feedback loop. For example, to use information related to surface temperature, Tsu, R could be generated as the sum of two contributions, one proportional to Tmed minus a reference level, and the other proportional to Tsu minus another reference level.

The control of skin blood flow in the neutral zone is likely to be at least as complex as the two examples above. Can we identify a Tset in a physiologic temperature regulation system that might be this complex?

The answer would be yes if the system were a perfect feedforward system because Tmed would be maintained perfectly constant. But, where dual feedback loops are active, the question becomes meaningless unless specific peculiarities of control can be identified.

A SIMPLE DUAL-INPUT MODEL OF THERMOREGULATORY CONTROL IN HUMANS

Difficulties in identifying Tset can be illustrated with the simple model that has been used to describe both skin blood flow control and control of sweat rate (22–24). Skin blood flow changes in neutral zone conditions are consistent with this model, as will be discussed below. According to this model, effector output level, R, is the sum of contributions from Tc and Tsk, according to the following equation:

$$R - Ro = a \times (Tc - Tco) + b \times (Tsk - Tsko) \qquad [1]$$

In this relationship, the effector activity, R, is expressed relative to a constant, Ro, that can be interpreted as a reference, or baseline level. For sweating, it is appropriately set to zero; but both metabolic rate and skin blood flow rate are usually referenced to baseline levels. Net effector activity is expressed as the sum of two contributions derived from Tc and Tsk information, respectively. The constants a and Tco correspond, respectively, to the constant of proportionality (open loop gain) and the set point in the simple proportional control system described above. The constants b and Tsko determine the contribution to R from Tsk. Figure 4 schematically illustrates control of sweating as an example of effector output determined by the linear combination of inputs from Tc and Tsk.

If this model describes thermoregulatory effector activity reasonably well, is Tco the "real" core temperature set point? If you believe so, then you should also regard Tsko as a real skin temperature set point. Putting that aside, for the moment, one way to approach this question is to endure a little algebra.

For example, suppose Ro = 0, a = 10, b = 1, and the original choices for Tco and Tsko are 37.0 and 33.0, respectively. Then with Tc and Tsk at 37 and 35, respectively, R, without worrying about units, is 2:

$$2 = 10 \times (37 - 37) + 1 \times (35 - 33)$$

However, these Tco and Tsko values are arbitrary; you can pick any Tco you want. Choose 36.5 for Tco and you can make the combination add up to 2 with Tso as 38:

$$2 = 10 \times (37 - 36.5) + 1 \times (35 - 38)$$

By expanding the terms in Equation 1, the reference constants can be gathered into a single constant, K:

$$R = a \times Tc + b \times Tsk + K \qquad [2]$$

In this formulation, the three reference constants, Tco in particular, lose their individuality; it brushes away the appearance that a meaningful Tco might be defined.

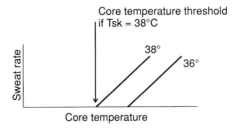

FIG. 4. Control in a dual-input proportional control system. In this schematic representation of the control of sweat rate, the relationship between Tc and sweat rate is shown for two levels of Tsk. With Tsk held steady at 38°C, SR is zero below a certain threshold level of Tc. If Tc increases above that level, SR increases in proportion to the difference between Tc and the threshold level. Similar behavior is seen with Tsk held steady at 36°C, with the same increase in SR per degree increase in Tc, except that the threshold level is higher. In terms of Equation 1, the slope of these lines is "a," the horizontal difference between them is determined by "b," and their threshold points are determined by the other constants and the constraint that SR cannot take on negative values.

On the other hand, the above focus on the arbitrariness of Tco may be obfuscation: true mathematically, but irrelevant physiologically. For example, note that the second summation of terms to add up to 2 includes a negative 3 from the Tsk contribution. That could be seen in physiologic terms as an inhibitory influence of Tsk, but it might stretch one's physiologic imagination to have to regard all Tsk levels below 38°C as inhibitory.

Experimental Approach in the Context of the Two-Input Model

In an experimental approach, we would look for features in control that might reveal a physiologically meaningful reference level. Conceivably, we might be able to identify a Tco on the basis of something special that happens at a particular Tc level.

What we are looking for is something that departs from the simple linear model. Suppose, for example, that all the SR:Tc lines for various levels of Tsk radiated from a common point. Then, the effect of Tsk would be seen as a moderating influence on proportional control driven from Tc relative to a set point appropriately defined as that particular value of Tc. Nadel et al. thought that SR lines for fixed Tsk might radiate from a fixed point (actually from a negative level of SR) and that the associated level of Tc would define a unique set point, but this intriguing possibility has not been pursued.

The lines that describe hypothetical SR in terms of Tc and Tsk in Fig. 4 do appear to have special features related to Tco. At a given Tsk, and below a particular Tc, SR is zero. With progressive elevation in Tc, a threshold point is reached beyond which SR increases in proportion to Tc. At a higher, fixed Tsk, the same pattern is seen, except that the threshold level is lower. It is tempting to interpret these threshold levels of Tc as a special feature that reveals a Tc reference level.

However, these apparent thresholds do not show some special peculiarity of control related to particular levels of Tc. In the model of Equation 1, the quantities (Tc − Tco) and (Tsk − Tsko) both take on negative values. Levels of Tc and Tsk below their respective reference levels result in negative contributions to R. The apparent threshold crossings in Fig. 4 are simply the point at which the sum of the two contributions first exceeds zero. No switch is activated by Tc level to turn off Tsk influence nor vice versa. The only deviation from the linearity expressed in the model is the necessary stipulation that SR cannot take on negative values. The argument that Tco and Tsko are arbitrary still holds.

However, threshold crossings are a reproducible feature of SR control, at least in the short term (25). Determining changes in Tc thresholds may be a practical way to assess various influences on thermoregulation quantitatively.

Perhaps experiments limited to measurements of Tc, Tsk, and effector output can be designed to discover peculiarities of control associated with Tc such as something akin to switching behavior, but so far we have no quantitative descriptions of behavior of any of the thermoregulatory effectors that require interpretation more complex than the simple two-input model. Identification of control mechanisms related to specific core temperature reference levels may not be possible in noninvasive experiments.

Significance of Altered Equilibrium Tc in a Two-Input System

Without belaboring the point, if we recognize that all of the "constants" a, b, Tco, Tsko, and Ro might be physiologic variables, it is clear that a change in equilibrium Tc in a fixed environment could be the consequence of change in any of them.

Conclusion

Thermoregulatory control in humans is at least as complicated as the two-input system described in Equation 1. In this context, apparent thresholds are of interest (25) but do not show a particular Tset, i.e., a set point for core temperature. Equilibrium Tc does not define Tset, and altered equilibrium Tc is not evidence of an altered Tset. Given the limitations of studying intact human subjects, i.e., without access to the nervous system, what would be necessary for validating a set point concept in relation to the influence of Tc would be some peculiarity of control apparent at a particular Tc.

EQUILIBRIUM TC IN THE NEUTRAL ZONE: "NORMAL BODY TEMPERATURE"

Another implication arises from study of the two-input models of thermoregulation. Equilibrium Tc must vary with Tsk within the neutral zone. Although we might intuitively expect that equilibrium Tc would simply increase in proportion to Tsk, the relationship might not be that simple.

Interaction Between Reflex and Physical Effects of Tc and Tsk and the Steady-State Relationship Between Tc and Tsk.

If both Tc and Tsk influence skin blood flow (SkBF) in the neutral zone in a manner similar to the way they influence SkBF and sweat rate (SR) in hyperthermia, then SkBF would increase in response to either, independently, as approximated in Equation 1. A change in either also interacts with the effector response.

This interaction is unique to control of SkBF. In control of SR, if Tc changes, a proportional, reflex-mediated change in SR occurs, but the Tc change has no effect on the heat loss rate associated with a given secretion rate. However, in control of SkBF, when a Tc change occurs, it not only causes a proportional,

reflex-mediated, change in SkBF, but it also alters the heat transfer rate associated with a given level of SkBF. For a given SkBF, greater Tc increases heat
transfer because arterial blood arrives at the skin warmer and loses more heat in
equilibrating with Tsk. Equally well, SkBF change elicited by change in Tsk
results in altered heat transfer rate per SkBF unit.

Imagine stable neutral zone conditions in which Tc and Tsk are fixed in an
equilibrium. Tc and Tsk jointly determine the associated level of SkBF as physiologic inputs to control. The equilibrium thermal balance depends on the rate at
which heat is transferred to the skin surface by SkBF (to a first approximation,
rate of heat transfer to the body surface is proportional to the product of SkBF
and the Tc:Tsk difference (8,26).

If Tsk then increases (remaining within the neutral zone range), both a physiologic control consequence (reflex-driven increase in SkBF) and a physical consequence (reduced heat transfer rate per unit of SkBF) follow: Three possibilities are offered:

1. These might balance perfectly so that the same heat transfer rate resulted
   from the matching of increased SkBF with reduction of heat flow per unit of
   SkBF. Tc would remain unaffected.
2. A minor reflex-driven increase in SkBF might be outweighed by the reduced
   Tc–Tsk difference, resulting in a net reduction of heat transfer. With accumulation of heat in the core, Tc would then tend to increase. The reflex
   effect, increased SkBF, and the physical effect, increased Tc–Tsk difference,
   would combine to tend toward an increased equilibrium Tc.
3. A large reflex response to the Tsk increase could result in SkBF increase so
   that heat flow increased despite the reduction in Tc–Tsk difference. With
   consequent reduction in Tc, the reflex and physical effects combine to tend
   toward a decreased equilibrium Tc.

According to this qualitative analysis, equilibrium Tc might remain unaffected
by Tsk changes or move in either direction, with or contrary to the Tsk change.
The implication that Tc might move in the "wrong" direction, i.e., contrary to
Tsk changes is not far-fetched.

Wrong-Way Tc Changes in After-Rise and After-Drop

We know that Tc typically increases during a short period after Tsk is dropped
from the neutral range to levels that eventually result in shivering (8). In the light
of the present analysis, this "after-rise" may be interpreted as evidence that the
reflex consequence of the Tsk change is an immediate reduction of SkBF to a
fraction of its former value and that that fraction is greater than the reciprocal of
the fractional change in the Tc–Tsk difference. In other words, heat loss from the
core is immediately reduced below the previous equilibrium level. Of course,
this cannot prevent the eventual progressive accumulation of heat debt through

loss of heat from the periphery via residual skin blood flow and conduction, but, transiently, Tc increases.

Wrong-way Tc change also occurs in "after-drop," the decline in Tc that follows immediately upon rapid increase in Tsk after development of hypothermia in a long period of exposure to Tsk below the neutral zone range (27). Clearly, the sudden increase in the rate of decline of Tc is due to increased convective cooling. The Tsk increase elicits an SkBF increase large enough to result in increased heat loss despite reduced Tc–Tsk gradient.

Those who have attempted to ascribe the afterdrop to the simple physics of conductive cooling—temperature deep within a solid will continue to decrease for a while after surface temperature is elevated to a new level after a period of cooling—have overlooked the fact that it is physically impossible in that setting for the rate of internal temperature decline to increase in response to increased surface temperature (28).

Influence of Other Variables on Equilibrium Tc in the Neutral Zone

The above implications do not depend on the specific formulation of the two-input model according to the prototypical relationship of Equation 1, only that SkBF increases more or less proportionally to Tc and Tsk, independently, that increased Tc for a given level of SkBF increases heat transfer, and that increased Tsk for a given level of SkBF decreases heat transfer (Tsk is always less than Tc in the specified neutral zone conditions). Without risking the absurdity of stretching a model beyond its possible applicability (29), we can discuss ways that the equilibrium Tc–Tsk relationship might be altered in terms of the parameters in Equation 1.

The basic shape of the Tc–Tsk equilibrium relationship would relate strongly to the a:b ratio. The greater the sensitivity of SkBF to Tsk changes, the more the likelihood that equilibrium Tc will decrease in response to a Tsk increase. Accordingly, we can expect that any influence that altered the sensitivity of SkBF to changes in either variable would alter the equilibrium relationship not only in the level of Tc associated with a given Tsk, but also in the shape of the relationship.

As to the significance of the other constants, we can avoid the stretch of speculating about them individually by again lumping them together as a single constant, K, and simply recognize that any influence that has the effect of altering SkBF for fixed Tc, Tsk and fixed ratio of Tc and Tsk sensitivities, i.e., the effect of changing K, will also alter equilibrium levels of Tc. In a particular equilibrium, the level of SkBF is exactly that which achieves the correct heat transfer rate for the particular Tc and Tsk. After change in K, SkBF is displaced from that level and a new equilibrium will be sought.

For example, dehydration reduces SkBF (30). Suppose, for the moment, that the effect is only to reduce K, so that for the same Tc and Tsk, SkBF will be reduced correspondingly [in reality, dehydration seems to influence both baseline

SkBF and reflex sensitivity (30,31)]. Also assume that this change can be induced instantaneously and that Tsk can be held fixed. In a thermal equilibrium before the change, Tc is at a particular level compatible with Tsk. SkBF, determined by current levels of Tc and Tsk, is at the level that results in thermal balance for that Tc–Tsk difference. Now turn on the effects of dehydration, i.e., reduce SkBF. Consequently, heat loss is reduced. With Tsk fixed, Tc tends to increase, causing SkBF increase on the way until the combined effect of the increased Tc–Tsk gradient and the increased SkBF restore heat loss to the equilibrium level. The equilibrium levels of Tc previously associated with each Tsk in the neutral range is affected similarly.

Another example of a nonthermal influence that might act through altering baseline SkBF rather than sensitivity of the thermal reflex responses is the effect of posture. A change in posture changes SkBF (32,33), presumably because of the influence on blood pressure regulation of the altered distribution of the venous volume. Lying down increases SkBF. With fixed Tsk, that should result in a reduced equilibrium Tc. Indeed, Tc decreases when a person lies down (33).

These two examples, couched in terms of an altered SkBF baseline rather than altered sensitivity of the reflex sensitivities, are intended to emphasize that anything that influences SkBF will alter equilibrium Tc for a given Tsk. According to the preceding discussion of the effect of influences on reflex sensitivity of SkBF to Tc or Tsk changes, we see that these can be expected to change the shape of the relationship as well. If dehydration, for example, were to reduce SkBF sensitivity to Tc, but not to Tsk, the consequence might be to convert the Tc–Tsk relationship from a right-way shape to a wrong-way shape. That is, before, equilibrium Tc would trend upward with Tsk increase; after, equilibrium Tc would decrease with Tc decrease.

Conclusion: The Tc–Tsk Relationship and the Set Point for "Normal" Tc

With a crude model, we can see that equilibrium Tc could be nearly independent of Tsk or could follow a relationship sloped one way or the other. If the relationship is not nearly independent of Tsk, then to specify Tc we also have to specify Tsk. Whatever the equilibrium Tc–Tsk curve looks like in the neutral zone for a given state of the various variables that influence baseline SkBF or the sensitivities of SkBF to Tsk or Tc, it changes if one of those variables changes. To proceed further than these theoretical considerations, experimental work on characteristics of thermoregulation in the neutral zone is necessary.

EXPERIMENTAL INVESTIGATION OF CONTROL OF SKBF IN THE NEUTRAL ZONE

A study of SkBF control in the 33–35°C Tsk range was recently published (17). Tsk was set at 33 or 35°C by means of water sprayed over most of the body surface except for one arm and the head and neck. In this way, Tsk uniformity was achieved without the interference with SkBF control that would be expected from immersion. Also, Tsk changes could be made rapidly. The authors expected that the responses to stepwise Tsk changes would show reflex SkBF changes due to Tsk change, uncomplicated by appreciable Tc change.

Their measure of Tc was esophageal temperature Tes, recorded from the region of contact between the esophagus and left atrium. This position was verified by the characteristic changes in the atrial waveform in electrocardiograms obtained from an electrode near the temperature sensor. They recorded forearm blood flow (FBF) in both the forearm that was sprayed with water and the other, which was exposed to room air. In this way, they hoped to resolve the contribution of local temperature to reflex-driven SkBF changes, i.e., flow in the "dry arm" would be influenced by reflex only, whereas "wet arm" flow changes would include any influence of local temperature. The sensitivity of cutaneous vascular tone to local temperature is well known (34).

The choice of FBF in a study devoted to SkBF control was based on findings that only the cutaneous vasculature is influenced in thermoregulatory reflexes (16,35) and the assumption that nonthermoregulatory reflex influences on the vasculature of the muscle of the forearm would be fixed in a supine subject, i.e., changes in FBF would reflect changes in SkBF (36). FBF was recorded by means of venous occlusion plethysmography.

Details of methods and experimental results can be found elsewhere (17). The chief findings are illustrated in Fig. 5.

The clearest finding is confirmation that SkBF is under the reflex influence of Tsk in this range of temperatures. FBF changed as rapidly as Tsk in both arms. Generally, the FBF changes were compatible with the two-input model described above in Equations 1 and 2, as indicated by linear regression analysis. However, the correspondence between the prediction from the regression parameters was little improved by the two-input model compared with regression on Tsk alone. The role of Tc is undoubted, however. In unpublished experiments, the investigators used a brief period of high Tsk to elevate Tc to hyperthermic levels and then observed FBF recovery during a subsequent period of neutral zone Tsk. FBF recovered along with Tc to previous equilibrium levels.

Also clear was an overall wrong-way pattern in the Tc–Tsk relationship. Tes decreased when Tsk was elevated to 35°C and increased when Tsk was decreased to 33°C. The Tes excursion was approximately 0.1°C. According to the logic developed above, this indicates that the reflex influence of Tsk on SkBF overcompensates for the thermal influence of Tsk on heat transfer, so that net heat loss temporarily decreases below the equilibrium level. However, the details are difficult to resolve.

Presumably, the initial heat loss imbalance is corrected in the reflex response to Tc, e.g., the Tc increase after Tsk decrease acts to elicit SkBF increase that corrects the overcompensation due to the reflex-driven decrease in Tsk. However, the observed changes in Tes, if any, during periods of constant Tsk did not

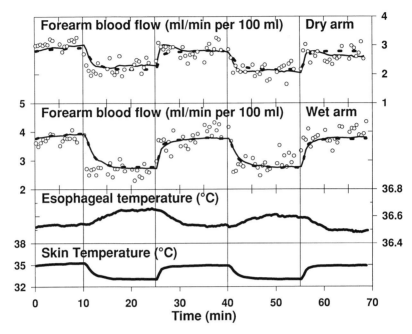

FIG. 5. Responses of eight subjects in whom Tsk over most of the body, including one forearm (wet arm), was cycled between 33 and 35°C by a water spray system. Skin blood flow changes are seen as changes in forearm blood flow, recorded in both forearms. The "dry arm" forearm and the head and neck were exposed to room air. Differences in the wet versus dry arm records show a slight influence of local Tsk on forearm blood flow, superimposed on the reflex driven by whole-body Tsk and Tc. Solid lines in the forearm blood flow records are from the linear regression analysis of the raw data with esophageal temperature and skin temperature as independent inputs (i.e., the relationship in Equations 1 and 2). Dashed lines are from regression analysis on skin temperature only. Reprinted with permission (17).

show this correction, even when Tsk was held at 33°C for an hour. Nothing in the features of the responses can resolve the question of whether the response to Tsk change reflects a feedforward connection, as opposed to influence via a second negative feedback loop.

Finally, slight differences between the responses in the wet versus dry forearm are of interest, particularly for questions about how these results might apply to real situations in which Tsk is not uniform. An influence of local temperature was indicated by the observation of lower overall FBF average in the dry arm, on which local Tsk, through exposure to room air, was near 31°C. But no influence of local Tsk in the 33–35°C range could be observed in separate experiments when whole-body Tsk was fixed and neutral and only one forearm was sprayed with water. Evidently, sensitivity to local temperature is minimal in the 33–35°C range, but lower levels of Tsk are effective in reducing SkBF. In any case, in a person with Tsk generally in the neutral range but with some cooler regions of skin, e.g., the distal extremities, SkBF in those regions is likely to be reduced below the reflex-set level.

Space does not permit addressing in detail some critical issues that arise on close inspection of these experimental results. One that should be mentioned, however briefly, is the implied treatment of Tc as representing temperature of a single, rapidly responding, thermal compartment served by a heat exchanger, the cutaneous vasculature. The experimenter need merely fix Tsk at a particular level and, shortly after, the associated equilibrium Tc can be recorded.

Reality differs. In additional experiments with Tsk held at 33°C for an hour, most subjects exhibited a trend in Tes after the initial response to setting Tsk at 33°C. Some cooled, some warmed, two out of seven remained at fixed Tes.

Indeed, the core organs—heart, brain, kidneys, and splanchnic system—may be considered a single thermal compartment of reasonably uniform temperature and overall thermal lag relative to arterial blood temperature of only a few minutes. The temperature of this compartment is well represented by Tes (2,37). In a resting person, however, this compartment exchanges heat with larger compartments in terms of mass (skeletal muscle and bone).

The former is characterized by a ratio of mass to blood flow 50 times or more greater than the well-perfused core organs and a correspondingly greater thermal lag relative to arterial blood temperature. In active skeletal muscle, the mass:perfusion rate soars and the active mass rapidly warms (38,39), but on completion of exercise, the mass:flow ratio quickly returns to previous levels and stored heat leaves the compartment with lag times of tens of minutes (39).

The large mass, variable dynamics, and influence of environmental conditions on the peripheral regions make this compartment affect Tc with long-lasting trends. A subject arrives in the laboratory for a study on thermoregulation in the neutral zone with a long thermal history written into his or her slow thermal compartments. To analyze trends, some means of observing heat content within at least the muscle compartment is necessary.

CONCLUSION

The experimental findings confirm expectations of how Tc might vary with Tsk in the range of Tsk in which thermal steady states are possible in a resting person through thermoregulatory effector activity limited to control of skin blood flow. The range spanned by equilibrium Tc within the Tsk boundaries of the neutral zone may be the best definition of normal Tc, or perhaps, the Tc–Tsk relationship itself is the best reference for normality.

Centuries of practical experience tell us that all this makes not much difference when studying a reading on a clinical thermometer and thinking about taking an aspirin, but the issue becomes germane when we closely scrutinize Tc levels and Tc changes for research purposes.

It is obviously no time to be thinking in terms of a core temperature set point when you observe a change in neutral zone equilibrium Tc.

ACKNOWLEDGMENTS

We gratefully acknowledge support of the University of Washington Research Royalty Fund Program in the preparation of this chapter.

REFERENCES

1. Adams WC, Fox RH, Fry AJ, Macdonald IC. Thermoregulation during marathon running in cool, moderate, and hot environments. *J Appl Physiol* 1975;38:1030–1037.
2. Brengelmann GL. Dilemma of body temperature measurement. In: Shiraki K, Yousef MK, eds. Man in stressful environments: thermal and work physiology. Springfield, IL: Charles C Thomas; 1987: 5–22.
3. Ramanathan NL. A new weighting system for mean surface temperature of the human body. *J Appl Physiol* 1964;19:531–533.
4. Mitchell D, Wyndham CH. Comparison of weighting formulas for calculating mean skin temperature. *J Appl Physiol* 1969;26:616–622.
5. Hensel H. *Thermoreception and temperature regulation.* London: Academic; 1981:1–321.
6. Hardy JD, DuBois EF. Basal metabolism, radiation, convection and vaporization at temperatures of 22 to 35°C. *J Nutr* 1938;15:477–497.
7. DuBois EF. *The temperature of the human body in health and disease.* New York: Reinhold; 1941: 24–44.
8. Burton AC, Bazett HC. A study of the average temperature of the tissues, of the exchanges of heat and vasomotor responses in man by means of a bath calorimeter. *Am J Physiol* 1936;117:36–54.
9. Bligh J, Johnson KG. Glossary of terms for thermal physiology. *J Appl Physiol* 1973;35:941–961.
10. Craig AB, Dvorak M. Thermal regulation during water immersion. *J Appl Physiol* 1966;21:1577–1585.
11. Cabanac M, Massonnet B. Thermoregulatory responses as a function of core temperature in humans. *J Physiol (Lond)* 1977;265:587–596.
12. Mekjavic IB, Sundberg CJ, Linnarsson D. Core temperature "null zone." *J Appl Physiol* 1991;71: 1289–1295.
13. Hey EN, Katz G. The optimum thermal environment for babies. *Arch Dis Child* 1970;45:328–334.
14. Sauer PJJ, Dane HJ, Visser HKA. New standards for neutral thermal environments of healthy very low birthweight infants in week one of life. *Arch Dis Child* 1984;59:18–22.
15. Sekins KM, Lehmann JF, Esselman P, et al. Local muscle blood flow and temperature responses to 915mhz diathermy as simultaneously measured and numerically predicted. *Arch Phys Med Rehabil* 1984;65:1–7.
16. Detry J-M, Brengelmann GL, Rowell LB, Wyss C. Skin and muscle components of forearm blood flow in directly heated resting man. *J Appl Physiol* 1972;32:506–511.
17. Savage MV, Brengelmann GL. Control of skin blood flow in the neutral zone of human body temperature regulation. *J Appl Physiol* 1996;80:1249–1257.
18. Cooper KE, Cranston WI, Snell ES. Temperature regulation during fever in man. *Clin Sci* 1964;27: 345–356.
19. Cabanac M, Massonnet B. Temperature regulation during fever: change in set point or change of gain? A tentative answer from a behavioural study in man. *J Physiol (Lond)* 1974;238:561–568.
20. Nielsen M. Die regulation der körpertemperatur bei muskelarbeit. *Scand Arch Physiol* 1938;79: 193–229.
21. Gisolfi CV. Temperature regulation during exercise: directions—1983. *Med Sci Sports Exerc* 1983; 15:15–20.
22. Wyss CR, Brengelmann GL, Johnson JM, et al. Control of skin blood flow, sweating, and heart rate: role of skin vs core temperature. *J Appl Physiol* 1974;36:726–733.
23. Wenger CB, Roberts MF, Stolwijk JAJ, Nadel ER. Forearm blood flow during body temperature transients produced by leg exercise. *J Appl Physiol* 1975;38:58–63.
24. Nadel ER, Bullard RW, Stolwijk JAJ. Importance of skin temperature in the regulation of sweating. *J Appl Physiol* 1971;31:80–87.
25. Brengelmann GL, Savage MV, Avery DH. Reproducibility of the core temperature threshold for sweating onset in humans. *J Appl Physiol* 1994;77:1671–1677.

26. Burton AC. The application of the theory of heat flow to the study of energy metabolism. *J Nutr* 1934;7:497–533.
27. Savard GK, Cooper KE, Veale WL, Malkinson TJ. Peripheral blood flow during rewarming from mild hypothermia in humans. *J Appl Physiol* 1985;58:4–13.
28. Webb P. Afterdrop of body temperature during rewarming: an alternative explanation. *J Appl Physiol* 1986;60:385–390.
29. Brown AC, Brengelmann GL. The interaction of peripheral and central inputs in the temperature regulation system. In: Hardy JD, Gagge AP, Stolwijk JAJ, eds. *Physiological and behavioural temperature regulation.* Springfield, IL: Charles C Thomas; 1970:684–702.
30. Nadel ER, Fortney SM, Wenger CB. Effect of hydration state on circulatory and thermal regulations. *J Appl Physiol* 1980;49:715–721.
31. Fortney SM, Wenger CB, Bove JR, Nadel ER. Effect of hyperosmolality on control of blood flow and sweating. *J Appl Physiol* 1984;57:1688–1695.
32. Johnson JM, Rowell LB, Brengelmann GL. Modification of the skin blood flow-body temperature relationship by upright exercise. *J Appl Physiol* 1974;37:880–886.
33. Nielsen M, Herrington LP, Winslow CEA. The effect of posture upon peripheral circulation. *Am J Physiol* 1939;127:573–580.
34. Barcroft H, Edholm OG. The effect of temperature on blood flow and deep temperature in the human forearm. *J Physiol (Lond)* 1943;102:5–20.
35. Rowell LB. *Human cardiovascular control.* New York: Oxford University Press; 1993:1–500.
36. Johnson JM, Brengelmann GL, Hales JRS, et al. Regulation of the cutaneous circulation. *Fed Proc* 1986;45:2841–2850.
37. Shiraki K, Sagawa S, Tajima F, et al. Independence of brain and tympanic temperatures in an unanesthetized human. *J Appl Physiol* 1988;65:482–486.
38. Äikäs E, Karvonen MJ, Piironen P, Ruosteenoja R. Intramuscular, rectal and oesophageal temperature during exercise. *Acta Physiol Scand* 1962;54:366–370.
39. Thoden J, Kenny G, Reardon F, et al. Disturbance of thermal homeostasis during post-exercise hyperthermia. *Eur J Appl Physiol* 1994;68:170–176.

Physiology, Stress, and Malnutrition: Functional Correlates, Nutritional Intervention,
edited by J.M. Kinney and H.N. Tucker.
Lippincott–Raven Publishers © 1997.

Thermoregulation in Severe Exercise

Bodil Nielsen Johannsen

August Krogh Institute, Copenhagen University, DK 2100 Copenhagen, Denmark

REGULATION OF CORE TEMPERATURE

During exercise the metabolic processes liberate heat in the muscles that increase in temperature. During brief intense bouts of exercise, muscle temperature can increase by 4–5°C from 34–35° to approximately 39°C within a few minutes (Fig. 1). However, due to the large convection by the circulation— muscle blood flow may reach values of up to 7–10 L/min in one exercising leg—the heat is dispersed quickly by the blood flow to the rest of the body core. The core temperature measured, for instance, by esophageal temperature will therefore increase also. Most daily activities are intermittent, so the work intensity varies from minute to minute and the muscle and core temperature fluctuate accordingly.

However, in prolonged continuous exercise lasting for more than 40 minutes, heat liberated by the metabolism is stored in the body, which results in an increase in body temperature. The heat-dissipating mechanisms are activated by the increased core temperature, and after 20–30 minutes a balance between heat liberation and heat loss is achieved and the core temperature is maintained at a new elevated level. This was first shown by Marius Nielsen in 1938 (1), who further pointed out that this was a regulated increase because it was independent of environmental condition within wide limits. These limits were later defined as "the prescriptive zone" (2).

The mean skin surface temperature, $\overline{T}_{sk}$, on the other hand, varies with ambient temperature, whereas it is independent of work load and rate of heat liberation in conditions under which thermal balance can be achieved (1,3). This is indicative of coupling between the heat transfer to the skin and the evaporative heat loss (3).

The increase in core temperature has later been shown to be regulated in proportion to the relative load on the individual (4), i.e., to the percentage of $\dot{V}O_2max$, the maximal aerobic capacity of the individual.

The core temperature during exercise is therefore independent of the rate of heat liberation. Two persons with different $\dot{V}O_2max$ working both at 50% of $\dot{V}O_2max$ will have the same core temperature, $\approx 38°C$, in steady state, whereas

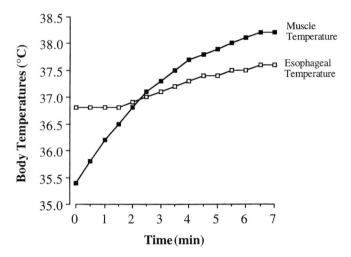

FIG. 1. Temperature changes in muscle (m. vastus lateralis) and in the deep esophagus at the start of exercise (200 W, subject JG).

the person with the highest $\dot{V}O_2$max will produce and dissipate more heat in this condition. Similarly, it has been shown that during eccentric exercise, e.g., walking/running downhill, potential energy is absorbed in the stretching active muscles and converted to heat, which is dissipated by sweating while core temperature is maintained in proportion to the metabolic rate (3,5).

Severe Exercise

Few have studied thermoregulation at exercise intensities above 75% of $\dot{V}O_2$max. Davies et al. (6) did, and found that the core temperature/$\dot{V}O_2$max relationship becomes curvilinear (Fig. 2). But also at such high relative work loads the core temperature was more closely related to the relative than to the absolute energy expenditure, and $\overline{T}_{sk}$ was independent of the metabolic rate for a given environment. Thus, the relationship between exercise core temperature and relative work load (4) was confirmed, and the range of work intensities extended to include relative work loads up to almost 90% of $\dot{V}O_2$max. These high intensities can be sustained for 1 hour by highly trained endurance individuals (6,7). The relationship was explained as follows. To achieve thermal equilibrium at a given absolute work load, both the high $\dot{V}O_2$ and low $\dot{V}O_2$ individual must obtain a balance between the heat delivered to the skin by the blood flow and the evaporative heat loss from the skin surface. This must be the case because $\overline{T}_{sk}$ and E are the same. Because metabolic rate and cardiac output are related and independent of relative load, it follows that for a given absolute metabolic rate the low $\dot{V}O_2$ individual is taxing his or her cardiac capacity to a larger degree. The

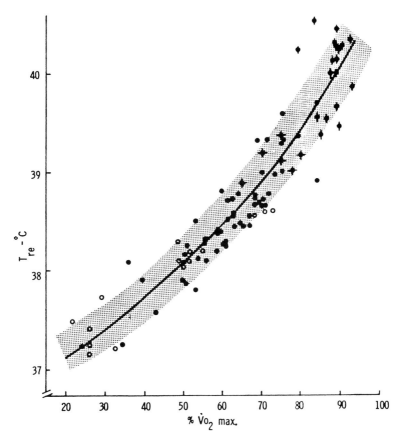

FIG. 2. The relationship between relative work load (%$\dot{V}O_2$max) and steady-state rectal temperature (○). Data from Saltin and Hermansen (4). Reprinted with permission (6).

higher core temperature and a higher core to skin temperature gradient in the low $\dot{V}O_2$max individual is an indication of a lower K (conductance of the peripheral tissues) (8,9) and peripheral blood flow. For a given work load, the low $\dot{V}O_2$max individual needs the same blood flow to the exercising muscles as a high $\dot{V}O_2$max subject, but when increasing the core–skin temperature gradient, the produced heat can be transported by a smaller volume of blood flow. This is illustrated by the conductance (8,9):

$$K = H_{skin}/(T_c - \overline{T}_{sk}) \, A_{Dub} \text{ or}$$

$$H = K{\downarrow}(T_c{\uparrow} - \overline{T}_{sk}) \, A_{Dub},$$

where T_c and $\overline{T}_{sk}$ are core and skin temperature, respectively, and A_{Dub} is the body surface area.

Thus, in the competition between the metabolic need of the exercising muscles and the thermoregulatory demand for skin blood flow, the result is an increased core temperature that allows for a transport of the heat by a smaller blood flow.

At high absolute work loads and at higher environmental temperatures near the upper limit of the prescriptive zone, the same strategy will become necessary in the high $\dot{V}O_2$ individual. The relationship of $\overline{T}_{sk}$ to T_a becomes steeper at 85% $\dot{V}O_2$max compared with 65% $\dot{V}O_2$max, indicating a vasoconstriction and a decrease in $\overline{T}_{sk}$ (Fig. 3). This could have an inhibitory effect on sweating and force the core temperature to increase above the equilibrium of the prescriptive zone and reach the upper limit when the environmental temperature is above 20°C (7). A similar observation of lower $\overline{T}_{sk}$ at very high work intensities was presented for one subject who could exercise for 2 hours at 88% ·O2 (10).

The reason for the increase in core temperature during exercise is still a matter for discussion. It may be (a) a resetting of the thermostat, as in fever, caused by neuromotor activation or reflexes, sympathetic activation, etc. due to exercise activity, (b) a necessity for activation of the heat dissipation (sweating and skin blood flow), (c) due to chemical or hormonal changes, activated by metabolic processes related to the relative severity of the work, or (d) due to cardiovascular limitations in the competition between metabolic requirements and thermoregulatory needs for skin blood flow.

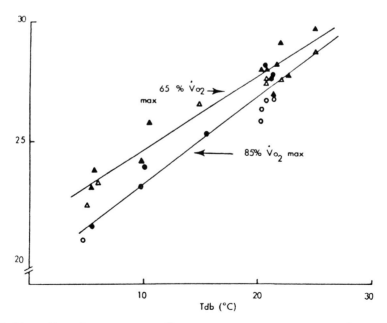

FIG. 3. Mean skin surface temperature, $\overline{T}_{sk}$, during exercise at 65% and 85 %$\dot{V}O_2$max at different environmental temperatures. Abscissa, dry bulb temperature (Tdb); ordinate, $\overline{T}_{sk}$. One subject. Reprinted with permission (7).

HEAT LOSS IN SEVERE CONDITIONS OF EXERCISE AND HEAT STRESS

One of the challenges of severe exercise is to dissipate the heat produced. This problem becomes worse the higher the environmental temperatures. The heat loss from the body surface takes place by convection, radiation, and evaporation. At increasing environmental temperature the skin temperature approaches that of the environment, and at approximately $35°T_a$ the two become equal. This means that at higher temperatures the heat that can be lost by convection and radiation decreases, and an increasing amount of the heat loss must take place through evaporation of sweat. The environmental conditions in which heat balance can be attained—the prescriptive zone—varies with the exercise intensity (2). Both upper and lower critical temperatures move to lower values with increasing heat production (10). The upper critical limit depends not only on the absolute heat liberation but also on the sweating capacity of the subject (Fig. 4). Furthermore, with the core–skin gradient decreased in warm environments, a greater skin blood flow is called for in more severe environmental conditions.

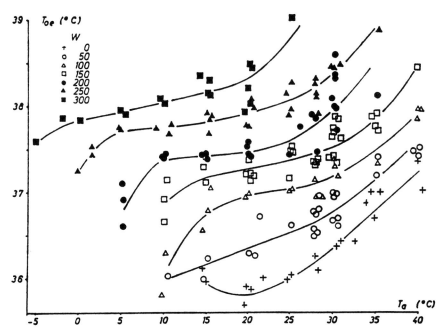

FIG. 4. Esophageal temperature after 2 hours at environmental temperatures between -5°C and 40°C at rest and at exercise intensities of 50, 100, 150, 200, 250, and 300 W (one subject). Reprinted with permission (10).

Control of Sweating

The sweating rate increases with increasing work load during exercise and environmental temperature (1,11). The stimulus for this is thought to be the increase in core temperature and skin temperature (3,12). The sweating response to these thermal stimuli, E_{sw}, are often described in mathematical form:

$$E_{sw} = \alpha \, (T_{core} - T_{set}) + \beta \, (\overline{T}_{skin} - T_{set}) \ldots \text{ or}$$

$$E_{sw} = \alpha \, (T_{core} - T_{set}) \times \beta \, (\overline{T}_{skin} - T_{set}) \ldots$$

However, such control equations cannot fully account for the relationship between heat liberation in the body and sweating. It is not clear why the "sensitivity" of the temperature center depends on the $\dot{V}O_2max$, why some individuals sweat more for the same temperature stimulus (the high compared with the low $\dot{V}O_2max$ person), or how such change in sensitivity is brought about by aerobic training in an individual (7).

Heat acclimation also leads to increases in the sweating rate (Fig. 5). (13–16). Due to reduction in set point, the same increase in core temperature induces a higher sweating rate after than before acclimation (17). But what is the mechanism for this change? In our studies (16) we hypothesized that the repeated elevations in core temperature during the acclimation could be responsible. The increasing core temperature and prolonged exercise in heat activate endocrine factors, which could change the activity of the sweat glands.

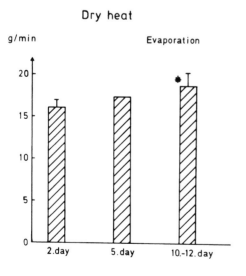

FIG. 5. Rate of sweat loss the second and final (8–12) day of acclimation to 40°C dry heat. Average ± SE, eight subjects. Data from Nielsen et al. (27).

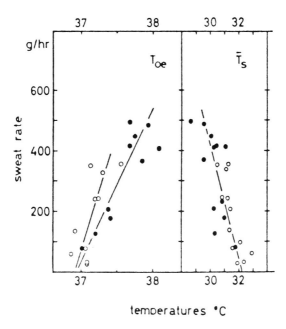

FIG. 6. Esophageal temperature (**left panel,** T_{oe}) and mean skin temperature (right panel, $\bar{T}_s$) after 1 hour of bicycling 10° uphill, concentric exercise (●), and downhill, eccentric exercise (○). Subject BJ. Reprinted with permission (3).

However, despite the fact that the hormones we have studied—catecholamines, aldosterone, arginine vasopressin, atrial natriuretic peptide, growth hormone—are strongly activated and increased during exercise and heat stress, the increase is the same for the same increase in core temperature after acclimation as before (Nielsen et al., unpublished observations). So the functional changes at the sweat gland with heat acclimation remains open for speculation. It could be speculated that the increased sensitivity might be caused by an increase in receptor density for neural and humoral stimuli, or perhaps by an increase in size and number of active sweat glands.

The controller for sweating responds "watt by watt" to the heat load on the subject (3,5,18,19). During eccentric exercise, heat is absorbed in the stretching muscles and sweating is increased by the same amount of energy as that absorbed without $\bar{T}_{sk}$ being changed (Fig. 6). Thus, the subject sweats more for the same Tcore during eccentric work (3,5). The same is the case if external heat radiation (heat radiation from the sun) is imposed (20). It is not known how heat (watts) is sensed by the temperature control system.

Also, nonthermal stimuli affect the temperature control, e.g., inputs from volume and osmoreceptors. This is discussed below.

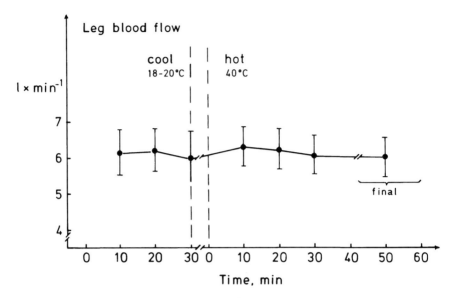

FIG. 7. Leg blood flow during uphill walking 60% $\dot{V}O_2$max 30 minutes in neutral and 60 minutes in 40°C dry heat. Final esophageal temperature was 40°C in the hot room. Reprinted with permission (27).

CARDIOVASCULAR REGULATION DURING SEVERE EXERCISE

The increase in metabolic requirements due to exercise is met by an increase in cardiac output and a redistribution of blood flow from the visceral organs. The reduction in splanchnic blood flow was found to be proportional to relative work load, i.e., to the percentage of $\dot{V}O_2$max (21). In hot environments there is an additional thermoregulatory demand for skin blood flow. The diversion of blood flow to the skin may be obtained by an increase in cardiac output in hot conditions (22,23) and through a further reduction in blood flow to the splanchnic organs (21). It is a question of discussion whether the blood flow to the exercising muscles is reduced in conditions of heat stress during severe exercise. This has been studied in various ways: by biopsy studies, measurements of metabolites, or recently by direct blood flow measurements. Indirect evidence implies that at high work load, 75–80% $\dot{V}O_2$max, glycogen breakdown is increased during exercise at 45°C as compared with 9°C (24). However, in studies with direct measurements of leg blood flow at exercise intensities between 40% and 75% of $\dot{V}O_2$max (16,26,27; and unpublished observations), we find no reductions in muscle blood flow, even at core temperature increasing to approximately 40°C in uncompensable heat stress in euhydrated subjects (Fig. 7). Therefore, is seems to be that the metabolic requirements have priority over thermoregulation.

DEHYDRATION BY SWEATING: EFFECTS OF LOSS OF VOLUME AND ELECTROLYTES

Another complication in severe exercise that influences thermoregulation is the large fluid loss due to sweating. In dehydrated subjects (5% of body weight), cardiac output decreased during 120 minutes of exercise at 65% $\dot{V}O_2$max in hot conditions (35°C) with 50% relative humidity (28). These conditions also led to a lower blood pressure and a higher core temperature than in euhydrated condition. The stroke volume was decreased despite a higher heart rate. Skin circulation and sweating rate were reduced. It is not known whether the blood flow to the exercising muscles is reduced under such circumstances. However, in a cold (2°C) environment, the reduced cardiovascular load permitted, even at 4% hypohydration, exercise intensities of 70% max $\dot{V}O_2$max to be sustained. T_{core} temperature equalled that found during the same exercise in a euhydrated state (Gonzales-Alonso et al., unpublished observations).

The large fluid loss during severe exercise, especially in warm conditions, also affects sweating and skin circulation. With increasing fluid loss there is a concomitant increase in core temperature during exercise (29). Sweat loss leads to loss of water and electrolytes. Because sweat is hypotonic, the remaining body fluid compartments become hyperosmotic.

Both the loss of volume and the increased osmolality has an effect on sweat gland function and skin circulation (30–32). Fortney et al. (33) found that dehydration increased the temperature threshold for sweating but had little effect

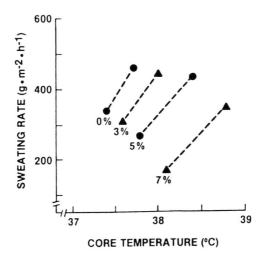

FIG. 8. Plot of total body sweat rate and core temperature during exercise in euhydrated state and when hypohydrated to various percentages of body weight. Reprinted with permission (35).

on sensitivity. Both slope and threshold for skin blood flow was changed to lower and higher values, respectively. The thermoregulatory control of sweating at different levels of hydration and exercise intensities was studied (34,35) (Fig. 8). Hypohydration decreased sweating sensitivity and increased the threshold for onset of sweating in a graded manner with increasing body water loss. Experiments in which blood volume and tonicity were varied independently show that changes in osmolality have the most effect on the sweating response. High osmolality reduces sweating and increases core temperature during exercise (31,33), whereas volume changes have the greatest effect on skin blood flow. Hypovolemia reduces heat loss by increasing the threshold for vasodilatation and decreases sensitivity to the temperature stimulus (30,32,33).

CONCLUSIONS

Severe exercise represents a challenge for thermoregulation. The load on the cardiovascular system of both metabolic and thermal requirements is balanced in favor of the metabolic needs. The large fluid loss by sweating induces a further load on the thermoregulation by the effects on both central circulation and skin circulation and by the effect on the function of sweating mechanism.

During exercise, heat is liberated by the metabolic processes in the muscles. Part of this is stored in the body, thus the body temperature increases. The core temperature during exercise is regulated linearly in proportion to the relative load on the individual, i.e., to the percentage of $\dot{V}O_2max$ (maximal aerobic capacity). For exercise intensities above 75% $\dot{V}O_2max$, the relationship of core temperature to $\dot{V}O_2max$ becomes curvilinear, and T_{core} increases more. This is the case within the prescriptive zone, where the core temperature is independent of the environmental temperature up to the upper critical limit. This upper critical limit is determined by the metabolic rate and by sweating capacity and can be changed by training and acclimation. In hot environments, a further stress to thermoregulation is added due to the increased skin circulation. The result is a displacement of blood flow and volume to the periphery and a reduction in central blood volume. Cardiac output is maintained in the hot environment (or even increased) through a compensatory increase in heart rate.

It is concluded that metabolic demands have priority over thermoregulatory function when cardiac output must be shared, e.g., during intense exercise, and during exercise in the heat, when core temperature is increasing toward critically high values.

REFERENCES

1. Nielsen M. De Regulation der Körpertemperatur bei Muskelarbeit. *Skand Arch Physiol* 1938;79: 193–230.
2. Lind AR. A physiological criterion for setting thermal environmental limits for every day work. *J Appl Physiol* 1963;18:51–56.

3. Nielsen B. Thermoregulation in rest and exercise. *Acta Physiol Scand Suppl* 1969;323:1–74.
4. Saltin B, Hermansen L. Esophageal, rectal and muscle temperature during exercise. *J Appl Physiol* 1966;21:1757–1762.
5. Nielsen B. Regulation of body temperature and heat dissipation at different levels of energy and heat production in man. *Acta Physiol Scand* 1966;68:215–227.
6. Davies CTM, Brotherhood JR, ZeidiFard E. Temperature regulation during severe exercise with some observations on effects of skin wetting. *J Appl Physiol* 1976;41:772–776.
7. Davies CTM. Influence of skin temperature on sweating and aerobic performance during severe work. *J Appl Physiol Respir Environ Exerc Physiol* 1979;47:770–777.
8. Burton AC. The application of the theory of heat flow to the study of energy metabolism. *J Nutr* 1934; 7:497–533.
9. Hardy JD. The physical laws of heat loss from the human body. *Proc Natl Acad Sci U S A* 1937;23: 631–637.
10. Kitzing J, Behling K, Bleichert A, Scarperi M, Scarperi S. Antriebe und effektorische Massnahmen der Thermoregulation bei Ruhe und während körperlischer Arbeit. *Int Z Angew Physiol* 1972;30:119–131.
11. Nielsen B, Nielsen M. On the regulation of sweat secretion in exercise. *Acta Physiol Scand* 1965;64: 314–322.
12. Nadel ER, Mitchell JW, Saltin B, Stolwijk JAJ. Peripheral modifications to the central drive for sweating. *J Appl Physiol* 1971;31:828–833.
13. Eichna LW, Park CR, Nelson N, Horvath SM, Palmes CD. Thermal regulation during acclimatization in a hot dry (desert-type) environment. *Am J Physiol* 1950;163:585–597.
14. Chen WY, Elizondo RS. Peripheral modification of thermoregulatory function during heat acclimation. *J Appl Physiol* 1974;37:367–373.
15. Mitchel D, Senay LC, Wyndham CH, van Rensburg AJ, Rogers GG, Strydom NB. Acclimatization in a hot humid environment: energy exchange, body temperature and sweating. *J Appl Physiol* 1976;40: 768–778.
16. Nielsen B, Hales JRS, Strange S, Christensen NJ, Warberg J, Saltin B. Human circulatory and thermoregulatory adaptations with heat acclimation and exercise in dry heat. *J Physiol* 1993;460:467–485.
17. Nadel ER, Pandolf KB, Roberts MF, Stolwijk JAJ. Mechanisms of thermal acclimation to exercise and heat. *J Appl Physiol* 1974;37:515–520.
18. Snellen JW. Mean body temperature and the control of thermal sweating. *Acta Physiol Pharmac Neel* 1966;14:99–174.
19. Webb P. The physiology of heat regulation. *Am J Physiol* 1995;268:R838–R850.
20. Nielsen B, Kassow K, Aschengreen FE. Heat balance during exercise in the sun. *Eur J Appl Physiol* 1988;58:189–196.
21. Rowell LB, Blackmon JR, Martin RH, Wazarella JA, Bruce RA. Hepatic clearance of indocyanine green in man under thermal and exercise stresses. *J Appl Physiol* 1965;20:384–394.
22. Williams CG, Bredell GAG, Wyndham CH, et al. Circulatory and metabolic reactions to work in heat. *J Appl Physiol* 1962;17:625–638.
23. Rowell LB. *Human circulation, regulation during physical stress.* New York: Oxford University Press; 1986.
24. Fink WJ, Costill DL, Van Handel PJ. Leg muscle metabolism during exercise in the heat and cold. *Eur J Appl Physiol* 1975;34:183–190.
25. Kirwan JP, Costill DL, Kuipers H, et al. Substrate utilization in leg muscle of men after heat acclimation. *J Appl Physiol* 1987;63:31–35..
26. Savard GK, Nielsen B, Laszczynska I, Larsen BE, Saltin B. Muscle blood flow is not reduced in humans during moderate exercise and heat stress. *J Appl Physiol* 1988;64:649–652.
27. Nielsen B, Savard G, Richter EA, Hargreaves M, Saltin B. Muscle blood flow and muscle metabolism during exercise and heat stress. *J Appl Physiol* 1990;69:1040–1046.
28. González-Alonso J, Mora-Rodríguez R, Below PR, Coyle EF. Dehydration reduces cardiac output and increases systemic and cutaneous vascular resistance during exercise. *J Appl Physiol* 1995;79: 1487–1496.
29. Adolph EF, Brown AH, Goddard DR, et al. *Physiology of man in the desert.* New York: Interscience; 1947.
30. Nadel ER. Effect of hydration state on circulatory and thermal regulations. *J Appl Physiol* 1981;49:715–721.
31. Nielsen B. Effects of changes in plasma volume and osmolality on thermoregulation during exercise. *Acta Physiol Scand* 1974;90:725–730.

32. Sawka MN. Physiological consequences of hypohydration: exercise performance and thermoregulation. *Med Sci Sports Exerc* 1992;24:657–670.
33. Fortney SM, Wenger CB, Bove JR, Nadel ER. Effect of hyperosmolality on control of blood flow and sweating. *J Appl Physiol* 1984;57:1688–1695.
34. Montain SJ, Latzka WA, Sawka MN. Control of thermoregulatory sweating is altered by hydration level and exercise intensity. *J Appl Physiol* 1995;79:1434–1439.
35. Sawka MN, Young AJ, Francesconi RP, Muza SR, Pandolf KB. Thermoregulatory and blood responses during exercise at graded hypohydration levels. *J Appl Physiol* 1985;59:1394–1401.

Physiology, Stress, and Malnutrition: Functional Correlates, Nutritional Intervention,
edited by J.M. Kinney and H.N. Tucker.
Lippincott–Raven Publishers © 1997.

Thermoregulation, Exercise, and Nutrition in the Cold: Investigations on a Polar Expedition

Mike A. Stroud

*Department of Nutrition, Southampton General Hospital,
Southampton S016 6YD, United Kingdom*

Expeditions and other feats of human endurance provide opportunities to study physiologic responses to a variety of stresses, including prolonged endurance exercise and cold exposure. This chapter on the interaction of thermoregulation, exercise, and nutrition in the cold is based around measurements and observations made on two men who attempted to walk across Antarctica without the help of other men, animals, or machines. Although the observations are restricted to changes in only two subjects, they are of interest in understanding the effects of stress and malnutrition in more conventional contexts.

THE EXPEDITION AND BASIS OF RESEARCH

During the southern summer of 1992–1993 two men ("A," 48 years of age and "B," 37 years of age) set out from the Atlantic coast of the Antarctic, aiming to perform the first crossing of the continent unaided by other men, animals, or machines. Each man towed a sledge weighing 222 kg that contained a 100-day supply of food, fuel, and essential survival equipment. In the first 20 days they traveled across the 350-km Filchner ice shelf (a region of glacial ice covering the sea bed) before reaching the coast of mainland Antarctica. From there they followed a 340-km, 14-day ascent to the polar plateau at an altitude of around 3,000 m and a further 550 km across the plateau to the South Pole, which was reached on day 68. After leaving the Pole, they traveled another 480 km over the plateau before a descent through the Trans-Antarctic Mountains to the far side of the continent and the Ross ice shelf, which was reached on day 90. An attempt to cross this second ice shelf in order to reach the open water of the Pacific was abandoned on day 95. The walk was the longest self-contained journey ever made (1).

Overall, the expedition entailed extremely prolonged endurance exercise, which was performed for 10–12 hours every day for 95 days. However, in physiologic terms the exercise would have been of only moderate intensity when compared with the work rates involved in, for example, running a marathon. Cold exposure was very marked because still air temperatures ranged from $-10°$ to $55°C$ and there was frequently additional cooling from strong winds. Nevertheless, for most of the time the men stayed warm due to their high work-associated heat production. However, there were two occasions on day 67 and day 91 when B apparently became hypothermic with marked confusion. Despite high dietary intakes during the expedition, weight loss in both men early on was extremely rapid due to the very high exercise-related energy expenditures, and both men became extremely malnourished.

The expedition permitted the study of men losing weight through the performance of high levels of exercise, despite a high dietary energy intake. Because the diet was prepackaged and repetitive, it was possible to obtain accurate estimates of energy and macronutrient intake, and these dietary records, linked with measurements of body weight and composition changes, provided good estimates of overall energy expenditure. These estimates were then compared with measurements of energy expenditure using the doubly-labeled isotope water technique. Measurements of resting metabolic rate, thermogenic responses to food, protein synthesis, exercise performance, skeletal muscle enzyme activities, and biochemical markers of nutritional status were also made, which give interesting insights into the physiologic responses to the multiple stresses of the expedition.

DIETARY INTAKE, BODY COMPOSITION, AND ENERGY EXPENDITURE

Work performed on a previous Antarctic expedition of similar nature had shown that daily energy expenditure when manhauling in polar conditions was likely to be around 25 MJ (2). However, an intake of only 23 MJ/day was planned for this expedition because it was felt that weight losses of up to 10 kg would be tolerable over the anticipated 100-day duration of the journey. The nature of manhauling expeditions dictates that food should weigh a minimum; therefore, rations with a high energy density have advantages. However, this conflicts with the need to maintain optimal endurance performance, which is enhanced by high-carbohydrate intakes both during exercise and particularly after prolonged exertion, when they help to restore intramuscular and hepatic glycogen stores. A compromise diet containing 23 MJ/day as 57% fat, 35% carbohydrate, and 8% protein was therefore selected, a decision supported by the successful use of a similar diet on the earlier Antarctic expedition (2). Although this diet contained a high proportion of fat, the carbohydrate content was still quite high at 480 g and there is evidence suggesting that humans can adapt to high-fat intakes with improved exercising muscle utilization of free fatty acids (3).

The diet consisted of freeze-dried meals, chocolate bars, biscuits, soups, and hot chocolate drinks, all supplemented with dehydrated butter in order to increase energy density. Dietary analysis was performed before departure, and because all food was weighed and packaged into daily ration bags and no food was wasted, unusually accurate estimates of daily energy intakes could be made. Measurements of body weights were made before, during, and after the expedition, with body composition measured using underwater weighing (UWW) 10 days before and 6 days after the expedition; skinfold thickness (SFT) 10 days before, 6 days after, and on days 0 and 95 of the expedition; and deuterium distribution space data on days 0, 50, and 95 of the expedition.

For a variety of reasons, the planned 23 MJ/day diet was not always consumed, and the final intake provided an average over the whole journey of 21.3 MJ/day, of which 56.7% came from fat, 35.5% from carbohydrate, and 7.8% from protein. Over the first 50 days, the average daily intake was 19.9 MJ, consisting of 95 g protein, 293 g fat, and 425 g carbohydrate, whereas during the period from days 50–95 the average daily intake was 22.2 MJ, consisting of 103 g protein, 338 g fat, and 557 g carbohydrate. Despite the high dietary energy intakes, changes in the measurements of body weight and composition were extreme, and both men became very debilitated toward the end of the journey. The results are shown in Table 1.

The deuterium data indicated that whereas A lost 22.9 kg of fat and gained 0.1 kg lean tissues during the first 50 days, B lost both fat (9.8 kg) and lean tissues (5.7 kg). A similar pattern was also seen for the last 45 days, when A lost 2.2 kg fat and gained 0.4 kg of lean tissue, whereas B lost 5.5 kg fat and gained 0.8 kg lean tissues. At the end of the expedition, the isotope data in both men suggested that fat content was zero, but the isotope dilution spaces were exceptionally large, suggesting that there had been considerable increases in the water content of the lean body mass. The UWW values for body fat at 7 days postexpedition, after considerable food intake and weight gain, suggested body fat levels of around 2% compared with around 18.7% before departure. However, these results assume an unchanging density of lean tissues as weight is lost, an assumption that may be untrue in these extreme circumstances. Nevertheless, the UWW results support the fact that fat stores were essentially zero on the last day of the journey and hence confirm that the changes in body composition during

TABLE 1. *Changes in body weight and body composition measured by underwater weighing (UWW), skinfold thickness (SFT), and isotope dilution spaces*

| | | | % Fat body composition | | | | | |
| | Body weight (kg) | | A | | | B | | |
Day	A	B	UWW	SFT	Isotope	UWW	SFT	Isotope
−10	89.9	69.0	17.4	25.0	—	16.3	16.80	—
0	95.6	74.8	—	26.2	22.3	—	20.1	22.8
50	72.8	59.3	—	—	—	—	—	—
95	71.0	53.0	—	12.2	0.0	—	9.6	0.0
+7	76.2	58.8	1.9	14.4	—	2.5	11.8	—

this expedition were extreme. Even the Minnesota experiment of Keys et al. (4) only described changes of 70% in fatness and 20% in muscle mass after 52 weeks of chronic undernutrition.

In view of the UWW and isotope body composition data, the relatively normal postexpedition estimates of body fat made from SFT measurements seem very unlikely, probably due to edema of the skin making the measurements inaccurate. Certainly both men showed marked gravitational edema in the legs at that time, which was probably due to malnutrition with inadequate microvascular repair and leakage of intravascular fluid to the extravascular space (5). However, it is also possible that subcutaneous fat was preserved due to the cold, either through a genuine adaptive response or due to difficulties in mobilizing subcutaneous fat in the face of cold-induced subcutaneous vasoconstriction.

Interestingly, even before the expedition, the SFT estimate of body fat in A was markedly different from the estimates based on UWW and isotope dilution, and I suspect that this was due to his having an unusual pattern of fat distribution for his age. The estimates of body fat from the SFT measurements were made according to the equations of Durnin and Womersley (6), which were derived from average U.K. population data. As with all such equations, the different regression lines anticipate the normal increase in internal to subcutaneous fat ratio with age, and there is no doubt that this phenomenon does occur in most members of the population. However, A was an extremely active man for someone of his age and had maintained high levels of activity throughout his adult life. It therefore seems likely that he maintained a pattern of fat distribution similar to that in a younger man; indeed, his pre-expedition UWW estimate of body fat relative to his measured subcutaneous fat values fit the pattern of a man in his 20s rather than in his late 40s. I therefore suspect that the accepted increase in internal fat with age is, at least in part, a reflection of habitual activity rather than an age-related phenomenon per se.

Mean daily energy expenditures during the expedition were estimated for the first 50 days and the last 45 days of the expedition by combining dietary intake data with daily energy deficits calculated from the isotope estimates of lean and fat losses for each period. Lean tissue losses were assumed to be 73% water and 27% protein, whereas fat losses were considered to be 100% fat. The calorific value of protein was taken as 18.39 kJ/g, and fat was taken as 39.7 kJ/g. The results are shown in Table 2.

It was hoped that the unusually accurate energy balance data would allow a validation study of the isotope-labeled (D_2O^{18}) water technique because, although well established, it has mostly been used at sedentary or low levels of activity, and when studies have examined its use at higher activity levels, the alternative assessments of energy expenditure were probably unreliable (7,8). However, application of the method during this expedition had to be modified because Antarctic snow is depleted in both the D and O^{18} isotopes. There would therefore be a change in isotopic background levels during the walk, so the normal method of applying predose background levels to the evaluation of postdose isotope disappearance curves

TABLE 2. *Energy expenditure (MJ/day) from energy balance and the isotope-labeled water technique*

Subject	Days 0–50		Days 51–95	
	Energy balance	Isotope	Energy balance	Isotope
A	38.1	35.5	26.6	23.1
B	28.3	29.1	23.9	18.8

would be misleading. This problem had been identified on an earlier Arctic expedition study that suggested that true background levels could be better assessed by extrapolating the isotope exponential decay curves to infinite time, which should equate to the new background (9). This technique was therefore applied with doses of D_2 ^{18}O taken on days 0 and 50 and isotope disappearance measured from daily urine samples analyzed at the Dunn Nutritional Laboratories, Cambridge. However, although the isotope exponential decay curves were as anticipated after the first dose, the curves after the second dose showed an unexpected increase in both D and ^{18}O enrichments between days 80 and 95 for both men. Because it is difficult to envisage why a change in enrichments of the natural background water source should have occurred at this point, the increases in D and ^{18}O in both men can only be explained by the re-entry of labeled isotopes from the breakdown of body tissues that do not usually exchange freely with body water and which contained either a "memory" of the higher background enrichments of the United Kingdom or which had taken up isotope and become "labeled" after the first dosing, e.g., a labeled cohort of red cells. In view of this problem, it was only possible to perform decay curve analysis for the second dose between days 51 and 80, assuming that any effects of isotope re-entry were largely swamped by the steepness of the decay curves at this time and that the energy expenditures for this period were typical for the whole of the last 45 days of the expedition. The resulting estimates of energy expenditure from the isotope studies are also shown in Table 2, whereas Table 3 shows the results of further analysis of the first dose decay curves to give estimated energy expenditures for 10-day periods during the first 50 days.

TABLE 3. *Variation in energy expenditure (MJ/day) measured using the isotope method during the first 50 days*

Day	A	B
1–10	39.8	26.8
11–20	26.9	22.0
21–30	44.6	48.7
31–40	36.4	26.7
41–50	29.9	23.3

ENERGY EXPENDITURE AND THERMOREGULATION

The very high energy expenditures recorded on this Antarctic journey sustained over such a long period are most unusual and must lie close to what is physiologically possible. Obviously, they may simply be due to the very high levels of motivation involved in such expeditions, and even the highest levels recorded between days 20 and 30 are credible because they correspond to the period when the heavy sledges were dragged uphill from the ice shelf to the plateau, and they fall well short of the theoretical energy expenditure ceiling of 58.5 MJ/day that it has been calculated could be attained by ultra-long distance runners (10). However, it would also seem possible that they might be partly explained by thermoregulatory or other metabolic responses to the cold.

Many studies of men working in the cold have concluded that heat production from the exercise is nearly always adequate to prevent any thermoregulatory responses from being needed and that observed increases of 5–15% in the energy cost of tasks can be ascribed to the restrictive effect of polar protective gear (11) or the increased workloads entailed when walking on snow (12). However, some studies do suggest that cold exposure alters metabolic efficiency, and O'Hara et al. (13) reported that fat losses in men on an Arctic military exercise were much higher than would be anticipated. These fat losses were accompanied by persistent ketonuria, and the investigators suggested that their observations might be explained by a cold-induced switch from carbohydrate toward fat utilization, with some energy lost as ketones on the breath and in the urine. The same group then followed up their field observations with a study that demonstrated similar excessive fat losses for men living and exercising for 10 days in a cold chamber (14). Interestingly, however, the excess fat losses observed in these chamber studies occurred despite normal subject core temperatures and only minimal decreases in their skin temperatures.

Although not proposed by O'Hara et al., it seems that these findings of higher than anticipated energy use in the cold might reflect changes in exercise metabolism due to cooling of the face, which is not easily protected. Riggs et al. (15) found slightly elevated levels of oxygen consumption and lower respiratory exchange ratios in men exercising with their faces exposed to a 6.5 m/s wind at 10°C. This is only moderate facial cooling compared with that which might be met in the polar regions after observations of high-energy expenditures during earlier polar journeys (2). Stroud examined exercise metabolism during more intense facial cooling (16). In that study, men exercised on cycle ergometers at increasing work loads (0, 75, 100, 125, and 150 W) with and without the face exposed to a −20°C wind. However, despite this causing profound decreases in facial temperatures, there were only small increases in oxygen consumption, with the mean for all levels of exertion increasing from 0.82 L/min to 0.86 L/min ($p < 0.05$). Nevertheless, there were more marked changes in exercising respiratory exchange, which decreased with facial cooling from 0.94 to 0.85 ($p < 0.05$). This indicates that facial cooling does cause a switch in metabolism toward the utilization of fat.

However, it would seem unlikely that facial exposure had great influence on the exercise costs observed during the trans-Antarctic crossing.

The changes toward metabolic utilization of fat with facial cooling are the converse of those observed during exercise and whole-body cold exposure. In such studies, cooling during exercise has been found to lead to an increase in respiratory exchange ratios, indicating a cold-induced switch toward carbohydrate metabolism (17–19). However, the changes have only been observed when exercise levels have been inadequate to maintain normal skin and core temperatures, and there also has been a significant increase in metabolic rate. It therefore seems likely that the results can be attributed to simultaneous shivering, although the substrate used by shivering muscle is a matter for debate. Young (20) has reported that nutritional carbohydrate deprivation and consequent depletion of resting muscle glycogen levels does not effect shivering capacity in resting individuals and hence argues that free fatty acids (FFAs) must be the most important substrates for shivering muscles. He also supported this argument by pointing out that even violent shivering is equivalent to work at a level of around only 30% of maximal oxygen consumption, and so the muscle utilization of FFAs would be analogous to the predominant use of these substrates during low-intensity exercise. Conversely, however, Martineau and Jacobs (21) have reported that glycogen depletion does lead to a decline in shivering heat production at rest and argue that because shivering does not involve all muscle units equally, some may be working at high fractions of maximal oxygen uptake even if whole-body oxygen consumption is only 30% of maximal. Glycogen could therefore be expected to be the chief substrate in actively shivering units. The most likely explanation for these apparently opposing reports would seem to be that the subjects used by Martineau and Jacobs were markedly thinner than those used by Young and hence were exposed to more intense cooling. As with exercise, low-intensity shivering probably uses fat predominantly, whereas high-intensity responses mainly use carbohydrates.

All of these results suggest that general cooling could have contributed to the high-energy expenditure observed during the Antarctic walk. However, the highest energy expenditures were observed during the first half of the journey, when the high work loads kept the men warm, and it was only during the second half, after they had lost much of their subcutaneous fat protection, that they reported feeling very chilled. It therefore seems unlikely that the cold had a large effect on overall energy expenditure.

RESTING METABOLIC RATES AND DIET-INDUCED THERMOGENESIS

Measurements of resting metabolic rates (RMRs) were made in the week before departure on the expedition and 1 week after its conclusion, although logistic difficulties dictated that measurements were confined to oxygen uptake with metabolic rates calculated according to the equations of Weir (22). After the

RMR measurement, the two men consumed a 4.2-MJ liquid meal before six further metabolic measurements were made at 15-minute intervals to assess their diet-induced thermogenic (DIT) responses. The results of these metabolic measurements are shown in Fig. 1. The results showed a marked increases in the maximum DIT responses to the test meal from 16.8% to 75.4% of RMR in A and from 17.6% to 96.2% of RMR in B. Furthermore, if account is taken of the changes in body composition, there were also increases in RMR/kg lean tissue of 11.2% in A and 8.8% in B.

These results showing an increase in RMR and DIT in the face of marked weight loss are in marked contrast to those that would be expected if similar weight loss had been induced by starvation. After dietary weight loss, both parameters normally decline (23,24), although if dieting is accompanied by exercise, such reductions are limited (25), and if weight loss is achieved through increases in exercise while on a normal intake, there are probably no declines at all (26). The Antarctic data therefore support the idea of a spectrum of change, with RMR and

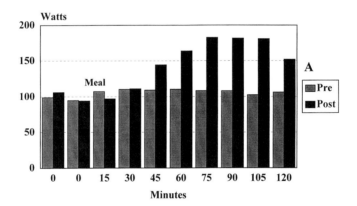

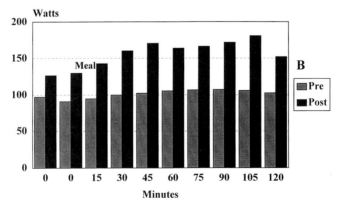

FIG. 1. Resting metabolic rate and dietary induced thermogenesis before and after the expedition.

DIT actually increasing if weight loss is induced by high levels of exercise during a period of high dietary energy intake.

Some of the reductions in RMR and DIT that are usually induced by undernutrition can be ascribed to losses of metabolically active tissue mass, although most authorities believe that there is also a genuine reduction in the metabolism of lean tissues per unit mass. Certainly, this would appear to be the case in frank starvation or cachexia, when there is a marked decline in RMR per kg lean tissue, despite their usually being some preservation of metabolically active viscera compared with less active skeletal muscle. Of course, in severe starvation this may be due to a partial breakdown in visceral organ function, and it is interesting to note that if daily energy deficits and weight losses of similar magnitude to those seen during the Antarctic expedition were induced by dietary restriction alone, it might have been expected that such organ breakdown would have occurred. However, in the case of this journey the large energy deficits were accompanied by normal to high intakes of protein, and it was probably these that maintained organ function despite the massive weight losses.

NITROGEN BALANCE AND PROTEIN TURNOVER

Studies of nitrogen balance were made once before, five times during, and twice after the expedition, with measurements of protein turnover using the [^{15}N] glycine single-dose end-product method (27). The results are shown in Table 4. Surprisingly, the smaller man, subject B, tended to be in negative nitrogen balance during the journey, whereas the larger subject A was not. Although the outputs took no account of fecal and some other nitrogen losses, these differences echoed

TABLE 4. *Nitrogen balance and protein synthesis*

Subject and Day	Nitrogen (g/day)			Protein synthesis (g/kg/12 h)
	Intake	Output	Balance	
A, Pre 7	34.1	12.0	22.7	4.01
A, Day 10	13.5	16.7	−1.7	3.82
A, Day 20	14.5	14.0	1.2	3.22
A, Day 50	15.5	12.9	3.3	[a]
A, Day 76	18.4	16.7	2.3	5.06
A, Day 96	5.7	12.4	−6.2	6.23
A, Post 14	29.6	19.5	10.6	3.51
A, Post 21	25.9	13.1	13.2	5.09
B, Pre -7	39.7	17.3	15.0	4.24
B, Day 9	14.1	12.2	−2.9	2.94
B, Day 19	15.4	15.6	−6.3	2.86
B, Day 49	16.0	14.9	−5.1	3.71
B, Day 77	18.4	12.4	2.1	[a]
B, Day 92	9.0	13.9	−10.3	3.58
B, Post 14	32.5	12.5	12.9	3.77
B, Post 21	23.0	20.3	−2.5	2.02

[a]Sample error.

the changes in the men's lean body composition described above, which can be expressed as equivalent changes in nitrogen balance. For the first 50 days of the expedition, lean losses in B were equivalent to −4.9 g N/day, whereas A showed gains equivalent to +0.7 g N/day, figures that are almost identical to the mean values of the nitrogen balance for the same period, which gave losses of −4.8 g N/day for B and gains of +0.9 g N/day for A. Similarly, during the latter 45 days of the expedition, the body composition data suggested losses of −0.8 g N/day for B and gains of +0.4 g N/day for A, whereas nitrogen balance gave mean losses of −0.9 g N/day for B and gains of +0.2 g N/day for B.

The remarkable similarity between these figures for nitrogen balance obtained by two completely independent methods suggests that nonurinary nitrogen losses during the period were small. This may be due to efficient colonic nitrogen salvage, which has been shown to occur during protein malnutrition and which would also have been favored by the expedition diet, which was low in nonstarch polysaccharides. However, there must have been some nitrogen losses in the feces, from the skin, and in nonmeasured urinary nitrogen, which only accounted for urea, ammonia, and creatinine. Gastrointestinal losses of nitrogen normally range from 1% to 10% of dietary intake, but in this case the low intake of fiber make it likely that losses were at the lower end of this scale. Skin losses are usually about 20 mg N/kg body weight, and the additional urinary losses would be on the order of 0.5 g/day. It therefore seems likely that total unaccounted nitrogen losses were actually around 3 or 4 g per day and that both men were therefore in significantly negative daily balance throughout the journey. The gains in lean tissue mass that were observed in subject A are therefore likely to be erroneous and are probably ascribable to increases in whole-body water content leading to errors in body composition assessments. Similarly, the losses of lean tissue in subject B may be underestimates. Nevertheless, even if there are some errors, one can be confident that the smaller man was still in more negative nitrogen balance with lower protein synthesis rates than was A.

Garrow (28) reported that when obese subjects lose weight through dietary restriction, approximately 25% of losses are lean, and hence it would appear that the exercise was tending to preserve lean body mass in both men. The dietary protein requirements for men undertaking endurance exercise of this nature are unclear. In a review, Lemon (29) concluded that protein requirements in very active individuals may be as high as 160% of the recommended dietary allowance, but he also noted that there is a decline in this exercise-induced protein requirement with continued training. Millward et al. (30) also concluded that in fully trained individuals, nitrogen losses associated with physical activity are minimal. However, both of these reviews assumed that individuals would be in energy balance, which was not the case during this expedition; therefore, it seems likely that nitrogen balance was dictated by the balance of exercise effects trying to maintain or enhance lean tissue mass while protein oxidation was needed to fuel exertion. During moderate- to high-intensity exercise, protein oxidation normally contributes 5–10% of energy supply, and because B, although much smaller, was pulling a sledge equal in weight to that of A, the difference in the nitrogen balance results might well reflect the relatively higher exercise intensities at which B must have worked during the journey.

Although the nitrogen balance figures may have underestimated the nitrogen losses by around 3–4 g/day, the resultant errors in the calculation of protein synthesis would only be on the order of +5%. The main purpose of measuring protein synthesis was to examine how the process responded to conditions of extreme stress and negative energy balance imposed over a long period. There is evidence that acute physical exercise leads to an increase in protein breakdown and a decrease in synthesis (31), but nothing is known about the effects of very long-term exertion. In subjects exposed to infection or trauma, both components of protein turnover, synthesis and breakdown, are increased, with breakdown predominating to produce a negative nitrogen balance (32,33). With undernourishment, the rate of protein turnover is reduced (34). The Antarctic expedition provided a scenario in which all three of these elements effecting protein turnover were combined: intense exertion, some degree of infection and trauma, and food deficit.

Mean values for protein synthesis in normal human subjects are between 2 and 3 g protein/kg/12 h (27,35) and hence the values for the pre-expedition tests were markedly increased in both men, probably due to overfeeding. This might also account for the high values seen in the first postexpedition assessments. However, average values for the measurements made during the course of the expedition were also higher than might have been expected, with means of 4.6 g protein/kg/12 h for A and 3.3 g/protein/kg/12 h for B. It would therefore seem that even in the face of great exertion, negative energy balance, and serious physical deterioration, the vital function of protein synthesis can be maintained, as long as adequate or nearly adequate dietary protein is provided.

MEASUREMENTS OF MUSCLE FUNCTION, AEROBIC CAPACITY, AND INTRAMUSCULAR ENZYMES

Although many studies have reported the effects of endurance training on both exercise performance and the enzyme systems of skeletal muscle, there are no reports describing the effects of prolonged exercise under conditions of inadequate food intake. Measurements were therefore made of maximal oxygen uptake 1 week before and after the expedition, along with measurements of maximal voluntary contraction (MVC) isometric force production in various muscle groups. On the same days as these tests, muscle biopsy samples were taken from the vastus lateralis to be assessed for four different enzyme activities, representative of different components of muscle energy metabolism (36): glyceraldehyde-3-phosphate dehydrogenase (Gly3PDH) from glycolysis; β-hydroxyacyl-CoA dehydrogenase (HAD) from β-oxidation of free fatty acids; citrate synthase (CS) from the citric acid cycle; and cytochrome-c oxidase (COX) from the electron transport chain.

TABLE 5. *Maximal voluntary contraction isometric force production (kg)*

	A			B		
	Pre	Post	% change	Pre	Post	% change
Elbow flexion	28.1	25.2	−10.4	27.4	16.3	−40.6
Elbow extension	23.2	18.6	−19.9	20.2	14.7	−27.2
Grip strength	46.1	45.4	−1.5	64.9	40.9	−27.0
Leg extension	121.0	113.8	−6.0	192.1	85.0	−55.8
Abdominal flexion	45.7	46.3	+1.3	52.5	42.7	−19.7
Upright pull	144.7	131.3	−9.3	183.2	113	−38.3

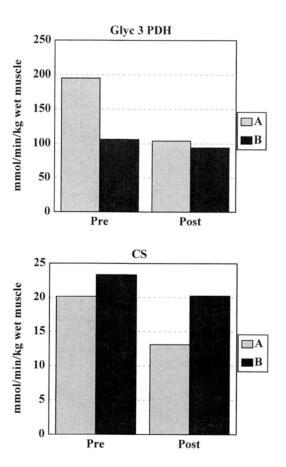

FIG. 2. Skeletal muscle enzyme activities before and after the expedition.

The changes in measurements of VO_2 max and strength are shown in Table 5, and the muscle biopsy enzyme activities are shown in Fig. 2. The decreases in the skeletal muscle enzyme activities would have directly affected peripheral oxygen utilization and so would partly explain the observed declines in VO_2 max. However, some of the decline in oxygen uptake also may have been due to losses of cardiac muscle and lowered cardiac output because such changes in the heart have been described during weight loss induced by dietary restriction with much smaller degrees of negative energy balance (37). The decline in the activity of the enzymes measured would not directly account for the observed losses of MVC force production, but it seems reasonable to assume that the declines were matched by losses on a similar scale of the contractile elements such as actin, myosin, and myosin adenosine triphosphatase.

Normally, the principal biochemical adaptation of skeletal muscle to training is an increase in aerobic capacity, reflected by increases in the mitochondrial

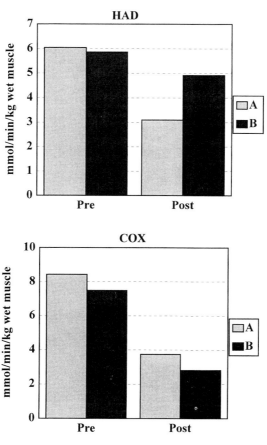

FIG. 2. *Continued.*

enzymes involved in β-oxidation, the citric acid cycle, and the electron transport chain (38). As a consequence, an increase in fat oxidation is seen during exercise with a decrease in carbohydrate oxidation and an increased work capacity (36,39). However, such studies have reported the effects of training combined with adequate nutrition, and it would seem likely that the changes seen in these expedition results can be attributed to the negative energy balance and the need for muscle protein oxidation to offset the energy deficit. The greater losses in strength seen in B would then reflect his greater negative nitrogen balance and lower rates of protein synthesis.

BIOCHEMICAL PARAMETERS

Blood samples were taken at 10-day intervals during the journey to assess a variety of hormonal and biochemical responses. Standard enzymatic and radioimmunoassays were used to measure glucose, insulin, growth hormone (GH), cortisol, testosterone, luteinizing hormone (LH), thyroid function, cholesterol, triglycerides, total protein, and albumin.

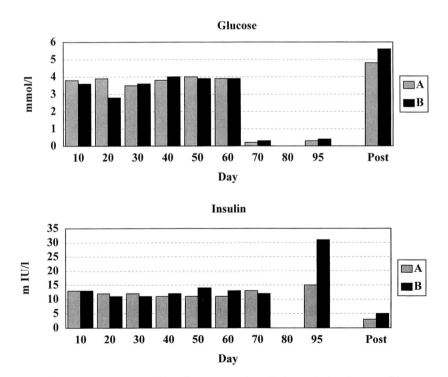

FIG. 3. Blood glucose and insulin concentrations during and after the expedition.

End-of-day blood glucose levels were low, with mean values of 3.0 mmol/L in A and 2.8 mmol/L in B, and on two occasions (days 70 and 95) both men were apparently grossly hypoglycemic, with values of around 0.3 mmol/L. Corresponding to these low values, end-of-day insulin levels were surprisingly high, with mean values of 12.7 mIU/L in RF and 14.6 mIU/L in MS, and an extraordinary value of 31 mIU/L in MS corresponding to the hypoglycemia of day 95. The glucose and insulin results are shown in Fig. 3. On the same occasion, B also had an elevated 6 pm cortisol value of 930 nmol/L and a massively increased growth hormone level of 70.5 mIU/L (Fig. 4). It would therefore appear that the low glucose values were not artifacts and that the combination of the prolonged exercise, relatively low carbohydrate intake, and undernutrition led to frank hypoglycemia, although the low levels may have been exaggerated by sampling in the cold, with low peripheral blood flow leading to greater peripheral glucose extraction. The insulin levels of around 11 to 14 mIU/L seen over the first 70 days of the expedition were rather high, considering that glucose levels were 4.0 mmol/L or less. This may have been due to a loss of insulin sensitivity secondary to the very high-fat diet, although the insulin levels of 15 and 30 mIU/L in A and B on day 95 would still seem totally inappropriate in the face of glucose levels

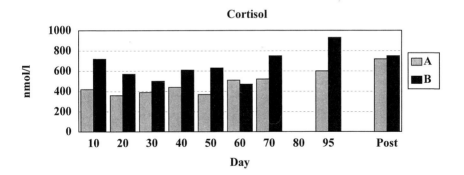

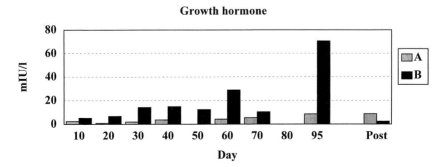

FIG. 4. Cortisol and growth hormone concentrations during and after the expedition.

of only 0.3 and 0.4 mmol/L. It therefore seems likely that this inexplicable hyperinsulinemia was causing the hypoglycemia.

Although the very low levels of glucose were associated with some subjective clouding of consciousness, the fact that the two men were conscious at all emphasizes the fact that it is the rapid changes in blood glucose levels seen in diabetics that cause such profound changes in conscious level, although the results are so low that the fact that the men had only mild symptoms does suggest that they had adapted to use ketones or other substrates in the central nervous system.

The low glucose levels may have contributed to the two occasions during the expedition when subject B apparently became hypothermic because the symptoms of hypothermia and hypoglycemia are indistinguishable. Furthermore, hypoglycemia has been shown to markedly impair the normal vascular and shivering responses to cold, presumably due to central neuroglypenic effects on the hypothalamus (40).

Testosterone levels in both subjects showed striking declines during the course of the experiment that were similar, although more marked, than those reported by Aakvaag et al. (41) in soldiers undergoing a combination of physical stress and near total sleep deprivation for 5 days. However, LH also declined during this expedition, whereas Aakvaag (41) reported little change or small increases in LH

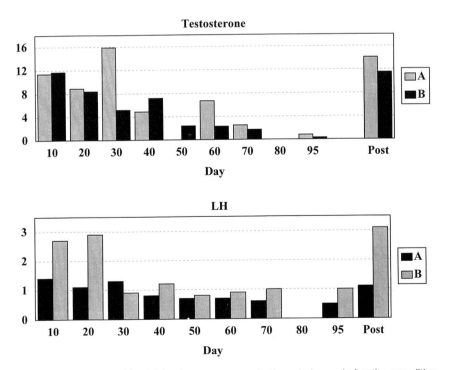

FIG. 5. Testosterone and luteinizing hormone concentrations during and after the expedition.

levels. The results are shown in Fig. 5. Changes in blood lipids were also interesting. Despite a daily intake of around 290 g of mostly saturated fat, total cholesterol values remained unchanged, whereas high-density lipoprotein cholesterol increased in both men from pre-expedition levels of around 0.9 mmol/L to post-expedition values of around 1.6 mmol/L, with low-density lipoproteins decreasing correspondingly. It would therefore seem that very high levels of exercise can offset the adverse effects of even the most abnormal of diets. Thyroid function remained normal throughout the expedition, and despite under-nutrition there were no significant changes in total protein or plasma albumin.

CONCLUSION

Overall, although there were only two subjects in the studies, the findings demonstrate that marked biochemical and physiologic changes can occur when men work hard in negative energy balance for a prolonged period. They therefore provide unique information regarding the body's capabilities to adapt under circumstances that were probably close to physiologic limits.

REFERENCES

1. Stroud MA. *Shadows on the wasteland.* London: Jonathan Cape; 1993.
2. Stroud MA. Nutrition and energy balance on the "Footsteps of Scott Expedition 1984–86." *Hum Nutr Appl Nutr* 1987;41:426–433.
3. Phinney SD, Bistrian BR, Evans WJ, Gervono E, Blackburn GL. The human metabolic response to chronic ketosis without caloric restriction: preservation of submaximal exercise capability with reduced carbohydrate oxidation. *Metabolism* 1983;32:769–776.
4. Keys A, Brozek J, Henschel A, Mickelson O, Taylor HL. *The biology of human starvation.* Vol. 1. Minneapolis, MN: University of Minnesota Press; 1950.
5. McCance RA. The history, significance and aetiology of hunger oedema. In: Studies of Undernutrition, Wuppertal, 1946-9. Special Report Series MRC no. 275. London: HMSO; 1951:21–82.
6. Durnin JGVA, Womersley J. Body fat assessed from total body density and its estimation from skinfold thickness, measurement on 481 men and women aged 16 to 72 years. *Br J Nutr* 1974;32:77–97.
7. Westerterp KR, Saris WH, Van Es M, Ten Hoor F. Use of the doubly labeled water technique in humans during heavy sustained exercise. *J Appl Physiol* 1986;61:2162–2167.
8. Forbes-Ewan CH, Morrisey BLL, Gregg GC, Waters DR. Use of doubly labelled water technique in soldiers training for jungle warfare. *J Appl Physiol* 1989;67:14–18.
9. Stroud MA, Coward WA, Sawyer MB. Measurements of energy expenditure using isotope-labelled water ($^2H_2{}^{18}O$) during an Arctic expedition. *Eur J Appl Physiol* 1993;67:375–379.
10. Davies CTM, Thompson D. Aerobic performance of female marathon and male ultramarathon athletes. *Eur J Appl Physiol* 1979;41:223–245.
11. Brotherhood JR. Studies on energy expenditure in the Antarctic. In: Edholm OG, Gunderson EKE, eds. *Polar human biology.* London: Heinemann Medical Books; 1973.
12. Pandolf KB, Haisman MF, Goldman RF. Metabolic energy expenditure and terrain coefficients for walking on snow. *Ergonomics* 1976;19:683–690
13. O'Hara WJ, Allen C, Shepard RJ, Allen G. Loss of body fat during an Arctic winter expedition. *Can J Physiol Pharmacol* 1977;55:1235–1241.
14. O'Hara WJ, Allen C, Shepard RJ, Allen G. Fat loss in the cold—a controlled study. *J Appl Physiol* 1979;46:872–877.
15. Riggs CE, Johnson DJ, Kilgour RD, Konopka RD. Metabolic effects of facial cooling in exercise. *Aviat Space Environ Med* 1983;54:22–26.

16. Stroud MA. Effects on energy expenditure of facial cooling during exercise. *Eur J Appl Physiol* 1991;63:376–380.
17. Weller A, Millard CM, Stroud MA, Greenhaff PL, Macdonald IA. The influence of cold-exposure on the metabolic and thermoregulatory responses to prolonged intermittent walking exercise in man. *J Physiol* 1995;483:123–124.
18. Jacobs I, Romet TT, Kerrigan-Brown D. Muscle glycogen depletion during exercise at 9°C and 21°C. *Eur J Appl Physiol* 1985;54:35–39.
19. Patton JF, Vogel JA. Effects of acute cold exposure on submaximal endurance performance. *Med Sci Sports Exerc* 1984;16:494–497.
20. Young AJ, Sawka MN, Neufer PD, Muza SR, Askew EW, Pandolph KB. Thermoregulation during cold water immersion is unimpaired by low muscle glycogen levels. *J Appl Physiol* 1989;66:1809–1816.
21. Martineau L, Jacobs I. Muscle glycogen availability and temperature regulation in humans. *J Appl Physiol* 1989;66:72–78.
22. Weir JB deV. New methods for calculating metabolic rate with special reference to protein metabolism. *J Physiol* 1949;109:1–9.
23. Finer N, Swan PC, Mitchell FT. Metabolic rate after massive weight loss in human obesity. *Clin Sci* 1986;70:395–398.
24. Morgan JB. Weight-reducing diets, the thermic effect of feeding and energy balance in young women. *Int J Obes* 1984;8:629–640.
25. Mole PA, Stern JS, Schultz CL, Bernauer EM, Holcomb BJ. Exercise reverses depressed metabolic rate produced by severe caloric restriction. *Med Sci Sports Exerc* 1989;21:29–33.
26. Tremblay A, Nadeau A, Despres JP, St-Jean L, Theriault G, Bouchard C. Long-term exercise training with constant energy intake. 2. Effect on glucose metabolism and resting energy expenditure. *Int J Obes* 1990;14:75–84.
27. Fern EB, Garlick PJ, McNurlan MA, Waterlow JC. The excretion of isotope in urea and ammonia for estimating protein turnover in man with ^{15}N-glycine. *Clin Sci* 1981;61:217–228.
28. Garrow JS. *Energy balance and obesity in man.* Elsevier and North Holland Press: Amsterdam; 1974.
29. Lemon WR. Does exercise alter dietary protein requirements? *Med Sport Sci* 1991;32:15–37.
30. Millward DJ, Botwell JL, Pacy P, Rennie MJ. Physical activity, protein metabolism and protein requirements. *Proc Nutr Soc* 1994;53:223–240.
31. Wolfe RR, Wole MH, Nadel ER, Shaw JHF. Isotopic determination of amino acid-urea interactions in exercise in humans. *J Appl Physiol* 1984;56:221–229.
32. Tomkins AM, Garlick PJ, Schofield WN, Waterlow JC. The combined effects of infection and malnutrition on protein metabolism in children. *Clin Sci* 1983;65:313–324.
33. Jeevanandam M, Peterson SR, Shamos RF. Protein and glucose fuel kinetics and hormonal changes in elderly and trauma patients. *Metabolism* 1993;42:1255–1262.
34. Waterlow JC. *Protein-energy malnutrition.* London: Edward Arnold; 1992:93.
35. Fern EB, Garlick PJ. The rate of whole body metabolism in the whole body of man measured with ^{15}N glycine and uniformly labelled ^{15}N wheat. *Hum Nutr Clin Nutr* 1983;37:91–107.
36. Wibom R, Hultman E, Johansen M, Matherei K, Constantin-Teodosiu D, Schantz PG. Adaptation of mitochondrial ATP production in human skeletal muscle to endurance training and detraining. *J Appl Physiol* 1992;73:2004–2010.
37. Ramhamadany E, Dasgupta P, Brigden G, Lahiri A, Rafferty EB, Mclean B. Cardiovascular changes in obese subjects on very low calorie diet. *Int J Obesity* 1989;13:95–99.
38. Holloszy JO. Enzymatic adaptations of skeletal muscle to endurance exercise. *Curr Prob Clin Biochem* 1981;11:118–121.
39. Hoppeler H, Howald H, Conley K, et al. Endurance training in humans: aerobic capacity and structure of skeletal muscle. *J Appl Physiol* 1985;59:320–327.
40. Gale EAM, Bennett T, Hilary Green J, Macdonald IA. Hypoglycaemia, hypothermia and shivering man. *Clin Sci* 1981;61:463–469.
41. Aakvaag A, Bentdal O, Quigstad K, Walstad P, Ronningen H, Fonnum F. Testosterone and testosterone bonding globulin in young men during prolonged stress. *Int J Androl* 1978;1:22–31.

*Physiology, Stress, and Malnutrition: Functional
Correlates, Nutritional Intervention,*
edited by J.M. Kinney and H.N. Tucker.
Lippincott–Raven Publishers © 1997.

An Analysis of Thermal Metabolism in Burned Patients

Charmaine Childs

*Regional Pediatric Burns Unit, Booth Hall Children's Hospital,
Blackley, Manchester M9 2AA, United Kingdom*

BURN INJURY AND THE ORIGIN OF ORGAN DYSFUNCTION

It is usually quite obvious that a person has been injured; an ugly wound, profound bleeding, or crushed limb are the outward signs of physical injury. Nociception, pain, and fear provide the initial stimulus (1), but the alarm becomes more widespread with activation of the hypothalamo-pituitary-adrenal axis (2). This is essentially adaptive, but it also may be destructive to the host if the stimulus persists. Some patients, of course, may be hopelessly injured, tissue damage and mutilation so great that normal defense mechanisms are inadequate and life is lost rather quickly. For those who survive their injuries, progress to recovery is dependent on a host of factors affecting the patient both before and after the accident. These include the patients pre-existing state of health as well as the quality of the facilities available and the expertise and knowledge of those caring for him or her.

Superficial burns heal spontaneously within about 7 to 10 days, but it takes much longer, weeks or even months, for deeper burns to heal. In the past it was not uncommon for some to remain unhealed long after the injury, and hypertrophic scarring, joint contractures, and physical and emotional disability were the inevitable consequences of delayed healing. Apart from the distressing cosmetic results that accompany wound contraction and scarring, there are other good reasons for closing the wound as soon as possible.

Burning the skin represents destruction of part of a very large organ, and if extensive, this could mean almost complete dysfunction of the skin organ. Regeneration can be slow, and time to healing represents the time the host must struggle to overcome the effects of this functional loss. Skin has both protective and regulatory functions, necrotic tissue can provide neither, and invasion by micro-organisms is always a possibility.

Bacteria do not normally make their way through an intact stratum corneum, although some fungi may do this and can live and reproduce both on the surface and in hair follicles or sebaceous ducts (3). Once the skin is destroyed, the immune system provides a secondary protective mechanism preventing bacterial spread to other organ systems (4), but this too may be compromised by a variety of inflammatory mediators suppressing immune function (5). Thus, from the outset the presence of a burn wound has deleterious affects on specialized tissues other than skin.

Heat damage has only to extend to the most superficial layers of the epidermis to destroy the waterproof barrier (6). There has been some debate about the nature and site of this barrier, but it seems to depend on a sphingolipid in the lowest level of the stratum corneum (7), which surrounds the keratin framework (6). Loss of the waterproof barrier represents just one of the regulatory functions disrupted by a burn. Water, electrolytes, and protein leak onto the surface as well as into tissue through heat-damaged vessels. With time this progressive leak of intravascular fluid becomes generalized, particularly if the burn is extensive, and is the primary cause of the decrease in blood volume and cardiovascular dysfunction that predisposes to clinical shock. Hypovolemia is exacerbated if fluid replacement is delayed or inadequate (8).

Evaporation of water from the open wound is inevitable unless covered by an impermeable membrane. Vaporization of water from the burn cools the surface according to the laws of physics (9). Some degree of insulation is provided by subcutaneous fat, but if this is destroyed, heat is conducted more easily to the surface. The patient cools, body temperature decreases, and compensatory thermoregulatory mechanisms are needed to maintain a normal body temperature; as would be expected in any other circumstances where individuals are exposed to cold (10). On the other hand, the ability to cool the skin in the warm is made impossible when sweat glands are burned, and vasomotor control of skin vasculature is lost as well. Thus the efferent mechanisms of thermoregulation are compromised by burn injury.

Within a short time the evaporation of water increases, even through a hard eschar (11), and if unabated, increased vaporizational heat loss leads to a disruption in the balance between heat production and heat loss, and the result is likely to be a decrease in deep body temperature. The relationship between evaporative water loss and metabolic rate was shown in the past to be fundamentally important to the development of burn-related disturbances of thermoregulation and metabolism (12). Nursed with wounds exposed to the air, extensively burned patients had a huge increase in both water and heat loss (13). Metabolic rate doubled in the most severely burned patients, and it is easy to see why these patients topped the list for the greatest increment in metabolic rate compared with any other injury or illness (14).

Modern treatment has changed all this. Patients' wounds are closed much sooner, and moderately burned patients are well on the way to recovery at 3 weeks. Historically this was the time corresponding to the flow phase (15) after injury, a period of intense metabolic activity, but a 3-week-old, unhealed, granulating wound is essentially a thing of the past. Today the evidence points to a much reduced metabolic response (16–19). It is doubtful if the metabolic state of the burned patient should be described as hypermetabolic today, yet patients are commonly described in this way.

More needs to be done to identify the stimuli, thermal or otherwise, that influence the demand for energy at all stages of the burn, and equally, we need to know the extent to which modern treatment may have modified this.

TREATING PATIENTS THE MODERN WAY

Modern treatment of the burned patient involves early removal of the wound and with it one hopes the illness and morbidity with which it is associated. Small superficial burns usually heal quickly but can still cause serious illness, particularly in young children (20).

Deep dermal burns are removed by tangential excision and closed with a split-thickness skin graft (21). If the burn is not too big, the patient may need just one skin grafting session, and, providing the split-thickness autograft takes, complete closure should be achieved within 5–7 days. With massive burns, donor sites may be scarce, so any unburned skin may need to be reharvested. Grafting is then performed in stages because each donor site needs time to heal. Complete closure may accordingly be delayed if the burn is extensive. If only a small area of donor skin is available, the skin can be meshed, widely if necessary, to increase the surface area of the graft (22). Once the meshed autograft is applied to the wound bed, it can be overlaid with a temporary physiologic dressing such as allograft (22). Because the fragile meshed autograft is prone to dehydration, shear forces, edema, and hematoma (22) the allograft gives protection during the early stages of attachment. Any excised, ungrafted areas also can be covered by allograft, and this is the best approach to massive skin loss (23). However, with allograft the take is only temporary. Tissue rejection, although delayed in the immunosuppressed burn patient, is inevitable after about 3 weeks (24).

In the past 10 years or so skin banks have flourished in an attempt to meet the demands for allograft skin. Temporary allograft retains many of the properties of a functional, waterproof barrier (7), so it is the best possible alternative to autograft, limiting water, protein, and electrolyte loss from the wound surface and preventing excessive heat loss. One would expect such a treatment, which in essence closes the wound and limits water and heat loss, to eliminate at least one important stimulus to the increased thermoregulatory demand for energy. By doing this, the increased calorie requirements of the burned patient, so well described in patients with exposed wounds, should be cut down, with a saving in the energy cost of the burn injury.

Allograft also lowers the number of bacteria under the graft, reduces pain, and generally improves the patient's condition (25). Temporary, physiologic wound cover, therefore, has a considerable advantage over a traditional petroleum jelly–impregnated gauze and dry dressing.

Cultured epithelial autografts (CEAs) also are used to close the wound, but the grafts take 3 to 4 weeks to culture, so immediate closure is inevitably delayed (26). When applied, the grafts are fragile and the take is often poor. Despite high hopes for its use, CEA has been rather disappointing. Tremendous efforts also are being made to develop an ideal skin substitute, but products are still being evaluated.

With early closure of the wound, patients go home sooner (27). Near-total excision of large burns (>30% total body surface area) in children within the first 24 hours reduces the need for blood during surgery (28) compared with excisions between the second and 16th days, and there is some suggestion, but no convincing evidence, that early surgery (within the first 7 days) may reduce morbidity (27). Random allocation of adult patients into early and late excision groups has shown that young adults with burns in excess of 30% (but without inhalation injury) have a lower mortality rate (29), but in older patients with inhalation injury mortality is largely unchanged (29). Excision and grafting after about 3 days is now fairly standard practice in the United Kingdom. Larger burns have bigger areas to be excised, so serial excision starting at about 2 days is performed in weekly stages until the wound is closed (30).

CHANGES IN BODY TEMPERATURE AFTER A BURN

Of all the disturbances in regulatory processes that accompany the burn, changes in body temperature are probably the most common. In the past, patients had raised body temperatures and an increased metabolic rate around the second to third week after the burn even in the absence of infection (31). Although there has always been controversy about the primary cause of the postburn hypermetabolism (31–33), increased evaporative water loss and surface cooling, as a stimulus to thermoregulatory heat production, seemed to provide a plausible explanation for the development of the hypermetabolic state. Whether this increased temperature should be termed fever or hyperthermia can be debated . Most probably it is a fever because it results from pathologic events, but until recently its cause had not attracted much attention (34,35).

Although modern treatment has reduced the metabolic response to injury, there seems to be little evidence of a corresponding effect on body temperature; there is a suspicion that it could even have made it worse. Recent studies in children have shown that elevated body temperature is a big problem, especially for clinicians preoccupied with the danger of febrile convulsions. In fact, the incidence of convulsions after burns in children is very low (C. Childs, unpublished observations). These data show that high temperatures develop during the early postburn period (34,35), and with the data already available in the literature describing pyrexia later on (31,33), it is clear that altered thermoregulation is an almost inevitable consequence of the injury. It would appear that body temperature is increased just hours after the burn (34) and in the absence of any obvious explanation—bacterial pyrogens (36,37), excessive heat production consequent on a massive obligatory water loss (38), or cold stimulus (39), for example—an explanation should be sought. The changes in body temperature are so early that the inflammatory response to the wound must be suspected as an important factor in the development of pyrexia, and it is to the origin of the early inflammatory-metabolic state that our attentions should now turn.

CHARACTERISTICS OF THE POSTBURN PYREXIA

Changes in Core and Surface Temperature

Unfortunately, the literature has been somewhat biased in its description of the metabolic and thermoregulatory response to injury, focusing more on the changes during the later development of the wound organ (40) and ignoring the acute changes that occur during the first day or so. This is when the wound is new and before the highly vascular, luxuriant bed of granulating tissue that makes up the regenerating wound has developed (41).

Children have been under-represented as subjects in burn studies, so it might be surprising to look to the young of our species to address a number of unanswered clinical questions, but this is now possible with recent evidence of the way children respond to thermal burns, particularly during the acute phase (34). We now know that there is a characteristic pattern to the thermoregulatory response to burn injury in children (34). Some similarities to this pattern are evident in the burned adult, but the response is a modest one and takes slightly longer to develop (42).

In the child, deep body temperature (T_b) measured in core tissues (T_c), rectum (T_r), tympanic membrane(T_{ear}), and bladder (T_{br}) and skin surface temperature ($\overline{T}_{sk}$) remain within the normal range during the first few hours after the accident (34), and there is a gradient between the inside and outside of the body ($T_r\overline{T}_{sk}$) of about 2–5°C (43) (Fig. 1). These data do not support the view that heat absorbed in the injury (44) contributes to early pyrexia in burned children because temperature measurements at this stage are essentially within the expected range. Over this same time period, T_r in the severely injured (non-burned) adult decreases in the usual conditions of the emergency room (45). The situation is different in the child. T_r does not decrease immediately after the accident. There is a period during which T_r remains stable (Fig. 1). The period of thermal stability does not last very long in children. By 5–8 hours, changes in skin and core temperature mark a point at which heat balance is shifted in the direction of heat storage, and this happens in a warm as well as a cool environment (46,47). The first sign of physiologic thermoregulation is a change in vasomotor tone. Acral skin blood flow starts to decrease and with it the temperature of the skin (48). This could be considered an inappropriate response to an increase in body temperature or even to a warm environment; nevertheless, it is a characteristic of the changes seen at this time and suggests a reduction in heat loss. The decrease in acral temperature is soon followed by an increase in rectal temperature. T_r increases to reach a peak, in excess of 40°C in many cases. Skin temperature reaches a nadir by about 10–12 hours after the burn (Fig. 1). At this time the gradient between core and surface temperature at the extremities can be as much as 13°C (43) (Fig. 1). T_c increases in a very characteristic way in almost all children studied irrespective of burn size, but peak T_c (measured in the ear) is highest in those with burns in excess of 10%, the group that receives intravenous resuscitation and intensive nursing care (Table 1). This is the case in a range of ambient temperatures from 22°C (cool) to 30–33°C (approximately thermoneutral). No such changes occur in the healthy child studied under the same environmental conditions. As for the burned adult, the modest increase in rectal temperature peaks much later, at about 24 hours (42).

During the first 24 hours after the burn, mean skin temperature, calculated using a modification of the methods of Ramanathan (49,50) in infants and children is variable but tends to increase and decrease with the pattern of deep body temperature (T_r, T_{ear}, T_{br}) (49,50). This also has been seen in the adult but at a much later stage after the burn (31,33). However, in acral regions skin tem-

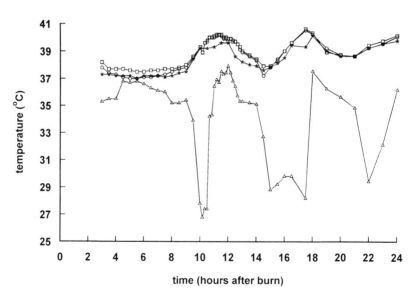

FIG. 1. Typical pattern of deep body and acral temperature in a 15-month-old girl with a burn of moderate severity (11% scald to back, shoulder, and neck). In an ambient temperature of 29.1 ±0.78°C (mean±SD), core temperature was monitored continuously and measured by thermistors placed into the bladder (□) and rectum (○). Hourly measurements of core temperature also were made using an infrared thermometer inserted into the external auditory canal toward the tympanic membrane (⋆). Acral temperature (△) was measured using a thermistor attached to the pulp of the great toe. All measurements were recorded at least hourly during the first 24 hours after the burn. There is a biphasic fever with the first peak between 10 and 12 hours and the second at 18 hours after the burn.

TABLE 1. *Peak tympanic temperature (T_{ear}) during the first 16 hours in patients with burns of different severities*

	Peak T_{ear} °C (mean ± SD)
≤5% tbsa	n = 6, 37.6 ± 0.34
6–9% tbsa	n = 10, 38.2 ± 0.57
≥10% tbsa	n = 5, 39.1 ± 0.56

T_{ear} in patients with the largest burns (≥10% tbsa) is significantly higher ($p > 0.05$, unpaired Student's *t* test) than in patients with smaller burns (≤5% and 6–9% tbsa). tbsa, total body surface area burned.

perature responds rather differently with a decrease in T_{ac}, preceding the increase in T_r and the subsequent pattern, almost the inverse of T_r (Fig. 1).

Some would argue that the increased air temperature of the intensive care room and the modern practice of wrapping the burn in bandages overinsulates the patient, making him or her hot. We have known for many years that skin temperature is higher than normal in burn patients during the later stage of the burn illness, and this is the case within a range of ambient temperatures, cool and warm, from 19 to 33°C (51). We now know that this is the case even during the first day or so. In a warm environment, $\overline{T}_{sk}$ of burned children is significantly higher than controls (Table 2), but in a cool environment, $\overline{T}_{sk}$ is comparable with healthy controls.

Effect of Warm Air and Bandaging

The legacy from earlier burns studies is that patients should be nursed in a warm environment (52,53). Under these conditions patients are comfortable and metabolic requirements can be minimized. This advice has been well

TABLE 2. *Skin temperature (°C) of patients and controls*

	Patients (n = 14; T_a 24.2 ± 0.43°C)	Controls (n = 5; T_a 21.3 ± 0.50°C)	Patients (n = 9; T_a 30.4 ± 0.36°C)	Controls (n = 14; T_a 30.1 ± 0.38°C)
$\overline{T}_{sk}$	32.7 ± 0.50	32.5 ± 0.29	35.5 ± 0.19	34.8 ± 0.11
Hand	32.9 ± 0.98	31.8 ± 0.66	36.5 ± 0.26	35.5 ± 0.14
Head	33.6 ± 0.51	33.1 ± 0.19	36.4 ± 0.23	35.8 ± 0.14
Limbs	31.8 ± 0.40	31.0 ± 0.25	35.0 ± 0.26	33.9 ± 0.22
Foot	31.6 ± 1.13	31.5 ± 0.69	36.0 ± 0.34	34.9 ± 0.21
Trunk	33.0 ± 0.43	34.0 ± 0.16	36.6 ± 0.19	35.3 ± 0.14

In cool conditions (T_a 21–24°C) mean skin temperature ($\overline{T}_{sk}$) of patients and controls is similar. In the warm temperature (approximately 30°C), $\overline{T}_{sk}$ and skin temperatures in each body region are significantly higher (Wilcoxon rank sum test for unpaired data) in the patients compared with controls ($p < 0.05$, $\overline{T}_{sk}$ and head; $p < 0.001$, hand, limbs, foot and trunk).

taken, and today most clinicians accept the principle that burn patients must be kept warm. The optimum temperature for the intensive care room appears to be open to interpretation, and clearly some centers do not keep their patients as warm as they might.

In the studies of young burned patients, infants and children are nursed from the outset in temperatures of approximately 30°C (54), and the burn is covered by dressings and crepe bandages. If the burn is a large one, this could involve covering an even larger part of the body with dressings and bandages, and an inability to lose heat could potentially become more of a problem than that of excessive heat loss. One has to consider whether the increase in T_r is due to fever or hyperthermia. In the latter case, high environmental temperatures and overwrapping or bundling should be considered as a possible cause, particularly because hyperpyrexia due to adverse environmental conditions is associated with sudden infant death syndrome in sleeping infants (55). An iatrogenic cause for the early pyrexia, as seen from the study of the heat content of burned children described below, was not found. Fever, even at this early stage after the injury, is a more plausible explanation.

Measurement of core and skin temperature can be used to calculate the body heat content. Heat content (kJ/kg) = $T_b \times 0.83 \times 4.18$, where T_b is mean body temperature, 0.83 the specific heat of body tissue, and 4.18 the conversion factor, kcal to kJ. For the first few hours after exposure to an ambient temperature of 30°C, body heat content was much the same in bandaged burned patients and similarly bandaged healthy children (47). By 12 hours, heat content of the patients started to increase. This phase of rapid heat storage was followed by a phase of thermal stability with a new but elevated plateau that was 7 kJ/kg above admission values, a significant increase (47). Burned children therefore respond differently from their healthy (bandaged) controls, storing more heat than normal in warm air (Fig. 2). If the conditions of the intensive care room and the bandages used as a temporary cover are not the main cause of the increased heat storage, what other factors could be involved?

We know from studies in animals that injury disrupts the normal efferent thermoregulatory mechanisms, widening the threshold temperatures for both the onset of heat production and heat loss (56). A central inhibition of heat loss, for example, would mean that the usual response to an increase in the heat content of the body was inhibited, so that vasodilatation of skin blood vessels, sweating, and adopting a more open posture would not be seen. We know that behavioral thermoregulation is altered after injury. In normal controls there is a good negative relationship between the preferred ambient temperature and the core temperature, but this relationship is lost on injury, and the injured patient prefers a high ambient temperature irrespective of the core temperature. This disturbance persists for some time after injury and is different from that seen in fever (57), where the normal relationship is displaced to the right. Adult burn patients will select a higher ambient temperature than controls, but the relationship between their choice and their core temperatures has not been investigated (58).

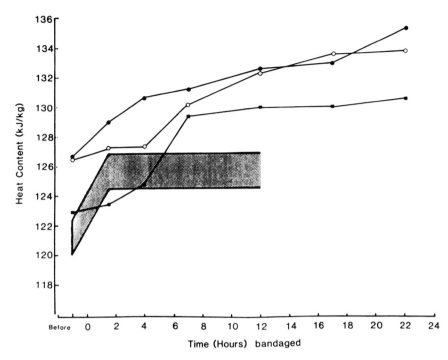

FIG. 2. Changes in heat content (kJ/kg) of healthy children, nude at T_a 20°C for a minimum of 60 minutes (before bandaging), and after 2–12 hours bandaged at T_a 30°C (shaded area represents mean ± SD of control data). Changes in heat content of bandaged patients with moderate (○; 10–12%) and extensive burns (•; 20–75%) nursed at T_a 30°C and in children with burns of 11–17% (■) nursed in a cooler environment (T_a 24°C). Reprinted with permission (47).

Relationship Between Evaporation Rate and Heat Loss

It might seem surprising to propose that heat loss may be inhibited after a burn when all the historical evidence points to the opposite: a massive obligatory water and heat loss from the exposed wound (9). It is now time to show that early removal of necrotic tissue brings the treatment of the burned patient in line with trauma surgery in general. Water and heat losses are not as great as shown previously. Modern treatment reduces the wasteful loss of both water and energy and thus lowers energy requirement in the burned patient (54,59,60).

At the time of admission, the wound is exposed. Within the range of ambient temperatures studied, 22–33°C evaporation rate in burned children was lowest over the area of full-thickness burn, ischemic, hard, and leathery and highest in partial-thickness areas that were red, edematous and wet. The evaporation rate (ER) was cut by half once bandages were applied (Fig. 3), and values were about the same as in a healthy child, sweating, at the same ambient temperature (61).

By 12 hours after the burn, there was evidence of an inhibition of heat loss from the unburned skin (43,61). Healthy skin is under central thermoregulatory control, and one would expect an appropriate response to a thermal stimulus. However, neither exposure to a warm environment nor an increase in the heat content of the body was a sufficient stimulus for burned patients to sweat. Dry heat loss (particularly by radiation), which is primarily dependent on the temperature gradient

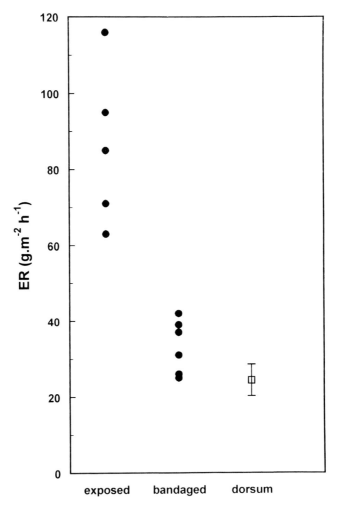

FIG. 3. Evaporation rate (g/m²/h) in seven patients (•) before (burn exposed) and after bandaging. Measurements were first made over the surface of the exposed burn during the first hour or so after admission to hospital (exposed) and over the bandages covering that same site (bandaged) at intervals during the first 24 hours after the burn. Mean ER for each paired set is given. For comparison, ER (median and range) measured over healthy skin of the anterior surface of the forearm (☐) of a child (control subjects) visibly sweating is also shown.

between surface (skin or bandages) and air was increased in the patients exposed to T_a 30°C compared with controls but evaporative heat loss in the two groups was much the same. Overall, total heat loss was not significantly different between the patients and controls. In cool conditions (T_a 22–24°C), ER was significantly higher in the burned compared with the healthy child and probably explained by the relatively greater ER from the body surface over the bandages. In healthy children, ER measured over the skin surface was at a minimum. Dry heat loss (principally by radiation and convection) was lower in the patients compared with the controls. Overall total heat loss was much the same in the two groups. Thus, under similar environmental conditions total heat loss in burned patients nursed in warm or cool conditions was about the same as their controls (61). These data are therefore in complete contrast to what has been reported in the past; for now, in the early period after a burn, excessive heat loss is not a feature of the injury. However, in view of the significant increase in stored heat, the rate of total heat loss could be interpreted as a relative reduction in heat loss compared with normal values. If ambient temperature is allowed to decrease (from 30°C to T_a 22°C, for example) the expected increase in total heat loss seen in the controls does not seem to occur particularly from T_a 30°C down to approximately 24°C (Fig. 4). In

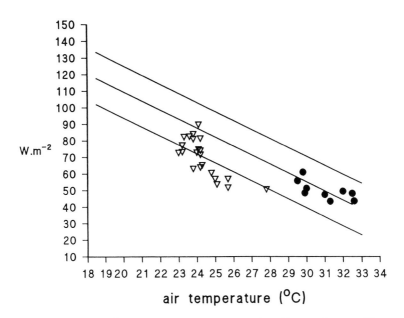

FIG. 4. Total heat loss (W/m²) of healthy children (bandaged) and burn patients at different environmental temperatures. Bandaged patients with moderate burns (•; 10–12%) nursed in a warm environment and patients with burns of 10–17% nursed in a cooler environment (∇) are shown superimposed on the control range (mean with 95% confidence interval). At T_a of approximately 30°C, patients had a comparable total heat loss to the control subjects, but patients nursed at a lower T_a had a total heat loss that was significantly lower than normal (p < 0.001, χ^2 test). Reprinted with permission (61).

this cool environment burned children did not look well and skin color was quite different. Unburned, unbandaged skin was marbled and bluish, and some of the burned children shivered. Core temperatures and heat content were significantly higher than normal. The changes seen in this group suggest reduced heat loss, particularly at the extremities (43,61), but it is unlikely this would be the only efferent thermoregulatory mechanism activated to achieve a higher body temperature because in a cool environment heat production would also have increased (62).

Relationship Between Tr and Heat Production

Studies of thermoregulation during the initial phase of thermal stability through the period of rapid heat storage shows at least one of the mechanisms activated to achieve a new and elevated thermal steady state.

In ambient conditions, simulating the intensive care room (T_a 30°C), healthy children are warm. Their hands and feet are pink, the face may be a little flushed, and they start to sweat at ambient temperatures above about 31°C. Dry heat loss, like total heat loss, is linear and lowest in ambient temperatures that bound the thermoneutral range (61).

In healthy children exposed to T_a 30°C, metabolic activity, measured as $\dot{V}O_2$, was studied during sleep and at rest, lying supine with eyes open. The measurements of $\dot{V}O_2$ were plotted against the child's age, and a range of measurements under these conditions produced two separate curves, best described by a parabolic regression because these data are curvilinear (54). Compared with the appropriate controls (63), $\dot{V}O_2$ in sleeping or resting patients with 10% or more burns (the resuscitation cases) was within the expected range for the child's age on about half the occasions when measurements were taken. $\dot{V}O_2$ was always highest at the time of the peak in rectal temperature (54). This was the point at which the temperature gradient (T_r-T_{ac}) was greatest (64) (Fig. 5).

As yet, the term hypermetabolism has not been defined, but it is unlikely that the increase in $\dot{V}O_2$ seen in these patients during the first few days (64) warrants such a description. This study, like other, modern studies, adds further evidence to the suggestion that the increase in metabolic activity after burn injury is not as great as it once was. In fact, some have failed to show a hypermetabolic response at all when compared with controls (65). It seems that with today's treatment a massive increase in metabolic rate is just not seen. The metabolic response to injury has been modified considerably by contemporary therapy, particularly early closure of the wound. Albeit initially temporarily closed by dressings, this method of surgical management ameliorates the demands on thermal metabolism. Nevertheless, there are clearly times when $\dot{V}O_2$ does increase well above normal, but this appears to be secondary to a concomitant increase in core temperature. If the increase in metabolic rate is not due to excessive heat loss, could the changes we see now be explained simply by an increase in core temperature?

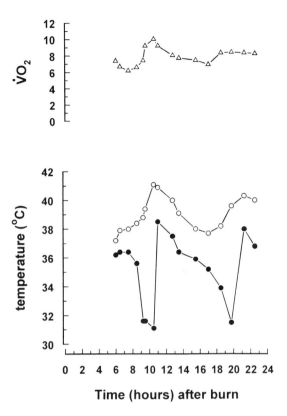

FIG. 5. Typical pattern of rectal temperature (T_r, $\bigcirc$), acral temperature (T_{toe}, $\bullet$), and oxygen consumption ($\dot{V}O_2$, $\triangle$) during the first 24 hours after the burn. The decrease in T_{toe} generally precedes the increase in T_r. $\dot{V}O_2$ reaches a peak, in this case 61% above the lowest value measured shortly after admission, at the time of the peak in T_r. In this example, the 11-month-old patient with a 10% scald was given paracetamol (acetaminophen) 11 hours after the burn.

EVIDENCE FOR A CHANGE IN HYPOTHALAMIC SET POINT TEMPERATURE

There are a number of reasons why body temperature increases in health as well as in disease. Whether hyperthermia or fever, the result is the same: core temperature goes up. But here the similarities end. In heat-induced disease, such as hyperthermia, the rate at which heat is lost from the body is insufficient to dissipate the heat stored within. Sweat glands function maximally when body temperature starts to increase, but sweat glands can fail to function optimally, particularly if the patient is dehydrated, and sweat production is reduced. Without this important route for heat loss, body temperature may increase even further. However, there is some evidence that heat stroke may occur even in patients who continue to sweat (66). Suggestions that the early postburn pyrexia may be due to overwrapping is a reasonable assumption, particularly if there were no avenues for heat loss, but the evidence so far rather refutes this. Fever is the more likely explanation. The difference between hyperthermia and fever is that fever is classically associated with an increase in the set point about which body temperature is regulated. The increase in body temperature is defended, and thermoregulatory control is optimal, operating at a higher level of core temperature. In the rising phase of fever, core temperature goes up rapidly, but efferent mechanisms are activated toward heat conservation, not heat loss. This would be the situation if the thermoregulatory set point were increased above the normal (37°C). As shown in Fig. 1, heat retention (as shown by a decrease in skin temperature) at the extremities occurs before there is any real change in core temperature. This is quickly followed by an increase in metabolic rate, but sweat rate remains about the same as the euthermic control. This is what would be expected in a warm environment from the experiments of Morimoto (62).

METABOLIC COST OF FEVER

It is now 75 years since DuBois (67) showed that metabolic rate was related to temperature so that there was, on average, a 13% increase in metabolic rate for each degree centigrade increase in rectal temperature. We continue to work with figures around this value, although 10% is often quoted (68). However, it is recognized that many other factors do influence metabolic rate, and cold, pain, and anxiety are just a few touched on already. We have used this approximation to examine the relationship between rectal temperature and oxygen consumption in burned children and can show that, corrected for temperature (69), the increase in metabolic rate during the early postburn period can be explained by the increase in body temperature (C. Childs, unpublished observation). The peak increase in metabolic rate, at approximately 12 hours, was less than predicted from a Q_{10} value of 2.3. This is the value most widely quoted with reference to the rate of biologic processes in homeotherms, but it has been suggested that under certain conditions in humans this value may be more variable (M. Ducharme, personal communication).

Some preliminary data have become available (C. Childs, unpublished observation) suggesting that even during the days and weeks that follow the burn, the values for oxygen consumption do not differ greatly from those values measured during the first day or so. The techniques of indirect calorimetry using modern flow-through systems (70) represent a major advance in the assessment of oxygen uptake and energy requirement at the bedside, but it does limit the measurement to a resting period, resting energy expenditure. Total energy expenditure (TEE) in the free-living burned patient, is perhaps the closest approximation to true energy expenditure, for such a measurement includes changes in energy expenditure associated with various activities that represent the person's true energy expenditure. Measurement is therefore not restricted to those times when the patient is at rest.

Measurement of TEE using the stable isotope method could be prone to errors during the rather unstable acute phase, but later and some days after the injury, studies have shown that total energy expenditure is indeed much lower in the patients treated by modern burn protocols (17) than in those patients studied 20 years ago.

INFLAMMATORY MEDIATORS OF THE ACUTE FEBRILE RESPONSE

Modern thinking about the generation of an acute phase response to injury provides the basis for tracing the origin of fever after a burn. Although the burn wound at first appears an isolated assault to the body, it does in fact represent a biologic integration between the brain and the immune system. The brain can modulate immune function in a number of ways via autonomic and neuroendocrine communication. Equally, the immune system may signal the brain via chemical messengers released from a variety of activated immune cells, locally at the site of the wound, but also from remote sites. If products of the immune system are responsible for the early post burn fever, it is clear that a bidirectional pathway is in operation.

With the exception of the elderly, most young accident victims are in good health before their injury. The influence of preexisting disease on the response to injury is always difficult to account for but in the child one would expect little in the way of developing or existing pathology. It is also possible to discount the influence of wound infection during the first 24 hours as a possible cause of fever because at this time wounds are not usually infected or colonized. Thus, during the first day, the interaction of neuroimmune mediators in acute postburn fever in children must be examined.

Burn injury is unlike other forms of tissue damage in that there is usually no bleeding, but blood flow is nevertheless grossly disturbed. Blood flow is absent in the area directly affected by the burn (the zone of coagulation necrosis), impaired in the zone of stasis, and increased in the minimally affected zone of hyperemia (71). From the outset, a variety of prostanoids and leukotrienes are produced once damage to the cell membrane phospholipids has occurred. By-products of burn-damaged tissue, such as collagen, thrombin, bradykinin and free radicals, lead to the production of arachidonic acid (via phospholipase A), vasoactivation, and chemoattraction to a variety of inflammatory cells. Heat-damaged protein also leads to activation of platelets and complement, particularly C5a (72) and intravascular neutrophil activation. The latter results in oxidative injury to a variety of cell membranes, erythrocytes in particular (73), through the production of free radicals that further exacerbate the inflammatory response by triggering the arachidonic cascade. Within a few hours the burn contains a coagulum of red cells, fibrin, fibroblasts, neutrophils, and, later, monocytes and macrophages (74). The cellular components of this inflammatory matrix produce a variety of growth factors and proinflammatory and inflammatory cytokines, and of these, interleukin-1 (IL-1), IL-6, and IL-8 appear in tissue fluid and plasma within a short time after the burn.

An increase in the thermoregulatory set point temperature, which is central to the development of fever, is associated with production of endogenous pyrogen, and IL-1 (alpha and beta), IL-6, IL-8, and tumor necrosis factor (alpha and beta) are pyrogenic in humans (75). It may eventually turn out to be a variety of cytokines alone or in combination with other molecules such as the prosta-glandins that eventually act upon thermosensitive neurones to alter the ther-moregulatory set point. At present the mechanisms are only partly understood.

At least some of these inflammatory cytokines have been identified in plasma of the burned patient (76) within a very short time after the accident. Although IL-1 is considered to be the most potent mediator of fever (77), it is difficult to detect in plasma (78). Its importance in tissue fluid (blister fluid in the burned patient) has yet to be determined in the overall sequence of inflammatory events, particu-larly the development of fever, but it seems unlikely that IL-1 in the periphery is likely to penetrate the blood–brain barrier (79). However, it may bind to specific receptors on astroglial processes in the perivascular space of the organum vascu-losum laminae terminalis, stimulating release of prostaglandin E2. Prostaglandins may well be the final pathway (80) in the genesis of the fever. However, produc-tion of IL-1 in the brain itself also may be stimulated by signals originating in peripheral cells, and certainly receptors for IL-1 have been found in the brain (81).

IL-1 has always been notoriously difficult to detect in blood, and this is also true after a burn, but in fluid from blisters the concentration is high and proba-bly reflects production from keratinocytes, endothelial cells, and fibroblasts at and around the site of the burn. The importance of IL-6 in plasma in burned patients is unclear, but studies in children show a positive and significant rela-tionship between IL-6 and rectal temperature. Maximum concentration of IL-6 occurred at the time of the peak in rectal temperature (78), 10 to 12 hours after the burn. Because IL-6 is a potent pyrogen in humans, it is likely that the appear-ance of these inflammatory molecules in the systemic circulation and in tissue fluid have some role in the induction of fever. The early increase in deep body temperature is therefore likely due to production of pyrogenic cytokines and, at this early period after the accident, an inflammatory response to a whole host of products released immediately after burning and cell death. Other sites distant from the burn also could be involved. The gastrointestinal tract has been inves-tigated as a potential source of pyrogenic and inflammatory material (82). In health, enterocyte integrity and barrier function retains all but the smallest of molecules within the gastrointestinal tract. However, after trauma and burns, enterocyte function is disturbed and cells become more permeable to molecules previously prevented from crossing the enterocyte (83). Markers of gut perme-ability appear in the circulation (84). Supported mainly by studies in animals (85), whole bacteria have been shown to cross the enterocyte to the circulation, and gut-derived organisms have been identified in mesenteric lymph nodes, spleen, and liver. In children, increased permeability to two specific probes (lactulose and mannitol) suggests that the gut of recently burned children does indeed become more permeable even at this very early stage (86). Whether this has any bearing on the early development of fever is unclear at present. The tight junction between enterocytes is also a potential site for passage of molecules, and with penetration of bacteria, cell products and endotoxin through the cell itself, the ability to protect the host from hazardous molecules is lost.

Initial priming of macrophages and neutrophils starts first with the formation of the wound, but repeated activation of immune cells, priming-activation sequences (87), produces an intense and exaggerated response with each new stimulus. Even routine treatments such as change of dressing could produce a bacteremia that then acts as a subsequent inflammatory stimulus. The cell products stimulated—cytokines, free radicals, proteases, and eicosanoids—produce autologous tissue injury and dysfunction. Later, inflammatory mediators and translocated bacteria or endotoxin originating within the gut represent a profound subsequent inflammatory stimulus, leading to clinical deterioration with each new stimulus. The septic inflammatory response syndrome (88), which is associated with infective as well as noninfective insults to the body, may have an important role in the development of multiple organ failure and this has a high mortality.

DISCUSSION

It is clear that recent changes in the treatment of the burned patient have had a major effect on the alterations in thermal metabolism seen after injury. The use of occlusive dressings followed by early excision and grafting has gone a long way to eliminate the enormous evaporative loss from the exposed burn. The change also has brought about many other benefits to the burned patient, and in children it is difficult to ignore the benefits to emotional well-being that early discharge from hospital can bring.

The change in the heat balance equation has exposed other differences in thermoregulation that had probably been obscured by the enormous heat drain from the exposed burn. One example is the early pyrexia seen in burned children and to a lesser extent in the burned adult. The differences between child and adult cannot yet be explained. The pyrexia is not iatrogenic.

Shortly after burn injury in the child, features of inhibition of thermoregulation observed after other forms of injury (1) and of cytokine-induced fever (75) are both found. The relative importance of these two influences, which could act in the same direction in the production of pyrexia, has yet to be determined. This fever, which is generally the rule in children with moderate to severe burns, does not seem to affect immediate outcome. A metabolic cost will, of course, be incurred because the increase in temperature will drive up the metabolic rate. The frequency of the fever and the rarity of convulsions in the burned children is surprising and merits further study.

One object of burn treatment must be to reduce the metabolic cost of the injury. This has not been entirely achieved by the newer methods of treatment, although it has led to a greater improvement. At least there is an explanation for it. Whether the energy cost of burn injury, at least in the early period, could be lowered further by nonsteroidal anti-inflammatory drugs is debatable. There is no convincing evidence as yet that fever is harmful, so aggressive steps to eliminate it may not have any particular advantage for the patient.

The changes in body temperature and heat content of burned children are largely independent of environmental temperature (20–30°C). However, the metabolic cost is greater at environmental temperatures below thermoneutral. Nursing burned patients at thermoneutrality lessens this cost. Morimoto et al. (62) have shown how the febrile response to a dose of pyrogen in the rabbit is mainly due to increased heat production in a cool environment, while the same effect is achieved by a reduction in heat loss in a warm one. There is evidence that both methods are used in the burned child to raise body temperature in a warm environment. Burned patients do seek a warm environment (39), and further work should be done to determine the changes in behavioral thermoregulation, as has been done for other injuries (89), in order to arrive at the optimum ambient temperature for treatment. Indiscriminate elevation of air temperature above the thermoneutral zone might be deleterious, particularly in the young child.

Despite these improvements, the burned wound still makes demands on the body: increased cardiac output, conversion of excess lactate to glucose, etc. (90). This is reflected in the loss of body weight that still occurs and is worsened when patients are not fed an adequate diet. This may be much less of a problem today because complete enteral preparations are now widely available. The benefits to the patient of supportive nutrient therapy is becoming appreciated by many clinicians, but nutritional complications have not been eradicated. Weight loss in the growing child is a real problem, and catch-up growth can be delayed for many years (91). As more and more clinicians recognize the importance of early enteral feeding, there is a pressing need to make sure that the dietary guidelines are appropriate in contemporary burn care. If they are not modified to accommodate the changes in energy requirement brought about by modern burn care, it may be overfeeding, rather than underfeeding, that becomes the dietary concern of the future.

REFERENCES

1. Stoner HB. A role for the central nervous system in the responses to trauma. In: Little RA, Frayn KN, eds. *The scientific basis for the care of the critically ill.* Manchester, England: Manchester University Press; 1986:215–229.
2. Barton RN, Cocks RA, Doyle MO, Chambers, H. Time course of the early pituitary–adrenal and metabolic responses to accidental injury. *J Trauma* 1995;39:888–894.
3. Blank, IH, What are the functions of skin lost in burn injury that affect short- and long-term recovery. *J Trauma* 1984;24(suppl):10–24.
4. Deitch AD, Gut failure: its role in the multiple organ failure syndrome. In: Deitch EA, ed. *Multiple organ failure.* New York: Thieme Medical; 1990:40–59.

5. Zhou D, Munster AM, Winchurch RA. Inhibitory effects of Interleukin 6 on Immunity. Possible implications in burn patients. *Arch Surg* 1992;127:65–69.
6. Crounse RG. Keratin and the barrier. *Arch Environ Health* 1965;11:522–528.
7. The epidermal barrier [Editorial]. *Lancet* 1987;1:1414
8. Muir IFK, Barclay TL, Settle JAD. *Burns and their treatment.* London: Butterworths; 1987.
9. Harrison HN, Moncrief JA, Duckett JW, Mason AD. The relationship between energy metabolism and water loss from vaporization in severely burned patients. *Surgery* 1964;56:203–211.
10. Gagge AP, Nishi Y. Heat exchange between human skin surface and thermal environment. In: Lee DHK, ed. *Handbook of physiology.* Section 9. Bethesda: American Physiological Society; 1977.
11. Cohen S. An investigation and fractional assessment of the evaporative water loss through normal skin and burn eschars using a microhygrometer. *J Plast Reconstruct Surg* 1966;37:475–486.
12. Neely WA, Petro AB, Holloman GH, et al. Researches on the cause of burn hypermetabolism. *Ann Surg* 1974;179:291–294.
13. Horn L, Converse JM. Heat loss as a factor in the fatal outcome from extensive burns. *Am J Physiol* 1964;207:861–864.
14. Wilmore DW. *The metabolic management of the critically ill.* New York: Plenum; 1977.
15. Cuthbertson DP. Post-shock metabolic response. *Lancet* 1942;1:433–437.
16. Carlson DE, Cioffi WG, Mason AD, et al. Resting energy expenditure in patients with thermal injuries. *Surg Gynecol Obstet* 1992;174:270–276.
17. Goran MI, Peters EJ, Herndon DN, Wolfe RR. Total energy expenditure in burned children using the doubly labelled water technique. *Am J Physiol* 1990:259;E576–E585.
18. Cunningham JJ, Lydon MK, Russell WE. Calorie and protein provision for recovery from severe burns in infants and young children. *Am J Clin Nutr* 1990;51:553–557.
19. Childs C, Little RA. Acute changes in oxygen consumption and body temperature after burn injury. *Arch Dis Child* 1994;71:31–34.
20. Childs C, Edwards-Jones V, Heathcote DN, et al. Patterns of S. aureus colonisation, toxin production, immunity and illness in burned children. *Burns* 1994;20:514–521.
21. Janzekovic Z. A new concept in the early excision and grafting of burns. *J Trauma* 1970;10: 1103–1108.
22. Muller MJ, Nicolai M, Wiggins R, et al. Modern treatment of a burn wound. In: Herndon DN, ed. *Total burn care.* London: WB Saunders; 1996:136–147.
23. Tompkins RG, Burke JF. Alternative wound coverings. In: Herndon DN, ed. *Total burn care.* London: WB Saunders; 1996:164–172.
24. Brown JB, Fryer MP, Randall P, Lu M. Post mortem homografts as biological dressings for extensive burns and debrided areas. *Ann Surg* 1953;138:618–623.
25. Zaroff LI, Mills W, Duckett JW, et al. Multiple uses of a viable cutaneous homograft in the burned patient. *Surgery* 1966;59:368–372.
26. Teepe RGC. *Cultured keratinocyte, implications for wound healing* [Ph.D. Thesis]. Leiden, The Netherlands: CIP-Data Koninklijke Bibliothek, Den Haag, 1993.
27. Pietsch JB, Netscher DT, Nagaraj HS, Groff DB. Early excision of major burns in children: effect on morbidity and mortality. *J Paediatr Surg* 1985;20 :754–757
28. Desai MH, Herndon DN, Broemling L, Barrow RE, et al. Early burn wound excision significantly reduces blood loss. *Ann Surg* 1990;211:753–759.
29. Herndon DN, Barrow RE, Rutan RL, et al. A comparison of conservative versus early excision, therapies in severely burned patients. *Ann Surg* 1989;209:547–553.
30. Herndon DN, Parks DH. Comparisons of serial debridement and autografting and massive excision with cadaver skin overlay in the treatment of large burns in children. *J Trauma* 1986;26:149.
31. Wilmore DW, Long JM, Mason AD, et al. Catecholamines: mediator of the hypermetabolic response to thermal injury. *Ann Surg* 1974;180:653–669.
32. Caldwell FT, Bowser BH, Crabtree JH. The effect of occlusive dressings on the energy metabolism of severely burned children. *Ann Surg* 1981;193:579–590.
33. Wilmore DW, Mason AD, Johnson DW, Pruitt BA. Effect of ambient temperature on heat production and heat loss in burn patients. *J Appl Physiol* 1975;38:593–597.
34. Childs C. Fever in burned children. *Burns* 1988;14:1–6.
35. Childs C, Little RA. Paracetamol (acetaminophen) in the management of burned children with fever. *Burns* 1989;14:343–348.
36. Atkins E, Bodel P. Fever. *N Engl J Med* 1972;286:27–34.
37. Cooper KE, Veale WL, Kasting N, Pittman QJ. Ontogeny of fever. *Fed Proc* 1979;38:35–38.

38. Barr PO, Liljedahl S-O, Birke G, Plantin L-O. Oxygen consumption and water loss during treatment of burns with warm dry air. *Lancet* 1968;January 27:164–168.
39. Danielsson U, Arturson G, Wennberg L. The elimination of hypermetabolism in burned patients. *Burns* 1976;2:110–114.
40. Wilmore DW. The wound as an organ. In: Little RA, Frayn KN, eds. *The scientific basis for the care of the critically ill.* Manchester, England: Manchester University Press; 1986:45–59.
41. Linares HA. Pathophysiology of the burn scar. In: Herndon DN, ed. *Total burn care.* London: WB Saunders; 1996:383–397.
42. Martineau L, Little RA, et al. Changes in core temperature during the early post burn period in adults. *Circ Shock* 1991;34;10–18.
43. Childs C, Stoner HB, Little RA. Evidence of a central inhibition of heat loss during the acute phase of burn injury in children. *Arch Emerg Med* 1990;7:303–304.
44. Davies JWL. *Physiological responses to burning injury.* London: Academic Press; 1982.
45. Little RA, Stoner HB. Body temperature after accidental injury. *Br J Surg* 1981;68:221–224.
46. Childs C. *Changes in heat content and heat loss during the acute phase of burn injury* [Ph.D. thesis]. Manchester, England: University of Manchester, 1989.
47. Childs C, Stoner HB, Little RA, Davenport PJ. A comparison of some thermoregulatory responses in healthy children and in children with burn injury. *Clin Sci* 1989;77:425–429.
48. Wright IP, Griffiths M, Childs C. A microprocessor based photoplethysmograph for use in clinical practice. *Anaesthesia* 1995;50:875–878.
49. Ramanathan NL. A new weighting system for mean surface temperature of the human body. *J Appl Physiol* 1964;19:531–533.
50. Henane R, Bittel J, Bansillon V. Partitional calorimetry measurements of energy exchanges in severely burned patients. *Burns* 1981;7:180–189.
51. Wilmore DW, Mason AD, Johnson DW, Pruitt BA. Effect of ambient temperature on heat production and heat loss in burn patients. *J Appl Physiol* 1975;38:593–597.
52. Caldwell FT, Wallace BH, Cone JB, Manuel L. Control of the hypermetabolic response to burn injury using environmental factors. *Ann Surg* 1992;215:485–491.
53. Davies JWL, Liljedahl S-O. The effect of environmental temperature on the metabolism and nutrition of burned patients. *Proc Nutr Soc* 1971;30:165–172.
54. Childs C. Studies in children provide a model to re-examine the metabolic response to burn injury in patients treated by contemporary burn protocols. *Burns* 1994;20:291–300.
55. Stanton AN. Overheating and cot death. *Lancet* 1984;2:1199.
56. Stoner HB. The burned patient's response to the environment: the 1991 Everett Idris Evans memorial lecture. *J Burn Care Rehabil* 1991;12:402–410.
57. Stolwijk JAL, Hardy JD. Temperature regulation in man—a theoretical study. *Pflugers Arch* 1966;291: 129–162.
58. Cabanac M, Massonnet B. Temperature regulation during fever: change of set-point or change of gain? A tentative answer from a behavioural study in man. *J Physiol* 1974;238:561–568.
59. Hildreth MA, Herndon DN, Parks DH, et al. Evaluation of a caloric requirement formula in burned children treated with early excision. *J Trauma* 1987;27:188–189.
60. Ireton CS, Turner WW, Hunt JL, Liepa GU. Evaluation of energy expenditures in burned patients *J. Am Diet Assoc* 1986;86:331–333.
61. Childs C, Stoner HB, Little RA, Davenport PJ. Cutaneous heat loss shortly after burn injury in children. *Clin Sci* 1992;83:117–126.
62. Morimoto A, Murakame, N Nakamori, Watanabe T. Ventromedial hypothalamus is highly sensitive to prostaglandin E2 for producing fever in rabbits. *J Physiol* 1988;397:259–268.
63. Childs C. Metabolic rate at rest and during sleep in a thermoneutral environment. *Arch Dis Child* 1993;68:658–661.
64. Childs C, Little RA. Acute changes in oxygen consumption and body temperature after burn injury. *Arch Dis Child* 1994;71:31–34.
65. Cone JB, Wallace BH, Caldwell FT, Bond PJ. Absence of postburn hypermetabolism in a group of children with serious burns. *J Burn Care Rehabil* 1993;14:9–11.
66. Shibolet S, Lancaster MC, Danon Y. Heat stroke a review. *Aviat Space Environ Med* 1976;47: 280–301.
67. DuBois EF. The basal metabolism in fever. *JAMA* 1921;77:352–355.
68. Baracos VE, Whitmore WT, Gale R. The metabolic cost of fever. *Can J Physiol Pharmacol* 1987;65:1248–1254.

69. Arturson G, Danielsson U, Wennberg L. The effects on the metabolic rate and nutrition of patients with severe burns following treatment with infrared heat. *Burns* 1978;5:164–168.
70. McGuinness K, Childs C. Development of an indirect calorimeter for use in infants and young children. *Clin Phys Physiol Measure* 1992;12:343–351.
71. Williams WG, Phillips LG. Pathophysiology of the burn wound. In: Herndon DN, ed. *Total burn care.* London: WB Saunders; 1996:63–70.
72. Ward PA. How does the local inflammatory response affect the wound healing process? *J Trauma* 1984;24(suppl):18–24.
73. Solomkin JS. Neutrophil disorders in burn injury: complement, cytokines, and organ injury. *J Trauma* 1990;30(suppl):80–85.
74. Hunt TK. Basic principles of wound healing. *J Trauma* 1990;30(suppl):122–128.
75. Kluger MJ. Fever revisited. *Pediatrics* 1992;90:846–850.
76. Nijsten MWN, DeGroot ER, Ten Duis HJ, et al. Serum levels of interleukin-6 and acute phase responses. *Lancet* 1987;2:921.
77. Dinarello CA. Interleukin-1. *Rev Infect Dis* 1984:6;51–95.
78. Childs C, Ratcliffe RJ, Holt I, et al. The relationship between interleukin-1, interleukin-6 and pyrexia in burned children. In: Dinarello CA, Kluger M, Powanda M, Oppenheim J, eds. *Physiological and pathophysiological effects of cytokines. Progress in leucocyte biology.* Vol. 10b. New York: Wiley Liss; 1990:295–300.
79. Morimoto A, Sakata Y, Watanabe T, Murakami N. Characteristics of fever and acute-phase response induced in rabbits by IL-1 and TNF. *Am J Physiol* 1989;256;R35–R41.
80. Blatteis CM, Bealer SL, Hunter WS, et al. Suppresion of fever after lesions of the anteroventral third ventricle in guinea pigs. *Brain Res Bull* 1983;11:519–526.
81. Farrar WL, Hill JM, Harel-Bellan A, Vinocour M. The immune logical brain. *Immunol Rev* 1987; 100:361–378.
82. Deitch EA. Intestinal permeability is increased in burn patients shortly after injury. *Surgery* 1990;107: 411–416.
83. Wilmore DW, Smith RJ, O Dwyer ST, et al. The gut: a central organ after surgical stress. *Surgery* 1988;104:917–923.
84. Carter EA, Tompkins RG, Schiffrin E, Burke JF. Cutaneous thermal injury alters macromolecular permeability of rat small intestine. *Surgery* 1990;107:335–341.
85. Alexander JW, Boyce ST, Babcock GF, et al. The process of microbial translocation. *Ann Surg* 1990; 212:496–512.
86. Childs C, Watson SB, Fisher MI, et al. Gut permeability in the acutely burned child. *Proceedings of the association of Clinical Biochemists,* June 1992:52.
87. Anderson BO, Harken AH. Multiple organ failure: inflammatory priming and activation sequences promote autologous tissue injury. *J Trauma* 1990;30(suppl):44–48.
88. Borre RC. Sepsis, sepsis syndrome, and the systemic inflammatory response syndrome (SIRS) [Editorial]. *JAMA* 1995;273:155–156.
89. Little RA, Stoner HB, Randall PE, Carlson G. An effect of injury on thermoregulation in man. *Q J Exp Physiol* 1986;71:295–306.
90. Wilmore DW, Stoner HB. The wound organ. In: Cooper G, Dudley H, Gann D, et al, eds. *Scientific foundations of trauma.* Boston: Butterworth Heinemann (in press).
91. Childs C, Hall T, Davenport PJ, Little RA. Dietary intake and changes in body weight in burned children. *Burns* 1990;16:418–422.

Physiology, Stress, and Malnutrition: Functional Correlates, Nutritional Intervention,
edited by J.M. Kinney and H.N. Tucker.
Lippincott–Raven Publishers © 1997.

Impaired Thermoregulation in Malnutrition

Simon P. Allison

*Department of Medicine, University Hospital, Queens Medical Centre,
Nottingham NG7 2UH, United Kingdom*

Over hundreds of millions of years, animals evolved in a relatively constant marine environment. To enable them to emerge onto land, they faced a number of physiologic obstacles: first, gas exchange; second, maintenance of salt and water balance; and third, the control of body temperature at an optimal level for physiologic function. They moved from an environment where they could depend on the constancy of the *milieu exterieur* to one where the *milieu interieur* became more important for survival and evolutionary progress. The poikilotherms, or reptiles, depended largely on passive means of thermoregulation, moving from water to land or from shade to sun as needed. This may be one reason why the reptiles reached the limits of evolutionary development and why most of them died out. The dinosaurs, for example, may well have fallen victim to a sudden climatic change, with decreases in environmental temperature that defeated their thermoregulatory reserve as well as destroying their food supply. The homeotherms, on the other hand, developed physiologic mechanisms for adjusting their internal environment and were thus able to survive fluctuations in climate. They also developed strategies to reduce heat loss, such as layers of fat, fur, or feather, which enabled them to colonize colder climates. Some also survived extreme cold by developing hibernating mechanisms for reducing metabolic rate and body temperature during the colder months.

It is no accident that the earliest traces of human origins have been found in the tropical regions of Africa because man is truly the "naked ape," with only a modest covering of fat and no fur. Humans' internal mechanisms are sufficient to maintain core temperature in the face of modest climatic fluctuation around their thermoneutral zone, but not to cope with low environmental temperatures. Paradoxically, although human brains grew in size until they consumed 20% of total energy expenditure, thereby increasing heat loss from the head, it also allowed development of the intellectual capacity to invent fire and clothing and to adopt protective behavioral responses, enabling humans to colonize temperate climates. The wall paintings and blackened remains of fires, found in the caves of southern Spain and dating from 20,000 BC, bear witness to the use of animal skins as clothing and of fire for both cooking and warmth, as humans migrated from Africa to the northern land mass. Human thermoregulatory physiology must be seen and understood against this background. A human's first and most important line of defense against cold is a behavioral response, which may be impaired when cognition is blunted, as in old age, illness, or with moderate hypothermia itself (see below). Internal mechanisms provide the fine tuning or adjustments to meet modest environmental fluctuations, but are quickly overwhelmed by severe conditions, such as exposure on mountainsides or immersion in cold water.

IMPORTANCE OF CORE TEMPERATURE

Normal core temperature in humans is maintained within very narrow limits between 36 and 37°C, albeit with a superimposed circadian rhythm (1). In healthy subjects 20–30 years of age, studied in the postabsorptive state at rest in a constant temperature room at 25°C and wearing a liquid conditioned overall perfused with fluid at 35.2°C, their core temperatures remained between $36.8 \pm 0.06°C$ and $36.85 \pm 0.07°C$ for 1 hour (2). In a similar study (3) in eight normal elderly women, core temperature was found to be $37.3 \pm 0.1°C$. In another series of studies on young individuals, baseline core temperatures all lay within the $36.37 \pm 0.21°C$ to $36.64 \pm 0.12°C$ range. The consequences of small reductions in core temperature may be considerable. After concern over the excessive numbers of apparently accidental deaths among deep sea divers, Keatinge et al. (4,5) examined the possibility that such accidents might be caused by a loss of judgment secondary to minor degrees of hypothermia. They found that, when body temperatures of volunteers were lowered experimentally by immersion in cold water at 36°C or below, memory was impaired and there was a marked slowing of the speed at which complex reasoning tasks could be performed. They also showed the protective effects of subcutaneous fat (6). Pugh and Edholm (7), studying cross-channel swimmers, found that, despite a water temperature of 15°C, most swimmers were able to maintain a normal core temperature. The two major factors responsible for this were a thick layer of fat preventing heat loss and the increased heat production from exercise. An examination of those who failed to complete the race found that they had less body fat and that their core temperature had decreased to 35–35.5°C. This small decrease in temperature was sufficient to cause confusion, loss of judgment, and hallucinations. Similar effects on cognitive function have been found with reductions of core temperature between 1 and 2°C (8) in hill walkers affected by exposure (9,10) and in motorcyclists wearing insufficient clothing to prevent heat loss due to the wind/chill factor (11). Central nervous system function is therefore crucially dependent on maintenance of a normal core temperature. Muscle strength and function are impaired when limbs are cooled. Berg and Ekblom (12), relating peak torque during knee extensions, maximal speed during cycling, and height of the vertical jump at different vastus lateralis temperatures, found a linear relationship with significant decline in muscle function in the range of 37–35°C and lower. These clinically significant changes in neuromuscular function could well explain (a) the blunting of appropriate behavioral responses to cold and (b) a predisposition to accidents and falls.

NORMAL PHYSIOLOGY

Thermoregulation depends on a balance between heat production and heat loss to maintain core temperature within a narrow range and body function at its optimal level (1). In addition to basal metabolism, thermogenesis may be increased by exercise, by the effect of food ingestion, and by the response to cold through shivering and nonshivering mechanisms. It is also increased by the febrile response to illness. Heat loss may be diminished by appropriate behavioral responses and by cutaneous vasoconstriction (13) to conserve heat in the core, rather than losing it from the skin by the physical processes of radiation, convection, conduction, and the latent heat of evaporation of sweat. An adequate covering of fat provides additional insulation and protection, as shown in studies on divers and swimmers. Conversely, heat loss may be increased by cutaneous vasodilatation and by sweating. These responses are dependent not only on the mental appreciation of a change in environmental temperature, but also on reflex mechanisms. Cold sensors in the exposed hands and face provide afferent stimuli to the autonomic center in the hypothalamus, both to increase thermogenesis and to cause vasoconstriction. These afferents are thought to be the major stimulus to peripheral cutaneous vasoconstriction in response to cold, mediated by sympathetic alpha-adrenergic receptors (1). To increase heat loss, cutaneous blood flow in the hands and feet is increased by release of sympathetic noradrenegic tone (14), mediated by the sympathetic nervous system and an unknown neurotransmitter (13). Skeletal muscle blood flow does not appear to be involved in thermoregulatory reflexes (13,15,16). The arteriovenous anastamoses in the hands and feet, controlled by beta 2 adrenoreceptors mediating vasodilatation, are important in some animals, but their significance in humans is dubious (17). In an extremely cold environment, cutaneous vasoconstriction may be paralyzed as the terminal arteries lose their responsiveness to noradrenalin (18,19).

The last bastion of thermoregulatory defense is provided by the temperature sensors in the carotid artery territory. A decrease in core temperature of as little as 0.1°C may initiate both increased thermogenesis and vasoconstriction via the sympathetic nervous system. Conversely, an increase in core temperature may inhibit the responses to external cold and prevent vasoconstriction, so-called central warm inhibition (20). The central coordinating mechanisms are situated mainly in the hypothalamus. Animal studies by Benzinger (20) and McLean and Emsley-Smith (1) have showed that the afferent neurons from peripheral neuroreceptors synapse in the spinal cord and that the postsynaptic fibers radiate both to the cerebral cortex and to the posterior hypothalamus. The cortical afferent neurons probably serve to mediate conscious perception of temperature change and the initiation of appropriate behavioral responses. The area of the posterior hypothalamus that also receives thermoreceptor afferents has been termed the "heat maintenance center," controlling both heat production and conservation. Heat dissipation by vasodilatation and sweating, on the other hand, is controlled by a temperature-sensitive area of the anterior hypothalamus, termed the "heat loss center." Although the posterior hypothalamus is not temperature sensitive, inhibitory fibers run to this region from the anterior hypothalamus, which is. Efferent signals from the posterior hypothalamus may be inhibited by heating or by direct electrical stimulation of the anterior area, the mechanism of central warm inhibition described above. In humans, the limited anatomic information available is consistent with the studies in animals (20–23). Current ideas concerning thermoregulation in humans are based on the concept of a central thermostat, the set level of which may be modified by factors such as nutritional status. In teleologic terms, it can be seen as protecting the function of the central nervous system at its optimum level. A concept central to the study of thermoregulation is that of the thermoneutral zone, or the zone of least thermoregulatory effort. In healthy nude male subjects, this was found to be in the range of 29–32°C (24) but may be increased during acute illness or injury, particularly in burned patients (25). It may be defined as "the range of environmental temperature in which, for a given level of feeding, the metabolic rate of an individual resting animal is at a minimum and in which evaporative heat loss is not increased as a result of sweating or increased respiratory ventilation" (24). Below this range there is a progressive increase in thermogenesis, and above it, although body temperature can be maintained by sweating, beyond a certain point higher temperatures lead to hyperthermia and an increase in metabolic rate. These studies emphasize the importance of defining environmental temperature during thermoregulatory studies and may account for apparently differing results between studies in which environmental temperature was not properly controlled.

Thermogenesis

Basal Metabolism

This has already been discussed by Marinos Elia at this meeting. It is affected by thyroid and sympathoadrenal function, as well as by intrinsic metabolic processes.

Response to Exercise

Apart from basal metabolism, this is the major component of total daily energy expenditure. In the daily life of most individuals, it increases energy expenditure by 50–100% over basal, but during intense athletic activity, it may increase by four- to fivefold. As shown in the studies by Stroud (26) of his and Fiennes' extraordinary march across the Antarctic, exercise may have important consequences for thermoregulation, not merely by increasing heat production, vasodilatation, and sweating, but by decreasing body weight and fat content, when prolonged exercise over many days increases energy expenditure over energy intake. Their planned dietary intake of 5,000 kcal daily underestimated their average daily energy expenditure by 1,500 kcal, resulting in a 30% weight loss over 93 days. Because fat is more energy dense than carbohydrate, it is logistically easier to drag sledges containing food higher in fat rather than carbohydrate content, but as studies have shown (27), severe exercise on a low-carbohydrate diet results in exhaustion of both hepatic and muscle glycogen and may cause hypoglycemia. Stroud and Fiennes not only became thin, losing much of their insulating body fat, but also hypoglycemic, their blood glucose levels decreasing to less than 2.0 mmol. All these factors predispose to hypothermia, as I shall discuss later.

Shivering and Nonshivering Thermogenesis

Shivering is mediated by somatic motor neurons and skeletal muscle fibers (23) but is initiated autonomically via the hypothalamus and spinal cord. In adult humans, it can cause a three- to fivefold increase in metabolic rate in cold environmental conditions but is a relatively inefficient method of increasing body heat content because some heat is dissipated to the environment because of insufficient insulation around the muscles involved and the associated increase in limb blood flow and increased conduction of heat to the skin. Therefore, although a threefold or greater increase in heat production can occur during shivering, it compensates for only 11% of the heat loss caused by the associated cooling (28).

Nonshivering thermogenesis has been shown in animals to be mediated by the sympathetic nervous system acting on brown adipose tissue (29), which is also present in human neonates (30). However, more recent work (31,32) has suggested that brown fat plays a minimal role in adult humans and that the respiratory capacity of adult human brown adipose tissue accounts for less than 0.2% of the whole body response to infused adrenalin. If nonshivering thermogenesis occurs in adult humans in response to cold, as seems probable, its nature is more diffuse than in rats or neonates and may involve several organs, including liver and muscle. Astrup (33) showed that ephedrine caused increased oxygen uptake in leg muscle and that this could contribute approximately 50% of the increase in whole body metabolic rate observed with the drug. Thermogenesis in white adipose tissue can increase by up to 50% with the administration of catecholamines, but because this tissue contributes less than 3% of total basal energy expenditure, it plays a comparatively unimportant part in the thermogenic response (34). The administration of catecholamines also leads to an increase in cardiorespiratory work, but again this only accounts for a small fraction of the associated thermogenesis. Jessen et al. (35) showed a significant increase in splanchnic thermogenesis in only one of four unconscious curarized human subjects during cold exposure, despite increases in whole body oxygen consumption and in plasma noradrenalin. Studies by Bearn et al. (36) and Sjostrom et al. (37) showed that an adrenalin infusion rate of 100 ng/kg/min caused an increase in oxygen consumption in the splanchnic area from 43 to 93 ml/m^2/min, with a doubling of hepatic blood flow. At a slightly greater infusion rate of 100 ng/min/kg fat-free mass, there was an increase in whole-body oxygen consumption of about 33 ml/m^2/min. Skeletal muscle and the splanchnic bed appear therefore to be the major sites of catecholamine-induced thermogenesis in adults.

Diet-Induced Thermogenesis

Diet-induced thermogenesis was formerly known as the "specific dynamic action of food," described largely in relation to protein ingestion and consisting of the energetic cost of digestion, absorption, and storage, as well as the postulated *luksuskonsumption* or adaptive diet-induced thermogenesis associated with states of overfeeding. The minimum energy cost of the disposal of nutrients may be calculated and expressed as a percentage of their total energy content (3). The theoretical postabsorptive energy cost of disposal is lowest for fat at 2%, 5.3% for glucose being stored as glycogen, and approximately 25% for amino acids (38,39). The figure for amino acids is similar whether they are being oxidized or stored as protein. There is an additional small theoretical energy cost of intestinal absorption of less than 2% of the energy content if nutrients are administered by the gastrointestinal tract, although this may be undetectable in practice (39,40). Studies of the thermic effect of nutrients may be difficult because with oral intake there may not only be a cephalic effect on thermogenesis with the ingestion of palatable food, but the thermogenic effect of a mixed meal may last for up to 8 hours, making studies of metabolic rate by measurement of oxygen consumption problematic. It also makes it difficult to calculate the thermic effect of food from measurements of oxygen consumption because such studies presuppose that the resting level of oxygen consumption would have remained steady during that period, which may not be the case. Indeed, in many studies, resting metabolic rate increases slightly with time in the absence of any intervention (41). For these reasons, many studies have depended on the use of parenteral nutrients, bypassing the cephalic and gut effects and producing a shorter and more manageable response. The infusion of glucose produces an increase in metabolic rate that exceeds the obligatory minimum cost of nutrient storage (42–44). This is not the case for fat (45), and the evidence concerning protein is inconclusive (39). The thermic effect of glucose is probably mediated by enhancement of sympathoadrenal activity because it is associated with an increase in plasma noradrenaline concentration (44,46). Astrup et al. (47) confirmed these findings, as well as a considerable increase in arterial plasma adrenaline concentration after a delay of 2 hours, which was associated with an increase in forearm oxygen consumption after forearm glucose disposal had decreased to basal levels. This increment of diet-induced thermogenesis over the obligatory requirement for storage, has been termed "the facultative response." It is proportional to the rate of glucose infusion and, in sick patients, may cause clinical problems. As Kinney's group (48) has shown, the normal response to a mixed intravenous feed may be a 10% increase in metabolic rate. Using high-carbohydrate loads, noncatabolic nutritionally depleted patients showed an increase in respiratory exchange ratio to 1, with a moderate increase in both oxygen consumption and carbon dioxide production. In catabolic patients, although the respiratory exchange ratio did not increase to 1, reflecting continuing fat oxidation, there was nonetheless an exaggerated increase in oxygen consumption and carbon dioxide production of an order that may be lethal in patients with respiratory failure requiring ventilation. Burke et al. (49) showed, in burned patients, that with a progressive increase in the rate of glucose infusion, there was little increase in CO_2 production up to an infusion rate of 6 mg/kg/min. Above this rate there was an inflection in the curve with a rapid increase in CO_2 production. We have observed striking shortness of breath induced by excessive intravenous carbohydrate loads in both catabolic and under-nourished patients. An increase in body temperature also has been described under these circumstances (50). As a consequence of such studies, the administration of glucose intravenously during parenteral nutrition has been restricted to lower rates than described formerly with hyperalimentation regimens and restricted to 50% of the total energy supply, or less than 6 mg/kg/min.

STUDIES ON UNDERNUTRITION AND THERMOREGULATION

Historical Perspective

The association between chronic undernutrition and hypothermia has been noted on many occasions during famine conditions (51). In 1921, Talbot (52) discussed the predisposition of undernourished children to hypothermia and the difficulties experienced by clinicians in elevating the body temperature of such children. McCance and Widdowson (53) described a similar predisposition in starving piglets, and Baric (54) showed that the well-fed young rat behaves like a normal homeotherm, whereas the starved animal responds like a poikilotherm to changes in environmental temperature. In two studies of chronic underfeeding and weight loss in young adult subjects, the experiment by Benedict in 1919 (55) and Key's Minnesota Study of 1950 (56), there was a reduction in deep body temperature. In the Minnesota experiment, measurements were made at a room temperature of $25.6 \pm 1.1°C$ and 50% relative humidity. In 32 subjects oral temperature decreased from control values of $36.18 \pm 0.26°C$ to $35.43 \pm 0.6°C$ after 12 weeks of semi-starvation. In a study of Nigerian children with kwashiorkor, Morley (57) found a high incidence of hypothermia. Brooke (58) also found a core temperature $1°C$ lower among undernourished Jamaican children compared with normal individuals. He showed that they behaved as poikilotherms, responding to diurnal variations in ambient temperature. Core temperature and thermoregulatory responses returned to normal after a period of refeeding. He and his colleagues (59) conducted further studies in these children 4–16 months of age (49% of expected weight for age and 77% of expected weight for height) and showed that when the ambient temperature was reduced from 33 to 24°C, there was unimpaired peripheral vasoconstriction in the hand, but, despite a decrease in central body temperature, there was a decrease in metabolic rate rather than a compensatory increase in thermogenesis. These responses again returned toward normal after a few weeks of refeeding. In another study on West Indian children with kwashiorkor, Brenton et al. (60) found a morning rectal temperature of $35.6°C$ or less in 21 of

45 children with kwashiorkor at some stage during their hospital admission. Most episodes of hypothermia occurred on the second or subsequent days after admission, despite a minimum ambient temperature of 16°C. The Jewish physicians of the Warsaw ghetto (61), describing their children with advanced hunger disease, reported, "Body temperature was usually low. Even in infectious diseases such as measles, diphtheria or chicken pox, the temperature was only mildly elevated. We saw many cases of tuberculosis, some with severe symptoms, but the temperature was normal or even below normal." In describing their adult subjects who had lost more than 30% of their body weight, they reported, "The general body temperature is lower than normal; instead of 36.6°, it is 35.2 to 35.3°C. For example, in typhus, usually characterized by high fever among other symptoms, the temperature often remains low. Patients complain of feeling cold." They also measured metabolic basal rate from gas exchange measurements: "After carefully examining 70 adults and children, we have concluded that resting metabolism was never elevated. In not very advanced cachexia, the deviations from normal were within the error of the method (usually around the lower limits of normal minus 10%). In the second and third levels of cachexia, with or without edema, resting metabolism was very low (−40%), lower than in myxedema. In two terminal patients, resting metabolism reached −60%." They also examined the responses to food ingestion: "Our team studied the effects of isodynamic and isocaloric amounts of ingested protein and sugar on 20 adults and 20 children with hunger disease…In our patients, contrary to what occurs in normal people, within two hours of ingesting 200 grams of cane sugar, resting basal metabolism increased by 20–50%, demonstrating increased burning of carbohydrate. Feeding 4–6 hard-boiled eggs does not affect, or sometimes even lowers the basal metabolic rate, demonstrating the lack of a specific dynamic effect of protein in hunger disease."

Experimental studies have addressed the possible mechanism of reduced thermogenesis in undernutrition. Several investigators have shown that a reduction in energy intake leads to a decrease in sympathetic nervous activity (62–65). In rats, the turnover of adrenaline in the heart and other organs is reduced after 48 hours or even 15 hours of starvation (66) but returns to normal after refeeding. Thyroid hormone levels are also affected by undernutrition, with an increase in reverse T3 and a reduction in T3 levels (65,67,68). There also may be interaction between the thyroid and sympathetic nervous system. Landsberg and Young have suggested that the decrease in plasma T3 level with underfeeding may lead to a decrease in tissue sensitivity to catecholamines.

Effects of Illness and Injury

Among patients, the superimposition of illness or injury on the starved state may have additional effects. Little and Stoner (69,70) measured core and skin temperatures in 82 patients shortly after accidental injuries of different severity and found decreases in these parameters commensurate with the severity of injury. They suggested that the initial decrease in skin temperature was caused by vasoconstrictor responses to injury and was unrelated to treatment. Decreases in core temperature appeared to be a feature of particularly severe injury and to be related to interference with central control mechanisms, causing inhibition of thermogenesis. Despite decreases in core temperature, severely ill patients failed to shiver, suggesting a raised threshold for this response in such patients. In a series of studies, Carli et al. (71–73) described the tendency of patients, particularly those who were undernourished, to become mildly hypothermic during surgery. Conversely, nursing patients at their thermoneutral zone diminished energy requirements and improves protein synthesis. The combination of undernutrition and injury therefore puts patients doubly at risk of hypothermia.

Effects of Aging

In a review in 1967, Wollner (74) drew attention to the fact that shivering and vasoconstriction in response to cold may occur less readily among some elderly individuals compared with younger subjects. Wagner et al. (75) studied responses to cold in young and old people 10–74 years of age. On exposure to an ambient temperature of 16–17°C for 10 minutes, the younger subjects reacted promptly with increased thermogenesis and peripheral vasoconstriction. The older men had a smaller increase in thermogenesis and a decreased vasoconstrictor response. Similar results were obtained in some elderly people by Collins et al. (76–78), who found that five of 17 old people studied had poor temperature discrimination and poor control of ambient temperature, perceiving peripheral temperature changes inaccurately. This problem was also reviewed by Keatinge (79). Age is therefore an additional risk factor for hypothermia in some segments of the elderly population.

NOTTINGHAM STUDIES

Effects of Underweight

Our own interest in the relationship between undernutrition and thermoregulation sprang from a study conducted between 1979 and 1981 on 700 elderly women admitted to our hospital with fractured femurs (80,81). We set out to recruit thin individuals for entry into a randomized controlled trial of the effect of overnight nasogastric tube feeding on clinical outcome. Michael Bastow examined all patients on admission and divided them into three groups by measuring mean arm circumference and triceps skinfold thickness, relating these measurements to reference values from a British population of the same age and sex (82). Those who were within one standard deviation of the mean of the reference range were assigned to group 1 and called "well-nourished" or "normal." Those who lay between one and two standard deviations below the mean were termed "moderately malnourished" or "thin" (group 2). Those who were more than two standard deviations below the mean were assigned to group 3, "severely malnourished" or "very thin." This screening was conducted in order to select only undernourished patients for entry into the prospective trial of nutritional support. Starting at the beginning of the summer of 1980, we were discouraged to find, after 3–4 months, that few thin patients had been admitted. However, by the month of December, not only had the total number of admissions increased, but the proportion of those who were very thin rose strikingly (Fig. 1). Whereas the well-nourished patients of group 1 showed a 30% increase in admission over the summer level, the very thin group 3 showed a 300% increase. In a more detailed study between December 1981 and February 1982, we related the weekly admission rates of the three nutritional groups of fractured femur patients to the daily range of ambient temperature, which we obtained from the local meteorological office. We were helped by the fact that in the winter of 1981–1982 there were two sharp decreases in temperature to −15°C, one before Christmas and one after. We were able to show a clear relationship between the increase in fractured femur rate and the decrease in ambient temperature (Fig. 2). This was particularly striking in the very thin group.

The increase in fractured femur rate during winter is well known and has always been ascribed to subjects slipping on the ice and snow. However, when we inquired as to where the injury had taken place, we found that among the very thin patients, 80% of the accidents had occurred indoors. As a result of these unexpected findings, we postulated that hypothermia may be predisposing to injury, particularly among the very thin patients. Accordingly, Michael Bastow measured the core temperature of the patients on admission using the aural thermistor technique (83), excluding from measurement those patients who had sustained their injury more

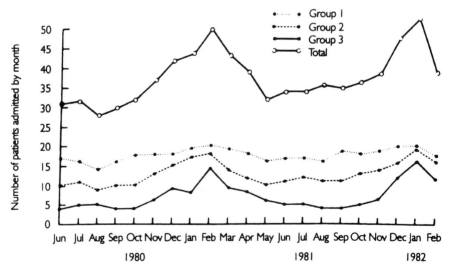

FIG. 1. Monthly admission rates in whole sample and in each group (group 1, well nourished; group 2, moderately malnourished; group 3, severely malnourished).

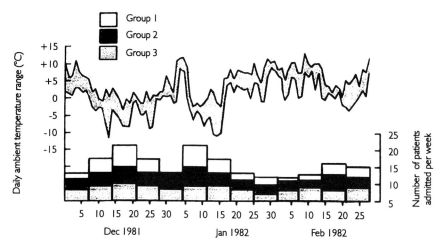

FIG. 2. Weekly admission rates in whole sample and in each group during winter 1981–1982, plotted with daily ambient temperature range (see legend to Fig. 1).

than 4 hours before admission. This was done in an attempt to exclude those who might have become cold subsequent to their injury. The results (Table 1) showed that, whereas the majority of patients in group 1 had a body temperature on admission of greater than 36°C, the majority of patients in group 3 had a temperature of less than 36°C and half of them less than 35°C. We therefore extended our hypothesis to suggest that not only might hypothermia have predisposed to injury, but that this might be explained by a thermoregulatory defect in those who were particularly undernourished. Such patients would have few problems in the summertime, exposed to the more tropical circumstances in which humans originated, but a cold winter would be sufficient to overwhelm their thermoregulatory responses, behavioral and physiologic. Fellows et al. (2,84) then undertook carefully controlled studies to address the question of whether undernutrition was associated with an impairment in thermoregulation in thin elderly women with fractured femur. The studies were conducted in a temperature-controlled laboratory with an ambient temperature set at 25°C. The subjects wore a liquid conditioned overall in a nylon suit with 120 m of plastic tubing sewn into the lining. This allowed studies to be conducted at perfusion temperatures varying from 35°C down to 23°C next to the

TABLE 1. *Core temperature on admission in the three groups of patients with fractured femurs*

Nutritional group	No. of patients with core temperature on admission			
	>36°C	35–36°C	<35°C	Total
Well nourished	36	7	3	36
Moderately malnourished	8	23	10	41
Severely malnourished	3	8	23	34

patient's skin. Venous occlusion plethysmography was used to measure total blood flow in the hands, forearm, and calf, and pulse and blood pressure were continually recorded. Mean skin temperature was measured as the arithmetic mean of eight thermistors applied in pairs to the skin of the anterior aspect of the shoulders, abdomen, thighs, and feet. Metabolic rate was measured by indirect calorimetry using a canopy method. Samples of arterialized venous blood were taken for levels of catecholamines, glucose, glycerol, lactate, and 3-hydroxybutate. Baseline studies were conducted to ascertain the stability of these measurements during the proposed 60 minutes of study. Fourteen elderly women recovering from fractured femurs participated, of whom eight were normally nourished and six belonged to the undernourished groups 2 and 3. Anthropometric and metabolic data are shown in Table 2, which also shows the subjects' dietary intake for the 7–10 days before the study. Particular care was taken to avoid starvation to ensure that only the effects of low weight were being measured.

Core temperatures were initially similar in the two groups (37.3 ± 0.1°C for normal individuals and 37.1 ± 0.2 °C for the undernourished group), at a suit inlet temperature of 35°C. As the suit inlet temperature was lowered from 35 to 28°C, the consequent vasoconstriction was associated with a median change of +0.1°C in both groups, However, on lowering the temperature from 28 to 23°C, the normally nourished group showed no change in core temperature, whereas the undernourished group showed a change of −0.1°C. Despite this decrease in core temperature, the undernourished group showed no significant increase in metabolic rate, whereas among those who were normally nourished, there was an increase of 10.3% ($p = 0.05$, Table 3).

TABLE 2. *Details of anthropometric indices, dietary intake, and hematologic and biochemical data of eight normally nourished and six undernourished elderly women*

	Normally nourished	Undernourished
No. of patients	8	6
Age (yr)	79 (68–85)	83 (80–89)[a]
Height (m)	1.57 (1.40–1.67)	1.46 (1.35–1.52)[a]
Weight (kg)	52.3 (47.2–69.6)	39.3 (30.1–42.7)[b]
Midarm circumference (cm)	25.0 (21.9–32.2)	19.2 (17.7–20.6)[b]
Sum of four skinfold thicknesses (mm)	47.5 (27.7–70.2)	26.4 (12.6–32.2)[a]
Energy intake (MJ/day)	5.232 (4.726–7.038)	4.399 (1.673–5.307)[a]
Serum albumin (g/L)	35 (33–38)	35 (32–43)
Hemoglobin (g/dl)	10.8 (10.1–13.8)	11.5 (9.1–14.9)
Serum sodium (mmol/L)	139 (135–140)	136 (133–144)
Serum potassium (mmol/L)	4.1 (3.6–4.4)	4.2 (3.8–4.7)
Serum urea (mmol/L)	5.9 (4.3–7.9)	5.2 (2.7–9.4)
Serum creatinine (μmol/L)	80 (64–95)	80 (70–98)

Values are medians and ranges.
[a]$p < 0.05$.
[b]$p < 0.01$.

TABLE 3. *Values for metabolic rate divided by weight$^{0.75}$ in eight normally nourished patients and six undernourished patients at environmental temperatures of 35°C and 23°C*

	Metabolic rate by weight$^{0.75}$ (J/min/kg$^{0.75}$) at environmental temperature of		
Nutritional group	35°C	28°C	23°C
Normally nourished (n = 8)	193.6 ± 8.3	204.6 ± 6.0	212.6 ± 5.7
Undernourished (n = 6)	187.6 ± 15.4	190.8 ± 13.9	188.7 ± 13.1

Values are means ± SEM.

From these studies, it was clear that, as in the Jamaican children, undernutrition and low body weight were associated with a failure of thermogenesis in response to cooling, although vasoconstrictor responses to conserve heat were maintained. Mansell et al. (3,85) then addressed the question as to whether this was a reversible phenomenon. Because of the difficulty of obtaining substantial weight gain in the very elderly, they studied a group of younger patients with gastrointestinal disease who were receiving nutritional support in the nutrition unit, before and after regaining weight (Table 4). Ten patients were studied, three male and seven female, 30–68 years of age (median 44.5). The principal diagnoses were Crohn's disease (n = 4), anorexia (n = 2), pancreatitis (n = 1), peptic ulcer with pancreatic fistula (n = 1), gluten-sensitive enteropathy (n = 1), and diverticular disease (n = 1). The patients were fed parenterally, by nasogastric tube, or with oral supplements as appropriate, and all had been given nutritional support for several days before the first study was conducted but had received no nutrients for 12 hours before the study. This was to exclude the possible effect of prolonged food deprivation on the results. The perfusion suit was perfused at two temperatures, first at 28°C and sec-

TABLE 4. *Anthropometric measurements, hemoglobin concentration, serum sodium, potassium, albumin, and plasma T4 and T3 concentrations in patients before and after weight gain*

	Before[a]	After[a]	Laboratory reference range
Body weight	45.8 ± 3.5	53.0 ± 4.2[b]	
% desirable body weight	78.5 ± 3.6	92.9 ± 4.1[b]	
Midarm circumference (cm)	21.6 ± 0.9	24.5 ± 1.2[b]	
Sum skinfolds (mm)	30.4 ± 4.0	46.2 ± 5.9[c]	
Hemoglobin (g/dl)	11.9 ± 0.4	12.4 ± 0.5	
Sodium (mmol/L)	137.2 ± 1.4	137.7 ± 0.5	135–145
Potassium (mmol/L)	4.08 ± 0.15	4.08 ± 0.08	3.5–5.3
Albumin (g/L)	34.6 ± 2.7	39.2 ± 1.6	31–51
Plasma free T4	9.8 ± 0.9	11.0 ± 0.9	9.4–25.0
Plasma free T3	3.5 ± 0.6	6.2 ± 1.6	
T4/T3 ratio	0.35 ± 0.04	0.59 ± 0.15	

[a]Values are means ± SE.
[b]p < 0.01.[c]p < 0.001, paired *t* test.

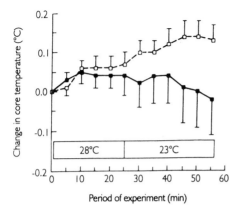

FIG. 3. Changes in core (auditory canal) temperatures from the baseline values during cooling at 28°C and then 23°C, before (■) and after (□) weight gain. Values are means with standard errors.

ond at 23°C. Figure 3 shows the change in core temperature from the baseline values during cooling, before and after weight gain, and Fig. 4 shows the corresponding values for metabolic rate. The differences in metabolic rate are unimpressive until one considers the degree of stimulus applied by a decrease in core temperature of 0.1°C in the undernourished state. Plotting the decreasing core temperature against the change in metabolic rate, the unresponsiveness of thermogenesis to the decrease in core temperature is shown more clearly (Fig. 5). In contrast, vasoconstriction in response to cold appeared to be well preserved (Fig. 6). They were able to conclude, therefore, that irrespective of age, undernutrition associated with a decrease in body weight is associated with a defect of thermogenesis in response to cold stimulus, whereas vasoconstrictor responses to conserve heat are unimpaired.

To determine whether failure of thermogenesis is a central phenomenon with resetting of the hypothalamic thermostat, or whether it is due to target organ unresponsiveness, Mansell went on to measure the response to infused adrenaline

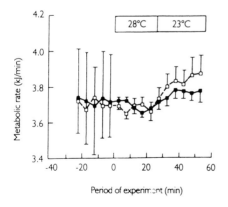

FIG. 4. Metabolic rate before and during cooling at 28°C and then 23°C, before (■) and after (□) weight gain. Values are means with standard errors. In the cooling period, the standard errors refer to changes from baseline and not to the absolute values.

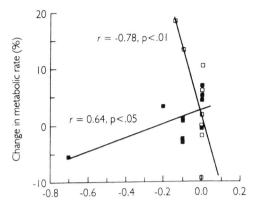

FIG. 5. Percentage change in metabolic rate from baseline during the final 10 minutes of cooling plotted against the decrease from the maximum core temperature achieved before (■) and after (□) weight gain.

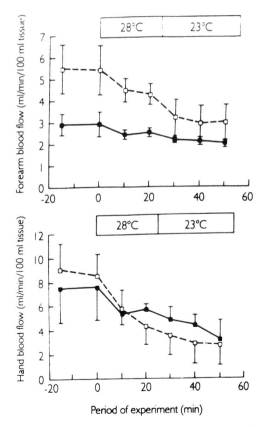

FIG. 6. Forearm and hand blood flow before and during cooling at 28°C and 23°C, before (■) and after (□) weight gain. Values are means with standard errors. In the cooling period, the standard errors refer to changes from baseline and not to the absolute values.

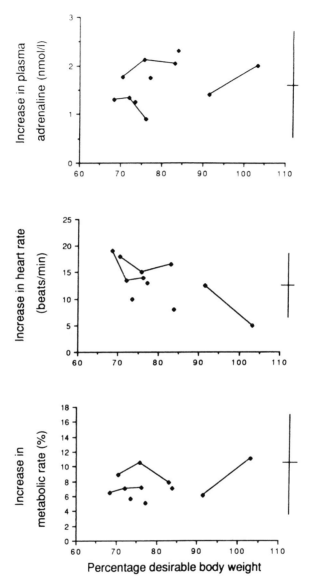

FIG. 7. Percentage increase in metabolic rate and increase in heart rate during an adrenaline infusion (25 ng/kg/min) plotted against percentage desirable body weight in patients experiencing weight loss. Three patients were studied on more than one occasion during weight gain. The increments in plasma adrenaline concentration induced by the infusions are also shown. To the right of each figure is shown the mean ±2 SD for the same variables in a group of 13 normal weight, healthy young females.

(25 ng/kg/min) in the same subjects. Three patients were studied on more than one occasion during weight gain. (Figure 7) shows the increments in noradrenaline, the corresponding increase in heart rate, and the increase in metabolic rate induced by the adrenaline infusion. To the right of the figure is shown the mean for the same variables in a group of 13 normal weight healthy young females. As far as could be concluded from this small number of studies, it seemed that target organ responsiveness to adrenaline was maintained and that the mechanism for the failure of thermogenesis in underweight patients most probably occurred via a central readjustment of the thermostat at hypothalamic level.

Effects of Food Deprivation in Normal Weight Subjects

The above studies were addressed specifically to the effect of weight loss on thermoregulation. The effect of short-term underfeeding was excluded by ensuring that all subjects had had a normal nutrient intake for several days before the studies were conducted. Macdonald et al. (86) studied separately the effects of various periods of starvation or underfeeding on the thermoregulatory responses of normal weight healthy subjects. In 1984 they found that, in young healthy subjects, a 48-hour fast caused a decrease in core temperature during exposure to cooling. In contrast, after a 12-hour fast, no abnormality was demonstrated. This defect of thermoregulation after a 48-hour fast was associated with a higher forearm blood flow than after a 12-hour fast. Although hand blood flow decreased and metabolic rate increased, these responses, particularly vasoconstriction, were inappropriately small when related to the decrease in core temperature. Therefore, it appeared that underfeeding as opposed to weight loss produces a defect of thermoregulation in response to cooling, but this is mainly due to a failure of appropriate vasoconstriction, with only a slight impairment of thermogenesis. A 48-hour fast also resulted in an enhanced thermogenic response to infused adrenalin but a diminished thermic effect of glucose infusion, due to reduced oxidative disposal (87,88).

Macdonald and Mansell (89,90) extended these studies to measure the effects on thermoregulation of 7 days on a hypocaloric diet as opposed to total starvation. Normal young subjects were given 60 kJ/day/kg ideal body weight, causing weight loss of 2 kg in a week. This had no significant effect on thermoregulation in response to cooling in contrast to total starvation or greater degrees of weight loss. Using the same model of 7 days of underfeeding, Gallen (91,92) found that the net thermic response to glucose and insulin was virtually abolished, although glucose disposal rates were unchanged. Glucose oxidation was slightly reduced, but glucose storage was maintained, although at only 2% of the energy cost of the glucose infused. This may well have been due to the concomitant reduction in other energy-consuming processes such as gluconeogenesis. Similar effects were shown by Webber (93–98) after total fasting for up to 72 hours. Again, this caused reduced glucose oxidation but did not impair glucose storage after glucose infusion. He was able to mimic this pattern of response by ketone body infusion and suggested that during fasting, hyperketonemia is important in mediating reduced glucose oxidation. He also found evidence that it inhibited lipolysis, preventing excess fat mobilization during fasting. Studies of prolonged fasting have shown reductions in metabolic rate (see Elia). However, Webber and Macdonald showed that fasting for 36 hours produced an increase in metabolic rate that had decreased by 72 hours of fast from that seen in the overnight fasted state. There was no relationship between the changes in metabolic rate and catecholamine levels, suggesting that they were mediated by intrinsic biochemical mechanisms, e.g., an increase in gluconeogenesis with its consequent energy costs. They also found increases in adrenoceptor sensitivity caused by fasting, as demonstrated by the response to an adrenalin infusion. Although cardiovascular responses were unaffected, the thermogenic and lipolytic responses were enhanced. This again suggests that the thermoregulatory changes with fasting are centrally rather than peripherally determined. Periods of fasting beyond 3 days cause a gradual reduction in metabolic rate, as shown by Cahill (99).

Effects of Hypoglycemia

Gale et al. (100) had observed that hypoglycemic diabetic patients were often admitted with a low body temperature. They subjected themselves to a cold stimulus using wet towels and cold fans until shivering started. Blood sugar was then reduced by insulin infusion. As blood sugar decreased below the normal range, shivering was switched off and core temperature decreased. Within seconds of an injection of glucose solution, shivering recommenced and core temperature was gradually restored. I have made similar clinical observations in a patient admitted to the hospital with hypoglycemia secondary to hypopituitarism. Fitzgerald (101) examined the case records of 22 patients admitted with hypothermia and found that, although some were hyperglycemic, nine had blood sugars below the normal range. In the Antarctic crossing study by Stroud, the travelers became hypoglycemic in the last week. Although they felt ill and cold, no formal temperature measurements were made. Clearly, diabetics, alcoholics, and those with liver disease and adrenal or pituitary disease are at risk in this respect, as are those who, undergoing feats of endurance without an adequate carbohydrate intake, deplete their glycogen supplies.

Alcohol and Hypothermia

Chronic alcoholism may predispose to hypothermia by undernutrition hypoglycemia and exposure to a cold environment while drunk. The acute administration of alcohol, given in the past to those rescued on mountainsides, has been criticized on the grounds that it might cause vasodilatation and increased heat loss, resulting in hypothermia (2). Haight and Keatinge (102) were unable to induce hypothermia in young healthy subjects by oral administration of ethanol alone; previous work had shown in fact that alcohol has very little vasodilator effect. Fellows (2,103) studied 10 healthy young subjects given ethanol 0.5 g/kg body weight diluted in 200 ml water and exposed in light underclothes to ambient temperatures of 21°C and 30°C on two separate occasions at least 1 week apart. Two subjects also were studied under the same conditions but were given 200 ml water without alcohol. A small decrease in core temperature was seen but was identical at the two environmental temperatures (−0.18 ± 0.6°C at 21°C and −0.17 ± 0.04°C at 30°C). A vasodilator effect of alcohol was seen at 30°C but was absent at 21°C, suggesting well-preserved vasoconstrictor responses to cold. These findings may have important implications for exposure victims. Providing that it is administered with food, it may contribute to the beneficial thermic effect of food without compromising normal vasoconstrictor responses to cold. On the other hand, in starved individuals whose glycogen reserves are low, ethanol may impair gluconeogenesis, causing hypoglycemia and consequent impairment of thermoregulation from that cause.

SUMMARY AND CONCLUSIONS

The normal mechanisms of thermoregulation to preserve core temperature within the narrow range of 36–37°C have been reviewed. A reduction in core temperature of as little as 1–2°C can impair cognition, judgment, and neuromuscular function, predisposing to accidents. Very low body weight and short periods of starvation both impair thermoregulation in response to cold, but by different mechanisms. With low weight, the predominant defect is failure of thermogenesis at the hypothalamic level, which may be restored by refeeding to a normal weight. Absence of an insulating fat layer is also contributory. With total starvation of 24–72 hours, there may be a transitory increase in basal metabolic rate at 36 hours, but the response to cooling is blunted, mainly by a failure of vasoconstriction but also a moderate blunting of the thermogenic response to the maximal stimulus of a decrease of 0.1°C in core temperature. In contrast to total starvation for 48 hours, a period of semi-starvation for 7 days caused no impairment of thermoregulation, although more prolonged periods of low intake leading to weight loss of more than 10% increasingly blunt the thermogenic response. Aging, injury, and hypoglycemia also impair thermoregulation and may be additive to the effects of undernutrition. Starvation for 48 hours also blunts the net thermic response to glucose, with reduced tissue oxidation. The energy expenditure of unimpaired storage is offset by reduced gluconeogenesis and lipolysis. Alcohol also has a thermic effect in normal individuals and does not appear to attenuate the normal vasoconstrictor response to cold exposure. These mechanisms explain the reports of mild hypothermia and accidents in children, adults, and the elderly in the presence of undernutrition or of overwhelming cold. The findings have important implications for both military and civilian medicine. They emphasize the importance of appropriate behavioral responses to cold and the frailty of physiologic responses when faced with a severe challenge. They also underline the potentially serious consequences of small decreases in core temperature of as little as 1–2°C and the factors such as undernutrition and periods of starvation that may predispose to such changes. The effects of starvation and of the thermic responses to substrates have implications for prevention and treatment.

ACKNOWLEDGMENTS

This chapter is based on work in which I was privileged to be associated with some outstanding colleagues who conducted the majority of the studies described. Without Professor Ian Macdonald, none of the physiologic studies would have been possible. Michael Bastow, Ian Fellows, Peter Mansell, Ian Gallen, and Jonathan Webber were outstanding colleagues and Research Fellows, to whom this chapter is dedicated.

REFERENCES

1. Maclean D, Emslie-Smith D. *Accidental hypothermia.* Oxford: Blackwell; 1977.
2. Fellows IW. The influence of nutrition upon thermoregulation [M.D. Thesis]. Nottingham, England: University of Nottingham, 1985.
3. Mansell PI. Undernutrition, thermogenesis and thermoregulation [M.D. Thesis]. Nottingham, England: University of Nottingham, 1989.
4. Hayward MG, Keatinge WR. Progressive symptomless hypothermia in water. Possible cause of diving accident. *Br Med J* 1979;1:1182.
5. Keatinge WR, Hayward MG, McIver NKI. Hypothermia during saturation diving in the North Sea. *Br Med J* 1980;1:280–291.
6. Keatinge WR. The effects of subcutaneous fat and of previous exposure to cold on the body temperature, peripheral blood flow and metabolic rate of men in cold water. *J Physiol (Lond)* 1960;153:166–178.
7. Pugh LGCE, Edholm OG. The physiology of Channel swimmers. *Lancet* 1955;2:761–768.
8. Coleshaw SRK, Van Someren RNM, Wolff A, et al. Impaired memory registration and speed of reasoning caused by low body temperature. *J Appl Physiol* 1983;55:27–31.
9. Pugh LGCE. Deaths from exposure in Four Inns walking competition. *Lancet* 1964;1:1210–1212.
10. Pugh LGCE. Accidental hypothermia in walkers, climbers and campers. Report to Medical Commission on Accident Prevention. *Br Med J* 1966;1:123–129.
11. Woods IR. Are motocyclists more likely to have accidents because they get cold? *J Appl Physiol* 1981; 320:77–78P.
12. Berg U, Ekblom B. Influence of muscle temperature on maximal muscle strength and power output in human skeletal muscles. *Acta Physiol Scand* 1979;1078:33–37.
13. Rowell LB. Cardiovascular aspecs of human thermoregulation. *Circ Res* 1983;52:367–379.
14. Roddie IC, Shepherd JT, Whelan RF. The contribution of vasoconstrictor and dilator nerves to the skin vasodilatation during body heating. *J Physiol (Lond)* 1957;136:489–497.
15. Detry JMR, Brenglemann GL, Rowell LB, Wyss C. Skin and muscle components of forearm blood flow in directly heated resting man. *J Appl Physiol* 1972;32:506–511.
16. Rowell LB. Reflex control of the cutaneous vasculature. *J Invest Dermatol* 1977;69:154–166.
17. Cohen RA, Coffman JD. Beta adrenergic vasodilator mechanism in the finger. *Circ Res* 1981;49: 1196–1201.
18. Lewis T. Observations upon the reactions of the human skin to cold. *Heart* 1930;15:177–208.
19. Keatinge WR. The effect of low temperature on the responses of arteries to constrictor drugs. *J Physiol (Lond)* 1958;142:395–405.

20. Benzinger TH. Heat regulation: homeostasis of central temperature regulation in man. *Physiol Rev* 1969;49:671–759.
21. Cross KW, Hey EN, Kennard DL, et al. Lack of temperature control in infants with abnormalities of the central nervous system. *Arch Dis Child* 1971;46:437–443.
22. Downey JA, Chiodi HP, Darling RC. Central temperature regulation in the spinal man. *J Appl Physiol* 1967;22:91–94.
23. Lloyd EC. *Hypothermia and cold stress.* London: Croom Helm; 1986.
24. Mount LE. The concept of thermal neutrality in heat loss from animals and man. In: Mokeith JL, Mount LE, eds. *The concept of thermal neutrality.* Boston: Butterworth; 1974:426–439.
25. Wilmore DW, Long JM, Mason AD, et al. Catecholamines: mediator of the hypermetabolic response to thermal injury. *Ann Surg* 1974;180:653.
26. Stroud MA, Brown NS, Macdonald IA. Plasma glucose, insulin, blood lipids and other biochemical parameters during 95 days of high endurance exercise on a high fat diet. *Clin Sci* 1994; 87(suppl):54.
27. Hultman E, Harris RC, Spriet LL. Work and exercise. In: Shils ME, Olson JA, Shike M, eds. *Modern nutrition in health and disease.* Philadelphia: Lea & Febiger; 1994:663–685.
28. Howarth SM, Spurr GB, Hutt BK, Hamilton LH. Metabolic cost of shivering. *J Appl Physiol* 1956;8:595–602.
29. Rothwell NJ, Stock MJ. A role for brown adipose tissue in diet-induced thermogenesis. *Nature* 1979;281:31–35.
30. Aherne W, Hull D. Brown adipose tissue and heat production in the newborn infant. *J Pathol Bacteriol* 1966;91:223–234.
31. Astrup A, Bulow J, Christensen NJ, Madsen J. Ephedrine induced thermogenesis in man: no role for interscapular brown adipose tissue. *Clin Sci* 1984;66:179–186.
32. Cunningham S, Leslie P, Hopwood D, et al. The characterisation and energetic potential of brown adipose tissue in man. *Clin Sci* 1985;69:343–348.
33. Astrup A. Thermogenesis in human brown adipose tissue and skeletal muscle induced by sympathonimetic stimulation. *Acta Endocrinol* 1986;12(suppl 278):1–30.
34. Hallgren R, Bergh C-H, Sjostrom L. Energy expenditure of adipose tissue. *Eur J Clin Invest* 1985;15: A3.
35. Jessen K, Rabol A, Winkler K. Total body and planchnic thermogenesis in curarized man during a short exposure to cold. *Acta Anaesthesiol Scand* 1980;24:339–34.
36. Bearn AG, Billing B, Sherlock S. The effect of adrenaline and noradrenaline on hepatic blood flow and planchnic carbohydrate metabolism in man. *J Physiol (Lond)* 1951;115:430–441.
37. Sjostrom L, Schutz Y, Gudinchet F, et al. Epinephrine sensitivity with respect to metabolic rate and other variables in women. *Am J Physiol* 1983;245:E431–E442.
38. Flatt JP. The biochemistry of energy expenditure. In: Bray GA, ed. *Recent advances in obesity research II.* London: Newman; 1978:211–228.
39. Jequier E. The influence of nutrient administration on energy expenditure in man. *Clin Nutr* 1986;5: 181–186.
40. Vernet O, Christin L, Schutz Y, et al. Enteral versus parenteral nutrition: comparison of energy metabolism in healthy subjects. *Am J Physiol* 1986;250:E47–E54.
41. Fellows IW, Bennett T, Macdonald IA. The effect of adrenaline upon cardiovascular and metabolic function in man. *Clin Sci* 1985;69:215–222.
42. Acheson KJ, Jequier E, Wahren J. Influence of beta-adrenergic blockade on glucose induced thermogenesis in man. *J Clin Invest* 1983;72:981–986.
43. Acheson KJ, Ravussin E, Wahren J, Jequier E. Thermic effect of glucose in man: obligatory and facultative thermogenesis. *J Clin Invest* 1984;74:1572–1580.
44. Welle S, Lilavivathana U, Campbell RG. Increased plasma norepinephrine concentrations and metabolic rates following glucose ingestion in man. *Metabolism* 1980;29:806–809.
45. Welle S, Lilavivathana U, Campbell RG. Thermic effect of feeding in man: increased plasma norepinephrine levels following glucose but not protein or fat consumption. *Metabolism* 1981;30:953–958.
46. Schwartz RS, Jaeger LF, Silberstein S, Veith RC. Sympathetic nervous system activity and the thermic effect of feeding in man. *Int J Obes* 1987;11:141–149.
47. Astrup A, Bulow J, Christensen NJ, et al. Facultative thermogenesis induced by carbohydrate. A skeletal muscle component mediated by epinephrine. *Am J Physiol* 1986;250:E226–E229.
48. Askanazi J, Rosenbaum SH, Hyman AI, et al. Respiratory changes induced by the large glucose loads of total parenteral nutrition. *JAMA* 1980;243:1444–1447.
49. Burke JF, Wolfe RR, Mullaney CJ, et al. Glucose requirements following burn injury. *Ann Surg* 1979; 190:274–285.

50. Askanazi J, Rosenbaum SH, Michelson CB, et al. Increased body temperature secondary to total parenteral nurition. *Crit Care Med* 1980;8:736–737.
51. McCance RA, Mount LE. Severe undernutrition in growing animals. *Br J Nutr* 1960;14:509–518.
52. Talbot FB. Severe infantile malnutrition. *Arch Dis Child* 1921;22:358–370.
53. McCance RA, Widdowson EM. The effect of lowering the ambient temperature on the metabolism of the new-born pig. *J Physiol* 1959;147:124–134.
54. Baric I. Contribution a la connaissance de l'intogenese du metabolisme de base. *Bull Acad Sci Math Nat* 1953;12:77–83.
55. Benedict FG, Miles WR, Roth P, Smith HM. *Human vitality and efficiency under prolonged restricted diet.* Publication No.280. Washington, DC: Carnegie Institute; 1919.
56. Keys A, Brozek J, Henschel A, Mickelson O, Taylor HO, eds. *The biology of human starvation.* Minneapolis: University of Minnesota Press; 1950.
57. Morley DC. Cold injury among children severely ill in the tropics. *Lancet* 1960;2:1170–1171.
58. Brooke OG. Influence of malnutrition on the body temperature of children. *Br Med J* 1972;331–333.
59. Brooke OG, Harris M, Salvosa CB. The response of malnourished babies to cold. *J Physiol* 1973;233: 75–91.
60. Brenton DP, Brown RE, Wharton BA. Hypothermia in kwashiorkor. *Lancet* 1967;1:410–413.
61. Winick M, ed. *Hunger disease: studies by the jewish physicians in the warsaw ghetto.* New York: John Wiley & Sons; 1979.
62. Landsberg L, Young JB. Fasting, feeding and the regulation of sympathetic nervous system. *N Engl J Med* 1978;298:1295–1300.
63. Landsberg L, Young JB. The role of the sympathetic nervous system and the catecholamines in the regulation of energy metabolism. *Am J Clin Nutr* 1983;38:1018–1024.
64. Landsberg L, Young JB. The influence of diet on the sympathetic nervous system in neuroendocrine perspectives. In: Muller EE, Macleod RM, Frohman LA, eds. *Neuroendocrine perspectives.* Vol. 4. Amsterdam: Elsevier Biomedical; 1990:191–217.
65. Jung RT, Shetty PS, James WPT. Nutritional effects on thyroid and catecholamine metabolism. *Clin Sci* 1980;58:183–191.
66. Rappaport EB, Young JB, Landsberg L. Initiation, duration and dissipation of diet induced changes in sympathetic nervous system activity in the rat. *Metabolism* 1982;31:143–146.
67. Vagenakis AG, Burger A, Portnay GI, et al. Diversion of peripheral thyroxine metabolism from activating to inactivating pathways during complete fasting. *J Clin Endocrinol Metab* 1975;41:191–194.
68. Suda AK, Pittman CS, Shimizu T, Chambers JB. The production and metabolism of 3, 5, 3′-triiodothyronine and 3, 3′, 5′-triiodothyronine in normal and fasted subjects. *J Clin Endocrinol Metab* 1978;47:1311–1319.
69. Little RA, Stoner HB. Body temperature after accidental injury. *Br J Surg* 1981;68:221–224.
70. Little RA, Randall P, Stoner HB. Modification of an autonomic component of thermoregulation by injury in man. *Arch Emerg Med* 1984;1:183.
71. Carli E, Emery PW, Freemantle CAJ. Effect of perioperative normothermia on postoperative protein metabolism in elderly patients undergoing hip arthroplasty. *Br J Anaesth* 1989;63:276–282.
72. Carli F, Gabrielczyk M, Clark MM, Aber VR. An investigation of factors affecting postoperative re-warming of adult patients. *Anaesthesia* 1986;41:363–369.
73. Carli F, Webster J, Pearson M, et al. Postoperative protein metabolism:effect of nursing elderly patients for 24 hours after abdominal surgery in a thermoneutral environment. *Br J Anaesth* 1991; 66:292–299.
74. Wollner L. Accidental hypothermia and temperature regulation in the elderly. *Gerontology* 1967;9: 347–359.
75. Wagner JA, Robinson S, Marino RP. Age and temperature regulation of humans in neutral and cold environments. *J Appl Physiol* 1974;37:562–565.
76. Collins KJ, Exton-Smith AN, Dore C. Urban hypothermia: preferred temperature and thermal perception in old age. *Br Med J* 1981;282:175–177.
77. Collins KJ, Exton-Smith AN. Thermal homeostasis in old age. *J Am Geriatr Soc* 1983;31:519–524.
78. Collins KJ. Low indoor temperatures and morbidity in the elderly. *Age Aging* 1986;15:212–220.
79. Keatinge WR. Medical poblems of cold weather. *J R Coll Physiol* 1986;20:283–287.
80. Bastow MD, Rawlings J, Allison SP. Undernutrition, hypothermia and injury in elderly women with fractured femur: an injury response to altered metabolism? *Lancet* 1983;1:143–146.
81. Bastow MD, Rawlings J, Allison SP. Benefits of supplementary tube feeding after fractured neck of femur: a randomized controlled trial. *Br Med J* 1983;287:1589–1592.

82. Vir SC, Love AHG. Anthropometric measurements in the elderly. *Gerontology* 1980;26:1–8.
83. Keatinge WR, Sloan REG. Deep body temperature from the aural canal with servo-controlled heating to the outer ear. *J Appl Physiol* 1975;38:919–921.
84. Fellows IW, Macdonald IA, Bennett T, Allison SP. The effect of undernutrition on thermoregulation in the elderly. *Clin Sci* 1985;69:525–532.
85. Mansell PI, Fellows IW, Macdonald IA, Allison SP. The syndrome of undernutrition and hypothermia—its pathophysiology and clinical importance. *Q J Med* 1988;69:842–843.
86. Macdonald IA, Bennett T, Sainsbury R. The effect of a 48 hour fast on the thermoregulatory responses to graded cooling in man. *Clin Sci* 1984;67:445–452.
87. Mansell PI, Fellows IW, Macdonald IA. Enhanced thermogenic response to epinephrine after a 48 hour starvation in humans. *Am J Physiol* 1990;253:R87–R93.
88. Mansell PI, Macdonald IA. The effect of 48 hr starvation on insulin sensitivity and glucose induced thermogenesis in man. *Q J Med* 1990;76:817–829.
89. Macdonald IA, Mansell PI. The effect of 7 days underfeeding on the thermoregulatory responses to cooling in lean women. *J Physiol* 1988;399:74P.
90. Mansell PI, Macdonald IA. The effect of underfeeding on the physiological responses to food in normal weight women. *Br J Nutr* 1988;60:39–48.
91. Gallen IW. Nutrition and the control of glucose and energy metabolism in man [M.D. Thesis]. Nottingham, England: University of Nottingham, 1990.
92. Gallen IW, Macdonald IA. The effects of underfeeding for 7 days on the thermogenic and physiological responses to glucose and insulin infusion (hyperinsulinaemic euglycaemic clamp). *Br J Nutr* 1990;64:427–437.
93. Webber J. The effects of acute starvation and of obesity on thermogenesis and substrate utilisation in man [M.D. Thesis]. Nottingham, England: University of Nottingham, 1994.
94. Webber J, Macdonald IA. The cardiovascular, metabolic and hormonal changes accompanying acute starvation in men and women. *Br J Nutr* 1994;71:437–447.
95. Webber J, Macdonald IA. The time course of the alterations of resting metabolic rate and insulin sensitivity during acute starvation. *Int J Obes* 1992;16(suppl):14.
96. Webber J, Macdonald IA. The relationship between changes in metabolic rate, haemodynamic variables and plasma catecholamine levels during acute starvation [Abstract]. *Proc Nutr Soc* 1993;52:53.
97. Webber J, Macdonald IA. Changes in resting metabolic rate in acute starvation are not related to changes in plasma catecholamines. *Clin Nutr* 1992;11(suppl):82.
98. Webber J, Simpson E, Parkin H, Macdonald IA. The effects of acute hyperketonaemia on glucose metabolism. *Clin Nutr* 1993;12(suppl 2):P2.
99. Cahill GF. Starvation in man. *N Engl J Med* 1970;282:668–675.
100. Gale EAM, Bennett T, Green JH, Macdonald IA. Hypoglycemia, hypothermia and shivering in man. *Clin Sci* 1981;61:463–469.
101. Fitzgerald FT. Hypoglycemia and accidental hypothermia in an alcoholic population. *West J Med* 1980;133:105–107.
102. Haight JBJ, Keatinge WR. Failure of thermoregulation in the cold during hypoglycemia induced by exercise and ethanol. *J Physiol* 1973;229:87–97.
103. Fellows IW, Macdonald IA, Bennett T. The influence of environmental temperature upon the thermoregulatory responses to ethanol in man. *Clin Sci* 1984;66:733–739.

Physiology, Stress, and Malnutrition: Functional Correlates, Nutritional Intervention, edited by J.M. Kinney and H.N. Tucker. Lippincott–Raven Publishers © 1997.

Overview: Thermoregulation in Human Stress

Matthew J. Kluger

Pathophysiology Division, Lovelace Respiratory Research Institute, Albuquerque, New Mexico 87108

Temperature exerts a profound effect on nearly all biological systems. For example, a change of 1°C causes an average change in metabolic activity of about 11%. The ability to maintain a relatively constant deep body temperature is a remarkable adaptation, which to a large extent freed an organism from the biochemical effects of increases and decreases in environmental temperature. Of course, deep body temperature is not constant, and as will be discussed in this review, these changes in temperature often have profound effects on a person's physiology and behavior.

The short presentations in this symposium provide excellent examples of the scope of adaptability of the humans to environmental stresses. Dr. George Brengelmann (this volume) provided an overview of thermoregulation in non-stressed humans (i.e., within their thermoneutral zone). Dr. Bodil Nielsen Johannsen (this volume) then described the thermoregulatoy adaptations we have to intense exercise on land. Dr. Michael Stroud (this volume) reviewed the physiologic and pathophysiologic changes that occurred with long-term intense exercise in a cold climate coupled with severe malnutrition. Dr. Charmaine Childs (this volume) then provided an analysis of thermal metabolism and temperature regulation in burn patients, and Dr. Simon Allison (this volume) ended the session with a provocative discussion of the effects of malnutrition on thermoregulation.

These are but a few of the thermal stresses we encounter. Table 1 contains a partial listing of the stresses reviewed in this symposium, as well as other types of stresses that impact on the regulation of body temperature. Some of these stresses are externally imposed on the individual (e.g., exposure to the cold). Others are internally imposed (e.g., exercise on land, which tends to increase core temperature, even at fairly low ambient temperatures). Others may appear to be externally imposed, yet the changes in core body temperature are the result of changes in the regulated body temperature (i.e., the thermoregulatory set point has been changed). For example, infection often results in fever (1). This increase in body temperature is not the direct result of the pathogen on body temperature, but rather the result of the release of endogenous mediators of fever (endogenous pyrogens), which reset the thermoregulatory set point in

TABLE 1. *What stresses do humans encounter that impact on their ability to thermoregulate?*

Externally imposed
Low or high ambient temperatures
Burns (insofar as integument is damaged)
Malnutrition (to extent that subcutaneous insulation is lost)
Internally imposed
Exercise
Hypoxia
Infection-induced fever
Psychological stress
Malnutrition (to extent that decrease in body temperature is regulated)
Selective brain tumors (e.g., in hypothalamus)
Metabolic diseases (e.g., hypothyroidism)
Peripheral vascular disease
Malignant hyperthermia
Burns (insofar as fever develops)

the hypothalamus at a higher level. Exposure to psychological stress also causes an increase in deep body temperature, which appears to be the result of a regulated increase in thermoregulatory set point (1). Hypoxia, on the other hand, causes a regulated reduction in set point in a number of species (2). Some stresses (e.g., malnutrition) may result in a lowered body temperature as a result of the loss of subcutaneous insulation, which may make a mild ambient temperature appear to be cold. As discussed below, the reduction in body temperature during malnutrition may actually be regulated.

A BRIEF OVERVIEW OF THERMOREGULATION

In reality, we are almost always under some form of thermal stress. As described by Brenglemann and Savage (this volume), within the thermoneutral zone these stresses can be easily handled by subtle changes in skin blood flow. Increasing skin blood flow tends to facilitate heat loss to the environment; decreasing skin blood flow conserves heat. Because heat flow between any two objects goes from the higher temperature to the lower temperature, when we are exposed to very high ambient temperatures (i.e., $T_{ambient} > T_{skin}$), the increase in skin blood flow actually facilitates an increase in body temperature. Fortunately, most endotherms (organisms that generate significant amounts of endogenous heat) regulate their deep core temperature at levels (e.g., about 36–40°C, depending on the species) that are usually higher than the environmental temperatures encountered.

When organisms are exposed to ambient temperatures that are above core body temperature, the only way to maintain a relatively constant deep body temperature is to rely on evaporative heat loss. Many species pant (e.g., dogs) or salivate and lick their fur (e.g., rats) to cool themselves. Others, such as humans, rely on sweating. The evaporation of 1 g of sweat from our skin removes about 600 calories. Because the average human can sweat 1 L or more per hour, this allows for the removal of about 600 Kcal of heat. This is roughly 10 times the normal metabolic heat production of a person. With repeated exposure to a hot environment, particularly during periods of exercise, a person can increase his capacity to sweat, thus increasing the potential for evaporative heat loss (3).

Of course, the loss of heat via evaporation is a viable option only when the air is not saturated with water (i.e., the relative humidity is less than 100%). As the relative humidity approaches a saturation point, we may continue to sweat, but this sweat does not contribute to evaporative heat loss.

The regulation of body temperature in the heat often involves behavioral thermoregulation. It is no accident that so many desert-dwelling animals are active at night when air temperature is much cooler. Human beings are superb behavioral thermoregulators, selecting microclimates that generally place them within their thermoneutral zone.

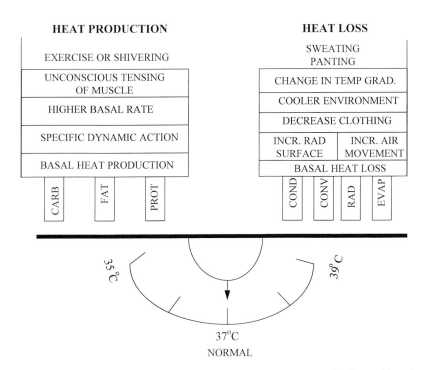

FIG. 1. The regulation of body temperature is a balance between heat production and heat loss. Carb, carbohydrate; Prot, protein; Cond, conduction; Conv, convection; Rad, radiation; Evap, evaporation. Adapted with permission (4).

Most thermal biologists assume that what is regulated is not total body temperature but rather core temperature. Brengelmann and Savage (this volume) argue that not only is core temperature regulated, but so is skin temperature. In a cold climate we are usually able to maintain core temperature relatively constant by decreasing skin blood flow, behavioral adjustments (e.g., avoidance, wearing suitable cloths), as well as by increasing metabolic heat production. However, average skin temperature generally does not decrease below about 33°C. Unlike many small mammals, humans have a limited capacity for generating additional heat via nonshivering thermogenesis. We rely on shivering, the contraction of skeletal muscle without doing external work, as the primary means to increase heat production.

Figure 1 shows the balance between heat production and heat loss, which generally results in the maintenance of core body temperature at relatively constant levels. At any given time, body temperature is maintained within normal limits by a balance between the many factors listed in this figure.

NOT ALL INCREASES IN BODY TEMPERATURE ARE THE RESULT OF A REGULATORY FAILURE

Although Brengelmann and Savage argue against the use of the term thermoregulatory "set point," I believe that it has some usefulness. Admittedly, this term is, as they state, "only vaguely defined" and probably bears no resemblance to any actual engineering model. One can substitute the term "set point" for "threshold around which we regulate body temperature," but "set point" is, in my opinion, not inaccurate. However, it must be acknowledged that there may be multiple set points for temperature regulation (e.g., skin and core) and that the system does not operate as a simply on-off switch but has a large degree of proportional control, and in some cases anticipatory control.

The concept of set point allows one to distinguish between fever (occurs when there is an elevated thermoregulatory set point) and hyperthermia (occurs when core body temperature is above the thermoregulatory set point). Thermal biologists define several categories of thermoregulation:

Normothermia, where $T_{core} = T_{set}$
Hyperthermia, where $T_{core} > T_{set}$
Hypothermia, where $T_{core} < T_{set}$
Fever, where $T_{core} = T_{set}$, but at an elevated core temperature
Anapyrexia, where $T_{core} = T_{set}$, but at a reduced core temperature

The relationship between set point and body temperature is shown graphically in Fig. 2. During the rising phase of fever, the individual is actually hypothermic, and this results in physiologic and behavioral responses (e.g., shivering, peripheral vasoconstriction, warming or heat-conserving behaviors), which lead to an increase in core body temperature. Once this elevated body temperature is

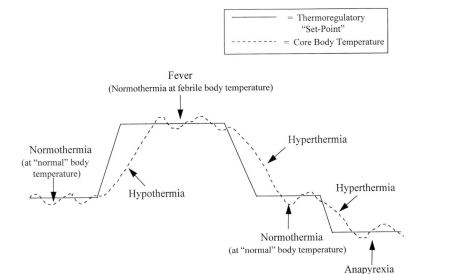

FIG. 2. A model of thermoregulation using the set-point concept. Normally body temperature is similar to the set point (normothermia). Generally subtle changes (e.g., vasomotor) are sufficient to maintain body temperature close to set point. During infection resulting in fever, the set point increases and the individual is hypothermic until T_{core} increases to T_{set}. Shivering, peripheral vasoconstriction, and behavioral responses are initiated to increase T_{core}. When a fever breaks, the individual is hyperthermic until T_{core} is once again similar to T_{set}. Anapyrexia is a reduction in set point and occurs during some disease states as well as during menopausal hot flashes. It is important to note that even during health, the set point for body temperature is not rigidly fixed. For example, body temperature varies on a circadian basis, and this is generally attributable to a change in the thermoregulatory set point.

reached, the individual is again normothermic, but at a febrile body temperature. When the fever breaks, the individual is hyperthermic, and appropriate effector responses (e.g., sweating, peripheral vasodilation, cooling behaviors) are now used to lower body temperature to once again achieve normothermia. Some diseases are associated with regulated reductions in body temperature or anapyrexia. As shown by Stroud (this volume) and by Allison (this volume), malnutrition predisposes individuals to having a lowered core body temperature. It is not known whether this lowered body temperature is regulated (i.e., anapyrexia) or unregulated (hypothermia).

Fever and anapyrexia, both regulated changes in body temperature, should not be considered thermoregulatory stresses. What is stressful to the febrile patient, for example, is being physically cooled (i.e., lower T_{core} below T_{set}). As core temperature decreases below the T_{set} temperature, the individual increases his or her rate of shivering and generally feels miserable.

In the rest of this review, I summarize some of the high points of the review articles presented by the specialists working in the area of human thermoregulation during stress. I attempt to point out whether the changes observed in body temperature are regulated or unregulated.

THERMOREGULATION IN THE NEUTRAL ZONE

As described above, Brengelmann and Savage (this volume) are not fans of the concept of thermoregulatory set point. They point out that it is often difficult to determine whether an increase in core temperature is due to a change in the set point for thermoregulation. For example, during exercise, the core body temperature of humans (and most other organisms) increases. Is this due to a change in set point? Jim Heath raised a similar question over 30 years ago when he evaluated field studies of reptilian thermoregulation (5). Field biologists were concluding whether a lizard, for example, was thermoregulating simply by measuring its body temperature. Heath showed that beer cans filled with tap water, when strewn about the desert, would appear to be thermoregulating because their core temperature was often markedly different from ambient temperature (this was due simply to the physics of heat exchange between a metal fluid-filled container and its environment). He argued that in order to study thermoregulation, particularly in behavioral thermoregulators, one must observe the behavior of the animals being studied.

The same argument holds true for human thermoregulation. To conclude whether there is a change in set point or whether the increase (or decrease) in body temperature is simply due to a load error, one needs to observe the thermoregulatory effector responses. For example, when body temperature increases during exercise, is the person sweating or peripherally vasodilated (heat-dissipating response) or is the individual shivering and peripherally vasoconstricted (heat-generating and -conserving responses)? Does the individual feel warm or cold? If the thermoregulatory set point had increased, it is probable that the effector responses would be similar to those observed during the rising phase of fever. That is, the individual would not be sweating, would be peripherally vasoconstricted, and would feel chilled. Because what happens is generally just the opposite, it is probable that the increase in core temperature is due to a load-error signal necessary to generate the appropriate thermoregulatory effector responses to reduce core body temperature.

Brengelmann and Savage point out that there are set points for core and for skin temperature and that they operate either in an additive or multiplicative fashion. The reality is that there may be even more set points, as Evelyn Satinoff demonstrated in her classic article (6). What Satinoff argued for is not a single thermostat, nor two thermostats, but multiple ones. Multiple integrators are postulated to be present at different levels of the central nervous system. Generally the effector responses appear to be coordinated around a single thermoregulatory set point, but under a variety of experimental conditions, one can observe apparently opposing thermoregulatory effector responses, which are not compatible with the concept of there being a single thermostat.

THERMOREGULATION IN SEVERE EXERCISE

During exercise most of the energy generated by skeletal muscle is liberated as heat. As a result, core temperature generally increases. Most investigators believe that the increase in core temperature generates an error signal, which results in effector responses that limit the further increase in core temperature. The more rapidly the core temperature increases (i.e., the greater the work-load), the more the core temperature increases. In most cases, eventually heat production equals heat loss, and body temperature levels off at some level higher than before the onset of exercise. Thus, set point has not changed. Bligh (7) summarized this as follows:

> The characteristics of mammalian thermoregulation are predominantly those of a proportional controller. In such a system a maintained effector function would depend on a maintained load-error, i.e., a deviation from the set-point. Since the re-establishment of thermal equilibrium at an increased level of body temperature during exercise depends on the maintained stimulation of heat loss effectors, and since exercise exerts only a small effect on skin temperature, the drive to the heat loss effectors is presumed to be derived principally from a maintained load-error between the set-point and the controlled body temperature.

As Johannsen (this volume) points out, the problem with the above theory is that as first shown by Marius Nielsen (8), within wide ambient temperatures, the increase in core temperature is independent of ambient temperature and is simply dependent on work-load or exercise intensity. These data are consistent with the hypothesis that thermoregulatory set point has increased during exercise. Because heat loss is dependent on the difference between skin and ambient temperature, at lower ambient temperatures heat loss should be facilitated and the core temperature of the exercising subject should not increase as much as during exercise in a warm environment. Of course, as pointed out in the recent review by Sawka et al. (9), core temperature during exercise does increase more in a warm environment (e.g., 35°C) than in a cool environment (e.g., 20°C). Lind (10) called the environmental temperature at which steady-state core temperature is independent of environmental temperature, but dependent on exercise intensity, the prescriptive zone.

Mrosovsky (11) listed several reasons why the prescriptive zone is not due to an increase in the thermoregulatory set point during exercise. One argument is that there is more sweating when one exercises in a warm environment, even when core temperatures are the same (12). This is because skin temperature is higher in the warm climate, creating a greater drive for sweating [see the dual-input model described by Brengelmann and Savage, this volume]. This greater production of sweat results in increased evaporative heat loss, resulting in a lower core body temperature. Another factor that may argue against a change in set point is that exercise results in a change in thermal sensation (alliesthesia), with cooler skin temperatures becoming more pleasant as internal temperature begins to increase (13). Thus, exercise in a cooler environment would be expected to result in a relatively higher body temperature than exercise in the heat. See Mrosovsky (11) for a more detailed discussion of this topic.

So, is core temperature regulated at a higher level within this prescriptive zone? Most investigators argue that most, if not all, of the increase in body temperature during exercise is not due to a regulated increase in body temperature (i.e., T_{set} has not increased).

One additional point that should be made is that the concept of core temperature during exercise being dependent on relative exercise load but independent of ambient temperature in the prescriptive zone probably only holds for exercise on land. During swimming, core temperature is dependent on exercise intensity, water temperature, and insulation of each subject (14). Thus, under these conditions there seems to be no clear relationship between exercise intensity and the increase in body temperature. These data also support the hypothesis that the thermoregulatory set point does not change during exercise.

THERMOREGULATION, EXERCISE, AND NUTRITION IN THE COLD: INVESTIGATIONS ON A POLAR EXPEDITION

Stroud (this volume) presents a remarkable, perhaps foolhardy, study of human performance in a cold climate in which two men attempted to walk across Antarctica without the help of other humans, animals, or powered machines. These subjects lost 26% and 29% of body weight during this 95 day trek, and despite the high level of physical exertion (generally associated with elevated core temperature), one of the subjects (Stroud) became hypothermic (anapyrectic?) on at least two occasions. This was associated with "marked confusion." The large loss of body mass and resultant loss of subcutaneous fat, coupled with the starvation diet, undoubtedly both contributed to this decrease in core temperature. Associated with this reduction in body mass was a marked reduction in blood glucose concentrations (about 0.3 mmol/L), values that are not generally thought to be compatible with life. These extraordinarily low plasma glucose concentrations were associated with "inexplicable hyperinsulinemia." Stroud suggests that the decrease in blood glucose concentrations may have been gradual, presumably providing time for adaptations to allow the brain to use ketones or other substrates.

Unfortunately, no measurements of deep body temperature were reported, and it would have been interesting to have correlated core temperature changes (e.g., via telemetry) over the course of the expedition. For example, is a circadian rhythm in body temperature maintained? How low did core temperature decrease? Symptoms of infection were described (e.g., muscle aches and pains, coughs). Were these associated with fever, or was the malnutrition severe enough to suppress this classical sign of infection? For example, Hoffman-Goetz and Kluger (15) showed that protein-calorie malnutrition led to a marked attenuation in the ability of rabbits to develop fever. Presumably this was attributable to a suppression in the production of endogenous pyrogens, which we now believe to be IL-1, IL-6, and possibly other cytokines (1). Similar data were then obtained in human subjects (16).

ANALYSIS OF THERMAL METABOLISM IN BURNED PATIENTS

Severely burned patients often experience a marked increase in metabolic rate. As described by Childs (this volume), the most probable explanation for this increase in metabolic rate is that the patients have developed fevers. It is known that tissue damage can result in the release of proinflammatory cytokines, which ultimately can lead to fever (1). The cytokines released from local burn sites may travel to the central nervous system to induce fever or may be inducing fever via nerves.

The evidence that peripheral nerves may transmit information from peripheral sites of inflammation to the central nervous system has been generated within the past few years. Bluthé et al. (17) demonstrated that intraperitoneal (i.p.) injection of lipopolysaccharide (LPS) failed to suppress investigatory behavior in rats that were subdiaphragmatically vagotomized. Sham-vagotomized rats showed the normal reduction in exploratory behavior after an injection of LPS. Goehler et al. (18) generated similar data on conditioned taste aversion. They found that i.p. administration of either IL-1β or tumor necrosis factor led to avoidance of novel tastes with which they were paired. However, subdiaphragmatic vagotomy led to an attenuation in this aversion. In a subsequent study, Watkins et al. (19) showed that subdiaphragmatic vagotomy blocked fevers caused by i.p. injection of IL-1β. In a follow-up study from Dantzer's group, Layé et al. (20) showed that subdiaphragmatic vagotomy blocks the induction of IL-1β messenger RNA in the mouse brain in response to peripheral injection of LPS. Therefore, even though burn patients may not show marked increases in circulating concentrations of IL-1, one of the important endogenous mediators of fever, this cytokine may be stimulating nerves at or near the site of burn, which transmit this information to the brain.

Burned patients appear to be most comfortable in a warm environment, and this may facilitate the development of fever, particularly in immobilized patients. According to one burn expert (Dr. I. Feller), the prognosis for survival is considered better in patients developing a fever of 1°C to 2°C than in patients who remain at the normal level or afebrile (21). This is not surprising because there are numerous data supporting the hypothesis that fever is an important host defense mechanism (22–24).

In view of the greater patient comfort in a warm environment and the clinical impression that fever is a strong indicator of survival, burn wards might consider allowing the patient to manually select his or her own microclimate (within a safe thermal boundary). Many other diseases are associated with patients experiencing chills (e.g., patients with kidney disease during dialysis), and this type of patient-controlled thermal environment should, at the very least, improve patient comfort.

IMPAIRED THERMOREGULATION IN MALNUTRITION

Allison (this volume) points out that even small reductions in core body temperature can lead to memory impairment, confusion, loss of judgment, and hallucinations. The conclusion is drawn that normal cerebral functions are extremely vulnerable to a 1 or 2°C reduction in temperature. This cause of hypothermia may be physical cooling (e.g., swimming in cold water) or initiated as a result of malnutrition (Stroud, this volume). Allison provides numerous examples of the effects of undernutrition on body temperature. As noted earlier in this chapter, Hoffman-Goetz and Kluger (15) have shown that fever is markedly suppressed due to depressed production of the protein mediators of fever. These data in an animal model of disease support the clinical impression of reduced fevers in diseases normally associated with large increases in body temperature.

In a fascinating study, Allison describes the effects of body mass on fractured femurs. Three groups of patients were recruited: (a) normally nourished, (b) thin but not malnourished, and (c) undernourished. During the winter months the incidence of fractured femurs increased markedly for group 3. To their surprise, they found that most of the injuries occurred indoors (rather than outside the home by slipping on ice or snow). Although a majority of the patients who were well nourished entered the hospital with relatively normal body temperatures, the majority of the undernourished patients had body temperatures of less than 35°C. These data led to the following intriguing hypothesis:

$$\text{Hypothermia} \rightarrow \text{disorientation} \rightarrow \text{falls} \rightarrow \text{fractured femur}$$

If the above hypothesis is correct, it would mean that mild hypothermia is a major risk factor for fractured femurs (as well as presumably other serious injuries). This hypothesis should be tested prospectively because it is possible that the malnourished subjects may simply have responded to the stress of femur breakage by mounting an anapyretic, rather than febrile, response. From numerous studies it is clear that during infection, injury, or trauma both endogenous mediators of fever (endogenous pyrogens) and endogenous cryogens or antipyretics are released (1). It is the balance between these factors that results in the typical febrile pattern. In some cases the balance of these pyrogens and cryogens results in a reduction in body temperature (e.g., during severe sepsis). For a more recent review on this topic, see Kluger et al. (24).

If Allison's hypothesis is correct, then patients at risk for hypothermia could be outfitted with biotelemetry devices to monitor core temperature to provide warming signals when T_{core} decreased below some critical temperature (e.g., 36°C). This could result in fewer debilitating injuries and improved quality of life.

Clearly, change in body temperature exerts a profound effect on human beings. When body temperature is below the normal range, individuals become disoriented and confused, which may contribute to marked increases in injuries to themselves and to others. When body temperature increases, this can facilitate host defenses (if at normal febrile temperatures) or can result in dehydration and excessive cardiovascular stress, as during hyperthermia. Kurz et al. (25) have recently shown that maintenance of body temperature during colorectal surgery led to lower incidence of surgical wound infections. In view of the profound effect of body temperature on human physiology and behavior, it is somewhat surprising that there are currently relatively few clinical studies being conducted in this area.

REFERENCES

1. Kluger MJ. Fever: role of endogenous pyrogens and cryogens. *Physiol Rev* 1991;71:93–127.
2. Malvin GM, Havlen P, Baldwin C. Interactions between cellular respiration and thermoregulation in the paramecium. *Am J Physiol* 1994;267:R349–R352.
3. Lind AR, Bass DE. Optimal exposure time for development of acclimatization to heat. *Fed Proc* 1963;22:704–708.
4. Gagge AP, Gonzalez RR. Mechanisms of heat exchange: biophysics and physiology. In: Fregly MJ, Blatteis CM, eds. *Handbook of physiology.* Section 4: Environmental physiology. Vol. 1. Oxford, NY: 1996:45–84.
5. Heath JE. Reptilian thermoregulation: evaluation of field studies. *Science* 1964;146:784–785.
6. Satinoff E. Neural organization and evolution of thermal regulation in mammals. *Science* 1978;201:16–22.
7. Bligh J. Temperature regulation in mammals and other vertebrates. In: *North-Holland research monographs. Frontiers of biology.* Vol. 30. Amsterdam: North-Holland; 1973:436.
8. Nielsen M. De regulation der körpertemperatur bei muskelarbeit. *Skand Arch Physiol* 1938;79:193–230.
9. Sawka MN, Wenger CB, Pandolf KB. Thermoregulatory responses to acute exercise-heat stress and heat acclimation. In: Fregly MJ, Blatteis CM, eds. *Handbook of physiology.* Section 4: Environmental physiology. Vol. 1. Oxford, NY 1996:157–185.
10. Lind AR. A physiological criterion for setting thermal environmental limits for every day work. *J Appl Physiol* 1963;18:51–56.
11. Mrosovsky N. *Rheostasis: the physiology of change*. Oxford, England: Oxford University Press; 1990:183.
12. Davies CTM. The effects of different levels of heat production induced by diathermy and eccentric work on thermoregulation during exercise at a given skin temperature. *Eur J Appl Physiol* 1979;40:171–180.
13. Cabanac M, Cunningham DJ, Stolwijk JAJ. Thermoregulatory set point during exercise: a behavioral approach. *J Comp Physiol Psych* 1971;76:94–102.
14. Nadel ER, Holmér I, Bergh U, Åstrand P-O, Stolwijk JAJ. Energy exchanges of swimming man. *J Appl Physiol* 1974;36:465–471.
15. Hoffman-Goetz L, Kluger MJ. Protein deprivation: its effects on fever and plasma iron during bacterial infection in rabbits. *J Physiol (Lond)* 1979;295:263–272.
16. Hoffman-Goetz L, McFarlane D, Bistrian BR, Blackburn GL. Febrile and plasma iron responses of rabbits injected with endogenous pyrogen from malnourished patients. *Am J Clin Nutr* 1981;34: 1109–1116.
17. Bluthé RM, Walter V, Parnet P, et al. Lipopolysaccharide induces sickness behaviour in rats by a vagal mediated mechanism. *C R Adac Sci [III]* 1994;317:499–503.
18. Goehler LE, Busch CR, Tartaglia N, et al. Blockade of cytokine induced conditioned taste aversion by subdiaphragmatic vagotomy: further evidence for vagal mediation of immune-brain communication. *Neurosci Lett* 1995;185:163–166.
19. Watkins LR, Goehler LE, Relton JK, et al. Blockade of interleukin-1 induced hyperthermia by subdiaphragmatic vagotomy: evidence for vagal mediation of immune-brain communication. *Neurosci Lett* 1995;183:27–31.
20. Layé S, Bluthé RM, Kent S, et al. Subdiaphragmatic vagotomy blocks induction of IL-1b mRNA in mice brain in response to peripheral LPS. *Am J Physiol* 1995;268:R1327–R1331.
21. Kluger MJ, Ringler DH, Anver MR. Fever and survival. *Science* 1975;188:166–168.

22. Kluger MJ, Kozak W, Conn C, Leon L, Soszynski D. The adaptive value of fever. *Infect Dis Clin North Am* 1996;10(1):1–20.
23. Kluger MJ, Kozak W, Conn C, Leon L, Soszynski D. The adaptive value of fever. In: Mackowiak PA, ed. *Fever. Basic mechanisms and management.* New York: Lippincott-Raven; 1997;255–266.
24. Kluger MJ, Kozak W, Leon LR, Soszynski D, Conn CA. Cytokines and fever. *Neuroimmunomodulation* 1996;2:216–223.
25. Kurz A, Sessler DI, Lenhardt R. Perioperative normothermia to reduce incidence of surgical-wound infection and shorten hospitalization. *N Engl J Med* 1996;334:1209–1215.

Physiology, Stress, and Malnutrition: Functional
Correlates, Nutritional Intervention,
edited by J.M. Kinney and H.N. Tucker.
Lippincott–Raven Publishers © 1997.

Shortened Length of Stay Is an Outcome Benefit of Early Nutritional Intervention

Hugh N. Tucker

Nestlé Clinical Nutrition and Baxter Healthcare Corporation, Deerfield, Illinois 60015

Every living organism must balance energy and nutrient intake with expenditure to maintain existence. This basic fact has been documented vividly in human experiences that are easily repeatable but should never again be condoned. The heroic work of the Jewish physicians in Warsaw during World War II describe a direct cause and effect between malnutrition, morbidity, and mortality (1). Studies documenting the effects of malnutrition by Benedict (2), Keys et al. (3), and others on the maintenance of lean body mass are well known. Mortality is associated with a loss of lean tissue approaching 50% of normal. More direct evidence that physiologic and functional deficits result from undernutrition cannot be imagined.

Unfortunately, even in the face of the accumulated knowledge, standard hospital care knowingly produces energy and nutrient deficits while otherwise attempting to provide acceptable care. A false sense of clinical security seems to be derived from the statement that "there have been no randomized controlled clinical trials proving the benefit of providing nutrition support." This reasoning is generally provided to excuse the lack of attention to the nutrition status of individuals at all stages of their treatment in the health-care setting and as a defense for malpractice. Disregard for the effect of malnutrition on care seems primarily due to both undergraduate and post-graduate medical training programs that present only limited aspects of nutritional care in a fashion that makes unclear any relevance to medical practice.

Due to both knowledge and technological barriers, malnutrition was a common finding in the acute care setting in the United States 10–20 years ago (4–11). Published findings over the past decade have generated a great deal of attention to, and the recognition of, poorer patient outcome and increased cost of care related to undernutrition (12–14). The increasing mandate for control of escalating health-care costs has focused outcome research on the cost penalties associated with malnutrition and on the relationship of malnutrition to poor patient outcome (15–18), longer than average stays (19), and higher costs (20–23). However, even with the accumulated body of information, there have been only marginal improvements in nutritional care since those original reports (24).

Alan Berg's commentary (25) concerning the awareness of chronic malnutrition in disadvantaged countries with a continuing lack of response is mirrored perfectly by the continuing debate over nutrition support for patients in the hospitals, long-term care institutions, and for the free-living elderly in industrialized nations. Berg describes two main problems. The first problem is the continued emphasis on the wrong research and research directions that can no longer provide the data required.

> We know enormously more now about the causes and consequences of malnutrition, and about who and where the vulnerable groups are. It is reasonable to question whether we are getting adequate return on investment in more nutrition-status surveys—that often measure for the sake of it. We also know what to do in many circumstances, because of numerous techniques (including economic techniques) and technologies in today's nutrition arsenal. Yet, almost no one seems to be trying to unlock the question of how to reach the payoff. Research needs have changed but we continue to do what we know how to do. Remarkably little intellectual attention has been given to getting to the end of the chain. There is a chasm between all we have learned through basic research and actions needed to cause something basic to happen. So much knowledge build up. So little benefit.

The second problem discussed by Berg is negligence in preparing individuals to work operationally in the field of nutrition. The stark parallel of Berg's comments on malnutrition in developing countries to medical practice in acute care institutions is painfully obvious. A lack of emphasis on nutrition training of medical students, in particular, and health-care professionals in general is universal. Practical therapeutic issues of nutrition support are never made relevant to medical practice in undergraduate medical school curriculum or in post-graduate medical training. With this educational backdrop, it should not be astounding that nutritional intervention is not considered as an imperative adjunct in caring for those individuals in the health-care system.

THE CLINICAL STUDY DEBATE

Study Premise

A major dilemma has been the misperceived inability to produce evidence-based clinical outcome data that can be universally respected. The ubiquitous and chronic nature of nutrient intake and the extreme variability of both subjects and care plans confound the usual approaches to clinical study design. When considering the design of experiments to demonstrate therapeutic efficacy, the scientific method is applied to compare the usual or norm to the test or changed condition. In other fields this has been a useful method for forming and testing hypotheses. In the field of clinical nutrition, the current obsession is with research designed to prove that nutrition support "is beneficial." Proof of the converse hypothesis—that withholding energy or nutrient intake at any time during the provision of health care improves outcome—must be the required test if the standard scientific methods are to be applied. This is not a valid scientific premise and would not be acceptable to most nutritionists. It seems only a paradox of the field of clinical nutrition that it is a necessity to prove that essential nutrient intake is beneficial.

Limitations of Prospective Randomized Clinical Trials

There is a widespread but unfounded belief that prospective randomized clinical trials (PRCTs) are the only credible tool (the standard) for providing evidence-based support of any benefit defined as "improved outcome." There are many types of hypotheses can be tested using this well-established tool. However, some aspects of clinical care cannot be studied adequately using only PRCTs to the exclusion of other equally valid observational techniques.

Alvan Feinstein has provided an excellent discussion on the limitations of clinical trials in his four part series in *Annals of Internal Medicine* (26–29). Although useful for evaluating the spectacular achievements of medical research, the fundamental paradigms characteristic of "hard science" cannot capture the crucial "soft" information about clinical and personal phenomena. Feinstein describes clinical medicine as containing at least two distinctly different sets of decision: the "explicatory" decisions that provide diagnoses, as well as etiologic and pathophysiologic explanations for the underlying causes and for mechanisms of disease, and "managerial" decisions to create plans for intervention and follow-up.

> Although the experiments conducted as randomized clinical trials have been scientifically helpful, the improved methods will have to include evidence obtained in the often unplanned "experiments" of ordinary clinical practice.

Feinstein groups therapies into three different types and explains the difficulties with clinical evaluation of each. Randomized clinical trial methodology lends itself only to physiologic endpoints and defined clinical outcomes that are characteristic of the first type or "remedial" therapy. Here a treatment is tested based on changes in a target state, and the progress of therapy to remove or relieve the target can be directly measured. This is classic remedial therapy that is familiar from drug efficacy evaluation, i.e., PRCT.

On the other hand, "prophylactic" therapies are aimed at preventing something that has not yet occurred. Prophylactic therapies may be either primary or secondary prevention. These two types comprise the second and third therapies. Primary prevention is given to persons who have no evidence of a condition or have a risk factor. In secondary prevention the treatment is provided to those already compromised to prevent progression of the condition or complications due to the condition. Nutritional support could not fit this definition more perfectly. Clinical evaluation of prophylactic therapies must involve large numbers of patients and multiple sites, and they require long periods of observation to detect differences in endpoints that are only indirectly affected by the therapy. Drawing any meaningful conclusion, even from these large trials, is difficult to impossible when the expected endpoints are broad outcome events such as lowering hospital costs or changes in length of stay (LOS). These types of outcomes are affected by many other coexisting (confounding) factors with more potent action than the adjunctive intervention of nutritional support. Any expectation of powerful evidence from an RPCT is naïve, at best. Soeters described a change in hospital LOS as a "questionable (and maybe suicidal) end point" for human clinical trials (30).

Feinstein continued by describing a further limitation of clinical trials based on the conflicting goals of basic study design. The two extremes of design—from fastidious to pragmatic—create nonreconcilable debate. The desire for a "clean" answer by careful screening and strict entry criteria to exclude any coexisting condition or treatment that might interfere is confounded by the realities of clinical care, especially in the critical care arena. The pragmatic trial designer complains that pure results are useless to the real world and are not representative of clinical practice. Clinical trials that are analyzed with one or the other of these two opposing viewpoints have, as Feinstein proposed, continued "to provoke dissatisfaction and dissent." This statement better than any other describes the state of the clinical nutrition literature.

It is thus clear that other types of data and observational experience must be included in any generalized discussions of efficacy based on broad health-care outcome benefits. A broader awareness of the essential and complementary nature of evidence from all other modes of research—animal, clinical, epidemiologic—is mandatory to enhance the information available regarding the functional benefit of providing nutrition support. As reported for techniques that document the benefit of combination therapies in rheumatoid arthritis (31), approaches incorporating longitudinal databases collected over 3–5 years are required to augment the data generated by prospective randomized clinical trials. Henry Blackburn expressed the same concern over ignoring all of the data, including animal and epidemiologic evidence regarding the Food and Drug Administrations deliberations concerning the clinical evidence for safety of fat substitutes (32).

EPIDEMIOLOGIC DATA COLLECTION AND FINANCIAL AUDITS

Smith and Smith evaluated the results of 22 published studies and reports encompassing more than 70 hospitals over the past 15 years (33). The objective was to determine a numeric range for malnutrition prevalence by various hospital categories. Prevalence was estimated from the reported percentages of medical and surgical patients who had one or more known risk factors for malnutrition at hospital admission or shortly thereafter. Although the risk factors varied from study to study, they were typically determined by three categories of routine medical information: medical and diet history; anthropometric measurements such as height, weight, and recent weight loss; and selected laboratory values such as serum albumin, hemoglobin, hematocrit, and total lymphocyte counts. Hospital categories included small-town community, urban public teaching, Veterans Administration, and pediatric (Fig. 1).

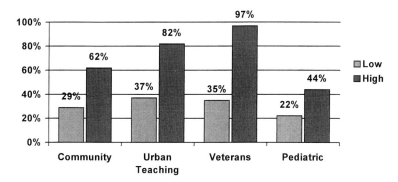

FIG. 1. Prevalence of malnutrition in U.S. hospitals presented as low and high reported incidence.

Although the data in Fig. 1 were generated from a variety of studies involving different institutions, patient conditions, and quality care standards, they support the general conclusion that malnutrition is a significant comorbidity among patients in U.S. hospitals. Moreover, two of the studies suggested that the situation may be worsening: the proportion of high-risk patients increased 70% between 1984 and 1987 in one community hospital (34), and in one university teaching hospital the percentages of at-risk patients grew from 33% in 1979 to 40% in 1985 to 43% in 1987 (14).

The causes of hospital malnutrition are multi-factorial. At-risk patients are among the sickest, and their malnutrition is partly due to prolonged stress responses to disease or trauma, to prior inadequate nutrition intake, or to the combination of all these factors. The failure of many hospitals to identify risk and deal with it early can result in further deterioration of patient health, longer than average hospital stays, and higher costs.

PREDICTABLE PENALTIES OF HOSPITAL MALNUTRITION

Even mild malnutrition can affect the body's normal maintenance and repair systems. Malnutrition is known to impair the immune system and thus decrease the ability to fight infections (35,36). Certain vitamin and mineral deficiencies impair enzyme systems involved in tissue repair, reducing wound healing rates and predisposing the patient to the development of pressure ulcers (37). Deficiencies or excesses of certain dietary fats can either decrease or increase inflammatory or other immune responses (38). There are many other such examples whereby malnutrition affects the body's healing processes or stress responses. Therefore, it is not surprising that malnutrition has a negative impact on the clinical and economic outcomes of at-risk patients.

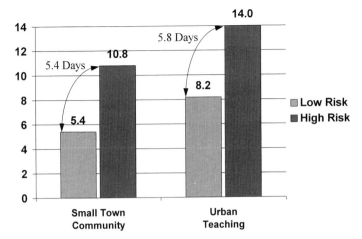

FIG. 2. Difference in ALOS between low- and high-risk patients in two types of acute care institutions.

Longer Average Length of Stay

Longer average length of stay (ALOS) is one identifiable consequence of hospital malnutrition. Figure 2 illustrates differences in ALOS between low- and high-risk patients in two hospitals included in the Smith and Smith review (33). Low-risk patients had no malnutrition risk factors, and high-risk patients had one or more. Data were collected from successive surgical and medical admissions and represent 500 patients from a small-town community hospital (39) and 100 patients from a large urban teaching hospital (12). Ninety-five percent of the patients from both institutions were under 65 years of age. The LOS penalty associated with risk of malnutrition is similar in both cases (5.4 vs. 5.8 days), although the penalty days are a higher percentage of the low-risk patients' LOS days in the small town (100% vs. 70%) when compared with the urban teaching hospital.

Higher Proportion of Total Patient Days

The Smiths used another method to evaluate the ALOS penalty by determining the proportion of total patient days accounted for by the at-risk patients. Figure 3 presents the results of this analysis for three hospital types. The first set of bars represents results from a survey of 217 consecutive hospital admissions (23), regardless of LOS. Patients with three or more malnutrition risk factors accounted for 26% of the sample and 42% of hospital days. The second set of bars represents data from 500 consecutive admissions, regardless of LOS, to a small-town community hospital. Here 31.5% of the

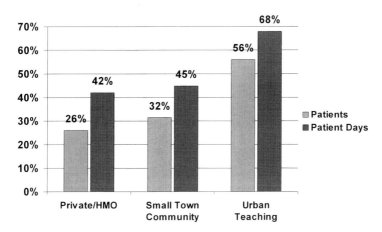

FIG. 3. Percentage of patients and the resulting hospital patient days found to be at risk for malnutrition.

patients were at risk for malnutrition and accounted for 45% of total patient days (40). The third set of bars is from a prospective audit of 100 consecutive admissions, regardless of LOS, to the acute medical service of an urban teaching hospital, where 56% of the patients were at risk for malnutrition and accounted for 68% of the patient days (12).

POOR OUTCOME AND EXTRA DAYS: HIGHER CHARGES

Although most studies infer higher hospital charges from longer ALOS, two studies have measured them explicitly and prospectively (12,40). The results provide a basis for calculating the unequal share of charges incurred by malnourished patients in two widely diverse hospital types: a 600-bed, urban teaching hospital and a small-town, 300-bed community hospital. These cost differentials are termed the "cost penalties for malnutrition" (33).

In the first example, a 1987 study reported that regardless of LOS, 56% of 100 consecutive patients admitted to a 600-bed urban teaching hospital had risk factors for malnutrition (12). When total patient charges were compared by risk group, there was a twofold ($8,624) increase for the at-risk patient (Table 1). The 56% of at-risk patients accounted for 72.5% of the total charges for the 100-patient sample.

When the tabulations were prospectively completed for the small-town community hospital, 32% of the 500 consecutive patient samples were malnourished and accounted for 45.2% of the total charges. There was a $1,296 per patient average difference in charges between malnourished patients and those without evidence of malnutrition (40).

TABLE 1. *At-risk patient costs at an urban teaching hospital*

	Patients at risk	Patients with no apparent risk	Total
No. of patients	56	44	100
Cost per patient	$15,956	$7,692	
Total cost (1987 dollars)	$893,536	$338,448	$1,231,984
Total costs (%)	72.5	27.5	100

Adapted with permission (12).

These two studies illustrate how the penalties of malnutrition add to the costs for everyone who has a financial stake in hospital care. Ten other studies have linked reduced ALOS with the provision of early nutritional care, and four of those have demonstrated cost savings as well (Table 2).

It seems rational to conclude that although the total costs for any institution will vary with the incidence of malnutrition and the average penalty cost for malnourished patients, nutritional intervention for malnourished patients will reduce the ALOS and consequently will bring down associated costs.

WHY THE COST PENALTIES REMAIN HIDDEN

Although the hospital charges used here as examples are not an accurate measure of malnutrition's cost from every group's perspective, they illustrate the magnitude of a problem that will find its way into every institution's bottom line. Unfortunately, in many institutions the cost penalties for malnutrition remain hidden:

TABLE 2. *Reduced ALOS and costs associated with nutritional intervention for at-risk patients*

Diagnosis/Procedure	Hospital days saved	% Decrease in ALOS	Annual per patient savings[a]	Ref.
Major abdominal trauma	3	11%	$3,356.00	16
Radical cystectomy	7	29%	—	41
Elderly hip fracture				
Thin patients	2	16%	—	42
Very thin patients	7	30%	—	42
Colorectal surgery	8	29%	—	43
Intestinal fistula	7	47%	—	44
Burns	7	24%	$6,400	73
Intractable diarrhea	26	37%	$14,750	66
Neonatal intensive care	7.5	14%	—	69
General pediatric	2	13%	—	67
Bone marrow transplant	3	8%	$1,436	70

[a]The dollar values are reported for the years during which the study took place and are not adjusted to 1996 values.

1. Conventional hospital accounting systems do not track severity of illness or nutrition risk. As a result, tracking the higher costs associated with malnutrition requires further investigation.
2. Published studies documenting the extra costs associated with nutrition risk are often highly technical and occur as isolated fragments in different journals and at irregular intervals. The information often does not reach the managers, and if it does the relevance of the studies may be questioned if not communicated in clear and concise financial terms that are understandable by nonclinicians.
3. Programs to screen for nutrition risk have been underdeveloped or nonexistent. Although the Joint Commission on Accreditation of Healthcare Organizations now mandates screening as part of routine patient care, the raw data are rarely aggregated to study the hospital-wide magnitude of malnutrition-related costs.

These and other factors mask the potential for demonstrating the power of nutrition to improve patient outcome and contribute to cost savings. Consequently, many hospital administrators and cost analysts may be drawn to the conclusion that nutrition is an added cost of questionable benefit and with low potential for increasing hospital revenue.

PATIENT BENEFITS OF EARLY NUTRITIONAL INTERVENTION

The above review of the literature is only presumptive support for the observation that when malnutrition is identified and treated early, hospital stay and associated costs go down. The presumptive evidence begs obvious questions. Can generalized conclusions be drawn from data collected from different institutions and under varying protocols? Can factors other than malnutrition explain the average longer hospital stay in the malnourished groups? Will the data stand up to rigorous statistical analysis that controls for confounding factors and isolate the independent effects of nutritional intervention? Can more precise cost estimates be derived from the association between malnutrition and longer hospital stay?

To address these questions, a financial audit tool [developed by Nutrition Care Management Institute (NCMI) and Clintec Nutrition Co.]—the Malnutrition Cost Survey (MCS)—was used to evaluate hospital malnutrition in terms of both patient outcome and total hospital costs.

MALNUTRITION COST SURVEY AUDIT METHODOLOGY

Data Collection

Data on nutrition risk, nutritional intervention, and length of hospital stay were collected by trained hospital staff from existing clinical records. The audit analyzed approximately 16,500 admissions at 20 different acute-care hospitals

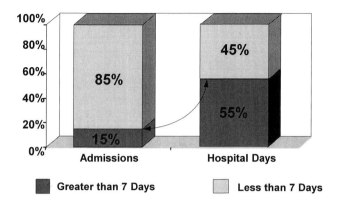

FIG. 4. Longer stay patient admissions consume a larger percentage of total hospital days.

across the United States. The records selected for analysis from these admissions were sequential medical and surgical patients ages 17 or older who were discharged after a stay in the hospital of greater than 7 days. Records of patients who died during hospitalization were excluded. The 8-day minimum LOS increased the efficiency of the audit by concentrating on the sickest patients, who (a) were likely to be at risk for malnutrition and (b) were hospitalized long enough for nutritional intervention to have taken place. These longer stay patients also account for a large proportion of total hospital days (Fig. 4) and therefore consume more of the hospital's resources.

Among the 20 participating hospitals were a total of 2,485 patient records that met the selection criteria for inclusion. Nutritional intervention was defined as providing a written order for nutrition therapy consisting of greater than 60% of

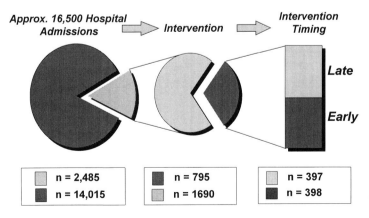

FIG. 5. Data summary for the Malnutrition Cost Survey.

a patient's caloric requirements. The method of intervention was not considered important for this analysis and could have been provided by parenteral nutrition (central line or peripheral), enteral nutrition (either total enteral nutrition or commercial protein/calorie supplements), or high protein/calorie food supplementation. The first day of administration of the product was considered the day of intervention. Intervention started after day 3 was considered late and intervention on or before day 3 was considered early. Figure 5 is a graphical summary of the audit scheme and includes the numbers of patients represented in each group.

Data Analysis: A Stepwise Approach

Data were analyzed in a three-step sequence by our clinical research group, the Nutrition Care Management Institute (NCMI) and Research Data Services Incorporated (RDSI; an independent data management and statistical analysis company). Each step applies progressively more rigorous statistical methods and stricter controls. Probing the data in this stepwise fashion assured the most stringent mathematical conditions under which fair observations may emerge and enabled the precise analysis of independent factors to determine the most important effects on hospital LOS.

The first level of analysis was designed to assemble data on nutritional intervention and to identify potential statistical relationships between nutrition and ALOS. For step one of the data analysis, NCMI completed tabulations, simple proportions, and *t* test group comparisons on the raw data from the 20 participating hospitals. In that way, the direction for further in-depth statistical analysis could be identified.

In step 2, RDSI created mathematical models based on standard methodology for stepwise multiple regression analysis. Those models defined the statistical significance of the influence of several factors of ALOS, including day of nutritional intervention.

Finally, the third step for data analysis involved another set of regression models that separated the specific effects of day of nutritional intervention apart and independent from all other significant factors identified in step 2. Once the quantitative relationships between day of nutritional intervention and ALOS were characterized, the potential cost savings could be calculated.

NUTRITION RISK AND ALOS

In this analysis the ALOS was selected as the measure of patient outcome. ALOS seemed an appropriate functional measure because it is clearly linked to the patient's hospital course, can be readily determined from the patient's clinical record, and is measurable in financial terms.

As noted above, many published hospital nutrition surveys show that malnutrition is associated with poorer patient outcome, longer hospital stay, and higher costs. Our data confirm those associations, but in order to strengthen a cause-and-effect relationship, it was necessary to demonstrate that delaying nutritional intervention in this higher acuity group has a direct effect on LOS.

NUTRITION RISK AND PATIENT DAYS

Within the select patient sample (n = 2,485) from the 20 hospitals, 94.4% of the patients had one or more risk factors for malnutrition. The results are similar to those reported in the many studies reviewed previously (5–11,14–20,22) in that they show a high proportion of patients at risk for malnutrition, who account for a large share of total hospital days. It should be obvious that the risk factors for malnutrition are also indicators of acuity. The relationship between ALOS and acuity is intuitive: the sick remain in the hospital longer than do the well.

EARLY NUTRITIONAL INTERVENTION AND ALOS

To support the hypothesis that nutritional intervention is beneficial, it is necessary to determine how the early nutritional intervention of one group affects their hospital stay compared with a later intervention group. The audit data were stratified as two subsets of admissions: those who received any type of nutritional intervention during hospitalization and those who did not. To demonstrate that timing of the nutritional intervention had a measurable effect on ALOS, the nutritional intervention group was subdivided into early and late groups for further analysis.

Despite the prevalence of risk factors, only about 32% of the total 2,485 patients received some type of nutritional intervention (food or commercial supplement, tube feeding, or parenteral nutrition) during their stay. Half (50.1%) of the interventions started on or before the patient's third hospital day (early), and the remainder occurred on or after the fourth day (late). The ALOS for the late subgroup was 3.0 days longer than that of the early subgroup, with the difference considered statistically significant according to a two-sample *t* test. Because there are several other possible intervening factors such as number of diagnoses, surgery, age, complications, etc. that could account for some if not all of the ALOS difference, the *t* test produces only presumptive results. It signals a likelihood but not the certainty of statistical correlation between early nutritional intervention and decreased average length of hospital stay. To determine whether such correlation could be demonstrated with more robust statistical models, RDSI applied stepwise multiple regression methods.

MULTIPLE REGRESSION MODELING: IDENTIFYING
SIGNIFICANT VARIABLES

The database was further refined, and analyses were confined to at-risk patients more than 17 years of age who survived their hospitalizations, stayed in the hospital at least 8 days but not more than 40 days, and had a body mass index (BMI) greater than the 5th percentile and less than the 95th percentile for age. A few patient records were excluded from analysis because they contained either incomplete or obvious original data recording errors. Five hundred three patient records met the selection criteria, and 95% of these patients had risk factors for malnutrition.

RDSI divided the entire hospital stay into two parts for each patient: days occurring before nutritional intervention (preintervention days) and days occurring after nutritional intervention (postintervention days). Eight variable factors were then identified, including the number of days before nutritional intervention, that potentially would influence the number of postintervention days. Malnutrition risk factors were not included as a variable because virtually all the patients had risk factors of malnutrition. Each of the eight variable factors were entered into a stepwise regression analysis equation to determine the degree of their individual influence on the number of postintervention days. The focus was on the postintervention time because nutrition can only affect hospital stay after it is applied, not before. Therefore, to create a fair comparison of the effects of all the variable factors, including the day of nutritional intervention, the length of the postintervention period was used as the outcome measure.

The RDSI stepwise regression model described in percentage points and statistical significance the strength of influence of each of the eight factors on the number of postintervention days (Fig. 6). Day of nutritional intervention, which was the only controllable factor, ranked second and accounted for 19% of the total variation in postintervention days for the average patient. Only total diagnoses ranked higher. The factors in aggregate described 15% of the total variation in LOS for the group. Total diagnoses, day of nutritional intervention, expected LOS, sex, and surgery were the five statistically significant factors. It

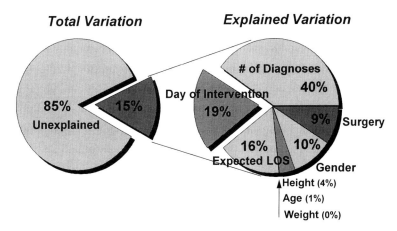

FIG. 6. Explained variation in observed LOS for the audited group receiving nutritional intervention.

is clear from these data that LOS is influenced by many uncontrollable events. These data show that 3% (19% of 15%) of the variation of LOS is explainable by the day of nutritional intervention.

It is imperative when designing clinical studies to recognize the enormous number of subjects that would be required in each group to demonstrate an effect of nutritional intervention on these types of general outcome indicators. It is not likely that any randomized controlled trial could be constructed with adequate numbers of subjects to demonstrate these differences; the uncontrollable variation is far too great compared with the measurable expected outcome difference. This does not mean that nutritional intervention is without important effect. Rather, nutrition is one of several factors affecting LOS.

INFLUENCE OF NUTRITIONAL INTERVENTION

Having identified the statistically significant variable factors, the next step was to determine the influence of nutrition preintervention days independent from the other factors. That was accomplished by setting a constant value for all other factors and then calculating the effects of day of nutritional intervention alone as its value was allowed to vary over a reasonable range. The calculations result in a mathematical formula that describes the relationship between day of nutritional intervention and the average number of days in the postintervention period. That relationship can then be used to predict the average number of days any at-risk patient would be expected to stay if they received nutritional intervention on days 1, 2, 3, etc. over the entire range of days.

For the MCS data the effects of early nutritional intervention become apparent when the relationship between day of nutritional intervention and LOS is graphed (Fig. 7). As days until intervention increased, so did the length of hospital stay in a ratio of 0.5. In other words, for each 2 days of earlier intervention, there was a decline of 1 day in LOS for the average patient.

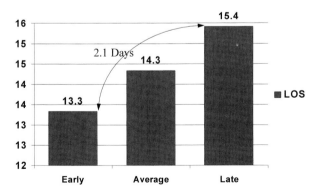

FIG. 7. Influence of nutritional intervention of ALOS.

EARLY VERSUS LATE NUTRITIONAL INTERVENTION: THE PATIENT DAY ADVANTAGE

In the NCMI first level of data analysis it was discovered that about half of the MCS patients who received nutritional intervention did so on or before the third hospital day. The other half received nutritional intervention on day 4 or later. The early subgroup had an ALOS of 3.0 days less than the late subgroup, but that estimate was probably higher than it should have been because it was uncorrected for the effects of non-nutritional factors shown in Fig. 6. Because the effects of nutrition can now be separated from the other factors, it is possible to calculate more precisely the LOS advantage between the early and late intervention subgroups. Figure 8 depicts the predicted LOS for the nutritional intervention groups resulting from the RDSI modeling. The three groups are the predicted LOS for early intervention, the predicted LOS regardless of intervention group, and predicted LOS for late intervention. The early intervention subgroup had a 2.1 day shorter LOS than did the late subgroup. Moreover, that estimate represents a corrected estimate of the influence of day of nutrition alone and is not confounded by the effects of other factors. It may thus be considered real.

Because sex was significant and contributed highly to the model, Fig. 9 examines LOS in early and late intervention groups while controlling for patient sex. The increase between early and late intervention was about 1.9 days for females and about 3.2 days for males.

Another prominent variable in the model was the presence of surgery. Figure 10 stratifies LOS within intervention group by both sex and surgery. For females and males without surgery, the increase in LOS across early and late intervention was about 1.8 and 2.0 days, respectively. For females and males with

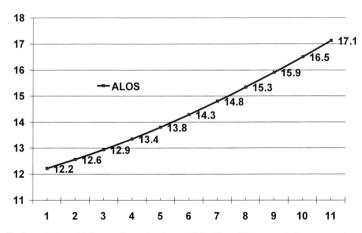

FIG. 8. Early nutritional intervention shortens LOS. The difference between early and late is 2.1 days.

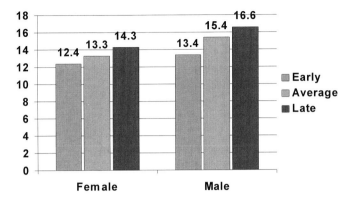

FIG. 9. Differences between sexes with early nutritional intervention.

surgery, the increase in LOS across early and late intervention was about 2.0 and 2.4 days, respectively.

The conclusion from the modeling described is that patients who receive early intervention, defined as intervention within the first 3 days of hospitalization, experience on average 2.1 days less time in the hospital than do patients who receive late intervention (day 4 or more). The size of this difference varies slightly, depending on gender, and whether the patient had surgery. In general, the difference is more pronounced among males.

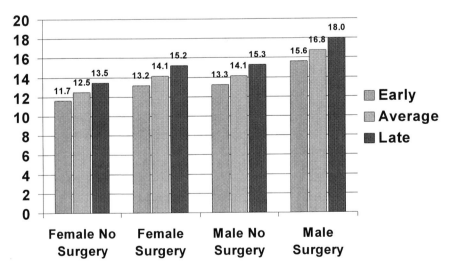

FIG. 10. Differences between sexes, the presence for surgery, and early or late nutritional intervention.

COST BENEFITS OF EARLY FEEDING OF PATIENTS AT NUTRITIONAL RISK

Nutrition has often been overlooked as a potential cost containment measure because its benefits are not always visible on the bottom line. Consequently, many hospital cost analysts may conclude that nutritional intervention is an added cost of questionable benefit.

Patient Day Savings and Potential Savings

The 2.1-day difference in corrected ALOS shown in Fig. 7 can be used to calculate the number of patient days saved during the MCS survey period due to early nutritional intervention. The calculation is straightforward: 2.1 days multiplied by the number of at-risk patients who received interventions on or before their third hospital day:

2,485 patients $\times$ 32% received intervention = 795 patients.
795 patients $\times$ 50.1% received early intervention = 398 early intervention patients.
2.1 days $\times$ 398 early intervention patients = 836 patient days saved.

The same calculation can be used to determine how many patient days were not saved due to late nutritional intervention:

2,485 patients $\times$ 32% received intervention = 795 patients.
795 patients $\times$ 49.9% received late intervention = 397 late intervention patients.
2.1 days $\times$ 397 late intervention patients = 834 additional patient days that might have been saved if nutrition had been applied earlier.

Thus, among the 795 patients who received nutritional intervention, early intervention had the potential to save a total of 1,670 patient days during the MCS survey period but realized less than 50% of that potential. The 50% remaining potential days represents future patient day savings available to the extent that institutions implement early nutritional intervention.

Potential Annual Dollar Savings

The estimates for patient day savings also can be used to predict how many total patient days might be saved in a typical month (or year) in the average institution in the MCS database. From that value and a cost estimate, an annual cost savings estimate can be projected, assuming that early nutritional intervention is provided to all at-risk patients.

It is not uncommon for a mid-size hospital to identify 60 at-risk patients per month who might have benefited from early nutritional intervention, and a resulting lower ALOS. Those are the patients who received nutritional intervention and those who did not, but had risk factors and stayed long enough that an early intervention would likely have had an effect. By applying the 2.1-day ALOS advantage for early versus late nutritional intervention, an estimate of total potential patient day savings per year for the average institution can be obtained: 2.1 days × 60 patients/month × 12 months = 1,512 potential patient days/year/institution.

To arrive at the projected annual dollar savings potential, multiply the potential annual patient days savings by an estimated variable daily patient cost. For the average institution in the MCS database, the reported daily variable cost estimate per patient was $697.00. Applying that figure to the results of the above calculation yields a projected total annual savings potential of $1,053,864.00: 1,512 patient days × 697 = $1,053,864.00 potential annual savings per average institution.

The potential annual savings on a per bed basis should be recalculated to adjust for differences in hospital size and to facilitate institutional comparisons. Each hospital's potential annual patient day savings were divided by the number of its medical and surgical beds per year. The average value for all the hospitals in the MCS database was 11.9 days per bed per year. Thus, 11.9 days saved per bed per year × 697 = $8,294.00 cost savings per bed per year for the composite MCS data.

FINAL COMMENTS

The past two decades have produced a substantial body of evidence that clinical nutrition can improve outcomes and reduce costs for malnourished and high-risk patients (41–73). Nevertheless, nutrition's power as a cost containment tool is generally overlooked for several reasons. First, the clinical studies tend to be highly technical, fragmented, and generally inaccessible to financial decision makers. Second, conventional hospital accounting systems track only the costs of products and services, and not their impact on patient outcomes. The fact that historic fee-for-service financial incentives have generally rewarded the providers that used the most billed services, sometimes at the expense of the most cost-effective resources, may explain this oversight.

The MCS presents a new financial perspective on hospital nutrition. Research results with the MCS show a significant gap between what is currently being saved by many institutions through early nutritional intervention and what might potentially be saved if nutrition care practices were improved. Those practice improvements are relatively simple to implement: identify at-risk patients upon admission and treat their malnutrition appropriately and early in their hospital course.

As the trends in managed care reverse the incentives to use more resources, providers that can demonstrate the ability to produce the best patient outcomes at the most efficient costs will thrive. This means that financial decisions have to take into account both the impact that products and services will have on patient outcomes, as well as their potential cost savings. Early nutritional intervention clearly improves outcomes and reduces costs.

Cost containment through nutritional intervention is a managed process. Its success depends on how much improvement in nutrition services occurs and how that improvement is documented through cost-sensitive evaluation and monitoring tools. And as with other practice modalities that improve outcome and reduce costs, early nutrition care fits well in continuous quality improvement processes.

REFERENCES

1. Winick M, ed. *Hunger disease: studies by the Jewish physicians in the Warsaw ghetto.* New York: Wiley; 1979
2. Benedict FG. *A study of prolonged fasting.* Publication No. 203. Washington, DC: Carnegie Institute; 1915:1–416.
3. Keys A, Brozek J, Henschel A. *The biology of human starvation.* Vols. 1 and 2. Minneapolis: University of Minnesota Press; 1950.
4. Butterworth CE. Skeleton in the hospital closet. *Nutr Today* 1974;9:4–8.
5. Bistrian BJ, Blackburn GL, Hallowell E, Heddle R. Protein status of general surgical patients. *JAMA* 1974;230:858–860.
6. Bistrian BJ, Blackburn GL, Vitale J, Cochran D, Naylor J. Prevalence of malnutrition in general medical patients. *JAMA* 1976;235:1567–1570.
7. Merritt RG, Suskind RM. Nutritional survey of hospitalized patients. *Am J Clin Nutr* 1979;32: 1320–1325.
8. O'Leary JP, Dunn GD, Basil S. Prevalence of malnutrition among patients admitted to a VA hospital. *South Med J* 1982;1095–1098.
9. Pollack MJ, Wiley JS, Kanter T, et al. Malnutrition in critically ill infants and children. *JPEN* 1982; 6:20–24.
10. Willard MD, Gilsdorf RB, Price RA. Protein calorie malnutrition in a community hospital. *JAMA* 1980;243:1720–1722.
11. Willcutts HD. Nutritional assessment of 1000 surgical patients in an affluent suburban community hospital. *JPEN* 1977;1:25A.
12. Robinson G, Goldstein M, Levine GM. Impact of nutritional status on DRG length of stay. *JPEN* 1987;11:49–51.
13. Shaw-Stiffel TA, Zarny LA, Pleban WE, Rosman DD, Rudolph RA, Bernstein LH. Effect of nutrition status and other factors on length of stay after major gastrointestinal surgery. *Nutrition* 1993;9: 140–145.
14. DeHoog S. Nutrition screening and assessment in a university hospital. In: *Nutritional screening and assessment as components of hospital admission. Report of the Eighth Ross Roundtable on Medical Issues.* Columbus, OH: Ross Laboratories; 1988:2–8.
15. Federer JG, Rane-Szostak, Blanford G. Evidence of malnutrition and prolonged recuperation in an extended care facility [Abstract]. American Dietetic Association 69th Annual Meeting, 1986:68.
16. Moore EE, Jones TN. Benefits of immediate jejunostomy feeding after major abdominal trauma. A prospective, randomized study. *J Trauma* 1986;26:874–879.
17. Mullen JL, Busby GP, Matthews DC, et al. Reduction of operative morbidity and mortality by combining preoperative and postoperative nutritional support. *Ann Surg* 1980;192:604–613.
18. Weinsier RL, Hunker EM, Krundiek GL, Butterworth DC. Hospital malnutrition: a prospective evaluation of general medical patients during the course of hospitalization. *Am J Clin Nutr* 1979;32: 418–426.
19. Messner RL, Stephens N, Wheeler WE, Hawes MC. Effect of admission nutritional status on length of hospital stay. *Gastroenterol Nurs* 1991;13:202–205.

20. Paulsen LM, Splett PL. Summary document of nutrition intervention in acute illness: burns and surgery. *J Am Diet Assoc* 1991;(suppl):15–19.
21. Pinchovsky-Devon G, Kaminski MV. Early nutrition intervention saves hospital days for patients with low serum albumen [Abstract]. American Society of Parenteral and Enteral Nutrition 10th Clinical Congress, 1986.
22. Ralph MK, Spurling S. Early nutrition screening documents costs of malnutrition [Abstract]. *J Am Diet Assoc* 1991;(Suppl.) A-12.
23. Smith PE, Smith AE. Nutrition intervention influences the bottom line. *Healthcare Financial Management* 1993;10:30–36.
24. Giner M, Laviano A, Meguid MM, Gleason JR. In 1995 a correlation between malnutrition and poor outcome in critically ill patients still exists. *Nutrition* 1996 12;1:23–29.
25. Berg A. Sliding toward nutrition malpractice: time to reconsider and redeploy. *Am J Clin Nutr* 1992;57:3–7.
26. Feinstein AR. An additional basic science for clnical medicine: I. The constraining fundamental paradigms. *Ann Intern Med* 1983;99:393–397.
27. Feinstein AR. An additional basic science for clinical medicine. II. The limitations of randomized trials. *Ann Intern Med* 1983;99:544–550.
28. Feinstein AR. An additional basic science for clnical medicine. III. The challenges of comparison and measurement. *Ann Intern Med* 1983;99:705–712.
29. Feinstein AR. An additional basic science for clinical medicine. IV. The development of clinimetrics. *Ann Intern Med* 1983;99:705–712.
30. Soeters PB. Glutamine: the link between depletion and diminished gut function? *J Am Coll Nutr* 1996;15195–196.
31. Pincus T. Rationale for combination therapy in rheumatoid arthritis: limitations of randomized clinical trials to recognize possible advantages of combination therapies in rheumatic diseases. *Semin Arthritis Rheum* 1993;23:2–10.
32. Blackburn H. Sounding board: Olestra and the FDA. *N Engl J Med* 1996;334;15:984–986.
33. Smith PE, Smith AE. In: Tucker GA: *Superior nutrition care cuts hospital costs.* Chicago, IL: Nutritional Care Management Institute; 1988.
34. Litton SE. Nutritional screening and assessment in a community hospital. In: *Nutritional screening and assessment as components of hospital admission. Report of the Eight Ross Roundtable on Medical Issues.* Columbus, OH: Ross Laboratories; 1988:2–8.
35. Redmond HP, Gallagher HJ, Shou J, Daly JM. Antigen presentation in protein-energy malnutrition. *Cell Immunol* 1995;163:80–87.
36. Grimble RF. Malnutrition and the immune response. Impact of nutrients on cytokine biology in infections. *Trans R Soc Trop Med Hyg* 1994;88:615–619.
37. Gilmore SA, Robinson G, Posthauer ME, Raymond J. Clinical indicators associated with unintentional weight loss and pressure ulcers in elderly residents of nursing facilities. *J Am Diet Assoc* 1995;95:984–992.
38. Andrassy RJ, Pizzine RP, Nirgiotis JG, Hennessey P. Linoleic acid enhances mitogen response and survival of septic weanling rats. *J Pediatr Surg* 1994;29:317–315.
39. Christensen KS, Gstundtner KM. Hospital-wide screening improves the basis for nutrition intervention. *J Am Diet Assoc* 1985;85:704–706.
40. Christensen KD. Hospital-wide screening increases revenue under prospective payment system. *J Am Diet Assoc* 1986;86:1234–1235.
41. Askanazi J, Hensie T, Starker PM, et al. Effect of immediate postoperative nutritional support on length of hospitalization. *Ann Surg* 1993;203:236–239.
42. Bastow MD, Rawlings J, Allison SP. Benefits of supplementary tube feeding after fractured neck of femur: a randomized controlled trial. *Br Med J* 1983;287:1589.
43. Collins JT, Oxby CB, Hill GL. Intravenous amino acids and intravenous hyperalimentation as protein sparing therapy after major surgery. *Lancet* 1978;1:788–791.
44. Deitel M. Nutritional management of external small bowel fistulas. *Can J Surg* 1976;19:505.
45. Delmi M, Rapin C-H, Bengoa J-M, Delmas PD, Vasey H, Bonjour J-P. Dietary supplementation in elderly patients with fractured neck femur. *Lancet* 1990;1335:1013–1016.
46. Gram JW, Zadrozny JB, Harrington T. The benefits of early jejunal hyperalimentation in the head-injured patient. *Neurosurgery* 1989;25:729–735.
47. Grimes CJC, Younathan MT, Lee WC. The effect of preoperative total parenteral nutrition on surgery outcomes. *J Am Diet Assoc* 87;87:1202–1206.

48. Heatley RV, Williams RP. Preoperative intravenous feeding. A controlled trial. *Postgrad Med J* 1979;55:541–545.
49. Hedberg A, Garcia N, Weinmann-Winkler S, et al. Nutritional risk screening: development of a standardized protocol using dietetic technicians. *J Am Diet Assoc* 1988;88:1553–1556.
50. Hunt DR, Mazlovitz A. Rowlands BJ, et al. A simple nutrition screening procedure for hospital patients. *J Am Diet Assoc* 1985;85:332–335.
51. Kamath SK, Lawler, MK, Smith AE, et al. Hospital malnutrition: a 33-hospital study. *J Am Diet Assoc* 1986;86:203–206.
52. Karp RJ. The use of the "at-risk" concept to identify malnourished hospital patients. *Nutr Clin Pract* 1988;3:150–153.
53. Kwong C, Wirth J, Avera E. Improved quality assurance through admission screening. *Nutr Suppl Serv* 1984;4:48–50.
54. Laven GT, Cowan AG, Green J. Nutrition in hospitalized children [Abstract]. *Am J Clin Nutr* 1980; 33:319.
55. Maillet JO. Evaluating your assessment program. *Nutr Suppl Serv* 1982;4:19–23.
56. Mullen JL, Buzby GP, Waldman MT, Gertner MH, Hobes CL, Rosato EF. Prediction of operative morbidity and mortality by preoperative nutritional assessment. *Surg Forum* 1979;30:80–82.
57. Muller JM, Dienst C, Pichmaier H. Peroperative parenteral feedings in patients with gastrointestinal carcinoma. *Lancet* 1982;1:68–71.
58. Nelson S, Bottsford JE, Long JM III. Finding malnourished patients in a community hospital. Development of a nutritional assessment service. *J S C Med Assoc* 1983;79:9–13.
59. Newmark SR, Sublett D, Black J, et al. Nutritional assessment in a rehabilitation unit. *Arch Phys Med Rehabil* 1981;62:279–282.
60. Reilly J, Hull SF, Albert N, Waller A, Bringardener S. Economic impact of malnutrition: a model system for hospitalized patients. *JPEN* 1988;12:371–376.
61. Reilly J, Mehta R, Teperman L, et al. Nutritional support after liver transplantation: a randomized prospective study. *JPEN* 1990;14:386–391.
62. Rombeau JL, Barol LR, Williamson CE, Mullen JL. Preoperative total parenteral nutrition and surgical outcome in patients with inflammatory bowel disease. *Am J Surg* 1982;143:139–143.
63. Roubenoff R, Roubenoff RA, Preto J, et al. Malnutrition among hospitalized patients: a problem of physician awareness. *Arch Intern Med* 1987;147:1462–1465.
64. Seltzer MH, Bastidas JA, Copper DM, et al. Instant nutritional assessment. *JPEN* 1979;3:157–159.
65. Smale BF, Mullen JL, Buzby G, et al. The efficacy of nutritional assessment and support in cancer surgery. *Cancer* 1981;47:2375–2381.
66. Smith AE, Powers CA, Copper-Meyer RA, et al. Improved nutritional management reduces length of hospitalization in intractable diarrhea. *JPEN* 1986;10:479–481.
67. Smith AE, Smith PE. Nutritional screening and impact of dietetic services on length of stay of pediatric patients at risk for malnutrition. In: *Nutrition screening and assessment as components of hospital admission. Report of the Eighth Ross Roundtable on Medical Issues.* Columbus OH: Ross Laboratories; 1988:21–26.
68. Smith PE, Smith AE. *Screening for hospital malnutrition: implications for the management and marketing of nutritional care.* Deerfield, IL: Clintec Nutrition; 1989.
69. Stave VS, Robbins S, Gletcher AB. A comparison of growth rates of premature infants prior to and after close nutritional monitoring. *Clin Proc Child Hosp Nat Med Center* 1975;35:171.
70. Szeluga DJ, Sutart RK, Brookmeyer R, et al. Nutritional support of bone marrow transplant recipients: a prospective, randomized clinical trial comparing total parenteral nutrition to an enteral feeding program. *Cancer Res* 1987;47:3309–3316.
71. Thompson JS, Burrough Ca, green JL, et al. Nutrition screening in surgical patients. *J Am Diet Assoc* 1984:84:337–338.
72. Weisdorf SA, Lynse J, Wind C, et al. Positive effect of prophylactic total parenteral nutrition on long-term outcome of bone marrow transplantation. *Transplantation* 1987;43:833–838.
73. Weinsier RL, Heimburger DC, Samples CM, Dimick AR, Birch R. Cost containment: a contribution of aggressive nutritional support in burn patients. *J Burn Care Rehabil* 1985;6:436–441.

Physiology, Stress, and Malnutrition: Functional Correlates, Nutritional Intervention,
edited by J.M. Kinney and H.N. Tucker.
Lippincott–Raven Publishers © 1997.

A Physiological Basis for the Clinical Improvements Produced by Nutritional Support

Ian A. Macdonald

Departments of Physiology and Pharmacology, University of Nottingham Medical School, Nottingham NG7 2UH, United Kingdom

It is now clear that the association of malnutrition with illness, trauma, or surgery leads to longer periods of hospitalization and increased morbidity and mortality. The provision of nutritional support to such patients at an early stage of hospitalization appears to improve their prognosis and reduce the length of hospital stay, but the mechanisms underlying this effect are not clear. The purpose of this chapter is to explore the physiologic basis for the beneficial effects of nutritional support.

The demonstration that nutritional support is of benefit in a wide variety of clinical situations indicates that it is highly unlikely that a single physiologic process is involved. It is more probable that one or more of a number of effects of malnutrition are of clinical importance and that nutritional support is of benefit for different reasons in different situations. The effects of malnutrition that are most likely to be of importance in this context are on immune function and wound healing, on skeletal (including respiratory) muscle function, and on more generalized physiologic and behavioral aspects. The demonstration in a number of studies that nutritional support has a beneficial effect within 1–3 weeks in individuals chronically malnourished indicates that any benefit cannot be dependent on complete restoration of normal body composition.

IMMUNE FUNCTION, INFECTION, AND WOUND HEALING

Protein-energy malnutrition in children has been associated for many years with impaired immune function and increased susceptibility to infection (1). This impairment of immune function may not be simply due to inadequate macronutrient supply. Good et al. found in experimental studies in animals that micronutrients such as zinc were of major importance for the maintenance of normal cell-mediated immune function (2). However, there is no information of the time course of improvement in immune function that might be achieved by supplementary intake of micronutrients such as zinc.

Aging is associated with alterations in immune function, such that in healthy elderly individuals circulating T-lymphocyte concentrations may be approximately 10% lower and immunoglobulin (Ig)G and IgA concentrations somewhat higher than healthy young subjects (3). In addition, the elderly have reduced antibody responses to some viral and toxin antigens. It is of interest that otherwise healthy elderly subjects with a low serum albumin concentration (30–35 g/L), suggestive of protein malnutrition, have markedly altered T-lymphocyte and IgA concentrations in plasma, and more marked impairment of the antibody response (3). Linked with this impaired immune function in the elderly are the demonstrations that neutrophils taken from elderly subjects display reduced responses when challenged in vitro (4–6). This may be related to an increase in the production of prostaglandins such as PGE_2, which inhibit white blood cell function (7). These prostaglandins are synthesized from arachidonic acid and act with other products of arachidonic acid metabolism, such as platelet-activating factor, to produce an inflammatory response to tissue damage. Cannon et al. (8) recently undertook an experimental study in healthy elderly subjects that attempted to modify the inflammatory response to tissue damage by dietary supplementation. They provided subjects with a fish oil supplement for 4 months before the study, increasing the intake of n-3 fatty acids (including eicosapentaenoic acid), which reduce the production of prostaglandins of the 2 series (e.g., PGE_2 from arachidonic acid) and increases the production of the less active 3 series compounds. Muscle damage was induced in supplemented and control elderly subjects and in young subjects, with eccentric exercise, and indices of the neutrophil response were measured. Control elderly subjects had no increase in plasma elastase (an index of neutrophil degranulation), whereas young subjects and the elderly receiving fish oil supplement had a substantial elastase response.

Thus, aging appears to be associated with alterations in immune function, some of which may be affected by dietary supplementation. Substantially more work is needed to determine the time course of any improvement in immune function in the elderly, during nutrient supplementation, and also whether substantial improvement can be achieved in the undernourished elderly. Nevertheless, the potential clinical significance of such aging and undernutrition-associated changes in immune function in relation to recovery from infection and injury should be recognized.

The time course of the changes in immune function during dietary energy restriction and subsequent refeeding have been studied in healthy obese subjects. Field et al. (9) fed a diet low in energy, but adequate in protein and micronutrients, to obese subjects for 6 weeks and observed reductions in total leukocyte, neutrophils, lymphocytes, and monocyte concentrations and a small reduction in the T-helper (CD4) lymphocyte subset concentration. Underfeeding also reduced the in vitro functional responses of monocytes to some mitogens. It is of interest that 1 week of refeeding normalized the lymphocyte and CD4 count and improved the in vitro functional response of the monocytes, although there was no recovery of the numbers of the other white blood cells. Although this study was conducted in healthy subjects, the findings are of value in relation to nutritional support because they provide evidence that undernutrition-induced impairments in immune function may be significantly improved by 1 week of refeeding. However, one must be a little cautious in interpreting this study because the subjects had received adequate intakes of protein and micronutrients during the underfeeding period, and the immune impairments produced were of minor clinical significance.

An indication of the clinical benefit of early nutritional support was provided by Collins et al. (10) in a study of patients undergoing major abdominal surgery who had a reported preoperative weight loss of approximately 10%. Patients were randomized to control [no intravenous (i.v.) nutritional supplementation], i.v. amino acids, or total parenteral nutrition (TPN) starting on the second postoperative day. The TPN group had significantly fewer postoperative complications, tended to have a lower rate of sepsis (two of 10 patients compared with four and five of 10 in the other groups), and more had been discharged home by 30 days postoperation than in the other groups. Thus, this study provided evidence that nutritional support is of benefit in shortening hospital stay and reducing complications. The tendency for less sepsis is an indication that this may have been affected by improved immune function, but this has not yet been confirmed by any subsequent, prospective studies.

A number of studies have investigated the effects of refeeding subjects who were chronically undernourished on phagocytic function of white blood cells and the occurrence of infection. Vaisman et al. (11) refed patients with anorexia nervosa who had been restricting their energy intake for at least 4 months. The phagocytic function of polymorphonuclear cells is, in part, dependent on superoxide production by stimulated cells. In the undernourished state, the anorectic subjects had normal rates of superoxide production. However, during the early stages of refeeding, the superoxide production by polymorphonuclear cells was reduced, with the maximum effect occurring at 3–4 weeks of refeeding, before returning to normal values by 2–3 months. Such an apparently paradoxical effect of refeeding also was observed in famine victims during the early stages of increased nutrient intake. Murray et al. (12) recorded the occurrence of infections in over 4,000 famine victims and measured plasma C-reactive protein concentrations (a marker of the acute phase response to infection) in a subgroup of them, before and during refeeding. Initially, 5% of the study population had clinical or laboratory evidence of infection before refeeding, whereas after 2 weeks of feeding this had increased to 30% before it then decreased slowly over the subsequent 7 weeks. The majority of these cases are attributable to reactivation of previous infections (such as malaria or tuberculosis) rather than completely new infective events. Thus, one would not expect such an effect in the majority of undernourished patients receiving nutritional support in the developed world. Nevertheless, these observations represent potential hazards associated with refeeding of the malnourished patient, and they should be taken into account.

There is widespread concern that providing nutritional support via the i.v. route may alter intestinal function, compromising its role in normal immune function, possibly leading to translocation of bacteria from the gut into the bloodstream. A recent, rather preliminary study in healthy subjects provides evidence that such concern may be unfounded (13), although more detailed studies are undoubtedly needed. Buchman et al. (13) studied healthy subjects during 14 days of TPN, with no oral intake. They found no reductions in intestinal immune function during TPN, and rather than a decrease in plasma IgA (which would be expected if intestinal immune function were reduced), there was actually a slight increase.

Most of the clinical benefit of nutritional support has been observed in patients who were previously malnourished. However, there are some examples of beneficial effects in normally nourished patients subjected to major trauma or surgery. Moore and Jones (14) demonstrated that early commencement of postoperative enteral feeding in patients with major abdominal trauma improved nitrogen balance. Enteral feeding did not alter the overall complication rate, but it significantly reduced the occurrence of sepsis in the first 5 days from 29% in the control group to 9% in the enterally fed group. If the patients in each group with the most severe abdominal trauma were removed from the analysis, the benefits of enteral feeding in reducing sepsis were even more marked (26% vs. 4%).

RESPIRATORY FUNCTION AND SKELETAL MUSCLE FUNCTION IN UNDERNUTRITION

One would expect undernutrition to affect muscle function because of reductions in lean body mass (due to negative energy balance) and a shortage of metabolic fuels for muscle contraction. However, the time courses of some of the changes in muscle function during experimental underfeeding, and during refeeding of malnourished patients suggest that factors other than body composition are important.

Adequate respiratory function is important in the recovery from illness and injury, both specifically in relation to respiratory infection and the need to expectorate, and also in the re-establishment of spontaneous respiration in the ventilated patient (15). It has been known for over 20 years that experimental underfeeding (500 kcal per day for 10 days) reduces the ventilatory response to hypoxia, but not hypercapnia (16). The decreased response to hypoxia was correlated with the underfeeding-associated decrease in resting metabolic rate, and both were normalized after 5 days of refeeding. During underfeeding, two of the subjects studied by Doekel et al. (16) effectively lost their ventilatory response to hypoxia. The investigators made the interesting comment that such a lack of respiratory function is also seen in myxoedema (17), and given the reduced thyroid function that occurs during undernutrition, this highlights a potential role for thyroid hormones in some of the functional changes seen in malnutrition.

Similar results were obtained by Baier and Somani (18), who gave either amino acids alone (550 kcal/day) or amino acids plus lipid (total energy 1,650 kcal/day) i.v. to healthy subjects for 10 days. Nitrogen balance was maintained in both groups, and the amino acid alone group lost slightly more weight (4.45 kg) than did the other group (2.97 kg). The group receiving amino acid plus lipid showed no alteration in the ventilatory response to hypoxia, either during the 10 days of infusion or the subsequent period of normal feeding. By contrast, the underfed group (amino acids alone) had a marked reduction in response to hypoxia, which was only partially restored by 7 days of normal diet. This study also found that the ventilatory response to hypercapnia was not affected by 10 days of undernutrition. Thus, it would appear that short periods of experimental undernutrition affect the sensitivity to hypoxia, but not hypercapnia, indicating an alteration in peripheral chemoreceptor function. Furthermore, inspiratory muscle strength and maximum voluntary ventilation are not affected by 7 days of underfeeding (19), providing further evidence that the change in hypoxic response is due to altered chemoreceptor function. Chronic undernutrition affects the respiratory system to a greater extent than would be expected from the loss of body weight. Patients with approximately 29% weight loss, due to nonrespiratory disease, had a 37% reduction in forced vital capacity and more marked decreased in respiratory muscle strength and maximal voluntary ventilation (20). Such impairments in respiratory muscle function would further compromise the response to hypoxia and hypercapnia and could seriously impede the recovery from illness. Major improvements in respiratory function would depend on replacement of muscle mass, but it is not known whether short-term nutritional support improves the functional responses to hypoxia in such patients, and further studies would be worthwhile.

A series of studies from Jeejeebhoy et al. have shown impaired skeletal muscle contractile function, both in chronically undernourished patients and after short-term undernutrition of healthy subjects. An early study of patients with gastrointestinal disease, who had lost a mean of 15% of body weight over the previous 1–6 months, showed altered contractile responses to electrical stimulation of the adductor pollicis muscle (21). The undernourished patients had slower muscle relaxation rates after electrical stimulation, a tendency for a lower maximal response to high-frequency stimulation, and a greater response to low-frequency stimulation. These results are consistent with undernutrition reducing the functioning of the type II, fast-twitch muscle fibers, thus increasing the reliance on the slower type I fibers. A small number of the patients received TPN for 4 weeks, at the end of which their muscle relaxation rate had returned to normal values. Unfortunately, no measurements were made at an early stage during the period of TPN, so it is impossible to tell how long a period of nutritional support is needed before improvements occur.

A subsequent study of undernutrition (2 weeks of 400 kcal/day) followed by complete starvation for 2 weeks in obese subjects showed a similar phenomenon, with an increase in force production at low stimulation frequency and a slower

muscle relaxation rate (22). It is of interest that all of these abnormalities of muscle function were normalized after 2 weeks of refeeding, although again it is not
known how quickly the effect occurred. Further evidence that improvement in
nutritional status can improve muscle function is provided by a study of patients
with anorexia nervosa (23). These patients were approximately 60% of ideal
body weight and had a history of weight loss over the previous 2–9 years, with
marked impairments of muscle function at baseline. After 4 weeks of refeeding,
the muscle relaxation rate and indices of fatiguability had returned to normal,
and by 8 weeks the proportion of total force produced by low-frequency stimulation was also normalized. These improvements in muscle function occurred in
association with increases in body nitrogen and potassium content, with proportionally larger changes in the latter. Russell et al. suggested that the restoration
of intracellular potassium may be more important than increasing body nitrogen
in improving muscle function during refeeding.

There is some disagreement in the literature concerning the effect of short
periods of underfeeding of obese subjects on the contractile responses to electrical stimulation of the adductor pollicis. Newham et al. (24) fed obese patients
with a 450 kcal/day diet for 12 days and found no change in the muscle relaxation rate, fatiguing, or proportion of maximal force produced by low-frequency
stimulation. Their results for normal subjects were similar to those observed by
Russell et al. (22,23), and Newham et al. also found profound impairments of
muscle function in three malnourished patients with a history of weight loss.
There is no obvious explanation for the different effects of short-term underfeeding in these studies, but it may relate to the absolute degree of undernutrition and the compliance of the patients. However, a separate study of the effects
of 48-hour starvation in normal weight subjects confirmed increased fatiguing
and delayed recovery during prolonged muscle stimulation (25). It is of great
interest that this impairment was reversed only 6 hours after the subjects had
resumed their normal diet.

Further evidence of impaired muscle function in undernourished patients is
provided by Chan et al. (26). They studied patients who had lost 10–18% of body
weight and were about to undergo gastrointestinal surgery. These patients had a
slower muscle relaxation rate and increased proportion of maximal force produced by low-frequency stimulation compared with healthy controls. After these
measurements, for the 48 hours before surgery the patients received an i.v. infusion of glucose (6.7 g/kg body wt/24 h) and potassium (1.3 mmol/kg/24 h). This
infusion produced an almost threefold increase in muscle glycogen and significantly changed both muscle relaxation rate and the force produced by low-frequency stimulation such that both variables were then similar to those seen in
healthy controls.

A more extensive study of the effects of nutritional support on muscle function in undernourished patients was reported by Brough et al. (27). They
observed that TPN improved total force production and muscle relaxation rate
and tended to reduce the force produced by low-frequency stimulation before

substantial changes in body composition occurred. The degree of initial malnutrition of these patients was not stated, although their estimated arm muscle circumference and triceps skinfold thickness were two thirds of normal. The time course of the improvements in muscle function produced by TPN is rather difficult to determine, but although some changes were apparent within a few days, normalization may have taken up to 10 weeks of intravenous feeding.

An intriguing feature of the effects of nutritional status and nutritional support on muscle function is the possible mechanisms that might link them. There is no doubt that muscle structure and composition must affect function, but it is clear from the studies reviewed above that improvements that occur with introduction of nutritional support are often dissociated from changes in muscle mass. The maintenance of intracellular potassium content is important for ensuring nerve and muscle excitability. The demonstration that potassium and glucose administration for 48 hours normalizes muscle dysfunction (26), and the suggestion from Russell et al. (23) that increases in whole-body potassium were of major importance in improving muscle function of anorectic patients during refeeding, point to this as a potential mechanism. This hypothesis is developed at some length by Pichard and Jeejeebhoy (28), with some experimental evidence of depletion of intracellular potassium in rats during starvation. They suggest a number of possible endocrine factors that may contribute to loss of potassium during underfeeding, including reduced insulin concentrations and increased sympathoadrenal activity. However, the latter seems unlikely because sympathetic nervous system activity decreases with undernutrition. Furthermore, important endocrine factors affecting membrane Na^+/K^+–adenosine triphosphatase (ATPase) activity and the resting membrane potential (and not mentioned by Pichard and Jeejeebhoy) are the thyroid hormones. The thyroid gland releases substantially more thyroxine (T_4) than the much more potent triiodothyronine (T_3), but under normal conditions much of this T_4 is converted to T_3 in peripheral tissues. Thus, the major physiologic effects of thyroid hormone are produced by T_3. It has been known for some time that starvation or a low-carbohydrate diet alters the peripheral metabolism of T_4, such that instead of producing the active T_3, the inactive reverse-T_3 is produced. Thus, dietary factors (i.e., undernutrition) can reduce thyroid status. One consequence of this would be reduced Na^+/K^+–ATPase activity and reduced excitability of nerve and muscle.

In addition to possible effects of undernutrition on muscle structure and potassium content, there will undoubtedly be effects on fuel supply. Thus, undernourished subjects have low muscle glycogen contents and reduced fuel stores in fat and protein. Furthermore, studies of 2 days of starvation or 7 days of underfeeding in rats showed reductions in the phosphocreatine, and to a lesser extent total creatine, content of skeletal muscle, indicating an abnormality of muscle energy metabolism (29). Although extrapolation from rat skeletal muscle to human muscle should be undertaken with caution, this does point to a possible explanation for the early effects of refeeding on muscle function. It is clear that studies are needed of the effects of creatine supplementation on muscle function in the undernourished.

GENERALIZED PHYSIOLOGIC AND BEHAVIORAL ASPECTS OF UNDERNUTRITION

The classical study of experimental, prolonged undernutrition undertaken by Keys et al. (30) identified a number of important physiologic and behavioral changes during the 6 months of underfeeding. In particular, subjects' physical work capacity was reduced, they were apathetic and depressed, and they had a general malaise and a number of other psychological disturbances. These symptoms of undernutrition are similar to those seen in famine victims and in undernourished patients admitted to the hospital. Keys et al. showed that all of the changes they observed during underfeeding were reversed by refeeding. Unfortunately, measurements during refeeding were not made at appropriate intervals to determine whether the more behavioral impairments had a different time course of recovery to the physiologic ones. However, it is clear that restoration of lean body mass was a slow process. and many other variables were normalized more quickly. It seems highly probable that restoration of normal food intake will have early effects on thyroid hormone metabolism and central nervous system function that produce subjective improvement in advance of major changes in body composition.

Undernutrition affects a number of physiologic processes, including the control of blood pressure and body temperature, both of which are compromised in acute and chronic undernutrition (31,32). Thus, the undernourished have an increased susceptibility to postural hypotension and to a decrease in core temperature when in a cold environment, both of which will tend to cause them to remain in bed to reduce the risk of either problem occurring. This, together with the reductions in muscle function in undernutrition, reduces a patient's mobility and is likely to delay their recovery from illness by predisposing them to bed sores and thromboembolism (15). It is not known how rapidly the effects of undernutrition on the control of blood pressure and body temperature are reversed by nutritional support, but it is clear that normal thermoregulation is achieved before the complete restoration of body weight (32).

It seems most likely that one of the important effects of nutritional support in patients' recovering from illness or surgery is to provide sufficient nutrient intake to prevent or reverse the behavioral and physiologic changes associated with undernutrition. Such effects are by their nature nonspecific and difficult to quantify, but it is clear that improving a patient's sense of well-being and reducing feelings of apathy and depression are at least as important as providing fuel and electrolytes for skeletal muscle. This is exemplified in an article from Askanazi et al. (33), reporting an early study of the effects of nutritional support after major surgery. The patients being studied were not malnourished before surgery, and postoperatively they were randomized to receive either TPN or 400 kcal/day of glucose in water i.v. for the first 6–7 days. Subsequently, oral food intake was resumed. The TPN group had a shorter period of hospitalization (17 vs. 24 days), but this could not be explained on the basis of individual, clearly identifiable factors such as improved wound healing. However, Askanazi et al. commented that the glucose/water group "had a slower convalescence with a decreased rate of return of post-operative activity."

A similar observation on the effects of postoperative energy intake on recovery from surgery was made by Bastow et al. (34). They studied women requiring surgery for fractured femurs and found that rehabilitation time was shortest in previously well-nourished women who ate well postoperatively. The previously poorly nourished women had a low postoperative voluntary food intake, longer rehabilitation time, and higher rate of mortality. Nutritional support (by nocturnal tube-feeding) given to the undernourished women shortened their rehabilitation time and tended to decrease mortality. The nutritional support also produced improvements in biochemical and anthropometric indices of nutritional status, which could have contributed to the improved mobility and shortened rehabilitation time.

CONCLUSIONS

There is no doubt that malnutrition is associated with reduced immune function, impaired muscle function, and a series of behavioral and psychological effects that reduce an individual's motivation and mobility. In otherwise healthy subjects, these effects may be of survival benefit in ensuring that body fuel stores last longer at a time of inadequate food supply. However, in illness or after injury or surgery there is overwhelming evidence that malnutrition delays recovery, and may increase mortality.

The majority of experimental evidence indicates that providing nutritional support to malnourished patients at an early stage of illness or postoperative recovery is of clinical benefit. The benefit is most noticeable when nutritional support is provided within the first 3 days of the clinical event and typically reduces the hospital stay by 2–3 days in 15. The speed of such an effect is inconsistent with it being due to substantial changes in body composition, and the fact that improvements are noticed in both medical and surgical patients indicates that a factor such as improved wound healing cannot be the only explanation. It is feasible that some of the beneficial effects on nutritional support are due to improved immune function, but there is little direct evidence in malnourished patients to support this proposal. It seems likely that a major effect of nutritional support is to improve muscle function, by increasing substrate supply and intracellular potassium content, such that patients are able to become more mobile at an earlier stage. A contributing mechanism to this effect could be an increased peripheral production of T_3. However, the effect of nutritional support that would appear to be of major importance, and which is likely to apply in most of the clinical situations in which such support is given, is the reversal of the psychological and behavioral effects of chronic undernutrition. Relieving the apathy, depression, and lack of motivation that are characteristic of prolonged undernutrition will be of major importance in increasing a patient's mobility and facilitating rapid convalescence and recovery.

The main challenge in the immediate future is to design studies that directly test the above hypothesis. At the moment, the arguments in favor of early nutritional support of malnourished patients tend to focus on the financial benefits associated with reductions in hospital stay and reduced complication rates. These arguments would become much more persuasive if there was convincing evidence as to how nutritional support produced its effects because one could then incorporate monitoring the appropriate variables into the clinical care of the patient. On the basis of the factors considered in this review, it seems most likely that this monitoring will include indices of immune function, skeletal muscle function, mobility, and in particular a patient's psychological status.

ACKNOWLEDGMENTS

I thank Kirsty Hitt for her assistance in the preparation of the manuscript. I dedicate this chapter to the memory of my former colleague, Michael Bastow, whose early studies were among the first to demonstrate the benefits of nutritional support in the malnourished, and whose enthusiasm attracted me to this area of clinical nutrition. He made a substantial contribution and is sorely missed.

REFERENCES

1. Abassy AS, Badr El-Din MK, Hassan AI, et al. Studies of cell-mediated immunity and allergy in protein-energy malnutrition. I. Cell-mediated delayed hypersensitivity. II. Immediate hypersensitivity. *J Trop Med Hyg* 1974;77:13–21.
2. Good RA, Lorenz E. Nutrition and cellular immunity. *Int J Immunopharmacol* 1992;14:361–366.
3. Lesourd B. Protein undernutrition as the major cause of decreased immune function in the elderly: clinical and functional implications. *Nutr Rev* 1995;53(suppl):86–94.
4. Niwa Y, Kasama T, Miyachi Y, Kanoh T. Neutrophil chemotaxis, phagocytosis and parameters of reactive oxygen species in human aging: cross-sectional and longitudinal studies. *Life Sci* 1989;44: 1655–1664.
5. Suzuki K, Swenson C, Sasagawa S, Sakatani T, Watanabe M, Kobayashi M, Fujikura T. Age-related decline in lysosomal enzyme release from polymorphonuclear leukocytes after n-formyl-methiolyl-leucyl-phenylalanine stimulation. *Exp Haematol* 1983;11:1005–1013.
6. MacGregor RR, Shalit M. Neutrophil function in healthy elderly subjects. *J Gerontol* 1990;45: M55–M60.
7. Goodwin J, Messner R. Sensitivity of lymphocytes to prostaglandin E_2 increased in subjects over age 70. *J Clin Invest* 1980;332:260–270.
8. Cannon JG, Fiatarone MA, Meydami M, Gong JX, Scott L, Blumberg JB, Evans WJ. Aging and dietary modulation of elastase and interleukin-I β secretion. *Am J Physiol* 1995;268:R208–R213.
9. Field CJ, Gougeon R, Marliss EB. Changes in circulating leukocytes and mitogen responses during very-low-energy all-protein reducing diets. *Am J Clin Nutr* 1991;54:123–129.
10. Collins JP, Oxby CB, Hill GL. Intravenous amino acids and intravenous hyperalimentation as protein-sparing therapy after major surgery. *Lancet* 1978;1:788–791.
11. Vaisman N, Tabachnik E, Hahn T, Voet H, Guy N. Superoxide production during re-feeding in patients with anorexia nervosa. *Metabolism* 1992;41:1097–1099.

12. Murray MJ, Murray AB, Murray NJ, Murray MB. Infections during severe primary undernutrition and subsequent feeding: paradoxical findings. *Aust N Z J Med* 1995;25:507–511.
13. Buchman AL, Mestecky J, Moukarzel A, Ament ME. Intestinal immune function is unaffected by parenteral nutrition in man. *J Am Coll Nutr* 1995;14:656–661.
14. Moore EE, Jones TN. Benefits of immediate jejunostomy feeding after major abdominal trauma—a prospective, randomized study. *J Trauma* 1986;26:874–881.
15. Elia M. Artificial nutritional support in clinical practice in Britain. *J R Coll Phys Lond* 1993;27:8–15.
16. Doekel RC, Zwillich CW, Scoggin CH, Kryger M, Weil JV. Clinical semi-starvation: depression of hypoxic ventilatory response. *N Engl J Med* 1976;295:358–361.
17. Zwillich CW, Pierson DJ, Hofeldt FD, Lufkin EG, Weil JV. Ventilatory control in myxoedema and hypothyroidism. *N Engl J Med* 1975;292:662–665.
18. Baier H, Somani P. Ventilatory drive in normal man during semi-starvation. *Chest* 1984;85:222–225.
19. Bender PR, Martin BJ. Ventilatory and treadmill endurance during semi-starvation. *J Appl Physiol* 1986;60:1823–1827.
20. Arora NS, Rochester DF. Respiratory muscle strength and maximal voluntary ventilation in undernourished patients. *Am Rev Respir Dis* 1982;126:5–8.
21. Lopes J, Russell DMcR, Whitwell J, Jeejeebhoy KN. Skeletal muscle function in malnutrition. *Am J Clin Nutr* 1982;36:602–610.
22. Russell DMR, Leiter LA, Whitwell J, Marliss EB, Jeejeebhoy KN. Skeletal muscle function during hypocaloric diets and fasting: a comparison with standard nutritional assessment parameters. *Am J Clin Nutr* 1983;37:133–138.
23. Russell DMR, Prendergast PJ, Darby PL, Garfinkel PE, Whitwell J, Jeejeebhoy KN. A comparison between muscle function and body composition in anorexia nervosa: the effect of re-feeding. *Am J Clin Nutr* 1983;38:229–237.
24. Newham DJ, Tomkins AM, Clark CG. Contractile properties of the adductor pollicis in obese patients on a hypocaloric diet for two weeks. *Am J Clin Nutr* 1986;44:756–760.
25. Shizgal HM, Vasilevsky CA, Gardiner PF, Wang W, Quellette Tuitt DA, Brabant GV. Nutritional assessment and skeletal muscle function. *Am J Clin Nutr* 1986;44:761–771.
26. Chan STF, McLaughlin SJ, Ponting GA, Biglin J, Dudley HAF. Muscle power after glucose-potassium loading in undernourished patients. *Br Med J* 1986;293:1055–1056.
27. Brough W, Horne G, Blount A, Irving MH, Jeejeebhoy KN. Effects of nutrient intake, surgery, sepsis, and long term administration of steroids on muscle function. *Br Med J* 1986;293:983–988.
28. Pichard C, Jeejeebhoy KN. Muscle dysfunction in malnourished patients. *Q J Med* 1988;69:1021–1045.
29. Pichard C, Vaughan C, Struck R, Armstong RL, Jeejeebhoy KN. The effect of dietary manipulations (fasting, hypocaloric feeding and subsequent feeding) on rat muscle energetics as assessed by nuclear magnetic resonance spectroscopy. *J Clin Invest* 1988;82:895–901.
30. Keys A, Brozek J, Henschel A, Mickelsen O, Taylor HL. *The biology of human starvation.* Minneapolis, MN: University of Minnesota Press; 1950.
31. Macdonald IA, Bennett T, Fellows IW. Disturbances of autonomic function produced by dietary or metabolic alterations. In: Joseph MH, Fillenz M, Macdonald IA, Marsden CA, eds. *Monitoring neurotransmitter release during behaviour.* Chichester, England: Ellis Horwood Publishers; 1986:57–68.
32. Mansell PI, Fellows IW, Macdonald IA, Allison SP. Defect in thermoregulation in malnutrition reversed by weight gain. Physiological mechanisms and clinical importance. *Q J Med* 1990;76;817–829.
33. Askanazi J , Hensle TW, Starker PM, Lockhart SH, La Sala PA, Olsson C, Kinney JM. Effect of immediate post-operative nutritional support on length of hospitalization. *Ann Surg* 1986;203:236–239.
34. Bastow MD, Rawlings J, Allison SP. Benefits of supplementary tube feeding after fractured neck of femur: a randomized controlled trial. *Br Med J* 1983;287:1589–1592.

Subject Index